Managed Care Strategies
A Physician Practice Desk Reference

George B. Moseley III, MBA, JD
Lecturer in Health Law and Management
Harvard School of Public Health
Boston, Massachusetts

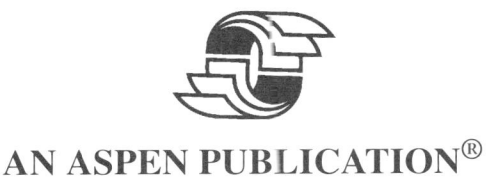

AN ASPEN PUBLICATION®
Aspen Publishers, Inc.
Gaithersburg, Maryland
1999

Library of Congress Cataloging-in-Publication Data

Moseley, George B.
Managed care strategies : a physician practice
desk reference / George B. Moseley III.
p.   cm.
Includes bibliographical references and index.
ISBN 0-8342-0735-4
1. Managed care plans (Medical care)—United States.
2. Group medical practice—United States.   I. Title.
R729.5.H43M67   1999
362.1'04258'0973—dc21
98-32278
CIP

Orders: (800) 638-8437
Customer Service: (800) 234-1660

About Aspen Publishers • For more than 35 years, Aspen has been a leading professional publisher in a variety of disciplines. Aspen's vast information resources are available in both print and electronic formats. We are committed to providing the highest quality information available in the most appropriate format for our customers. Visit Aspen's Internet site for more information resources, directories, articles, and a searchable version of Aspen's full catalog, including the most recent publications: **http://www.aspenpublishers.com**
Aspen Publishers, Inc. • The hallmark of quality in publishing
Member of the worldwide Wolters Kluwer group.

Editorial Services: Kathy Litzenberg
Library of Congress Catalog Card Number: 98-32278
ISBN: 0-8342-0735-4

Printed in the United States of America

1   2   3   4   5

To my Slovak grandfather, Daniel Dreveny,
and to my good friends, Dale and John.

Table of Contents

Acknowledgments

This book was the product of teamwork. In writing it, I received support from the following people. Kalen Conerly has been my contact person at Aspen Pubishers during the heaviest period of writing this book. She provided just the right balance of encouragement and prodding that kept me going when my motivation lagged. I always counted on her for clear thinking, affirmation, and positive reinforcement. Ellen Zane is Network President of the Partners Community Health Care System, a steadily expanding integrated delivery system based on the Massachusetts General Hospital and Brigham & Women's Hospital in Boston. She has spoken numerous times to the students in my class on an Introduction to the New American Health Care System: Law, Policy, and Management. From her, I have learned as much as the students about thoughtful and aggressive strategies for growing and consolidating physician practices into an efficient provider network. I have incorporated many of her ideas into my recommendations here. Neil Motenko is one of the top antitrust lawyers in the United States and a member of the Health Law Department of the law firm Nutter, McClennan & Fish. He, too, has been a guest lecturer for several years in my course on the New American Health Care System. Through his presentations, he has informed me of the nuances of antitrust law as they influence the strategic options I recommend to physicians in this book. His insights were particularly useful in writing Chapter 28 on physician collaboration and discussions throughout about price-fixing and deselection. Bob Blendon, who has been chairperson of the Department of Health Policy and Managemement at the Harvard School of Public Health, and Karen Donelan are leading gatherers and analyzers of survey data on American attitudes toward health care. They have generously allowed me the use of some of that data in the first four chapters of the book.

Introduction

Just about three years ago, I was gathering material for a new course I was planning to teach at the Harvard School of Public Health. It was entitled "Introduction to the New American Health System: Law, Policy, and Management." I was looking for articles and books that presented practical information on getting involved with managed care, from the viewpoints of all the key players—hospitals, physicians, employers, and health plans. The bulk of what I found seemed targeted at executives and managers who were either starting or already running managed care organizations (MCOs). There was very little help for the various parties that must interact with the MCOs. The periodical, *Business & Health*, offered some guidance to employers. The journal of the American Hospital Association, *Hospitals & Health Networks*, did a decent job of advising hospital administrators on the adjustments they should make to managed care.

Physicians were served primarily by occasional articles in *Medical Economics* magazine. The few more substantial articles or small books tailored to physicians dealt with one issue—how to evaluate a managed care contract. There is an entire range of organizational and operational options for physicians in adapting to their new roles in the health care system. There is an alphabet soup of institutions for organizing doctors: IPAs, PHOs, GPWWs, MSOs, and PPMCs, to name a few. There are numerous practice changes that a modern physician must make: information gathering, utilization management, quality assur-

ance, patient satisfaction, and clinical outcomes, among others. Nearly all the literature discussed these topics from the perspective of an MCO executive or hospital administrator who might be offering them to or imposing them on physicians.

There was almost no writing that assumed that physicians might be separately interested in these issues. No authors or journals seemed to believe that physicians might want to take charge of some of these care management initiatives, particularly those of a clinical nature. No one imagined that groups of doctors could form and manage some of these new delivery entities on their own. Few authors and publishers saw physicians as leaders, executives, and entrepreneurs. An audience of half a million doctors, in a state of confusion and anxiety, was being ignored.

I believe that, in the face of a substantial loss of autonomy and control, deselection from managed care provider panels, and declining incomes, a large proportion of physicians are willing to take bold new initiatives. I believe that, with guidance and supporting information, they will:

- begin to accumulate practice earnings for reinvestment to expand and improve the practice
- move aggressively to ally themselves with other physicians in larger, more powerful practice groups
- seriously examine new organizational models for those groups

- assume the risk of either forming or joining these new groups
- take leadership roles in organizing their physician colleagues, planning new groups, and eventually managing them
- make dramatic changes in their practice styles to deliver higher-quality, lower-cost medical care
- embrace managed care and use it to their advantage
- assert the authority that comes from their numbers and their clinical influence in all dealings with hospitals, other providers, MCOs, employers, other payers, and government regulators

My intention in writing this book is to give physicians the basic tools for determining their own futures in the health care system, rather than letting hospitals, MCOs, government regulators, or market forces do it for them.

I designed this book to accomplish several objectives:

- To give physicians the background data to assess the changes and forces they are facing.
- To lay out a step-by-step strategy for a physician to evolve from a solo or small group practice to a market-dominant, provider-sponsored delivery system.
- To describe the different types of organizational models they can use to implement that strategy.
- To provide methodologies for evaluating their alternative courses of action.
- To introduce them to the operational changes they will have to make to practice managed medicine.
- To explain the pros and cons of all the choices they must make, provide guidelines for the actions they will take, and warn of the pitfalls and risks in every strategy they might adopt.
- To, at every point, be as practical and action-oriented as possible.

I wish physicians to use the knowledge in this book to guide their strategic and operational practice decisions for at least the next three years. Toward that end, I have constructed the book according to the following plan. This is an explanation of why I have included each chapter topic that follows and have arranged them in their particular order. They are intended to fall into a natural progression.

From the beginning, I wanted the first chapter to be a set of facts about the changes sweeping the health care industry that would persuade physicians of the need to read the rest of the book. I expected to gather a few key pieces of data from a variety of sources, describing the inroads of managed care and the ways they have transformed the practice of medicine. Then I came upon the wonderful set of data reports published annually by Hoechst Marion Roussell. They are discussed more thoroughly in the Resource List at the end of Chapter 1. The reports gather in one place quantitative information from several sources, such as the Medical Group Management Association and the SMG Marketing Group. Two of my Harvard colleagues who do extensive survey work with Louis Harris and Associates, Bob Blendon and Karen Donelan, allowed me to use some of their excellent data. The data tables and quantitative reports that appear in almost every issue of *Medical Economics* magazine were a valuable resource.

When I was through, I found that I had enough solid facts to illuminate six aspects of the managed care transformation spread across the first four chapters. This is a lot of coverage. However, I feel that the data are so powerful and so useful—both as a foundation for this book and for later use in strategic market analysis—that I chose to include them.

The fifth chapter describes the strategic framework around which the rest of the book is built. It lays out a step-by-step program by which an ambitious single physician could conceivably move from a solo or small group practice all the way to a physician-sponsored, multiprovider integrated delivery system. It is a path that can take physicians from positions of impotence and frustration to careers of executive leadership, market strength, clinical freedom, and financial comfort.

The strategy is described literally as a series of steps, as follows:

- Step One: Preparing Your Practice for Operation under Managed Care
- Step Two: How To Analyze and Evaluate a Managed Care Contract
- Step Three: Forming or Joining a Small, Single Specialty Group Practice
- Step Four: Joining an Independent Practice Association
- Step Five: Growing into a Larger, Multispecialty Group Practice
- Step Six: Forming a Physician-Hospital Organization—An Affiliation between Your Group Practice and a Hospital
- Step Seven: Partnering with a Management Services Organization or Physician Practice Management Company
- Step Eight: Forming a Medical Foundation
- Step Nine: Selling Your Practice to a Hospital, Managed Care Organization, Or Physician Practice Management Company
- Step Ten: Increasing the Level of Integration in Your Provider Organization
- Step Eleven: The Final Step–Evolving into a Regionwide Vertically Integrated Delivery System

As a practical matter, it would not make sense for a physician or physician group to implement each of these steps, one after the other. There would not be enough time. By the time they got to steps eight or nine, the market would have passed them by long ago. It would be a waste of resources. Once the physicians have formed a large multispecialty group practice, integrated their practices and operations, and gained experience in managing care, they are ready to move to some kind of role in an IDS. It would be illogical for them to go through the PHO and medical foundation stages.

The reason that all of these initiatives have been discussed and designated as strategic steps

is that they all are possible way stations on the different paths physicians may take in reaching their best position in a managed health care system.

The sixth chapter is a quick look at a physician's professional life as her practice becomes more and more dominated by managed care. It is intended, along with the data in the first four chapters, to set the background for the strategic moves that this book urges her to consider and adopt.

The seventh chapter explains all the basic operational adjustments a physician must make to adapt his practice to managed care. These are changes and improvements that he can begin immediately, even in a solo practice, without altering its structure or strategic direction. They do not require talking with other physicians or affiliating with other provider organizations. However, in a small practice, they will be implemented on a small scale. It will take consolidation and integration with other physicians to execute these programs at a level that produces maximum benefits.

The first contact most physicians have with managed care is through a contract to provide services to an MCO. Chapter 8 explains how to examine those contracts and wind up with ones that are most rewarding for the physician. For many physicians, this knowledge alone will improve the quality of their professional lives. Chapter 9 follows up by offering ideas on how to effectively negotiate not only managed care contracts but also other transactions that physicians frequently face.

Chapter 10 introduces the physician to what may be her first overt strategic action—joining with other physicians in her specialty to begin practicing together in a small group. Some may already have reached this stage on their own. For the others, it presents the challenge of learning how to subordinate personal wishes to the common good of everyone in the group. It is good practice for what she must do in the coming years.

Chapter 11 raises the stakes only slightly by explaining how and why to participate in an IPA.

This organizational form is recommended as only a transitional strategic step, to give a physician experience in practicing, even partially and passively, as a member of a very large group of physicians trying to be a more influential player in the managed care game. With the right leadership, the IPA can also be the vehicle for steering the physicians toward greater integration with each other.

Chapter 12 talks about group practices without walls (GPWWs) because they get a lot of media attention and have been established successfully in a number of cases. They have not been recommended as a strategic step because of legal questions about how participating physicians collaborate with each other and because their lack of integration makes them a wasteful, delaying step. In some cases, a GPWW may serve as a viable alternative to an IPA.

The larger, multispecialty group practice described in Chapter 13 is the most important organizational form in the book. It can be a highly desirable strategic end stage for physicians who do not want to sell out to another entity and prefer instead to own and control their own delivery organization. Through virtual integration and arm's-length strategic affiliations, it is conceivable that physicians in one of these groups could be fully plugged into a good IDS without having to surrender their independence.

Chapter 14 could have been placed anywhere in the chapter sequence of this book. At some point or another in their strategic planning, physicians must analyze the market in which they practice for competitive opportunities. This chapter explains how to carry out that assessment.

Chapter 15 represents another major strategic move for a group of physicians—its first affiliation with a nonphysician provider and with a much larger, better-financed organization—a hospital. The physician-hospital organization (PHO) has been criticized nearly as much as the IPA as an unnecessary delaying step. This chapter argues that a PHO serves a purpose as an introductory step for hesitant physicians on the road to further integration, but only so long as the physicians join as a large, somewhat unified group.

The organizational option described in Chapter 16 is another strategic "end point" for physicians. Once they have sold their practice assets to a PPMC, it is somewhat difficult to turn back. Only with great difficulty could a physician extricate herself from a PPMC and restart an independent medical career. For that reason, this step and the commitment it entails must be carefully studied.

The formation of a medical foundation, as described in Chapter 17, may seem like a modest step, but it can be momentous for the right group of physicians. It is an essential organization form in states that vigorously enforce the "corporate practice of medicine" doctrine. As a nonprofit, charitable model, it can have great philosophic attraction for physicians who wish to avoid the trappings of commercialism. It may also be the corporate shell for that critical end-stage entity, the larger, multispecialty group practice.

Chapter 18 explains the basic principles of selling a physician's practice assets to almost any buyer, then becoming employed by that entity. The buyer may be a hospital, an MCO, or a PPMC. The chapter also discusses the transaction from the viewpoint of the buyer, in those cases where it may be a physician group. Many physicians are selling their practices in this way and, in the process, giving up aspirations for creating some kind of larger physician-driven organization.

In Chapter 19, the book explores the variety of sophisticated systems, procedures, and policies that have become the standard tools for integrating the clinical, financial, and business operations of physician practices. This is another omnibus topic that must be understood and acted upon in some fashion by every physician group.

Whereas Chapter 8 discusses the basic terms of a simple professional services contract between a physician and an MCO, Chapter 20 deals with the much more challenging matter of providing those services under a capitation arrangement. It looks not only at the unique provisions of capitated contracts, but also at some of their effects on the way the physician must practice medicine.

Chapter 21 presents the organizational form recommended by this book as the ultimate stage in a most ambitious physician practice development strategy—the IDS. Though there is much debate over the exact shape of an IDS and how integrated it should be, there is little doubt that a systemic multiprovider approach to health care delivery is the right path. This chapter helps to explain how physicians might travel that path.

One of the greatest sources of physician anxiety is their loss of control as the health care system evolves. In Chapter 22, they have a chance to learn about the design of governance structures that will enable them to retain maximum authority and to facilitate their decision making. This is an issue that arises in every kind of organization, even those controlled entirely by physicians.

Perhaps the second greatest source of physician anxiety is the possibility that they will not be "selected" to contract with an MCO or to join an existing provider group or, once having been selected, they will be "deselected." There is a very real concern that a physician could lose a major source of income if she is unfairly rejected by a payer or provider organization. Chapter 23 examines the circumstances under which physicians may be selected and deselected, and suggests ways for physicians to keep the contracts and affiliations they really want.

Almost every strategic recommendation in this book involves collaboration with another person or entity—physician, hospital, private investors, MCOs, and others payers. Chapter 24 offers guidelines for making the best choices of individuals and organizations that may become lifelong partners.

Chapter 25 explains the reimbursement systems that physicians are likely to encounter under managed care. It looks at the ways money flows to a physician organization, then at the methods the organization uses to allocate that money to individual physicians. A physician confused about how his compensation is determined is an upset physician. This chapter tries to alleviate some of that confusion.

Chapter 26 covers another foundation topic for nearly all physicians—the tools she needs to understand and manage risk. If she can apply these tools to effectively assume that risk, she stands a greater chance of keeping her managed care contracts and maximizing her managed care income.

This book makes only a nice wish list unless there is money to finance the strategic projects and enterprises it recommends. Lack of sufficient capital is one of the greatest barriers to physicians retaking the initiative in health care reform by forming their own delivery organizations. In Chapter 27, they can learn about the many varieties of capital financing and which sources are most suitable for each of their capital projects.

Physicians want very badly to collaborate with each other in responding to the overtures of much larger delivery systems and MCOs. They would prefer to do this without all becoming employees of a single organization. Chapter 28 explains the legal implications of physician attempts to collaborate for competitive reasons. It explains how and when they may talk to each other about what kinds of issues without running afoul of the law.

Lots of new businesses fail within just a few years. So do a lot of health care businesses, and even physician organizations. Chapter 29 describes some of the more common reasons that modern physician ventures never achieve profitability. By avoiding these pitfalls, a physician and her group improve their chances of long-term practice success. Chapter 30 is a hopeful attempt to offer a few alternatives to the physician who wants to hang on to the features of traditional medical practice as long as possible.

In Chapter 31, the several strategic steps in this book are bundled into complete multiyear strategic scenarios. Criteria are suggested for evaluating these scenarios. Then letter grades are assigned for the degree to which each scenario satisfies each of the criteria. An overall grade is given to the entire scenario. The result is a series of strategic score cards. The basic scoring methodology can be applied, with different criteria, weights, and scores, to any strategy that a physician may wish to consider.

The undertakings recommended in this book are ambitious, expensive, risky, and, in some cases, daring. However, they do not stretch the limits of what the boldest, most aggressive physicians might dream of achieving. There are additional steps in the possible strategic progression.

As leaders of large integrated delivery systems, physician groups may take over all the functions of the MCOs and may deal directly with payers. This is already happening where physicians have entered into direct service contracts with employers. The Medicare+Choice program encourages the formation of physician-sponsored organizations to deal directly with HCFA.

Once physicians have formed the most powerful physician group permitted by the antitrust laws in their market area, they are in a position to link up with similar organizations in other areas.

By building and connecting such groups in major markets across the country, it is possible to create a nationwide network of physicians with the resources and influence to deal on equal footing with the largest health plan or payer. Within the network, the physicians can deal with each other on whatever terms they choose. Such a national system also must comply with antitrust laws.

By using any combination of the strategic steps described in this book, physicians have the power to become a dominant force, if not the dominant force, in shaping and managing the U.S. health care system. It takes only two additional ingredients—boldness and determination.

## CHAPTER 1

Industry Trends That Are Forcing Physicians To Rethink Their Long-Term Strategies

Basic Facts about Physician Practices
Basic Facts about Integrated Delivery Systems

INTRODUCTION

The American system for delivering and financing health care is now called an "industry." It already looks very different from the way it did 20, or even 10, years ago. The dramatic and revolutionary changes are still continuing. It probably will take another 5 or 10 years for a new, more stable industry structure to take shape. In the meantime, the roles of all the players in health care are being transformed. Some are gaining authority; others are losing it. Everyone is performing new tasks and facing new challenges. This is most true for physicians.

The first four chapters summarize the industry changes and their impacts on physicians. A considerable body of data is used to demonstrate the changes. These changes are the reasons why proactive physicians must take steps now to restructure their practices, form alliances with other physicians and providers, and learn new operational skills. The remainder of the book describes those steps.

These data chapters are organized as follows:

- Chapter 1
  Basic Facts about Physician Practices
  Basic Facts about Integrated Delivery Systems
- Chapter 2
  Basic Facts about Managed Care Organizations

- Chapter 3
  Physician Involvement in Managed Care
  Effects of Managed Care on Physician Practice Operations and Strategy
- Chapter 4
  Physician and Patient Attitudes toward the New Health Care System

WHO SHOULD READ THIS CHAPTER

There can be few physicians who are not aware of the spread of managed care and capitated reimbursement, the implementation of cost and utilization control measures, the demise of solo and small group practices, and related trends. Many may not know the specific extent of these developments. In this chapter, they will see quantitative evidence of the most important industry trends. In most cases, they are likely to be surprised at how far managed care has taken over health care and the effect it is having on the way doctors practice medicine.

The data and analyses in these chapters are also good specific indicators of how quickly physicians must adapt. There are several breakdowns by geographic areas of the country. Physicians in some areas may see that they have more, or less, time to prepare for the changes taking place in their area. Other figures may tell them which changes are coming at which rates.

These chapters are a guide on exactly which practice changes physicians should think about making in order to stay competitive. In some cases, they will find that they have alternatives— different types of payers may offer different forms of reimbursement or require different controls on utilization. To an extent, the figures in these chapters will help doctors plan their practice change strategies over the next few years.

There is information here about some individual managed care organizations, their finances, and the scope of their operations. This may be useful to physicians who must evaluate and negotiate with them.

The extensive data on the performance of physician practices and MCOs, under a variety of circumstances, provide a basis of comparison with each reader's practice. For instance, a physician can see how much he will have to lower his utilization rates to participate in an MCO.

Physicians who are thoroughly persuaded of the threat of managed care, have a good sense of its impact on other physician practices, and feel qualified to analyze any MCO that comes along, may be able to move directly to the chapters that explain the strategic options that interest them.

BASIC FACTS ABOUT PHYSICIAN PRACTICES

This section provides background information on the current status of physician group practices, apart from their involvement in managed care activities.

There were nearly 6,738 medical group practices in operation in 1996, but this represented a decline of 2.4 percent from 1995 (Table 1–1). Notice that all of the decline occurred in the smallest groups—those with fewer than 11 full-time equivalent (FTE) physicians. All the other group size categories increased in number. In

fact, the number of the largest groups (over 50 FTE physicians) grew the most. This would suggest that doctors are consolidating into larger and larger groupings. While groups of under 11 FTE physicians still make up almost three-quarters of all group practices, that proportion is dwindling steadily.

The group practice growth trend is intriguing when looked at in terms of who owns the practices (Table 1–2). Physicians still own the vast majority (58 percent) of medical group practices.

Table 1–1 Number of Medical Group Practices by Number of Full-Time Equivalent (FTE) Physicians and Their Growth Rate from 1995 to 1996

Group Size (# of FTE Physicians)	Number of Medical Group Practices		Percentage of Groups (%)		Growth Rate (%)
	1995	1996	1995	1996	1995–1996
fewer than 11 FTEs	4,902	4,674	71.0	69.2	–4.7
11–25 FTEs	1,185	1,190	17.2	17.6	0.4
26–50 FTEs	423	439	6.1	6.5	3.8
51–75 FTEs	115	125	1.7	1.9	8.7
76–150 FTEs	122	138	1.8	2.0	13.1
over 150 FTEs	159	172	2.3	2.5	8.2
Total	6,906	6,738	100	100	–2.4

Source: Adapted with permission from Medical Group Practice Digest, p. 6, © 1997, Hoechst Marion Roussel.

Table 1–2 Number of Medical Group Practices by Owner Type, and Their Growth Rates from 1995 to 1996

Owner	Number of Medical Group Practices		Growth Rate (%)
	1995	1996	1995–1996
Government	13	12	−7.7
Hospital	519	443	−14.6
Employer	19	18	−5.3
Integrated Health System	111	91	−18.0
Management Company, For-Profit Investor	63	55	−12.7
Physicians	4,369	3,923	−10.2
University/Medical School	147	142	−3.4
Other	180	161	−10.6
Unknown	1,487	1,908	28.3

Source: Adapted with permission from *Medical Group Practice Digest*, p. 6, © 1997, Hoechst Marion Roussel.

But that figure reveals that over 40 percent are owned by nonphysicians. Hospitals are the second most common owners (7 percent). However, the numbers in every single ownership category declined, except those for "Unknown." These increased by over 28 percent.

The groups in that category obviously do not belong in any of the others, but it is unclear just who the owners might be. The best guess is that these group practices are owned by combinations of different parties, such as physicians and a hospital or physicians and a practice management company. If that interpretation is accurate, it would indicate that the movement in group practices is toward those new forms emerging in response to managed care.

Physician compensation increased from 1992 to 1996 in all specialties except diagnostic radiology (Table 1–3). The pay of primary care physicians grew three times as fast (16.92 percent) as did the pay of specialist physicians (5.49 percent). This reflects the greater market demand for primary care doctors to serve in gatekeeper and similar roles. Still, a few specialties (dermatol-

ogy, emergency medicine, and general surgery) did quite well, increasing their earnings even more than their primary care colleagues.

Keep in mind that the salary growth for even primary care physicians averaged little more than 4 percent a year, barely keeping ahead of the inflation rate. Certain specialties such as anesthesiology, ophthalmology, and urology actually earned fewer inflation-adjusted dollars in 1996 than they did in 1992.

The compensation for midlevel providers, including several categories of physician extender, have increased as well—at a rate midway between that of the primary care and specialist physicians. Their importance has grown as physician groups endeavor to increase their productivity without proportionately increasing the number and compensation of physicians in the groups.

The methods by which primary care doctors are compensated by their groups vary considerably. A great preponderance (83.7 percent, up from 79.7 percent in 1995) have their pay tied in some degree to their work productivity (Table

Table 1–3 Increases in Physician Pay, 1992–1996, by Physician Specialty

	1992	1996	% Change
All Primary Care	$115,646	$135,217	16.92
Family Practice	112,585	132,434	17.63
Internal Medicine	119,538	140,000	17.12
Pediatrics	116,637	132,039	13.21
All Specialties	$210,020	$221,544	5.49
Anesthesiology	235,000	237,749	1.17
Invasive Cardiology	320,476	353,769	10.39
Noninvasive Cardiology	243,912	247,133	1.32
Dermatology	153,347	181,774	18.54
Emergency Medicine	138,502	179,997	29.96
Gastroenterology	203,773	224,382	10.11
Hematology/Oncology	167,406	190,550	13.83
Neurology	153,140	161,310	5.33
Obstetrics/Gynecology	206,133	217,549	5.54
Ophthalmology	199,183	205,500	3.17
Otorhinolaryngology	199,583	226,554	13.51
Psychiatry	120,000	136,470	13.73
Pulmonary Disease	161,153	169,034	4.89
Diagnostic Radiology	271,723	269,404	−0.85
General Surgery	187,073	223,388	19.41
Orthopedic Surgery	289,323	310,475	7.31
Urology	215,721	222,236	3.02
All Midlevel Providers	$49,636	$55,459	11.73
Certified RN Anesthetist	77,461	79,002	1.99
Nurse Practitioner	42,500	50,910	19.79
Optometrist	68,950	77,450	12.33
Physician Assistant, Surgical	43,407	63,589	46.49
Physician Assistant, Primary Care	43,407	56,249	29.59
Psychologist	60,000	62,379	3.97

Source: Physician Compensation and Production Survey: 1997 Report Based on 1996 Data. Reprinted with permission from the Medical Group Management Association, 104 Inverness Terrace East, Englewood, Colorado 80112–5306; 303-799-1111. Copyright © 1997.

1–4). One-third are paid entirely on the basis of productivity. As a general rule, the smaller groups are more likely to employ simpler compensation methods, like equal shares, straight salary, or salary plus incentives. The larger groups lean more toward productivity systems that require more sophisticated information gathering.

Most of the growth in the salaries of family physicians occurred from 1994 to 1995 (Table 1–5). In other recent years, the annual increases

Table 1–4 Compensation Method for Primary Care Physicians, by Group Size

Group Size	Productivity (%)			Salary Plus Incentives (%)	Straight Salary (%)	100% Equal Shares	Other (%)
	100%	75–99%	50–74%				
10 or fewer	28.1	9.8	6.3	31.3	16.4	2.7	5.5
11–25	38.5	20.5	7.7	25.6	5.1	—	2.6
26–50	44.4	21.0	8.6	22.2	2.5	—	1.2
51–99	28.0	32.0	10.0	14.0	8.0	—	8.0
100 or more	33.3	21.2	12.1	18.2	15.2	—	—
All Groups	33.2	16.6	7.6	26.3	11.0	1.3	4.1

Compensation Methods:

100% Productivity – 100% of physician pay is based on individual physician productivity.
75–99% Productivity – 75% to 99% of physician pay is based on individual physician productivity; remainder is based on other factors.
50–74% Productivity – 50% to 74% of physician pay is based on individual physician productivity; remainder is based on other factors.
Salary Plus Incentives – 50% to 99% of physician pay is a guaranteed base salary. The balance is determined through other measures, such as productivity and proft sharing.
Straight Salary – 100% of physician compensation is attributable to fixed salaries.
100% Equal Shares – All physicians in the medical group are paid equal amounts based on the group's performance.
Other – Compensation levels determined by evaluating patient satisfaction, physician leadership roles, seniority, and involvement in community services.

Note: Sample size was 17,417 providers in 537 groups.

Source: Adapted with permission from *Medical Group Practice Digest*, p. 26, © 1997, Hoechst Marion Roussel.

barely exceeded 4.0 percent, hardly enough to keep up with inflation.

Physicians increasingly are asked to serve in positions of managerial leadership. Their compensation for assuming those responsibilities is substantial (Table 1–6). One out of every four chief executive officers (CEOs) of medical group practices earns well over $300,000 a year for the work. The average salary varies greatly by geographic region. In the West, where greater managed care pressures would seem to place a premium on physician executives, they earn the least—$144,000. In the South, where managed care penetration is generally lower, an average physician executive will be paid $233,000 a year.

One way a group practice makes itself more visible in the community and accessible to

Table 1–5 Family Physicians' Median Base Salaries and Annual Percentage Increases

	Median Base Salary	Annual % Increase
1993	$102,000	8.23
1994	$103,050	1.01
1995	$115,000	13.04
1996	$120,000	4.16
1997	$125,093	4.24

Source: Adapted with permission from *Managed Care Magazine*, Vol. 6, No. 7, p. 35, © 1997.

Table 1–6 Salaries of Physician as CEOs of Medical Group Practices

25th Percentile	$191,946
Median	$241,820
75th Percentile	$333,961
South	$223,358
East	$194,713
Midwest	$177,000
West	$144,000

Source: Management Compensation and Production Survey: 1997 Report Based on 1996 Data. Reprinted with permission from the Medical Group Management Association, 104 Inverness Terrace East, Englewood, Colorado 80112–5306; 303-799-1111. Copyright © 1997.

patients is through the creation of satellite offices (Table 1–7). Two-thirds of all groups have such branch operations. Of that number, over a quarter operate five or more satellite offices.

Many physician groups aim to make themselves more attractive to patients and managed

Table 1–7 Percentage of Groups with Satellite Offices

Have Satellite Offices	64.3
Do Not Have Satellite Offices	35.7

Number of Satellite Offices per Group (%) (of those groups with at least one satellite or branch office)

1–2 Satellites	51.9
3–4 Satellites	21.4
5–6 Satellites	11.6
7+ Satellites	15.1

Source: Adapted with permission from *Medical Group Practice Digest*, p. 11, © 1997, Hoechst Marion Roussel.

care organizations (MCOs), as well as bring in additional revenues, by offering a variety of supplementary services and facilities (Table 1–8). Two-fifths provided an on-site diagnostic X-ray capability; almost a third operated a clinical laboratory. About a quarter offered extended office hours and formal patient education programs.

Like most other areas of the economy, physician practices are applying computers in new ways to managing their operations (Table 1–9). These are some of the clinical applications. The multispecialty groups, which tend to be larger and more ambitious, are more likely to use computers for accessing the Medline database and clinical patient information. Over a quarter of them use computers to exchange clinical data with other physicians. As a general rule, single specialty groups employ computers more extensively than solo doctors, and multi-specialty groups are more computerized than any other practices.

Table 1–8 Some Facilities and Services Offered, by Group Practices

Facilities within the Practice

Ambulatory Surgery	14.5%
Audiology	10.7%
Clinical Laboratory	29.8%
Immediate Care	14.8%
Physical Therapy	11.4%
X-ray (Diagnostic)	40.7%

Patient Services Offered

Cardiology Stress Testing (Treadmill)	21.2%
Extended Hours for Patient Care	29.9%
Formal Patient Education Programs	24.3%

Source: Adapted with permission from *Medical Group Practice Digest*, p. 11, © 1997, Hoechst Marion Roussel.

Table 1–9 Physician Use of Computers for Practice Functions, by Practice Type

	Solo Practice (%)	Single Specialty (%)	Multispecialty (%)
Access information such as Medline via on-line services or the Internet	29	45	47
Access to clinical patient information	14	24	40
Record patient clinical information, such as medical histories	13	13	22
Transmit clinical information to other doctors, who may or may not work at other sites	10	7	27

Source: Courtesy of Louis Harris & Associates, Inc., New York, New York.

Physicians are not the only ones relying on their computers to access health information. Their patients are doing the same thing, using the Internet, often at the urging of their doctors. Here, too, the multispecialty groups are the most aggressive (Table 1–10).

LEADING TRENDS

- Number of medical group practices is declining.
- Average size of medical group practices is increasing.
- Growth in numbers of group practices may be among those types created in response to managed care.
- Primary care physician salaries are still much lower than specialist salaries, but are growing three times as fast.
- Over time, physician salary increases are barely keeping pace with inflation.
- Salaries of midlevel providers are increasing faster than specialist salaries but not as fast as primary care salaries.
- Compensation of most primary care doctors is tied to their productivity.
- Average annual increases in family physician salaries have been quite modest.

Table 1–10 Patient Use of the Internet for Health Information, by Practice Type

	Solo Practice (%)	Single Specialty (%)	Multispecialty (%)
Physician suggests that patient get health information from Internet	15	21	35
Patient gets health information from Internet on own initiative	65	73	76

Source: Courtesy of Louis Harris & Associates, Inc., New York, New York.

- Physician executives of medical group practices are earning substantial incomes.
- A majority of groups have satellite offices.

- Large proportions of both physicians and their patients are using computers to access and exchange medical information.

BASIC FACTS ABOUT INTEGRATED DELIVERY SYSTEMS

When different kinds of providers (e.g., primary care physicians, specialist physicians, hospitals) combine themselves into systems or networks in order to be able to deliver a wider range of the health care services required by a patient, they are creating an "integrated delivery system" (IDS). The coming together is called "integration" because the operational management and clinical information and decision making of the provider components tend to be merged. As a general rule, an IDS does not include a financing component. If it did, it would more truly be a managed care organization.

There were 570 systems at the end of 1996 that identified themselves as being in the process of integration. Of these, 189 (up from 159 in 1995) were the most highly integrated, which meant that they included at least three delivery components (a physician organization, an acute care hospital, and one other significant provider entity) and were operating under at least one systemwide managed care contract.

Table 1–11 Initiators of Integrated Health Systems

Hospital	66.7%
Combination	22.8
Physician	5.3
HMO/PPO	4.2
PHO	1.1
Total	100%

Source: Adapted with permission from *Integrated Health Systems Digest*, p. 16, © 1997, Hoechst Marion Roussel.

Provider entities include health care facilities such as hospitals, nursing homes, home health agencies, physician practices, diagnostic imaging centers, and free-standing outpatient surgery centers. A health care facility is not necessarily affiliated with only one IDS. It could contract with, or be owned in part by, more than one system.

Since the formation of an IDS is such a major undertaking, it is useful to note which providers or other entities take the initiative (Table 1–11). In two-thirds of the cases, it is a hospital that is the catalyst. Until now, physicians have been responsible for initiating only 5 percent of the integrated systems. Some combination of parties starts a quarter of the systems.

A key question to be answered in forming any business, and certainly a health care delivery system, concerns the geographic scope of its operations. This determines the market area and number of patients it will target and the competition it will encounter. In 1996, the delivery focus of over half the integrated systems was "regional" (Table 1–12). A region could encompass a large part of a state and even stretch across state lines. Most of the other half of the systems are servicing a "local" area, perhaps surrounding a small city or part of a large city.

The total number of provider units participating in integrated systems increased from 4,381 in 1995 to 5,328 in 1996, a jump of 22 percent (Table 1–13). Nearly 80 percent of these providers were connected with IDSs made up of more than 20 units each—truly large systems. These might include 2 or 3 hospitals, 10 to 12 physician organizations, and a variety of other units.

An interesting feature of an IDS is the kinds of relationships it has with its provider components. Generally, it can completely own the providers, or it can simply contract with or "rent" them. In the smallest systems (4–6 units), which tend to be

Table 1–12 Delivery Focus of Integrated Health Systems

	Number of Systems		1995–1996 % Change
Delivery Focus	1996	1995	
Local	70	58	20.7
Statewide	19	16	18.8
Regional	100	85	17.6
Total	189	159	

Source: Adapted with permission from *Integrated Health Systems Digest*, p. 7, © 1997, Hoechst Marion Roussel.

the newest or most tentative ventures, about 80 percent of the providers participate through contracts. In contrast, any system larger than 6 units owns over 40 percent of its providers. This follows the notion that, as systems become larger and more competitive, they feel the need to own their provider components—in order to control them more tightly.

In defining these relationships with their providers, IDSs tend to follow the 60–40 ratio between contracting and owning. There are

exceptions for certain types of provider units. In about 70 percent of the cases, an IDS contracts with home health agencies, hospices, and cancer centers. On the other hand, an IDS prefers to own a free-standing outpatient surgery center 55 percent of the time. These data may be broadly useful for system planners to see what kinds of units go into an IDS and the kinds of relationships they have with it (Table 1–14).

A physician may reasonably wonder what share of physician practices and other types of providers in the United States are tied into integrated systems. It may be an indication of how quickly he or she ought to consider doing the same thing. Approximately 10 percent of physician practices participate in some form of IDS (Table 1–15). This may not seem like much, but that figure grew by a full percentage point from the previous year. A little less than one-fifth (18.8 percent) of hospitals are part of an IDS, and that figure jumped three percentage points over 1995. Over 10 percent of health maintenance organizations (HMOs) have their organizational base in an integrated system. Sometimes, the HMO is a catalyst in forming a system; other times, the system develops the HMO.

The propensity for owning or renting provider units varies greatly depending on who initiated it (Table 1–16). An HMO that starts an IDS wants

Table 1–13 Number of Provider Units in Integrated Health Systems, by System Size and Relationship with the System

Units per System	Total # of Units		% Contracted	% Owned
4–6 Provider Units	49	(54)	79.6	20.4
7–10 Provider Units	212	(175)	56.1	43.9
11–20 Provider Units	884	(803)	54.5	45.5
21+ Provider Units	4,183	(3,343)	58.2	41.8
Total	5,328	(4,381*)	57.7	42.3

*This total includes six integrated health systems with three provider units per system.

Note: Figures in parentheses are from 1995.

Source: Adapted with permission from *Integrated Health Systems Digest*, p. 12, © 1997, Hoechst Marion Roussel.

Table 1–14 Number of Provider Units in Integrated Health Systems, by Unit Type and Relationship with the System

Unit Type	Total # of Units		% Contracted	% Owned
Physician Practice	2,072	(1,732)	57.4	42.6
Hospital	1,377	(1,093)	55.2	44.8
Home Health Agency	455	(372)	66.4	33.6
Nursing Home	232	(181)	53.0	47.0
HMO/PPO	159	(139)	58.5	41.5
Free-Standing Outpatient Surgery Center	134	(121)	44.8	55.2
Rehabilitation Center	86	(73)	57.0	43.0
Diagnostic Imaging Center	64	(51)	62.5	37.5
Hospice	50	(34)	72.0	28.0
Mental Health Center	42	(34)	54.8	45.2
Dialysis Center	38	(34)	55.3	44.7
Cancer Center	24	(19)	70.8	29.2
Other*	595	(498)	60.3	39.7
Total	5,328	(4,381)	57.7	42.3

*"Other" includes pharmacies, laboratories, chemical dependency centers, and blood banks.

Note: Figures in parentheses are from 1995.

Source: Adapted with permission from *Integrated Health Systems Digest*, p. 12, © 1997, Hoechst Marion Roussel.

Table 1–15 Percentage of All Provider Facilities Participating in Integrated Systems, by Facility Type

Facility Type	Total # of Facilities in U.S.	% of Them in Integrated Systems	
Hospital	5,497	18.8	(15.2)
HMO	556	13.2	(11.7)
Physician Practice	14,791	9.4	(8.5)
Free-Standing Outpatient Surgery Center	2,134	5.2	(4.3)
Home Health Agency	15,087	2.5	(2.0)
Diagnostic Imaging Center	2,156	2.2	(1.8)
Nursing Home	15,220	1.1	(1.0)

Note: Figures in parentheses are from 1995.

Source: Adapted with permission from *Integrated Health Systems Digest*, p. 17, © 1997, Hoechst Marion Roussel.

Table 1–16 Ownership vs. Rental of Provider Units by Integrated Systems by Type of Initiator

Initiator	Total # of Units		Contracted % ("Rented")		Owned %	
Hospital	3,477	(2,890)	57.6	(61.0)	42.4	(39.0)
Physician	318	(179)	64.2	(58.1)	35.8	(41.9)
HMO/PPO	375	(364)	7.5	(5.8)	92.5	(94.2)
PHO	14	(3)	92.9	(66.7)	7.1	(33.3)
Combination	1,144	(945)	57.7	(70.2)	42.3	(29.8)

Note: Figures in parentheses are from 1995.

Source: Adapted with permission from *Integrated Health Systems Digest*, p. 16, © 1997, Hoechst Marion Roussel.

to own the providers in over 90 percent of the cases. At the other extreme, over 90 percent of physician-hospital organizations (PHOs) that evolve into IDSs prefer to contract with their providers. This is not surprising since PHOs themselves are usually created in the hopes that a great deal of further integration will not be necessary. HMOs, on the other hand, have a natural preoccupation with controlling their costs as well as the providers who incur them. Integrated systems established by other entities gravitate toward the 60–40 rental/ownership ratio.

Where in the United States are integrated systems to be found? Approximately one-quarter each are located in the West, Midwest, and Southeast (Table 1–17). To show that integration does not always go hand in hand with managed care penetration, only 10 percent of the systems operate in the Northeast—an area with high levels of managed care enrollment.

Nearly half (47.2 percent) of the 159 most highly integrated health systems had their central offices located in just seven states: California (11.9 percent), Michigan (8.8 percent), Texas (6.9 percent), Georgia (5.7 percent), Florida (5.0 percent), Arizona (4.4 percent), and Tennessee (4.4 percent).

Physicians trying to assess their own need to integrate might like some more precise geographic information. The data in Table 1–18 describe the extent of integration in major metro-

politan statistical areas (MSAs) classified into four market stages.

The health care management consulting firm, APM Inc., classified cities by their degree of managed care market evolution, using the following structure:

• Stage 1 – Markets are unstructured, with independent hospitals, physicians, employers, and HMOs.

Table 1–17 Distribution of Integrated Systems by Region

Region	Number of Systems	Percentage of Systems
West	48 (40)	25.4 (25.2)
Southwest	30 (28)	15.9 (17.6)
Midwest	46 (39)	24.3 (24.5)
Northeast	20 (11)	10.6 (6.9)
Southeast	45 (41)	23.8 (25.8)
Total	189 (159)	100

Note: Figures in parentheses are from 1995.

Source: Adapted with permission from *Integrated Health Systems Digest*, p. 14, © 1997, Hoechst Marion Roussel.

- Stage 2 – Markets are those in which a loose managed care framework is forming, propelling the emergence of leading MCOs, coupled with weak provider networks and hospital affiliations.
- Stage 3 – Markets show MCOs consolidating, and extensive formation of group practices and hospital systems occurs.
- Stage 4 – Markets achieve managed competition, with strong employer coalitions and the emergence of integrated physician/hospital systems. There are only four MSAs classified in this stage.

The 21 MSAs were selected to represent each of the four market stages (Table 1–18). The 72 systems described are all among the 189 most highly integrated systems covered in previous tables.

Perhaps the most noteworthy figures are the average 31 percent of hospitals and nearly 11 percent of physician centers participating in integrated systems in these markets. Those are significant numbers. In the most highly evolved Stage 4 markets, at least 60 percent of the hospitals have integrated in three of the four MSAs (Minneapolis-St. Paul, San Diego, and Worcester). Physician integration in those cities ranges from a low of 23 percent (San Diego) to a high of 42 percent (Worcester). If these four stages represent points on a continuum, then perhaps physicians in less integrated markets should look forward to integration levels like these.

The extent of integration is quite high in even some of the less advanced markets. For instance, 30 percent of the physician centers and 47 percent of the hospitals are part of integrated systems in Detroit, a Stage 3 market. Hospital integration has reached 57 percent in Cleveland-Lorain-Elyria and 44 percent in St. Louis, both Stage 2 markets.

The numbers in most all of these MSAs show increases from the previous year. Hospital integration went from 33 percent to 42 percent in Chicago, 40 percent to 47 percent in Phoenix-Mesa, 11 percent to 32 percent in New York City, and 35 percent to 57 percent in Cleveland-

Lorain-Elyria. Physician integration grew from 4 percent to 9 percent in Boston, and 7 percent to 14 percent in Riverside-San Bernardino.

In one year (1995–1996), the average integration levels for hospitals in all 21 MSAs increased from 25.8 percent to 31.1 percent, for physician centers from 9.7 percent to 10.6 percent, for HMOs from 9.5 percent to 13.0 percent, and for nursing homes from 2.0 percent to 2.1 percent. These are significant increases for a 12-month period. They suggest that integration is being pursued aggressively in many market areas.

A physician contemplating forming or joining an IDS may wonder how many of his or her colleagues he or she is likely to encounter there. In other words, how many physicians participate in an average integrated system? The figures are not small and they vary by region (Table 1–19). The largest systems are in the Central Region of the country, where they include an average of 1,985 physicians each. Systems in the Eastern region get by with less than half that number (747). Notice also the ratio between primary care and specialist physicians. Nowhere does it come even close to the 50–50 balance that is often recommended as ideal for integrated systems.

Another aspect of the physician role in IDSs has to do with the number of physicians likely to be working together in a system-related practice, office, or center. The numbers vary by region, from as many as 24 in the West to as few as 7 in the Southeast. This probably reflects historical distinctions in practice culture. Even more interesting is the contrast with the average number of physicians in non–system-related practices and offices. In these figures, there is rather little variation from region to region. However, in four of the five regions, the system practices are much larger than the nonsystem ones, by factors of two or three. In the Southeast, the system physician centers are actually slightly smaller than their nonsystem counterparts. These data may give physicians a feel of how large a work group they are likely to be part of if they join an integrated system.

A natural question about integrated systems is whether they perform more efficiently than pro-

Table 1–18 Extent of Integration in Major Metropolitan Statistical Areas (MSAs) Percentage of Facilities in Integrated Systems, by Facility Type*

Metropolitan Statistical Area	# of Systems	Hospitals (%)	Physician Centers (%)**	HMOs (%)	Nursing Homes (%)
Stage 4 Markets					
Los Angeles-Long Beach, CA	5	18.7	9.4	11.1	0.0
Minneapolis-St. Paul, MN	5	57.1	32.8	57.1	5.0
San Diego, CA	4	59.3	23.1	20.0	5.8
Worcester, MA	2	85.7	41.7	50.0	8.3
Stage 3 Markets					
Chicago, IL	5	42.1	5.6	13.6	2.8
Washington, DC (MD-VA-WV)	2	14.3	3.9	0.0	2.4
Detroit, MI	6	47.2	30.5	42.9	7.1
Houston, TX	3	38.7	3.2	0.0	0.0
Boston, MA (NH)	4	24.1	9.4	7.1	0.0
Riverside-San Bernardino, CA	1	20.0	13.5	0.0	0.0
Orange County, CA	2	14.3	8.2	50.0	0.0
Phoenix-Mesa, AZ	7	46.7	12.1	23.1	3.8
Stage 2 Markets					
New York, NY (CT-NJ-PA)	8	32.3	3.3	10.0	2.9
Philadelphia, PA (NJ)	2	12.0	3.2	0.0	1.7
Atlanta, GA	5	27.7	6.6	10.0	0.0
Dallas, TX	1	17.4	1.3	0.0	0.0
St. Louis, MO	2	44.4	6.0	15.4	3.2
Baltimore, MD	2	37.9	1.7	9.1	1.8
Pittsburgh, PA	2	23.8	5.0	0.0	0.6
Cleveland-Lorain-Elyria, OH	4	56.8	6.5	18.2	0.0
Stage 1 Markets					
Nassau-Suffolk, NY	0	13.8	1.9	0.0	1.6
Total	**72**	**31.1**	**10.6**	**13.0**	**2.1**

*For instance, 13.1% of all the hospitals in the Los Angeles-Long Beach, CA, MSA are owned by or under contract with one or more of the four integrated systems operating in the area.

**"Physician Centers" includes free-standing ambulatory centers, medical group practices, and physician offices in which surgery is performed.

Source: Adapted with permission from *Integrated Health Systems Digest*, p. 18, © 1997, Hoechst Marion Roussel.

Table 1–19 Physicians per Physician Center* Inside and Outside Integrated Systems, by Geographic Region

Region	Physician Centers in Systems		Physician Centers Not in Systems	
	# of Centers	Average # of Physicians	# of Centers	Average # of Physicians
West	300	24.1	2,503	7.9
Southwest	223	11.4	1,949	7.0
Midwest	377	15.8	3,104	7.9
Northeast	89	17.9	2,145	6.3
Southeast	183	6.5	3,085	6.8
Total/Average	1,172	15.8	12,786	7.2

*A "physician center" includes free-standing ambulatory centers, medical group practices with five or more physicians, and physician offices in which surgery is performed.

Source: Adapted with permission from *Integrated Health Systems Digest*, p. 27, © 1997, Hoechst Marion Roussel.

vider organizations that are not part of such systems.

One possible measure of efficiency is the number of patients that physicians in these systems see in an average week. The common wisdom about IDSs is that they encourage more rapid turnaround of patients by their physicians. A physician might want to compare her current patients-per-week productivity with these numbers (Table 1–20). Almost 72 percent of primary care doctors see between 50 and 150 patients per week; another 17 percent are visited by over 150 patients. The numbers for specialists are a bit lower, as expected.

Two common criteria for assessing the operational efficiency of hospitals are their average occupancy levels and the average length of stay (ALOS) of their patients (Table 1–21). The data compare occupancy and ALOS for hospitals inside and outside IDSs in the 21 cities mentioned earlier. Several patterns are worth noting.

There is considerable variation among the cities. The system hospitals' ALOS ranges from a low of 4.1 days in Baltimore and Riverside–San

Bernardino to a high of 9.3 days in Pittsburgh. A doubling of the ALOS is hard to explain on clinical or demographic grounds. It may suggest room for improvement in the higher-scoring cities.

The same situation holds true for the occupancy rates. They vary from a low of 40.8 percent

Table 1–20 Number of Patients Seen by Physicians in Systems

Number of Patients per Week	Primary Care Physicians (%)	Specialist Physicians (%)
1–25	2.2	5.9
26–50	7.8	14.9
51–100	40.0	42.2
101–150	32.8	22.1
151+	17.1	14.8
	100	100

Source: Adapted with permission from *Integrated Health Systems Digest*, p. 25, © 1997, Hoechst Marion Roussel.

Table 1–21 Comparative Utilization Measures for Hospitals Inside and Outside Integrated Systems in Selected MSAs

Metropolitan Statistical Area	Average Length of Stay (ALOS) in Days		Average Occupancy (%)	
	System	Nonsystem	System	Nonsystem
Stage 4 Markets				
Los Angeles-Long Beach, CA	5.3	4.9	43.3	39.8
Minneapolis-St. Paul, MN	4.9	5.1	50.5	51.7
San Diego, CA	4.3	5.1	48.5	48.6
Worcester, MA	6.4	6.7	68.5	83.6
Stage 3 Markets				
Chicago, IL	5.5	6.1	62.8	60.4
Washington, DC (MD-VA-WV)	5.1	5.5	65.6	61.4
Detroit, MI	7.2	6.8	61.0	53.0
Houston, TX	4.7	8.9	51.1	45.0
Boston, MA (NH)	6.7	8.5	73.2	73.2
Riverside-San Bernardino, CA	4.1	4.3	52.6	43.7
Orange County, CA	4.6	4.4	40.3	40.0
Phoenix-Mesa, AZ	4.7	8.4	53.3	45.8
Stage 2 Markets				
New York, NY (CT-NJ-PA)	8.8	9.3	75.2	74.8
Philadelphia, PA (NJ)	7.1	7.0	61.7	70.8
Atlanta, GA	—	—	—	49.4
Dallas, TX	8.0	6.0	62.5	47.2
St. Louis, MO	—	—	—	45.5
Baltimore, MD	4.1	6.9	64.5	58.7
Pittsburgh, PA	9.3	6.7	64.9	66.5
Cleveland-Lorain-Elyria, OH	5.4	4.5	58.9	40.6
Stage 1 Markets				
Nassau-Suffolk, NY	7.9	7.8	73.0	73.9

Source: Adapted with permission from *Integrated Health Systems Digest*, pp. 20–21, © 1997, Hoechst Marion Roussel.

in Orange County to a high of 75.2 percent in New York City. Remember that a high occupancy rate is desirable.

If integrated systems work the way they are supposed to, they should produce lower ALOSs and higher occupancy levels. This is generally the case for ALOS. The figures for Stage 3 and 4 markets, the more integrated areas, are mostly in the four- to five-day range. On the other hand, hospitals in Stage 1 and 2 markets, the less integrated areas, tend to keep their patients for seven to eight days.

Table 1–22 Annual Utilization Measures for HMOs Inside and Outside Integrated Systems

Utilization Measure	HMOs in a System	HMOs Not in a System
# of HMO Enrollees per Plan	178,157	95,829
Hospital Days per 1,000 Non-Medicare Members	243	261
Hospital Days per 1,000 Medicare Members	1,477	1,599
Hospital Admissions per 1,000 Non-Medicare Members	66	68
Hospital Admissions per 1,000 Medicare Members	261	249
Physician Encounters per Non-Medicare Member	3.82	3.47
Physician Encounters per Medicare Member	9.72	7.69
Ambulatory Visits per Non-Medicare Member	1.51	1.34
Ambulatory Visits per Medicare Member	3.33	2.66
ALOS per Non-Medicare Hospital Admission	3.72	3.90
ALOS per Medicare Hospital Admission	5.91	6.18

Source: Adapted with permission from *Integrated Health Systems Digest*, p. 25, © 1997, Hoechst Marion Roussel.

A definite trend prevails with occupancy rates, but not quite as one would expect. Three of the four cities in Stage 4 have average occupancies at or below 50 percent, while all of the cities in Stage 1 and 2 markets have approximately 60 percent or more of their acute care hospital beds filled, on average. There seems to be an inverse correlation between integration and occupancy.

Regardless of how far an IDS has gone down the road of integration, one would expect a system hospital to operate more efficiently than a nonsystem hospital. In other words, even a moderately integrated system should work better than no system at all. This is just barely true here. The ALOS of system hospitals is lower in 11 of the 21 cities; the system occupancy rates are higher in 12 of the 21 cities. However, there is another predictable trend with regard to ALOS—9 of the 11 cities with more efficient hospitals are located in Stage 3 and 4 markets, showing a positive correlation between integration and lower ALOS.

A total of 88 HMOs were part of the most highly integrated health systems at the end of 1995, representing 13.2 percent of operating HMOs (an increase from 11.7 percent in 1994). Of the 67.7 million Americans in HMOs in 1995 (up from 55.0 million in 1994), 15 million of them (22.1 percent) were members of HMOs in the 189 most highly integrated systems.

HMOs are considered to be part of an IDS by virtue of either ownership or contractual arrangements. They are not considered part of an integrated system if they hold only provider network service agreements with the system.

In terms of enrollment, HMOs that belong to an integrated system are almost twice as large as those that do not—178,157 average versus 95,829. The comparative utilization data for HMO-connected hospital activities pretty much follow expectations (Table 1–22). Hospital days per 1,000 members, hospital admissions per 1,000 members, and ALOS were all lower for

HMOs in a system than for those not in a system. The only exception was a higher rate of hospital admissions for Medicare members.

As managed care–driven organizations are wont to do, the care for these member-patients was shifted to outpatient settings. Both physician encounters and ambulatory visits per member were decidedly higher within systems than they were outside.

LEADING TRENDS

- The vast majority of IDSs have been created by hospitals.

- Typically, IDSs have contractual relationships with three-fifths of their provider units and own the other two-fifths. The percentage of owner relationships is increasing.
- Approximately one-tenth of all U.S. physicians are participating in an IDS. Twice as many hospitals are part of such systems.
- Most physicians in integrated systems see between 50 and 150 patients per week.
- Hospital utilization rates are generally lower and physician utilization rates are higher for HMOs that are part of IDSs.
- Physicians that are part of an IDS practice in settings (e.g., group practice, outpatient clinic) with twice as many other physicians as those who are not in an IDS.

RESOURCE LIST

The bulk of the data in the first four chapters comes from the four-volume Managed Care Digest series published each year by Hoechst Marion Roussel. The topics of the four volumes are Integrated Health Systems Digest, Institutional Digest, Medical Group Practice Digest, and HMO-PPO/Medicare-Medicaid Digest. Each volume costs $95 and can be purchased by calling 1-800-529-9615 or writing Hoechst Marion Roussel, P.O. Box 9627, Kansas City, MO 64134-0627.

Much of the data appearing in several of the above digests was gathered by the Medical Group Management Association (MGMA). Many of the items in the resource lists for other chapters are published by the MGMA and available from them. It is an outstanding source of reasonably priced information of all kinds about the management and operation of group practices. Their Super Search Packets are top-notch, comprehensive collections of article reprints on many hot topics in physician practice management. Their Information Exchanges report the results of surveys on some of those same topics taken of their member group practices. Every physician group should be a member of the MGMA. Contact them

at the following address: MGMA, 104 Inverness Terrace East, Englewood, CO 80112-5306; Service Center (888) 608-5602; www.mgma.com

Another excellent source of data about developments in the health care industry is the journal, *Health Affairs*. In addition to peer-reviewed feature articles, each bimonthly issue includes numerous shorter data-intense reports in the Health Tracking and DataWatch sections. A one-year subscription costs $79 and may be ordered by calling 1-800-765-7514. The editorial offices of the journal may be found at the following address: Health Affairs, Suite 600, 7500 Old Georgetown Road, Bethesda, MD 20814-6133; (301) 656-7401; healthaffairs@projhope.org; www.projhope.org/HA/

The health care delivery and financing industry is highly restricted by federal and state laws, regulations, and court decisions. The most painless way of staying up-to-date on those legal developments is to join the American Health Lawyers Association (AHLA). Membership gives you monthly legal summaries, access to comprehensive multiday health law workshops on critical topics, and the opportunity to buy an excellent series of books, monographs, practice guides, and workshop binders. Contact the AHLA at: AHLA, Suite 950, 1120 Connecticut Avenue, Washington, DC 20036-3902; (202) 833-0766; www.healthlawyers.org

The American Medical Association (AMA) publishes a wide variety of materials to support their member physicians in carrying out both their clinical and managerial duties. Several items are referred to in the resource lists of the chapters in this book. There are four AMA publications that offer statistical data on the nature and scope of medical practices in this country.

Medical Groups in the US, 1998 Edition

Physician Marketplace Statistics, 1997/98 Edition

Physician Characteristics and Distribution in the US, 1997/98 Edition

Socioeconomic Characteristics of Medical Practice 1997

For these or any other publications of the AMA, contact them at: AMA, 515 North State Street, Chicago, IL 60610; (800) 621-8335; www.ama-assn.org

Medical Economics

Every March or April, this magazine publishes a large multipart section on developments and trends in managed care. This issue includes quite a bit of data and charts on the continuing changes in managed care and how physicians are responding to them. Reading this one issue is a good, quick way to bring yourself up-to-date on the health care system in which you must practice and compete.

Business and Health

During the first quarter of every year, this magazine publishes a special issue entitled "The State of Health Care in America." It is an excellent summary of developments over the past year in key areas of health care delivery and financing. The slant of the articles is toward the primarily employer audience of the magazine. Nonetheless, they offer a good, succinct survey of what is happening in American health care.

Managed Care Facts, Trends and Data: 1997–98, Atlantic Information Services, (800) 521-4323

"The Reconfiguration of U.S. Medicine," *JAMA*, 5 July, 1995

Industry Trends That Are Forcing Physicians To Rethink Their Long-Term Strategies

Basic Facts about Managed Care Organizations

INTRODUCTION

This chapter continues the quantitative portrayal of the trends in the health care industry that require new strategic thinking by physicians. Here, we look at the entities that are driving most of this change—the managed care organizations (MCOs). Not only will most physicians end up receiving the major share of their revenues from MCOs, many will see their professional lives largely under MCO control.

At the very least, an MCO provides the financing function in the process that gets health care services from providers to patients. In a sense, they serve the same purpose that insurance companies do under a fee-for-service (FFS) system. The patients sign up with and become members of an MCO. The patients' employer pays a premium to the MCO for a defined package of health care services. The MCO arranges with a group of providers to deliver those services. After deducting an amount from the employer's premium to cover its administrative costs (marketing, enrollment, billing, claims processing) and profit, the MCO pays the providers for their services.

There are two basic models of MCO—the health maintenance organization (HMO) and the preferred provider organization (PPO). There has been a blurring of the distinction between the two (particularly as HMOs offer point-of-service [POS] options), but generally an HMO requires its member-patients to see only those providers it

has contracted with, while PPO members are merely encouraged by financial incentives to visit the system's "preferred" physicians and hospitals. Compensation of PPO physicians has traditionally been on a discounted FFS basis.

In 1996, there were 749 HMOs in the United States serving over 77 million people (Table 2–1). HMO enrollments have been climbing steadily and dramatically for 10 years, more than

Table 2–1 Total Number of HMOs and Their Enrollments

Year	Number of Operating HMOs	Enrollment
1987	707	31,024,000
1988	659	33,715,000
1989	623	35,031,000
1990	610	37,538,000
1991	581	40,388,000
1992	562	44,373,000
1993	541	49,095,000
1994	556	55,006,000
1995	669	67,575,000
1996	749	77,339,000

Source: Adapted with permission from *HMO–PPO Digest*, p. 8, © 1996, Hoechst Marion Roussel.

Table 2–2 Number of HMOs and Their Enrollments, by Enrollment Size

Size of HMO	Number of HMOs		Total Number of Enrollees (millions)	
0–14,999	171	(26%)	0.9	(1%)
15,000–24,999	53	(8%)	1.1	(2%)
25,000–49,999	136	(20%)	6.0	(7%)
50,000–99,999	128	(19%)	9.0	(13%)
100,000–249,999	116	(17%)	17.7	(26%)
250,000+	65	(10%)	33.9	(50%)
Total	669	(100%)	68.6	(100%)

Source: Adapted with permission from the State of Health Care in America 1997, *Business and Health*, p. 33, Medical Economics Publishing Company, Inc.

doubling in that time. The number of operational HMOs today is actually lower than it was in 1987 (707). They are clearly becoming larger organizations.

There is tremendous variation in the size of individual HMOs. The top 10 percent accounted for 50 percent of total industry enrollments; the top 27 percent enrolled 76 percent of all HMO members (Table 2–2). At the other extreme, the bottom one-quarter of HMOs was responsible for only 1 percent of all enrollees—an average of 5,250 members per HMO.

By the year 2000, the SMG Marketing Group predicts that about 750 HMOs will be covering nearly 100 million people.

There are four distinctly different types of HMO. They are defined this way:

- *Independent Practice Association (IPA).* Physicians practicing in their own offices participate in a prepaid health care plan. They charge agreed-upon rates to enrolled patients and bill the IPA on a discounted FFS or capitated basis.
- *Network HMO.* This is an organizational form in which the HMO contracts for medical services with a network of independent medical groups.

- *Group HMO.* There are two variations of this model. In a "closed panel" plan, the medical services are delivered in HMO-owned health centers or satellite clinics by physicians who belong to a specially formed and legally separate medical group that serves only the HMO. In an "open panel" plan, the HMO contracts with an existing, independent group of physicians to deliver medical care, while being free to serve other plans and patients.
- *Staff HMO.* The HMO members receive care from a group of physicians who are either salaried employees of the HMO itself or of a specially formed professional group practice that is an integral part of the HMO plan.

The ebb and flow in the number of operating HMOs has been different for each of the four types (Table 2–3). While IPA, network, and group models declined slowly from 1991 to 1993, and then increased in number during 1994 and 1995, staff HMOs declined steadily throughout the five years. In 1996, the most impressive growth was among the IPA and group HMOs—14 percent and 19 percent, respectively. This pattern makes some sense. As physicians recently have become more aggressive in seeking practice models that maintain their clinical autonomy, they have

Table 2–3 Number of Operating HMO Plans, by Model Type

Model Type	1991	1992	1993	1994	1995	1996
IPA	365	363	352	359	439	502
Network	84	72	68	76	88	105
Group	73	71	68	70	92	96
Staff	59	56	53	51	50	46

Source: Adapted with permission from *HMO–PPO Digest*, p. 8, © 1996, Hoechst Marion Roussel.

moved away from the more inflexible staff model to the IPA and open panel network models that allow a greater degree of freedom in practicing medicine and affiliating with MCOs.

Roughly the same trend has occurred in the enrollments of each HMO model type (Table 2–4). The number of patients served by the staff HMOs has actually declined from 1993 to 1996. It has increased dramatically for the three other types, jumping 19.9 percent for group HMOs from 1995 to 1996 and 19.0 percent for IPA model HMOs. The looser the model, the greater the growth.

A more precise breakdown of HMO membership size reveals other differences among model types (Table 2–5). Group and staff HMOs tend to have the largest average memberships: 41.7 per-

cent of group models have over 100,000 members and 26.1 percent of staff models do the same. This probably can be attributed to the fact that many of them (e.g., Kaiser Foundation Health Plan, Group Health Cooperative of Puget Sound) were founded decades ago and have accumulated large memberships. The other two models are not unusually small—46.8 percent of IPAs and 38.1 percent of network HMOs have more than 50,000 members. On the whole, group HMOs are the largest in average number of members.

Although tax status makes less and less difference in the way HMOs compete for members, there are marked differences among the four model types (Table 2–6). As one moves from the looser to tighter models, the propensity for not-

Table 2–4 Enrollment in HMOs, by Model Type

Model Type	1996	1995	1994	1993
IPA	45,280,900	38,066,500	28,776,800	24,103,500
Network	8,361,900	8,939,700	7,334,900	6,123,100
Group	19,507,700	16,264,400	14,071,800	14,032,500
Staff	4,188,700	4,304,500	4,822,900	4,835,400
Total	77,339,200	67,575,100	55,006,400	49,094,500

Source: Adapted with permission from *HMO–PPO Digest*, p. 6, © 1996, Hoechst Marion Roussel.

Table 2–5 HMO Membership Size, by Model Type

	IPA		Network		Group		Staff	
Membership Size	# of HMOs	%	# of HMOs	%	# of HMOs	%	# of HMOs	%
Unknown	19	70.4	6	22.2	2	7.4	0	0.0
<15,000	112	64.7	33	19.1	18	10.4	10	5.8
15,000–24,999	53	72.6	9	12.3	5	6.8	6	8.2
25,000–49,999	83	66.9	17	13.7	12	9.7	12	9.7
50,000–99,999	106	71.6	17	11.5	19	12.8	6	4.1
100,000–249,999	82	63.1	17	13.1	23	17.7	8	6.2
250,000+	47	63.5	6	8.1	17	23.0	4	5.4

Source: Adapted with permission from *HMO–PPO Digest*, p. 13, © 1996, Hoechst Marion Roussel.

for-profit status increases. Only 22 percent of IPAs have that status, while 63 percent of staff HMOs are not-for-profit. This characteristic may also be related to the average ages of the model types. Most of the staff HMOs were formed at a time when the delivery of health care services was considered to be a charitable act, not a moneymaking opportunity. IPAs, on the other hand, are more recent innovations, at a time when health care has become more commercial.

The varying ages of the different types of HMOs is made plain by the following data: 87 percent of staff HMOs are 10 years of age or older, while 51 percent of IPAs are less than 10 years old (Table 2–7). Only six staff HMOs have been formed in the last nine years, in contrast with 256 IPAs created during the same period.

The consolidation in the health care industry has extended to HMOs. There are now "chains" of HMOs consisting of as many as 51, 55, and

Table 2–6 HMO Tax Status, by Model Type

	IPA		Network		Group		Staff	
Tax Status	# of HMOs	%	# of HMOs	%	# of HMOs	%	# of HMOs	%
Not-for-Profit	108	50.9	32	15.1	43	20.3	29	13.7
For-Profit	394	73.4	73	13.6	53	9.9	17	3.2

Source: Adapted with permission from *HMO–PPO Digest*, p. 13, © 1996, Hoechst Marion Roussel.

Table 2–7 Age of HMO Plan, by Model Type

Age	IPA # of HMOs	Network # of HMOs	Group # of HMOs	Staff # of HMOs
Under 5 Years	172	43	20	5
5–9 Years	84	18	7	1
10–14 Years	181	29	33	16
15+ Years	65	15	36	24

Source: Adapted with permission from *HMO–PPO Digest*, p. 13, © 1996, Hoechst Marion Roussel.

123 individual HMO plans each. Table 2–8 is a list of all the HMO chains operating in 1995 along with their enrollments. This information may help a physician or physician group evaluate an HMO with which it is considering a contract. Is it, in fact, part of a chain? If so, how many other plans are part of it and what is its total enrollment? The answers may indicate that the HMO is a dominant market force, worth being affiliated with, or is so large that decisions will be made in corporate headquarters for the benefit of the entire organization, not the local market in which the physicians practice.

The nation's 36 HMO chains accounted for 68.5 million enrollees in 1996, representing 88.6 percent of total HMO industry enrollment. Just five of those chains (Blue Cross/Blue Shield Association; Kaiser Foundation Health Plan, Inc.; United HealthCare Corporation, Aetna U.S. Healthcare; and Prudential Insurance) enrolled over half (57.2 percent) of all HMO members.

Similar information is offered by the next set of data (Table 2–9). This listing of the 25 largest individual HMO plans includes their age, model type, and tax status. If physicians prefer to ally with certain types of HMOs, with a certain tax status, this will help them identify the appropriate plan. Of course, because these are individual plans, they operate in narrower geographic areas and may not be available for the physicians who want them.

The consolidation of health care facilities, through merger and acquisition, is a hard fact (Table 2–10). The number of combinations increased by 54 percent from 1995 to 1996. Mergers and acquisitions among hospitals grew by 28 percent, among HMOs by 118 percent, and among physician medical groups by 63 percent.

One of the most powerful indicators of the spread of managed care is the growth in HMO market penetration by state (Table 2–11). "Penetration" refers to the percentage of population enrolled as HMO members. The top seven states, and the only ones with penetration over 40 percent in 1996, are Delaware, Massachusetts, Minnesota, California, Maryland, Oregon, and Arizona. In some states, the level of HMO market penetration has grown steadily over the last few years. Minnesota, Maryland, and Pennsylvania are good examples. The penetration rate has surged suddenly in other states like Delaware (36.9 percent to 59.4 percent), Utah (22.2 percent to 37.9 percent), and Virginia (18.6 percent to 27.1 percent). A bit inexplicably, the percentage of HMO enrollments has actually dropped in a few states—New Hampshire (44.3 percent to 33.7 percent) and North Carolina (16.3 percent to 13.7 percent).

A physician looking for an area in which to practice without substantial intrusions from managed care might begin the search with this list. The data make clear, however, how suddenly

Table 2–8 HMO Chains, Enrollments, and Number of Individual HMO Plans in 1996

Company Name	HMO Plans	Enrollment
Aetna U.S. Healthcare	56	6,336,938
Allina Health System	3	1,030,563
American Health Care Providers, Inc.	2	126,187
AvMed Health Plans	5	328,136
Blue Cross/Blue Shield Association	123	13,960,444
CIGNA Healthcare	51	3,276,128
Coventry Corporation	5	829,391
Exclusive Healthcare	8	146,409
Family Health Systems, Inc.	2	144,850
Foundation Health Systems	20	3,146,682
Group Health Cooperative of Puget Sound	3	911,032
Harvard Pilgrim Health Care	2	1,237,093
HMO Group, The	9	1,883,321
HealthPartners	2	708,799
Healthsource	16	1,091,933
Humana Health Care Plans	21	1,975,815
Independent Health Association Inc.	3	621,304
Intermountain Health Care	4	342,426
John Deere Health Care	2	332,850
Kaiser Foundation Health Plan, Inc.	15	7,791,264
Maxicare Health Plans, Inc.	7	402,409
Mercy Health Plans	2	179,087
Mid-Atlantic Medical Services	4	829,259
NYLCare Health Plans	9	1,671,402
Oxford Health Plans	4	1,535,500
PHP Healthcare Corporation	2	21,700
PacifiCare Health Systems	18	4,080,127
Physician Corporation of America	3	933,813
Principal Health Care	19	735,955
Prucare (Prudential Insurance)	35	4,420,989
Sentara Health Systems	2	208,152
Sisters of Providence Health System	2	314,014
United American Healthcare Corp.	3	116,149
United HealthCare Corporation	55	6,700,681
Vanderbilt Health Plans	2	46,597
Wausau Insurance Companies	4	120,403
Total	523	68,537,802

Source: Adapted with permission from *HMO–PPO Digest*, pp. 10–11, © 1996, Hoechst Marion Roussel.

Table 2–9 Summary Data on 25 Largest Individual HMO Plans (Enrollment, Age, Model Type, Tax Status)

Plan	1996 Enrollment	1996 Age	Model Type	Tax Status
Kaiser Permanente Health Plan-Oakland, CA	2,528,603	52	Group	NFP
Kaiser Permanente Health Plan-Pasadena, CA	2,447,843	52	Group	NFP
PacifiCare of California-Cypress, CA	1,417,239	19	Network	FP
Health Net-Woodland Hills, CA	1,260,657	18	Group	FP
Keystone Blue/Pittsburgh, PA	1,148,926	11	IPA	FP
Oxford Health Plan-New York, NY	1,142,800	11	IPA	FP
Harvard Comm. Health Plan-Dedham, MA	1,078,000	28	Staff	NFP
California Care-Woodland Hills, CA	939,655	11	Group	FP
PacificCare/FHP/California-Cerritos, CA	927,600	36	IPA	FP
HMO Blue-Boston, MA	876,845	15	Network	NFP
HIP of Greater NY-New York, NY	817,828	50	Group	NFP
US Healthcare/SE PA-Blue Bell, PA	788,038	21	IPA	FP
Medica Choice-Minneapolis, MN	754,765	22	IPA	NFP
Foundation Health/CA-Rancho Cordova, CA	740,434	20	Group	FP
HealthPartners-Minneapolis, MN	702,034	5	Group	NFP
Group Health Coop./Puget Sound-Seattle, WA	681,406	50	Staff	NFP
U.S. Healthcare/NJ-Fairfield, NJ	680,397	12	IPA	FP
Keystone Health Plan/East-Philadelphia, PA	657,798	10	IPA	FP
U.S. Healthcare/NY-Uniondale, NY	657,192	11	IPA	FP
Tufts Associated Health Plans-Waltham, MA	625,877	16	IPA	NFP
Health Options-Jacksonville, FL	599,108	12	IPA	FP
NYLCare/Mid Atlantic-Greenbelt, MD	587,140	19	IPA	FP
Humana Medical Plan/Florida-Miramar, FL	564,874	24	IPA	FP
Kaiser Foundation Health Plan-Rockville, MD	559,143	25	Group	NFP
HMO Illinois-Chicago, IL	552,000	20	Group	NFP
Total	23,736,202			

Source: Adapted with permission from *HMO–PPO Digest*, p. 12, © 1996, Hoechst Marion Roussel.

HMOs can make their appearance and begin to dominate a local market. There are still a few corners of the country where medicine can be practiced in the old-fashioned way, but they are disappearing fast.

As mentioned in the previous section on integrated delivery systems (IDSs), HMOs are showing up increasingly as components in integrated systems (Table 2–12). This is much more likely to be the case with group (37.5 percent) and staff (30.4 percent) model HMOs; IPA plans are the least inclined (20.3 percent) to get intimately involved with such systems. This follows naturally from the initial reason most physicians join

Table 2–10 Mergers and Acquisitions in the Health Industry, by Facility Type

	1996	1995
HMOs	61	28
Home health care	129	62
Hospitals	170	133
Labs/MRI/dialysis	77	51
Long-term care	118	67
Physician medical groups	205	126
Psychiatric care	35	47
Rehabilitation	60	66
Other	122	53
Total	977	633

Source: Adapted with permission from The State of Health Care in America, 1997, *Business and Health*, p. 32, © 1997, Medical Economics Publishing Company, Inc.

IPA—to reap the benefits of managed care contracts with a minimum of entanglements.

Tax status also makes a difference in which HMOs link up with IDSs. In 1996, over 30 percent of not-for-profit HMOs had such a linkage, compared to only 21 percent of for-profit HMOs.

Consumer and employer demands for more choice, plus greater competition from other provider networks, have prompted HMOs to offer a greater variety of coverage options (Table 2–13). Most of the change has occurred in the last five years. In 1994, nearly 60 percent of HMOs were offering a PPO option, up from 30 percent in 1990. A POS option, which allows members to decide at the time they need care whether they will stay inside or go outside the system for a provider, was available from three-quarters of all HMOs in 1994, compared to only 20 percent four years earlier. Sixty percent (60 percent) of HMOs had traditional indemnity plans, while 65 percent had gotten into the business of supporting self-insurance by employers.

Table 2–11 HMO Market Penetration and Number of HMOs by State (Ranked from highest penetration to lowest)

State	Penetration (% of population)			Number of HMOs		
	1996	1995	1994	1996	1995	1994
Delaware	59.4	36.9	25.6	15	12	11
Massachusetts	51.9	49.2	42.1	24	25	22
Minnesota	47.1	41.8	35.7	10	11	13
California	45.6	42.4	38.4	47	42	37
Maryland	43.6	35.9	29.7	24	22	24
Oregon	41.7	43.3	34.9	9	10	8
Arizona	40.0	33.5	30.4	20	18	13
Pennsylvania	38.9	31.0	21.0	36	28	21
Utah	37.9	22.2	21.2	10	10	9
Colorado	37.5	31.4	34.7	18	16	14
New York	35.6	32.7	26.1	45	43	37
Connecticut	34.3	34.0	21.0	20	19	18
Florida	33.8	26.3	18.0	64	51	40
New Hampshire	33.7	44.3	25.1	7	7	8
New Jersey	32.2	28.7	22.9	31	23	18

continues

Table 2–11 continued

State	Penetration (% of population)			Number of HMOs		
	1996	*1995*	*1994*	*1996*	*1995*	*1994*
Wisconsin	31.9	28.6	25.9	31	30	27
Rhode Island	30.3	27.9	22.3	6	6	7
Washington	30.2	24.3	24.9	19	19	18
Missouri	29.9	23.0	19.5	35	30	26
Hawaii	28.6	25.2	19.6	10	9	4
Virginia	27.1	18.6	14.1	26	26	25
Illinois	25.2	23.6	18.6	42	41	36
Ohio	25.0	21.9	21.4	47	42	37
Michigan	24.9	24.1	19.5	21	18	18
Tennessee	24.4	23.5	9.0	22	19	13
Vermont	23.6	22.6	17.4	4	4	4
Nevada	20.7	18.0	16.7	12	11	7
Texas	20.0	16.8	14.6	54	35	28
Maine	19.7	14.8	11.3	7	6	3
New Mexico	18.9	17.6	18.6	6	6	9
Louisiana	16.3	12.9	7.4	19	16	11
Kentucky	15.9	16.8	12.4	20	18	14
South Dakota	15.4	13.0	3.0	2	2	2
Indiana	15.3	14.0	12.5	31	30	27
Oklahoma	15.3	12.9	11.0	12	11	10
Georgia	15.2	12.5	10.9	18	15	15
Kansas	15.0	10.6	8.4	18	17	16
North Carolina	13.7	16.3	8.7	19	17	13
Nebraska	10.9	8.7	9.1	5	5	7
Iowa	10.8	9.8	9.4	11	11	11
South Carolina	10.2	7.5	5.4	14	11	11
Arkansas	8.3	5.2	6.4	7	7	8
Idaho	7.1	4.4	4.8	10	6	7
West Virginia	7.0	4.4	3.2	10	6	4
Alabama	6.7	10.4	7.6	14	13	9
North Dakota	6.2	4.0	2.4	5	5	5
Montana	2.6	2.2	2.1	3	2	4
Mississippi	1.8	2.0	0.8	15	8	4
D.C.	—	—	—	15	16	13
Total U.S.	29.2	25.7	21.1	749	669	556

Note: The 357,038 HMO enrollees in the District of Columbia were not used to calculate penetration for fear of double-counting residents of Maryland and Virginia. Alaska and Wyoming were served by one operating HMO in 1996, but neither had any members.

Source: Adapted with permission from *HMO–PPO Digest*, pp. 18–19, © 1996, Hoechst Marion Roussel.

Table 2–12 HMOs That Were Part of Integrating Health Care Systems, by Model Type and Tax Status

	Percentage of HMO Plans	
	1995	*1996*
Model Type		
IPA	18.0	20.3
Network	26.7	24.9
Group	41.9	37.5
Staff	32.3	30.4
Tax Status		
Not-for-Profit	42.6	31.6
For-Profit	16.7	20.7
Overall Average	23.8	7.3

Note: For the purposes of this table, "integrating health care system" was defined as an organization made up of two or more facilities that have a formal agreement to integrate or share the delivery of health-related services.

Source: Adapted with permission from *HMO–PPO Digest*, p. 23, © 1996, Hoechst Marion Roussel.

Table 2–13 Percentage of HMOs Offering Particular Options

	1994	*1990*
Point-of-service	74.0	19.8
PPO	58.5	28.0
Indemnity	59.1	25.0
Self-insurance	65.3	25.3

Source: Adapted with permission from The State of Health Care in America, 1997, *Business and Health*, p. 46, © 1997, Medical Economics Publishing Company, Inc.

What this means for physicians affiliating with an HMO is the opportunity to participate in several kinds of patient payment plans. Regardless of the plan covering the patient, however, the physician's compensation may be the same. The bigger danger is that a physician signing up to serve patients in a basic HMO plan may be expected to see members of PPO and self-insurance plans as well. That may be more than the physician bargained for.

The likelihood that an HMO offers open-ended options or POS plans varies according to the model type (Table 2–14). Both are more popular with IPAs than with staff HMOs.

A more recent innovation is the triple-option plan that allows the member a choice of an HMO, a PPO, or straight indemnity (Exhibit 2–1). Here, too, these are more likely to be available from an IPA or a group HMO.

It is worth examining the actual impact HMOs have had on patients and their employers (Table 2–15). Perhaps the first step is to look at where consumers go for advice on choosing a health care plan. Not surprisingly, half take the word of friends or family. Somewhat surprisingly, about a third pay attention to patient surveys. Nearly that many turn to individual doctors for their opinions on health plans. Only 12 percent of consumers find the health plans themselves to be "very believable."

Patients make their choice of plans from among those offered by their employers. That raises the question of what factors an employer considers in deciding to make a plan available to its employees (Figure 2–1). The matter of "cost" remains at the top of the list of items that give a health plan "value," commanding the attention of 51 percent of employers in 1997. However, this represents a decline from 59 percent in the previous year. Furthermore, "quality" is now ranked as important by just as many employers. The next four items are all quality related: HEDIS reports, other report card formats, measurement of treatment outcomes, and the use of plan-sponsored practice protocols. Each increased in importance from 1996 except the protocols.

This is refreshing news. It demonstrates a shift away from a myopic employer focus on costs and a new concern for the quality of what they are buying for their employees. Physicians pushing

Table 2–14 HMOs Offering Open-Ended Options or Point-of-Service Plans with Enrollments, by Model Type

Model Type	Open-Ended Options		Point-of-Service Plans	
	% of HMOs Offering	Enrollment	% of HMOs Offering	Enrollment
IPA	20.4 (37.8)	2,191,383	71.0 (57.1)	10,836,757
Network	14.3 (27.4)	366,932	59.4 (49.4)	1,540,128
Group	16.3 (27.1)	300,487	76.7 (58.1)	1,666,026
Staff	22.2 (25.0)	126,196	33.3 (25.6)	202,260

Note: Open-ended options allow members enrolled in an HMO plan to use the plan's provider network or go outside of the network to any physician of choice.

Point-of-service (POS) plans are separately licensed HMOs that allow their members to choose whether to use the plan's provider network or go outside the network to obtain services at the time that they need the service.

Both of these types of hybrid plans usually assess a higher fee to the member for going outside the provider network. Figures in parentheses are from 1995.

Source: Adapted with permission from *HMO–PPO Digest*, p. 16, © 1996, Hoechst Marion Roussel.

for greater autonomy in clinical decision making will benefit from this trend.

In response to the preferences expressed by employers, along with general criticism of their concentration on profits, MCOs have begun to provide their primary customers, the employers, with a variety of data on the quality of care being

Exhibit 2–1 HMOs Offering Triple-Option Plans, by Model Type

IPA	35.1%	(46.0%)
Network	28.8%	(25.0%)
Group	39.2%	(34.7%)
Staff	22.0%	(33.3%)
All HMOs	33.9%	(40.7%)

Note: Triple-option plans include a choice of an HMO, a PPO, or an indemnity plan. Figures in parentheses are from 1995.

Source: Adapted with permission from *HMO–PPO Digest*, p. 16, © 1996, Hoechst Marion Roussel.

delivered to the employee-patients (Exhibit 2–2). While cost and utilization information still rank at the top, results of member satisfaction surveys and report cards like Health Plan Employer Data and Information Set (HEDIS) are nearly as important. This is more evidence that physician voices demanding greater attention to issues of clinical quality are being heard.

Nonetheless, the cost-control mechanisms of managed care do seem to be working well to the advantage of employers. While the average cost per employee of health care obtained from HMOs and PPOs increased substantially from 1995 to 1996, they both were less expensive than the traditional alternatives of Blue Cross/Blue Shield, commercial insurance, and self-insurance (Table 2–16). The biggest surprise is the top cost of employer self-insurance, which is often touted as an economical source of health care coverage for those employers able to accept the risk.

The average premiums paid for family and individual coverage by HMOs differs greatly from one state to another (Table 2–17). In fact, the states at the two extremes, Maine with the

Table 2–15 Sources That Influence Consumers' Choice of Health Plan (Percentage of consumers who rate each source as "very believable")

Friends and family	50
Patient surveys	34
Individual doctors	29
Independent organizations that evaluate plans	19
Employers	19
Health insurance plans	12
Doctors' associations	9
Government agencies	7
The media	5

Source: Adapted with permission from The State of Health Care in America, 1997, *Business and Health*, p. 15, © 1997, Medical Economics Publishing Company, Inc.

highest monthly family premiums ($549.19) and Oregon with the lowest ($352.69), are often compared for lifestyle and demographics. If anything, this highlights the variety of factors that can affect premium levels, from local cost of living to intensity of health care market competition.

This state-by-state list might help physicians evaluate the premiums to be charged by a plan they are joining or forming. The figures might even give them a basis for comparison with the compensation they are receiving from an HMO or one of its provider organizations. However, because they are simply averages for many different HMOs, it would not be advisable to rely on them too closely.

The average premiums for the four HMO model types are a little more relaxing (Table 2–18). On the whole, the premiums charged by IPAs are the highest or among the highest. The lowest premiums are most often found with net-

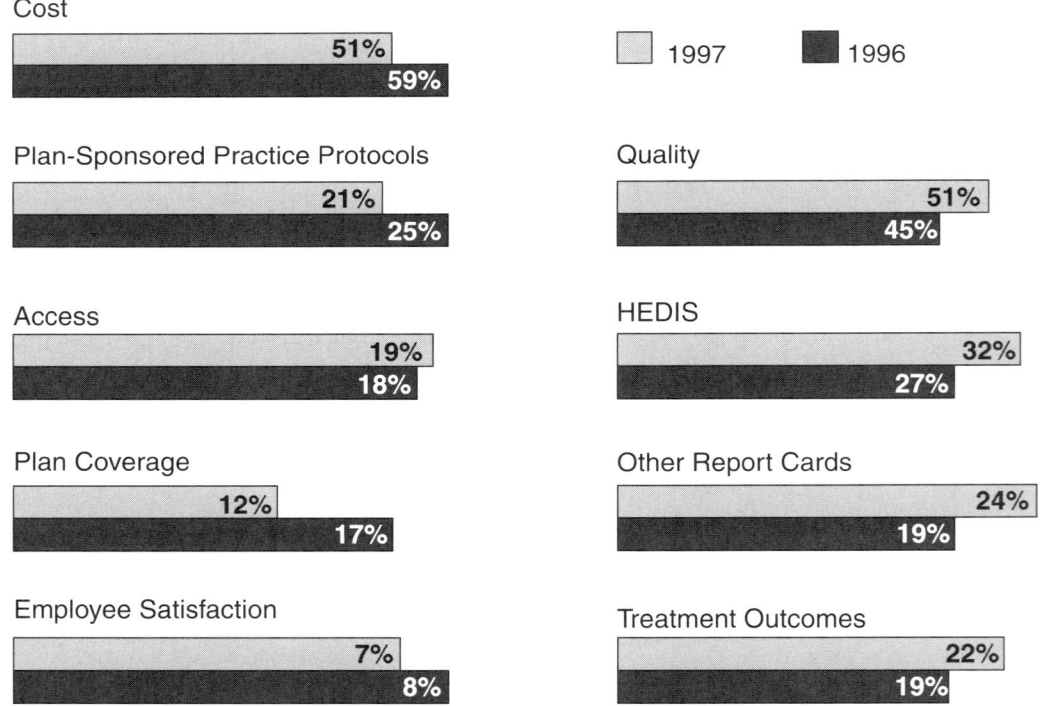

Figure 2–1 How Employers Define Value in a Health Plan. *Source:* Copyright © 1997 by Medical Economics Publishing. Reprinted by permission from *MEDICAL ECONOMICS Magazine.*

Exhibit 2–2 Types of Quality Information Provided by MCOs to Employers

Cost and utilization	89%
Member satisfaction	88%
HEDIS or other report cards	72%
Disease incidence	42%
Condition-specific health status	30%
Mortality rates	25%
Health status	24%

Source: Adapted with permission from *Competitive Edge, 5.1*, InterStudy Publications.

Table 2–16 Average Health Care Cost per Employee, by Health Plan Source

	1996 ($)	1995 ($)
HMO	3,125	2,824
PPO	3,235	2,687
BC/BS	3,258	
Commercial insurance	3,580	
Self-insurance	3,999	
All employers	3,261	2,907

Source: Adapted with permission from *Connecticut Hospital News*, Vol. 14, No. 5, p. 35, © 1997, Hospital News.

Table 2–17 HMO Individual and Family Premiums, by State

State	Average Family Premium ($)		Average Individual Premium ($)	
Alabama	420.09	(421.53)	144.76	(147.47)
Arizona	371.05	(393.59)	134.47	(133.47)
Arkansas	419.95	(391.00)	139.22	(124.57)
California	373.51	(390.63)	130.12	(134.18)
Colorado	408.95	(415.74)	141.73	(142.89)
Connecticut	545.41	(527.14)	183.65	(187.87)
Delaware	577.96	(581.61)	211.58	(202.63)
District of Columbia	464.25	(471.79)	154.75	(147.43)
Florida	439.66	(403.62)	150.20	(137.35)
Georgia	439.65	(430.98)	146.98	(143.21)
Hawaii	392.12	(394.17)	131.82	(132.51)
Idaho	357.39	(357.39)	140.71	(140.71)
Illinois	443.33	(431.68)	149.14	(144.12)
Indiana	447.78	(441.03)	154.34	(150.38)
Iowa	417.68	(381.93)	157.29	(144.65)
Kansas	431.83	(421.71)	148.44	(145.26)
Kentucky	425.77	(391.57)	145.62	(140.33)
Louisiana	407.42	(430.57)	148.71	(150.03)
Maine	559.03	(549.19)	177.39	(186.07)
Maryland	456.16	(421.03)	154.21	(142.44)

continues

Table 2–17 Continued

State	Average Family Premium ($)		Average Individual Premium ($)	
Maryland	456.16	(421.03)	154.21	(142.44)
Massachusetts	517.20	(511.87)	185.34	(180.34)
Michigan	416.46	(414.62)	148.89	(150.67)
Minnesota	429.14	(428.53)	130.90	(131.53)
Mississippi	431.63	(431.63)	148.84	(148.84)
Missouri	432.27	(429.19)	161.34	(158.80)
Montana	787.83	(—)	262.61	(228.68)
Nebraska	405.77	(421.35)	139.76	(144.21)
Nevada	436.18	(444.83)	146.01	(149.01)
New Hampshire	519.12	(441.75)	172.04	(162.14)
New Jersey	541.57	(519.81)	186.34	(175.85)
New Mexico	365.44	(365.13)	122.91	(122.75)
New York	436.90	(443.73)	152.99	(157.26)
North Carolina	435.12	(430.31)	146.37	(144.56)
North Dakota	431.10	(387.73)	155.93	(139.83)
Ohio	415.72	(389.86)	143.59	(134.40)
Oklahoma	383.26	(374.33)	135.12	(124.55)
Oregon	355.07	(352.69)	126.79	(125.77)
Pennsylvania	455.29	(425.15)	156.55	(147.65)
Rhode Island	384.39	(384.39)	140.93	(140.93)
South Carolina	455.90	(455.60)	152.05	(152.00)
South Dakota	518.32	(507.61)	172.78	(169.20)
Tennessee	406.24	(419.73)	149.75	(146.51)
Texas	442.72	(450.44)	148.97	(145.23)
Utah	385.97	(367.10)	127.36	(120.89)
Virginia	410.24	(426.18)	141.82	(142.96)
Washington	387.23	(397.92)	129.24	(126.75)
West Virginia	572.86	(513.06)	190.95	(165.23)
Wisconsin	446.60	(428.55)	158.34	(158.22)
National Average	$434.08	($425.87)	$150.22	($146.59)

Figures in parentheses are from 1995.

Source: Adapted with permission from *HMO–PPO Digest*, pp. 28–29, © 1996, Hoechst Marion Roussel.

work or staff HMOs. Because IPAs do not try to exercise tight cost controls over their providers, the higher premiums are predictable. Staff HMOs directly employ their physicians and often own their own hospitals, permitting closer supervision of their performance, so lower premiums are expected from them. The efficiency of the network HMOs is interesting since they are a looser form of HMO-provider relationship.

These premium levels have returned profits or surpluses for the vast majority of HMOs through the mid-1990s (Exhibit 2–3). For the first five

Table 2–18 HMO Individual and Family Premiums per Month, by Model Type (Both experience and community-rated)

Model Type	Average Family Premium		Average Individual Premium	
	Experience ($)	Community ($)	Experience ($)	Community ($)
IPA	412.29	448.67	145.39	154.87
Network	383.49	432.19	127.97	148.74
Group	414.87	435.28	139.85	147.74
Staff	332.01	426.80	143.05	147.87
All HMOs	403.20	443.69	139.70	152.75

Note: *Community rating* calculates premiums on the basis of actual and expected costs over a broad geographic area. *Experience-rated* premiums are based on the age, sex, and historical utilization of the population covered. Experience rating is not a permissible basis for premium calculation under federal HMO certification regulations. Experience rating is the primary method for determining premiums for most other kinds of health insurance coverage.

Source: Adapted with permission from *HMO–PPO Digest*, p. 28, © 1996, Hoechst Marion Roussel.

years of the decade, between 80 percent and 90 percent of HMOs were in the black. However, the pressures of steadily increasing administrative and medical costs, coupled with employer demands for lower premiums, abruptly cut the proportion of HMOs reporting positive net earnings to 38 percent, close to the levels of the 1980s.

Exhibit 2–3 HMOs That Had a Profit or Surplus

1988	36%
1989	60%
1990	83%
1991	83%
1992	86%
1993	89%
1994	88%
1995	61%
1996	50%
1997	38%

Source: Adapted with permission from *Competitive Edge*, 6.2 and telephone conversation with Richard L. Hamer on November 2, 1998, InterStudy Publications.

An HMO serves its members through a network of providers—employed, owned, or under contract (Table 2–19). When a physician joins an HMO network, she might be interested in knowing how many other providers will be working in partnership with her. On average, she will find over 800 primary care physicians, nearly 1,900 specialists, and just over 30 hospitals. The largest provider networks tend to be maintained by IPAs and network HMOs. Staff model HMOs get by with approximately half the number of providers of the other HMO types.

When the average number of providers is combined with the average enrollment for each type of HMO, some interesting ratios emerge (Table 2–20). Although they affiliated with the largest number of providers, IPAs and network HMOs had even larger enrollments, with the result that each individual provider was responsible for the smallest number of enrollees.

For instance, there were 170 enrollees per primary care physician and 3,763 enrollees per acute care hospital in network HMOs. By contrast, staff HMOs had an average of one primary care physician for every 763 enrollees and one acute care hospital for every 9,563 enrollees. Although the difference may be partially

Table 2–19 Number of Providers Used by an HMO, by Model Type and Provider Type

Provider Type	IPA	Network	Group	Staff	Average
Acute Care Hospital	34	36	33	16	32
Psychiatric Hospital	3	4	3	1	3
Primary Care Physicians	846	869	875	280	813
Specialists	2,010	1,717	1,781	861	1,864

Source: Adapted with permission from *HMO–PPO Digest*, p. 15, © 1996, Hoechst Marion Roussel.

explained by the greater efficiency of a staff type HMO, the main reason is that staff physicians see only patients who come to them through the HMO while network HMO and IPA physicians are seeing patients from other sources.

The size of an HMO does seem to be a factor in its operating efficiency (Table 2–21). As they increase in enrollment from less than 15,000 to over 250,000, there is an almost steady increase in the number of enrollees per primary care physician and acute care hospital. What is most intriguing is the rate of increase. Physicians in the largest HMOs see more than three times as many patients as do those in the smallest. For hospitals, the ratio is almost 11 to 1. These figures may be useful to physicians deciding which size HMO to contract with.

Sometimes, it can be helpful to know exactly how an HMO is dividing up its premium dollars.

Although the breakdown can vary greatly from one HMO to another, these are the proportions for an average HMO (Exhibit 2–4). Generally, hospitals and physicians each get about $.40 of a premium dollar, and the physicians' share is split almost evenly between primary care and specialist physicians. The HMO takes the remaining $.17 to cover its administrative expenses and profit.

The specific method of compensating physicians varies a lot among the four types of HMO (Table 2–22). Salaries are much more popular with staff HMOs (82.1 percent), since their physicians are direct employees. They use capitation

Table 2–20 HMO Enrollees per Hospital and Primary Care Physician, by Model Type

Model Type	Average # of Enrollees per Acute Care Hospital	Average # of Enrollees per Primary Care Physician
IPA	4,329	178
Network	3,763	170
Group	16,191	650
Staff	9,563	763

Source: Adapted with permission from *HMO–PPO Digest*, p. 15, © 1996, Hoechst Marion Roussel.

Table 2–21 HMO Enrollees per Hospital and Primary Care Physician, by Membership Size

Membership Size	Average # of Enrollees per Acute Care Hospital	Average # of Enrollees per Primary Care Physician
Fewer than 15,000	1,641	109
15,000–24,999	1,988	214
25,000–49,999	3,976	255
50,000–99,999	5,314	316
100,000–249,999	9,278	344
250,000 and over	14,621	404
Overall Average	6,257	281

Source: Adapted with permission from *HMO–PPO Digest*, p. 15, © 1996, Hoechst Marion Roussel.

Exhibit 2–4 How the MCO Premium Dollar Is Divided

Hospital	42%
HMO	17%
Primary care physicians	20%
Specialist physicians	19%

Courtesy of Deloitte & Touche.

much less often (56.4 percent) than the other three models (76.8 percent, 84.2 percent, and 83.3 percent). Roughly four-fifths of IPAs and network HMOs pay their physicians on a fee-for-service basis. Bonus programs are used by 20 to 30 percent of all HMOs. Profit sharing is a significant form of compensation only for group HMOs. These numbers may give physicians some idea of how they can expect to be paid when they affiliate with a particular kind of HMO.

HMOs use capitation contracts, to some degree, with all their providers (Table 2–23). At least 70 percent of all types of HMOs capitate their primary care physicians; for group HMOs, the percentage rises to 85 percent. The group HMOs also are more likely (68.6 percent) to pay their specialists on a capitation basis. Roughly

half of HMOs use capitation contracts with their ancillary providers. About a third do the same with hospitals. On the whole, IPAs are the least enthusiastic about capitation. This may be due to the legal restrictions on the negotiation of a single capitation rate with a group of independent practitioners.

Whether through bonuses or risk withholds under capitation schemes, a growing number of managed care organizations (MCOs) are linking their physician compensation to satisfaction of certain performance criteria (Table 2–24). Performance-based compensation is more common with HMOs than PPOs. For both, the most frequent criteria used are patient volume and specialty referrals. Physicians can expect to encounter such performance standards more and more in the future.

MCOs, particularly HMOs, are famous for employing a variety of mechanisms to control the utilization of resources and their associated costs (Table 2–25). They have achieved some impressive results. The average HMO has reduced its annual hospital days to 256.8 per 1,000 members. This is balanced by 3.5 annual physician encounters and 1.5 annual ambulatory visits per member. The utilization rates vary by HMO type, but not dramatically. The hospital days are in a fairly narrow range, 231.1 for group HMOs to 265.9 for staff HMOs. The highest physician encounter rate (4.2 for staff HMOs) is about a third more than

Table 2–22 Physician Reimbursement Methods Used by HMOs, by Model Type

Reimbursement Method	IPA (%)	Network (%)	Group (%)	Staff (%)
Salary	6.5	14.5	26.9	82.1
Profit Sharing	2.3	3.9	12.8	7.7
Fee-for-Service	81.5	78.9	51.3	46.2
Bonus Program	22.5	25.0	26.9	28.2
Capitation	76.8	84.2	83.3	56.4

Note: Because of multiple answers, the totals for each model type exceed 100%. Some other reimbursement methods used by HMOs include discounted FFS and return of risk withholds.

Source: Adapted with permission from *HMO–PPO Digest*, p. 14, © 1996, Hoechst Marion Roussel.

Table 2–23 Use of Capitation Contracts, by Model Type and Provider Type

Provider Type	IPA (%)	Network (%)	Group (%)	Staff (%)
Primary Care Physician	73.0	71.6	85.0	68.8
Specialist	31.4	52.4	68.6	43.4
Ancillary Provider	41.4	58.4	50.0	51.4
Hospital	28.6	38.8	47.2	36.2

Source: Adapted with permission from HMO–PPO Digest, p. 24, © 1996, Hoechst Marion Roussel.

the lowest (3.3 for IPAs). The highest ambulatory visit rate (1.6 for group HMOs and 1.7 for staff HMOs) is a third higher than the lowest rate (1.2 for network HMOs).

The variation in utilization rates is much greater among HMOs in different states (Table 2–26). Hospital utilization is almost three times higher in South Carolina (442.6 days) than in New Hampshire (175.8 days). Physician encounters in Idaho (5.3) are more than twice what they are in the District of Columbia (2.2). Ambulatory visits in Louisiana (0.2) are a fraction of the average in Maine (4.9). There can be many reasons for these differences and the effects of managed care are only one of them.

Another area of HMO influence over clinical decision making is the utilization of drugs (Table 2–27). A growing proportion of HMOs are

Table 2–24 Percentage of MCOs That Link Reimbursement to Physician Performance Criteria

Performance Criterion	PPOs (%)	HMOs (%)
Cardiac Catheterization	7	10
Endoscopies	7	16
MRIs	10	16
Patient Volume	15	25
Specialty Referrals	15	28

Courtesy of Louis Harris & Associates, Inc., New York, New York.

demanding some form of drug utilization review by their providers. By 1996, four-fifths of them had such a requirement.

After variations in premiums and in utilization rates, it is perhaps not surprising that there also are wide differences in clinical performance by MCOs across the country. The Quality Compass, a report by the National Committee for Quality Assurance, sifted data from its accreditation activities for 329 HMOs and other MCOs, which cover about 37 million of the 58 million Americans enrolled in managed care plans.[*] The report determined the average, highest, and lowest ratings for each of more than 50 quality measures.

These are some of the key measures and the ratings:

Advising smokers to quit
Average: HMO doctors advised 61 percent of smokers to quit
High: advised 85 percent to quit
Low: advised 30 percent to quit

Beta blockers prescribed to heart attack survivors
Average: prescribed to 62 percent
High: prescribed to 100 percent
Low: prescribed to 15 percent

---

*Source: Data from Quality Compass Paints a Mixed Picture of Health Plan Quality Nationally, Medical Management Network, Vol. 5, No. 10, pp. 8–9, © 1997.

Table 2–25 HMO Utilization Rates (Hospital Days, Physician Encounters, Ambulatory Visits), by Model Type

Utilization Criterion	IPA	Network	Group	Staff	All HMOs
Annual Hospital Days per 1,000 Members	260.9	257.4	231.1	265.9	256.8
Annual Physician Encounters per Member	3.3	3.7	3.9	4.2	3.5
Annual Ambulatory Visits per Member	1.5	1.2	1.6	1.7	1.5

Source: Adapted with permission from *HMO–PPO Digest*, p. 26, © 1996, Hoechst Marion Roussel.

Table 2–26 HMO Utilization Rates (Hospital Days, Physician Encounters, Ambulatory Visits), by State

State	Annual Hospital Days per 1,000 Members	Annual Physician Encounters per Member	Annual Ambulatory Visits per Member
Alabama	338.4	5.2	1.7
Arizona	204.9	2.8	1.5
Arkansas	315.7	5.1	2.7
California	193.5	3.5	1.2
Colorado	237.8	4.5	2.3
Connecticut	284.8	3.4	2.1
Delaware	364.6	3.3	0.6
District of Columbia	361.0	2.2	—
Florida	250.6	2.8	1.1
Georgia	236.5	4.2	1.3
Hawaii	220.8	4.4	0.4
Idaho	231.8	5.3	0.4
Illinois	246.5	3.2	1.3
Indiana	222.0	3.1	2.6
Iowa	258.0	2.8	0.1
Kansas	300.2	3.8	0.6
Kentucky	251.6	3.3	2.4
Louisiana	293.4	2.3	0.2
Maine	273.8	4.5	4.9
Maryland	277.4	3.6	1.4
Massachusetts	297.7	4.0	2.7
Michigan	264.5	3.2	1.5
Minnesota	274.3	3.4	1.2

continues

Table 2–26 continued

State	Annual Hospital Days per 1,000 Members	Annual Physician Encounters per Member	Annual Ambulatory Visits per Member
Mississippi	320.0	—	—
Missouri	264.4	3.0	1.9
Montana	242.0	4.7	—
Nebraska	220.6	3.0	1.9
Nevada	188.9	3.4	—
New Hampshire	175.8	3.6	—
New Jersey	279.4	4.3	0.4
New Mexico	193.9	3.9	0.6
New York	331.0	3.9	2.0
North Carolina	270.8	3.4	3.0
North Dakota	292.0	3.7	2.4
Ohio	263.3	3.7	1.6
Oklahoma	224.6	4.3	0.6
Oregon	177.9	2.7	0.4
Pennsylvania	264.2	3.7	0.7
Rhode Island	(380.0)	3.8	3.2
South Carolina	442.6	3.1	3.1
South Dakota	244.0	2.6	0.1
Tennessee	226.6	2.9	0.5
Texas	237.3	4.2	2.0
Utah	210.3	3.0	0.8
Virginia	234.4	2.6	1.9
Washington	177.6	3.7	0.7
West Virginia	236.6	3.9	—
Wisconsin	282.9	3.5	1.7
National Average	256.8	3.5	1.5

Note: Ambulatory visits differ from physician encounters. Ambulatory visits are visits by an HMO member to an HMO clinic or physician's office when a physician is not seen, usually for tests, prescription refills, injections, immunizations, and the like. During physician encounters, the patient is seen by a physician. The sum of the visits and encounters is the total patient encounters with the HMO.

Source: Adapted with permission from *HMO–PPO Digest*, pp. 26–27, © 1996, Hoechst Marion Roussel.

Breast cancer screening (mammograms) given to women aged 52 to 69
Average: gave them to 70 percent of women
High: gave them to 90 percent of women
Low: gave them to 30 percent of women

Cervical cancer screening (Pap smears) to women aged 15 to 34
Average: gave them to 70 percent of women
High: gave them to 100 percent of women
Low: gave them to 25 percent of women

Table 2–27 HMOs Requiring Drug Utilization Review, by Model Type

Model Type	1996 (%)	1995 (%)	1994 (%)	1933 (%)	1992 (%)
IPA	83	76	67	61	53
Network	81	79	68	59	56
Group	80	77	74	71	59
Staff	68	63	69	60	60
All HMOs	82	75	68	62	55

Source: Adapted with permission from *HMO–PPO Digest*, p. 33, © 1996, Hoechst Marion Roussel.

The report also revealed the average results of member satisfaction surveys at the accredited MCOs:

- 56 percent of the enrollees in all the MCOs were "completely" or "very" satisfied with their health plan.
- 82 percent of them said their care was not delayed by requests for approval.
- 80 percent of them had no trouble being referred to a specialist.
- 40 percent found their plan to be "good" or "excellent" regarding the number of doctors they had to choose from.

On nearly every measure, health plans in New England scored highest, while those in Arkansas, Mississippi, and other South-Central states did the worst. New England plans also had the highest member satisfaction ratings.

The other form of MCO, the PPO, is more numerous than the HMO (983 versus 749) and serves more employee-members (88.6 versus 77.3 million) (Table 2–28). The predominant owners of PPOs are insurance companies and independent investors, accounting for 64 percent of individual PPOs and 59 percent of their eligible employees-members. Investor-owned PPOs are much larger than any others, averaging 288,000 eligible employee-members each. The more numerous insurance company PPOs have an average of only 35,000 eligible employee-members each. The second largest PPOs are those owned by HMOs (106,877).

Like HMOs, many PPOs have been organized into chains (Exhibit 2–5). The top three are quite large, encompassing 120, 97, and 78 individual PPOs, respectively. Altogether, chains own 71.5 percent of PPOs.

A variant of the PPO is the exclusive provider organization or EPO. It is still set up as a loose network of physicians, with the difference that patients must remain within the network to receive health care benefits. They must pay out-of-pocket for services obtained from non-network physicians.

About a third of PPOs offer an EPO option to payers, but the proportion varies according to the ownership of the PPO (Exhibit 2–6). Two-thirds of the PPOs run by physician groups make this option available.

By a ratio of almost two to one, PPOs own the networks of physicians who provide the health care services that they promise to payers (Table 2–29). This means that the PPO directly employs the physicians. Otherwise, they are simply on contract with the PPO. The following figures also reveal that 66 percent of all PPO networks are the creation of insurance companies or independent investors. Physician groups or joint physician/hospital ventures account for only 113 of the total of 3,222 PPO networks.

Measured by the average number of contracts they have with providers, PPOs are quite large entities. The typical PPO contracts with 2,818 primary care physicians, 5,345 specialists, 118 hospitals, and 989 ancillary providers. Broken down by type of owner, there is a rough correlation between a PPO's number of provider contracts and its enrollment (Table 2–30).

It is noteworthy that none of these PPO data on physician contracts indicate a primary care/specialist ratio approaching the recommended 50–50 proportion. In most cases, the ratio is closer to 1 to 2.

The next set of data tie the number of providers under PPO contract directly to the number of eligible employees (Table 2–31). Those PPOs owned by HMOs and insurance companies use a much higher number of physicians and hospitals to serve each 1,000 eligible employees. Some of the other variation may be accounted for by differences in the range of health plan benefits provided by each PPO. Remember, too, that providers under PPO contract are usually paid a discounted FFS and can devote more or less of their practice to non-PPO patients. The fewer patients a PPO physician is willing or able to see, the more physicians the PPO must have under contract to serve a given patient population.

The vast majority (85.4 percent) of PPO doctors are paid on a FFS basis with a cap limiting the maximum payment (Exhibit 2–7). The only other payment method used to any significant degree is a discount from a physician's usual billed charges (8.0 percent).

The two most popular methods for PPO reimbursement of hospitals is per diem rates (44.0 percent) and a discount from the institution's usual and customary charges (39.9 percent) (Exhibit 2–8). The use of diagnosis-related groups (DRGs) is not yet a significant factor (7.7 percent).

About 40 percent of PPOs are using some form of risk contract (shared or full) with their providers (Table 2–32). Twenty-nine percent (29 percent) are sharing the risk between themselves; only 3 percent have evolved to the usage of full risk contracts. The PPOs most likely to enter into risk contracts are those owned by physician-hospital joint ventures, insurance companies, and hospitals.

Table 2–28 Number of PPOs, by Owner Type and Number of Eligible Employees

Type of Owner	Number of PPOs	Number of Eligible Employees	Average Eligible Employees per PPO
Employer/Employer Coalition	7	419,438	59,920
HMO	68	1,961,953	28,852
Hospital	19	892,029	46,949
Hospital Alliance	42	3,347,922	79,712
Independent Investor	120	34,546,236	287,885
Insurance Company	507	17,546,498	34,608
Multiownership	33	3,526,956	106,877
Physician-Hospital Joint Venture	42	2,370,393	56,438
Physician/Medical Group	23	1,744,230	75,836
Third-Party Administrator	23	412,540	17,937
Other[*]	99	21,881,410	221,024
Total	983	88,649,605	90,183

[*]"Other PPO owners" include: Managed care company, public corporation, health care corporation, not-for-profit corporation, private corporation, provider ownership, subscriber ownership, and utilization management company.

Source: Adapted with permission from *HMO–PPO Digest*, pp. 66–67, © 1996, Hoechst Marion Roussel.

When asked how they thought MCOs would develop in the future, the most common prognostication of a group of health system chief executive officers (CEOs) in the eastern United States was the continued growth of POS plans (Exhibit 2–9). Significant numbers also planned to improve their information systems, expand their provider networks to keep members happy, and invest heavily in outpatient centers. These developments would be good news for physicians,

Exhibit 2–5 Top PPO Chains and Number of PPOs Owned by Each

Company Name/Headquarters	Number of PPOs	
Aetna Life & Casualty Company (Hartford, CT)	120	(124)
Private Healthcare Systems (Waltham, MA)	97	(93)
United HealthCare Corporation (Minneapolis, MN)	78	(106)
Blue Cross/Blue Shield Association (Chicago, IL)	72	(52)
CIGNA Healthcare (Bloomfield, CT)	64	(63)
USA Health Network Company (Phoenix, AZ)	47	(47)
Prudential Insurance Company (Roseland, NJ)	45	(47)
Community Care Network, Inc. (San Diego, CA)	33	(20)
CRA Managed Care (Boston, MA)	27	(27)
Principal Health Care (Rockville, MD)	24	(22)
Humana Health Care Plans (Louisville, KY)	18	(17)
NYLCare Health Plans (New York, NY)	11	(11)
HealthStar Managed Care Corporation (Lincolnwood, IL)	10	(10)
Anthem Health Systems (Indianapolis, IN)	9	(6)
PacifiCare Health Systems (Cypress, CA)	9	(5)
Foundation Health Systems (Woodland Hills, CA)	7	(—)
Healthsource (Hookset, NH)	5	(—)
Equifax HAS (Dallas, TX)	5	(5)
Health Management Associates (Tempe, AZ)	5	(5)
Columbia/HCA Healthcare Group (Nashville, TN)	4	(4)
Maxicare Health Plan (Los Angeles, CA)	3	(—)
Emerald Health Network (Cleveland, OH)	3	(2)
Coventry Corporation (Nashville, TN)	2	(2)
North Mississippi Health Services (Tupelo, MS)	2	(2)
Sisters of Providence Health Systems (Seattle, WA)	2	(—)
Total	703	

Figures in parentheses are for 1995.

Source: Adapted with permission from *HMO–PPO Digest*, pp. 72–73, © 1996, Hoechst Marion Roussel.

Exhibit 2–6 PPOs Offering Exclusive Provider Organization (EPO) Options, by Owner Type

Physician/Medical Group	70%
Hospital Alliance	54%
Other	50%
Third-Party Administrator	48%
Hospital	47%
Independent Investor	45%
Physician-Hospital Joint Venture	45%
Multiownership	42%
Employer/Employer Coalition	40%
Insurance Company	18%
HMO	6%
All PPOs	31%

Source: Adapted with permission from *HMO–PPO Digest*, p. 68, © 1996, Hoechst Marion Roussel.

Table 2–29 PPO Use of Owned and Rented Networks, by Owner Type

Owner Type	Owned Networks	Rented Networks
Employer/Employer Coalition	6	—
HMO	89	2
Hospital	23	19
Hospital Alliance	52	38
Independent Investor	215	290
Insurance Company	1,174	433
Multiownership	250	50
Physician-Hospital Joint Venture	53	22
Physician/Medical Group	31	7
Third-Party Administrator	46	79
Other	192	151
Total	2,131	1,091

Source: Adapted with permission from *HMO–PPO Digest*, p. 71, © 1996, Hoechst Marion Roussel.

Table 2–30 Average Number of Provider Contracts per PPO, by Owner and Provider Type

Owner Type	Primary Care Physicians	Medical/Surgical Specialists	Ancillary Providers	Hospitals
Employer/Employer Coalition	776	1,572	678	30
HMO	1,233	2,688	260	59
Hospital	708	1,388	117	37
Hospital Alliance	1,425	2,715	514	55
Independent Investor	5,887	8,781	2,025	297
Insurance Company	2,263	4,441	691	76
Multiownership	3,079	4,860	505	126
Physician-Hospital Joint Venture	681	996	201	22
Physician/Medical Group	788	1,562	249	46
Third-Party Administrator	1,118	1,929	704	53
Other	7,836	15,607	2,375	280
Average	2,818	5,345	989	118

Source: Adapted with permission from *HMO–PPO Digest*, p. 83, © 1996, Hoechst Marion Roussel.

Table 2–31 Average Number of Providers under Contract (Per 1,000 Eligible Employees), by Owner Type

Owner Type	Primary Care Physicians	Medical/Surgical Specialists	Ancillary Providers	Hospitals
Employer/Employer Coalition	12	30	4	1
HMO	89	210	10	5
Hospital	26	49	4	2
Hospital Alliance	51	99	16	2
Independent Investor	55	95	18	3
Insurance Company	90	188	23	5
Multiownership	41	88	12	2
Physician-Hospital Joint Venture	19	30	3	1
Physician/Medical Group	46	117	6	3
Third-Party Administrator	80	140	30	5
Other	51	106	34	3
Average	69	143	19	4

Source: Adapted with permission from *HMO–PPO Digest*, p. 85, © 1996, Hoechst Marion Roussel.

offering increased practice opportunities within and without the MCOs' provider systems.

LEADING TRENDS

- There are slightly fewer HMOs operating now than 10 years ago, and they have enrolled twice as many people.

- One-quarter of the HMOs are responsible for three-quarters of the enrollees.
- Far and away the most common form of HMO is the one with the loosest relationship with its physicians—the IPA-type HMO. The oldest, most tightly knit form of HMO—the staff HMO—has been declining slowly in numbers.

Exhibit 2–7 Percentage of Physicians Reimbursed by PPOs through Various Methods

Fee Cap	85.4
Capitation	1.6
Package Price per Episode	0.7
Discount from Billed Charges	8.0
Other	4.2
	100%

Source: Adapted with permission from *HMO–PPO Digest*, p. 86, © 1996, Hoechst Marion Roussel.

Exhibit 2–8 Percentage of Hospitals Reimbursed by PPOs through Various Methods

Discounted Charges	39.9
Per Diem	44.0
Usual and Customary Charges	1.7
DRG-based	7.7
Capitation	0.2
Other	6.5
	100.0%

Source: Adapted with permission from *HMO–PPO Digest*, p. 86, © 1996, Hoechst Marion Roussel.

Table 2–32 PPOs Using Risk Contracts with Providers

Owner Type	Shared Risk (%)	Full Risk (%)	Shared and Full Risk (%)	No Risk Contracts (%)
Employer/Employer Coalition	—	—	—	100
HMO	2	—	2	96
Hospital	22	6	—	72
Hospital Alliance	10	—	5	85
Independent Investor	9	1	3	86
Insurance Company	44	3	11	41
Multiownership	7	3	7	84
Physician-Hospital Joint Venture	29	7	5	59
Physician/Medical Group	12	—	28	61
Third-Party Administrator	5	—	5	90
Other	46	2	6	47
Average	29	3	8	61

Source: Adapted with permission from *HMO–PPO Digest*, p. 87, © 1996, Hoechst Marion Roussel.

Exhibit 2–9 Survey of Health System CEOs in Eastern United States

95%   POS plans will continue to flourish.

75%   Health plans will include larger provider networks to keep members happy.

54%   Health plans will move away from gatekeeper model.

48%   Indemnity insurance will not disappear anytime soon.

88%   Plan to improve their information systems.

70%   Plan to invest heavily in outpatient centers.

32%   Plan to acquire Medicare HMO licenses.

27%   Plan to go after the Medicaid HMO market.

Courtesy of Arthur Anderson.

- About half of HMO members are enrolled in IPA models, and another third are in group-type HMOs.
- The pace of mergers and acquisitions in the health care industry is accelerating.
- The states most heavily penetrated by HMOs are Massachusetts, New Hampshire, Oregon, California, and Minnesota—all over 40 percent of their populations.
- Roughly three-quarters of all HMOs offer a POS plan, and about a quarter make open-ended options available.
- The primary influences over a consumer's choice of health plan are friends and family, patient surveys, and individual physicians.
- Employers claim to give equal weight to quality and cost in evaluating health plans, a distinct move away from the traditional cost focus.
- HMOs offer employers the lowest cost source of health care coverage, and self-insurance and indemnity coverage are the most expensive.
- The average HMO provides care through more than 800 primary care physicians

(PCPs), nearly 1900 specialists, and just over 30 acute care hospitals.

- Primary care physicians in group- and staff-model HMOs are responsible for approximately four times as many enrollees as those in IPA and network HMOs.
- In the average HMO, two-fifths of the premium dollar goes for hospital care, one-fifth each is paid to PCPs and specialists, and the last fifth is retained by the HMO.
- Capitation contracts are used most often by group-model HMOs and least often by IPA-type HMOs.
- The average HMO has reduced annual hospital days per 1,000 members to just under 260, combined with 3.5 annual physician encounters per member.
- The vast majority of PPOs are owned either by insurance companies or independent investors. They account also for well over half of all PPO-eligible employees.
- The average PPO has provider contracts with about 2,500 PCPs, 4,600 specialists, and 130 hospitals.
- Almost all PPO physicians are reimbursed on a "fee cap" basis.
- About one-fourth of PPOs use some form of risk contract with their providers.

## CHAPTER 3

Industry Trends That Are Forcing Physicians To Rethink Their Long-Term Strategies

Physician Involvement in Managed Care
Effects of Managed Care on Physician Practice
Operations and Strategy

INTRODUCTION

This chapter provides a statistical look at the interaction of physicians with the managed care movement and infrastructure in this country. The first set of tables examines the level of involvement of physicians with the managed care organizations (MCOs) and the forms of that involvement (e.g., capitation, number of managed care contracts, number of covered lives, share of capitated revenues, and income). The second set of tables is a closer study of how managed care has changed the way physicians deliver medical services.

PHYSICIAN INVOLVEMENT IN MANAGED CARE

Concerned and responsible physicians are interested in how many of their colleagues are participating in managed care and in what ways. These data may motivate and shape their own plans for becoming involved—or not.

From a survey conducted by Cambridge Associates of Cleveland, Ohio, for Medimetrix, as reported in *Medical Economics* (September 22, 1997), it was found that virtually all (94 percent) group practices owned or participated in managed care plans in 1996. This is an increase from 88 percent in 1995. The percentage of group practices that expected to get more than half their income in 1996 from managed care contracts rose to 41 percent from just 25 percent in the previous year. It cannot be ignored that managed care is the dominant force in the professional lives of most physicians.

The rates of participation in managed care, through health maintenance organizations (HMOs) and preferred provider organizations (PPOs), vary somewhat by physician specialty (Table 3–1). Most involved in HMOs are pediatricians (88 percent), thoracic and cardiology surgeons (88 percent), gastroenterologists (89 percent), obstetricians/gynecologists (88 percent), and ophthalmologists (86 percent). Least involved are psychiatrists (50 percent) and general practitioners (52 percent). At least three-quarters of all other specialties are participating in HMOs and PPOs.

The percentages of physicians engaged in capitation contracts with payers is lower and even more variable (Table 3–1). Over 60 percent of some specialists (family practitioners, internists, and pediatricians) are capitated. Involvement in capitation has barely reached one-fourth of many other specialties, like thoracic and cardiology surgeons, general surgeons, neurosurgeons, obstetricians/gynecologists (ob/gyns), ophthalmologists, and orthopedic surgeons. The reasons are that only primary care specialties are likely to

Table 3–1 How Participation Rates Vary by Specialty

	% of Physicians Participating In:		
	HMOs	*PPOs*	*Capitation*
Anesthesiologists	80	80	30
Cardiologists	79	80	37
Cardio/thoracic surgeons	88	88	26
Family practitioners	79	81	63
Gastroenterologists	85	89	37
General practitioners	52	59	48
General surgeons	76	82	23
Internists	79	83	62
Neurosurgeons	82	86	22
Ob/Gyns	84	88	26
Ophthalmologists	86	86	28
Orthopedic surgeons	82	85	23
Pediatricians	88	92	69
Plastic surgeons	74	75	18
Psychiatrists	50	62	13
Radiologists	79	76	32
All surgical specialists	82	84	25
All nonsurgeons	75	78	47
All fields	**77**	**80**	**40**

Note: Because participation may overlap, percentages total more than 100. Here HMO and PPO participation figures are for a typical week in early spring of 1997. The source throughout these charts and tables is the *Medical Economics* Continuing Survey. Figures are medians.

Source: Copyright © 1997, Medical Economics Publishing Company. Reprinted by permission from *MEDICAL ECONOMICS Magazine.*

perform enough services for a given patient population to permit calculation of accurate capitation rates.

Another way of looking at managed care involvement is in terms of the percentage of a physician's active patients who are covered by capitation arrangements (Table 3–2). The highest percentages here are also in the primary care specialties. The average of all physicians has one-fifth of their active patients under capitation. This figure is lower than the share of all physicians participating in capitation (40 percent) because a

physician is "participating" if only 5 percent of her patients are under capitation.

In 1996, the average doctor earned $120,000 in gross income from managed care. Gross income from capitated arrangements was $42,500. The following breakout (Table 3–3) shows the gross income levels from these managed care sources for the leading specialties. Ob/gyns receive the largest gross income from MCOs—over $200,000. Interestingly, it is orthopedic surgeons who get the most capitation income ($75,000). Although less than one-fourth of them participate in capita-

Table 3–2 Which Specialties Have the Highest Capitated Visit Rates

	Percent of Active Patients Who Are Capitated	Percent of Total Visits from Capitated Patients
Anesthesiologists	10	20
Cardiologists	10	10
Cardio/thoracic surgeons	12	20
FPs	28	25
Gastroenterologists	10	10
GPs	25	20
General surgeons	20	20
Internists	10	15
Neurosurgeons	10	15
Ob/Gyns	15	20
Ophthalmologists	10	12
Orthopedic surgeons	15	15
Pediatricians	25	25
Plastic surgeons	5	5
Psychiatrists	20	25
Radiologists	10	8
All surgical specialists	**15**	**20**
All nonsurgeons	**20**	**20**
All fields	**20**	**20**

Note: Figures are medians and exclude physicians with no capitation contracts.

Source: Copyright © 1997 by Medical Economics Publishing. Reprinted by permission from *MEDICAL ECONOMICS Magazine.*

tion contracts, when they do, the rates they are paid produce substantial incomes.

An interested physician might want to review these data on the physicians in his specialty participating in MCO plans and capitation (Table 3–1), receiving gross income from MCOs and capitation (Table 3–2), and patients under capitation (Table 3–3). Then, compare them with the figures on his own participation, income, and patients. The results will begin to indicate whether his practices are behind or ahead of the trends. Just remember that there are a lot of good reasons why one physician's involvement with managed care might vary from these averages.

One reason for different levels of managed care involvement does not seem to be practice group size (Table 3–4). Even solo doctors are participating at an 82 percent level. For all other groups, the participation rates are about 80 percent or higher.

On the other hand, the percentage of physicians receiving capitated income varies in an almost linear fashion by group size (Table 3–4). Except for the small anomaly of two-physician groups, the proportion earning capitation dollars rises steadily from about 30 percent to nearly 65 percent. The larger the group, the more likely it is to be receiving capitated income. The larger groups can better afford the systems necessary to practice efficiently under capitation.

A group's share of patients who are managed care members does not vary a lot by size (Table 3–4). Neither does the percentage of active

Table 3–3 Who Earns the Most From Managed Care and Capitation

	Median 1996 Gross Income* from:			Percent of 1996 Gross Income* from:		
	HMOs	PPOs	Capitation	HMOs	PPOs	Capitation
Anesthesiologists	$62,450	$56,450	$32,500	20%	20%	10%
Cardiologists	57,950	57,670	30,000	12	10	10
Cardio/thoracic surgeons	83,490	55,480	50,000	20	10	10
FPs	66,590	47,080	56,000	25	20	23
Gastroenterologists	77,140	70,760	32,500	20	20	10
GPs	42,680	35,000	40,000	20	20	20
General surgeons	64,710	62,240	56,250	20	20	20
Internists	45,610	39,290	32,500	20	15	10
Neurosurgeons	79,100	80,770	45,000	20	15	10
Ob/Gyns	100,000	103,600	55,000	25	25	15
Ophthalmologists	77,230	52,540	32,500	15	10	10
Orthopedic surgeons	87,160	95,660	75,000	20	20	15
Pediatricians	85,650	84,420	56,000	30	30	20
Plastic surgeons	57,420	63,730	24,000	15	14	5
Psychiatrists	33,790	33,000	48,000	20	20	25
Radiologists	70,000	52,970	37,500	15	15	10
All surgical specialists	**78,800**	**72,280**	**45,000**	**20**	**20**	**10**
All nonsurgeons	**55,860**	**48,340**	**42,000**	**20**	**20**	**15**
All fields	**63,280**	**56,240**	**42,500**	**20**	**20**	**15**

*Gross is the individual physician's share of 1996 practice receipts before professional expenses and income taxes. Figures exclude physicians with no HMO, PPO, or capitation contracts.

Source: Copyright © 1997 by Medical Economics Publishing. Reprinted by permission from *MEDICAL ECONOMICS Magazine*.

patients under capitation. Still, the highest figures in both categories are for the largest groups, of 50 or more physicians.

The share of a physician's gross income coming from MCOs and from capitation follows a similar pattern (Table 3–4). There is relatively little variation except for the largest groups, in this case those of 25 or more physicians.

The data become more interesting when broken down by type of geographic area (Table 3–5). The degree of physician involvement in managed care is highest in suburban and urban areas and

lowest in rural and inner city areas. In no area is it much below 80 percent.

The percentage of physicians receiving capitated income follows a rather different pattern. The highest number, by a significant margin, is for physicians practicing in the inner city. Physicians in rural and urban areas are least likely to be receiving capitated income.

A determined physician wanting to seek out or escape managed care opportunities might use these data to identify the kinds of areas in which to locate a practice.

Table 3–4 How Practice Size Correlates with Cap tation

	Percent of Doctors Reporting Capitation Income	Percent of Gross Income from Capitation*	Percent of Active Patients under Capitation*
Solo	34%	11%	15%
Expense-sharers	31	10	10
Partnerships of 2	39	20	20
Groups of:			
3	30	10	12
4	34	10	15
5–9	42	20	20
10–24	47	10	10
25–49	52	10	15
50 or more	64	20	24

and with Managed Care Participation

	Percent of Doctors Reporting HMO/PPO Participation	Percent of Gross Income from HMOs/PPOs**	Percent of Active Patients in HMOs/PPOs**
Solo	82%	48%	54%
Expense-Sharers	93	41	48
Partnerships of 2	93	45	51
Groups of:			
3	95	38	51
4	92	45	52
5–9	93	48	53
10–24	93	34	40
25–49	99	54	54
50 or more	89	56	56

*Excludes physicians with no capitation contracts.
**Excludes physicians with no HMO or PPO affiliations. Figures are medians.

Source: Copyright © 1997 by Medical Economics Publishing. Reprinted by permission from *MEDICAL ECONOMICS Magazine.*

There is virtually no difference in physician managed care involvement levels among areas of the country (Table 3–6). They range from 85 percent to 89 percent. The proportion of physicians reporting capitated income is noticeably higher in the Far West (51 percent) than any other part of the country. The very lowest areas for capitated income are the Mid-South (24 percent) and the Great Lakes (30 percent). The rest of the country hovers around the 40 percent figure. There is nowhere to flee the spread of managed care, but pervasive capitation is still a few years off in some parts of the country.

A physician's share cf patients who belong to MCOs is higher in three areas (Table 3–6)—the Far West (66 percent), the Rocky Mountain states

Table 3–5 Inner-City Doctors Are Way Ahead in Capitation

	Percent of Doctors Reporting Capitation Income	Percent of Gross Income from Capitation[*]	Percent of Active Patients under Capitation[*]
Urban	36%	15%	15%
Suburban	42	15	20
Rural	34	10	10
Inner-city	53	20	20

Managed Care Is Hardest To Escape in the Suburbs

	Percent of Doctors Reporting HMO/PPO Participation	Percent of Gross Income from HMOs/PPOs[**]	Percent of Active Patients under HMOs/PPOs[**]
Urban	87%	46%	51%
Suburban	92	52	58
Rural	79	33	37
Inner city	81	47	55

*Excludes physicians with no capitation contracts.
**Excludes physicians with no HMO or PPO affiliations. Figures are medians.

Source: Copyright © 1997 by Medical Economics Publishing. Reprinted by permission from *MEDICAL ECONOMICS Magazine.*

(61 percent), and New England (58 percent). Patients are least likely to be MCO members in the Mid-South (41 percent) and the Great Plains (45 percent). When it comes to capitated patients, look to the Far West (30 percent), the Mid-East (25 percent), and the Great Lakes (20 percent). Everywhere else is in the 10- to 15-percent range.

When a physician chooses to get involved in managed care, she has five choices of MCO (depending on the market area)—a PPO and four types of HMO. The popularity of different MCO models varies by the size and specialty composition of the physician group (Table 3–7).

Although the figures are not conclusive, the larger groups are more drawn to the tighter forms of MCO—network, group, and staff HMOs. The smaller physician groups lean toward looser models that permit them to remain small and independent—PPOs and IPAs.

Multispecialty group practices are often assembled for the purpose of attracting the attention of MCOs. They usually feel more comfortable with the more closely integrated structures of network, group, and staff HMOs. Single specialty groups are more likely to be composed of a small number of like-minded physicians, resulting in a preference for the more relaxed PPO and IPA forms.

Many physicians are more focused on the number of managed care contracts they have and the number of covered lives they are responsible for (Table 3–8) than the specific type of MCO that is their contract partner. Both those key indices increased dramatically for all groups from 1995 to 1996. The average number of contracts per group went from 6.6 to 16.3; the average number of lives covered by those contracts rose by a factor of seven, from 3,167 to 23,160.

Except for the very large groups, the number of contracts and lives were in a rather tight range. Groups with over 100 physicians stand out most clearly. They have approximately twice as many managed care contracts and are serving over three times as many covered lives. There is very little difference between single and multispecialty groups on these two matters.

A physician might want to compare his group with regard to the number of managed care contracts and the number of covered lives.

The share of revenue that a group derives from at-risk contracts is directly related to its size and specialty composition (Table 3–9). As a group grows from 10 physicians to over 150, its at-risk revenues go from 61 percent to 95 percent. Multispecialty groups receive an additional 20 percent of their revenue from at-risk contracts compared with single specialty groups (73 percent versus 55 percent). Notice, too, the big jumps in at-risk revenue shares experienced by all groups

Table 3–6 Physicians Participating in Managed Care and Receiving Capitated Income and Share of Active Patients under Capitation

	The Far West Leads in Capitation Income				Where Managed Care is Most Prevalent		
	Percent of Doctors Reporting Capitation Income	*Percent of Gross Income from Capitation**	*Percent of Active Patients under Capitation**		*Percent of Doctors Reporting HMO/PPO Participation*	*Percent of Gross Income from HMOs/ PPOs**	*Percent of Active Patients in HMOs/ PPOs**
EAST	**40%**	**20%**	**20%**	**EAST**	**89%**	**48%**	**55%**
New England	40	10	10	New England	88	58	58
Mid-East	40	20	25	Mid-East	89	46	53
SOUTH	**35%**	**10%**	**12%**	**SOUTH**	**87%**	**44%**	**48%**
South Atlantic	38	10	12	South Atlantic	88	45	50
Mid-South	24	5	10	Mid-South	85	36	41
Southwest	35	10	15	Southwest	86	47	47
MIDWEST	**39%**	**10%**	**15%**	**MIDWEST**	**88%**	**41%**	**46%**
Great Lakes region	30	15	20	Great Lakes region	85	51	51
Great Plains	42	10	12	Great Plains	89	39	45
WEST	**47%**	**20%**	**30%**	**WEST**	**86%**	**58%**	**65%**
Rocky Mountain region	37	10	15	Rocky Mountain region	87	56	61
Far West	51	25	30	Far West	86	58	66

*Excludes those physicians with no HMO or PPO affiliation or capitation. Figures are medians.

Source: Copyright © 1997 by Medical Economics Publishing. Reprinted by permission from *MEDICAL ECONOMICS Magazine.*

between 1994 and 1995. All physician groups need to understand the techniques for efficient practice of medicine under financial risk.

As the proportion of a group's managed care revenue increases, so does the likelihood that the revenue will come from at-risk fee-for-service (FFS) and, eventually, capitated contracts (Table 3–10).

As a multispecialty group with at-risk managed care contracts increases the proportion of its revenues coming from managed care, the median annual revenue per full-time equivalent (FTE) physician increases (Exhibit 3–1). This has two important implications. As the group's revenues and managed care involvement grow, the physicians increase their productivity. The

Table 3–7 Type of Managed Care Contract for Group Practices with HMO/PPO Contracts, by Group Size and Specialty Composition

			Type of Managed Care Contract		
	PPO (%)	IPA HMO (%)	Network HMO (%)	Group HMO (%)	Staff HMO (%)
Group Size					
10 or fewer	76.5	32.9	32.9	23.5	7.1
11–25	72.1	36.1	37.4	24.5	7.5
26–50	76.2	29.8	44.1	36.9	8.3
51–100	78.1	39.0	48.8	36.6	12.2
101 or more	74.2	25.8	45.2	29.0	19.4
Specialty Composition					
Single Specialty	80.5	34.9	33.3	23.4	6.5
Multispecialty	73.9	32.8	38.3	26.3	10.0
All Groups	74.4	33.3	35.3	24.7	7.9

Source: Adapted with permission from *Medical Group Practice Digest*, p. 27, © 1997, Hoechst Marion Roussel.

Table 3–8 Average Number of Managed Care Contracts and Covered Lives, by Group Size and Specialty Composition

	Average Number of HMO/PPO Contracts	Average Number of Covered Lives
Group Size (# of FTE Physicians)		
10 or fewer	15.8 (6.0)	15,329 (1,768)
11–25	13.2 (7.2)	24,493 (3,801)
26–50	15.9 (4.3)	21,821 (4,729)
51–100	25.1 (3.8)	22,507 (6,182)
101 or more	34.2 (3.9)	73,081 (15,616)
Specialty Composition		
Single Specialty	16.2 (5.7)	24,987 (3,183)
Multispecialty	17.7 (8.8)	21,897 (3,129)
All Groups	16.3 (6.6)	23,160 (3,167)

Note: Figures in parentheses are from 1995.

Source: Adapted with permission from *Medical Group Practice Digest*, p. 24, © 1997, Hoechst Marion Roussel.

Table 3–9 Share of Revenue from At-Risk Contracts, by Group Size and Specialty Composition

	1995 (%)	1994 (%)
Group Size (# of FTE Physicians)		
10 or fewer	60.6	50.5
11–25	67.4	52.1
26–50	75.0	67.5
51–75	75.8	83.8
76–150	94.7	75.0
151 or more	94.7	93.3
Specialty Composition		
Single Specialty	54.7	49.5
Multispecialty	73.1	65.9
All Groups	60.8	55.1

Source: Adapted with permission from *Medical Group Practice Digest*, p. 25, © 1997, Hoechst Marion Roussel.

increased revenues per physician mean that there is more money to invest in systems required by managed care and to raise physician compensation.

The ratio between FFS and capitated revenues per physician also changes as the size of the group grows (Table 3–11). The volume of FFS revenues does not fluctuate greatly; if anything, it seems to go up a bit with the group size. The most dramatic change is in the amount of capitated revenues. From groups with 11 to 25 physicians, to those with over 150 physicians, those

revenues quadruple ($42,506 to $174,454). After other medical revenues are added in, the average doctor can look forward to his revenues going from $370,000 in the smallest groups to $547,000 in the largest. These figures are good news for physicians facing the inevitability of managed care and capitation. For the time being anyway, FFS revenues do not decline while capitated revenues surge upward.

The shift in proportions between FFS and capitated revenues looks even clearer in simple percentage terms (Table 3–12). FFS revenues fall from 92 percent of the total for very small groups to 66 percent for the very large. This happens without the absolute FFS dollars decreasing. Instead, the capitated revenues grow enough to move from 6 percent to 31 percent. Figures like these suggest that a physician need not suffer economically as capitation becomes a bigger part of her practice life.

Some physician groups have chosen to acknowledge the importance of managed care by starting or acquiring an ownership interest in an HMO or PPO (Table 3–13). Once a group reaches 50 physicians, this option begins to look especially appealing. Sixteen percent of groups with 51 to 100 physicians own at least a piece of an HMO; 18 percent have bought into a PPO. Eleven percent each of groups of over 100 physicians are owners of HMOs and PPOs.

Six to seven percent of all multispecialty groups have MCO ownership interests. Single specialty groups do not have a lot of interest in HMOs, but 5 percent are invested in PPOs.

The decision to become an owner of an MCO, even in part, gives physician groups the opportu-

Table 3–10 Sources of 1995 Group Practice Gross Charges, by Managed Care Involvement

Revenue Category	No MC Revenue (%)	10% or Less MC Revenue	11–50% MC Revenue	51–100% MC Revenue
Capitated Contract	—	4.0	16.0	58.5
At-Risk FFS	15.0	9.7	10.0	—
Not-At-Risk FFS	16.7	16.4	19.5	—

Source: Adapted with permission from *Medical Group Practice Digest*, p. 25, © 1997, Hoechst Marion Roussel.

Exhibit 3–1 Total Revenue 1994 Median Annual Revenue per FTE Physician in Multispecialty Groups with At-Risk Managed Care Contracts, by Degree of Managed Care Involvement

Groups with No Managed Care Revenue	$440,353
Groups with 10% or Less Managed Care Revenue	$426,491
Groups with 11% to 50% Managed Care Revenue	$455,101
Groups with 51% to 100% Managed Care Revenue	$525,201

Source: Adapted with permission from *Medical Group Practice Digest*, p. 16, © 1996, Hoechst Marion Rous-

Table 3–11 Total Revenue from FFS and Capitated Sources; 1994 Median Annual Revenue per FTE Physician in Multispecialty Groups, by Group Size and Revenue Source

Group Size (# of FTE Physicians)	FFS Revenues ($)	Capitated Revenues ($)	Other Medical Revenues ($)	Total Medical Revenues* ($)
fewer than 11 FTEs	327,437	20,725	7,616	369,095
11–25 FTEs	345,515	42,506	9,657	417,003
26–50 FTEs	405,987	46,181	5,658	460,313
51–75 FTEs	383,857	66,462	10,534	480,944
76–150 FTEs	409,729	107,552	8,252	521,016
over 150 FTEs	375,587	174,454	17,652	547,067

*The revenues from each source are medians and usually do not add up to the total figure.

Source: Adapted with permission from *Medical Group Practice Digest*, p. 15, © 1997, Hoechst Marion Roussel.

Table 3–12 Shares of Revenue from FFS and Capitated Sources—1995 Median Annual Revenue per FTE Physician in Multispecialty Groups, by Group Size and Revenue Source

Group Size (# of FTE Physicians)	Fee-For-Service Revenue (%)	Capitated Revenue (%)	Other Medical Revenue (%)
fewer than 11 FTEs	92	6	2
11–25 FTEs	87	11	2
26–50 FTEs	89	10	1
51–75 FTEs	83	14	2
76–150 FTEs	78	20	2
over 150 FTEs	66	31	3

Source: Adapted with permission from *Medical Group Practice Digest*, p. 15, © 1997, Hoechst Marion Roussel.

Table 3–13 Group Practices with Ownership Interests in HMOs and PPOs, by Group Size and Specialty Composition

	HMO (%)	PPO (%)
Group Size (# of FTE Physicians)		
10 or fewer	3.6 (1.4)	4.3 (1.4)
11–25	2.9 (1.1)	5.1 (1.3)
26–50	3.7 (1.0)	4.9 (1.7)
51–100	15.8 (3.8)	18.4 (1.7)
101 or more	10.7 (4.2)	10.7 (2.3)
Specialty Composition		
Single Specialty	0.8 (1.2)	4.9 (1.5)
Multispecialty	6.3 (2.0)	6.5 (1.4)
All Groups	4.2 (1.4)	5.5 (1.5)

Note: Figures in parentheses are from 1995.

Source: Adapted with permission from *Medical Group Practice Digest*, p. 24, © 1997, Hoechst Marion Roussel.

nity to influence the practices of at least one of the payer organizations with whom it contracts.

LEADING TRENDS

- The proportion of group practices involved in some way with managed care is approaching 100 percent.
- The percentage of physicians receiving at least some capitated income is nearing 50 percent.
- The larger the group practice, the more likely it is to be receiving capitated income.
- Roughly one-fifth of the active patients of all physicians are under capitation arrangements; about half are covered by managed care contracts.
- Physician participation in managed care and receipt of capitated income does not vary significantly in different areas of the country.
- The proportion of patients with managed care coverage is highest in the Far West, the Rocky Mountain states, and New England.
- Physician groups are most likely, by a wide margin, to contract with the PPO type of MCO. Next most popular contract partners are network and independent practice association (IPA) forms of HMOs.
- The typical group practice has 16 managed care contracts covering 23,000 lives.
- The share of group practice revenues from at-risk contracts is climbing steadily toward the two-thirds mark.
- The annual revenue per physician is significantly higher in multi-specialty groups that receive a higher proportion of their revenue from at-risk contracts.
- Large multispecialty groups receive 5 to 10 times as much revenue per physician from capitation as small groups.
- The percentage of group practices with ownership interests in MCOs is small, but growing steadily.

EFFECTS OF MANAGED CARE ON PHYSICIAN PRACTICE OPERATIONS AND STRATEGY

One of the leading gripes physicians have about managed care is the changes it has caused or required in the way they practice medicine. This section looks at the nature and extent of those changes, usually from the viewpoint of the physician. Briefer attention is given to the managed care impacts on hospitals. Then, there is a review of the adjustments physicians have made in their practice systems to accommodate the demands of managed care.

Over three-quarters of doctors believe that it has become harder to practice medicine as a result of managed care (Figure 3–1). Half of all physicians report that their satisfaction with medicine, their

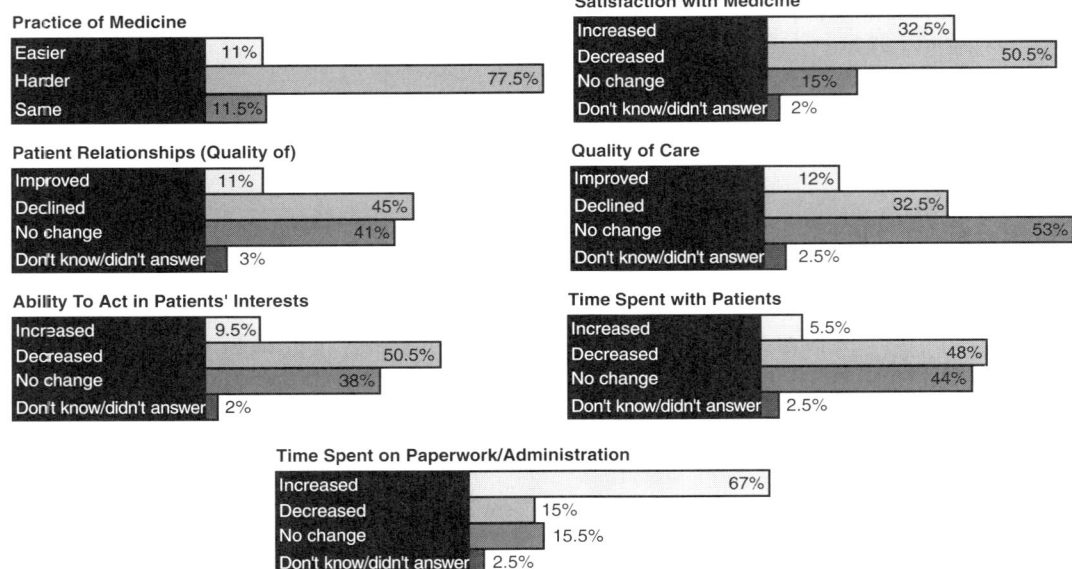

Figure 3–1 How Managed Care Has Affected Physicians. *Source*: Copyright ©1997 by Medical Economics Publishing. Reprinted by permission from *MEDICAL ECONOMICS Magazine*.

time spent with patients, and their ability to act in the patient's interests has decreased. The only thing that has gone up is the time they spend on paperwork and administration.

Fortunately, only one-third believes that the quality of care has declined due to managed care. Nearly half see a fall-off in the quality of patient relationships.

As discomforting as these opinions are, keep in mind that 50 percent of physicians claim that their satisfaction with medicine and the time spent with patients has improved or stayed the same. The same was true for their ability to act in the patient's interests and for the quality of their relationships with patients. Sixty-five percent of doctors think that the quality of care has improved or remained unchanged.

MCOs commonly require their physicians to refer patients to other physicians within the MCO network who were selected for their attention to quality and utilization (Exhibit 3–2). This can disrupt traditional and preferred referral relationships. Between 35 percent and 42 percent of physicians in all kinds of practice settings claim that

their referral patterns have been affected to a "great extent."

The same physicians were asked about some slightly less controversial effects of managed care on their clinical decision making (Table 3–14). These impacts were felt most strongly in multi-specialty group practices, which generally embrace managed care more completely. Over one-third of them felt encouragement from their

Exhibit 3–2 Effect of Managed Care in Changing Physician Referral Patterns, by Practice Type

	Affected to a "Great Extent"
Solo Practice	40%
Single Specialty Group	35%
Multispecialty Group	42%

Courtesy of Louis Harris & Associates, Inc., New York, New York.

Table 3–14 Effect of Managed Care in Changing Physician Clinical Decision Making, by Practice Type and Area of Decision Making

	Affected to a "Great Extent"		
	Solo Practice (%)	*Single Specialty (%)*	*Multispecialty (%)*
Fostering the use of clinical information technology in your practice/ hospital	2	1	11
Encouraging you to follow clinical protocols	13	7	13
Encouraging you to make more efficient use of diagnostic and laboratory tests	8	9	25
Encouraging you/primary care physicians to take overall responsibility for the care of patients	15	18	36

Courtesy of Louis Harris & Associates, Inc., New York, New York.

MCO partners to give overall responsibility for the care of patients to primary care doctors. One-quarter were pushed to make more efficient use of diagnostic and laboratory tests. A little more than 10 percent of those groups felt pressure to adopt clinical protocols and use information technology in their practice operations.

Both solo and single specialty practices experienced significantly less "encouragement" in all of these areas. Nonetheless, they probably represent future trends that all physicians ignore at their peril.

A great anxiety of physicians who have become dependent on managed care contracts is that they will be dropped from the MCO panel. Thirteen percent of all doctors have had managed care contract applications denied and another 6 percent have been subsequently dropped (Table 3–15). The numbers are not huge, but they are significant enough to give cause for worry.

The common wisdom is that MCOs have achieved much of their cost savings by shifting patient treatment from inpatient to outpatient settings (Table 3–16). Most of the data bear that out. Hospital average lengths of stay (ALOS) have

steadily declined while outpatient services per 1,000 covered lives have climbed. In the following data, the former decreased 22 percent between 1991 and 1995, while the latter increased 33 percent.

The changes in hospital utilization and charges can be tied even more directly to the effects of managed care (Tables 3–17 and 3–18). High managed care penetration is associated with a statistically significant decrease in ALOS in metropolitan areas of all sizes. Despite the shorter

Table 3–15 Percentage Denied or Dropped from Managed Care Contracts, 1995

	Denied	*Dropped*
General and family physicians	9	3
All physicians	13	6

Source: Adapted with permission from *Managed Care Magazine*, Vol. 6, No. 7, p. 35, © 1997, Stezzi Communications.

Table 3–16 The Shift from Inpatient to Outpatient Treatment of Many Patient Conditions

	Average Length of Stay (days)	Outpatient Services per 1,000 Covered Lives (services delivered)
1991	6.0	8,294
1992	5.7	9,492
1993	5.2	9,749
1994	5.0	10,926
1995	4.7	11,068

Source: Adapted with permission from The State of Health Care in America, 1997, *Business and Health,* p. 7, © 1997, Medical Economics Publishing Company, Inc.

Table 3–17 Effect of Managed Care Penetration on Hospital Utilization

	Average Length of Stay (severity adjusted)	
	Low Penetration (<25% population)	High Penetration (>25% population)
Small metro area (<250,000 people)	5.7 days	4.6 days
Medium metro area (250,000–999,999 people)	5.4 days	5.2 days
Large metro area (more than 1,000,000 people)	5.4 days	5.2 days

Note: For hospital care overall, high managed care penetration was associated with statistically significant decrease in ALOS in large and small metro areas, but not in medium-size metro areas.

Source: Adapted with permission from The State of Health Care in America, 1997, *Business and Health,* p. 10, © 1997, Medical Economics Publishing Company, Inc.

Table 3–18 Effect of Managed Care Penetration on Hospital Charges

	Hospital Charges per Admission (severity adjusted)	
	Low Penetration (<25% population)	High Penetration (>25% population)
Small metro area (<250,000 people)	$9,118	$7,872
Medium metro area (250,000–999,999 people)	$9,909	$9,535
Large metro area (more than 1,000,000 people)	$10,657	$11,761

Note: Despite shorter stays, large metro areas with high managed care penetration showed significantly higher hospital charges per admission than their counterparts with less managed care.

Source: Adapted with permission from The State of Health Care in America, 1997, *Business and Health,* p. 10, © 1997, Medical Economics Publishing Company, Inc.

stays, large metro areas with high managed care penetration showed higher hospital charges per admission than the same size areas with less managed care. Medium and small metro areas did experience lower charges when more managed care was present.

Managed care was cited as the cause of several changes noted in a recent survey of 5,300 urban and rural hospitals, conducted by the American Hospital Association and reported in *Hospitals & Health Networks* on July 5, 1997:

- Between 1994 and 1995, the number of rural hospitals forming networks increased almost 30 percent, while urban hospitals doing the same rose nearly 15 percent.
- Outpatient visits climbed 40 percent in rural hospitals during the first half of the 1990s, compared with 26 percent for urban hospi-

tals. Outpatient revenues as a percentage of total gross patient proceeds went up 27.3 percent in rural areas and 23.2 percent at urban facilities during the same period. Inpatient stays dropped almost 5 percent for city hospitals and 2.5 percent for their rural counterparts. The cost per case grew only 1.3 percent from 1994 to 1995 in rural hospitals and 3.1 percent in the urban versions.

- Rural hospitals launched a response to managed care during the first half of the '90s decade that went virtually unnoticed. They went on a boom of buying up physician practices, tripling the number of doctors working for them.

- Between 1985 and 1993, the states with the fastest growth in managed care penetration also had the highest rate of growth in primary care physician income and the lowest growth rate in the incomes of radiologists, anesthesiologists, and pathologists (RAP). The number of RAP physicians increased most rapidly in those states with the lowest rates of managed care growth.

- Primary care incomes grew 4.78 percent annually in states with the highest managed care growth, compared with 1.20 percent in the states in the lowest quartile of growth. The difference in income growth for medical and surgical subspecialty physicians between the highest and lowest quartiles was not statistically significant. The incomes of RAP physicians went up 0.14 percent in the highest quartile versus 4.14 percent in the lowest.

- Between 1985 and 1993, the number of family practice and pediatric residency positions that were filled rose 32 percent. The number of medical and surgical residencies filled remained constant, while the number of RAP positions filled decreased 14 percent.[*]

---

[*]Data on physician incomes and hiring are from "The Impact of Managed Care on the Physician Marketplace," by Simon, Dranove, and White, *Public Health Reports*, May 1997.

Either under pressure from their MCO partners or on their own initiative, physician groups have implemented a variety of mechanisms to help them practice medicine that is sensitive to quality and cost. One of those mechanisms is treatment protocols. Over one-third of all groups are using protocols; at least one-half of the largest groups (over 50 physicians) have introduced them into their practices (Exhibit 3–3). As group size increases, so does utilization of these protocols. As might be expected, multispecialty groups are somewhat more inclined to use them than single specialty groups.

Where do physician groups find the treatment protocols they use? Just about one-third of them develop the protocols themselves (Exhibit 3–4). Other common sources are MCOs and insurance companies, hospitals, and medical specialty societies.

The term "treatment protocols" is sometimes used interchangeably with "practice guidelines." A separate set of data also reports on the use of medical practice guidelines by group practices

Exhibit 3–3 Group Practices That Use Treatment Protocols, by Group Size and Specialty Composition

	Percentage Using Treatment Protocols
Group Size	
10 or fewer	35.3
11–25	33.1
26–50	43.4
51–100	52.9
101 or more	53.8
Specialty Composition	
Single Specialty	33.9
Multispecialty	39.8
All Groups	37.8

Source: Adapted with permission from *Medical Group Practice Digest*, p. 13, © 1997, Hoechst Marion Roussel.

Exhibit 3–4 Development Source of Treatment Protocols

Medical Group Practice	33.6
HMO/PPO/Insurance Company	6.5
Hospital	5.5
Medical Specialty Organization	4.5

Source: Adapted with permission from Medical Group Practice Digest, p. 13, © 1997, Hoechst Marion Roussel.

(Exhibit 3–5). In most cases, the guidelines are applied to specialists alone or in combination with primary care doctors. Nonphysician professionals are covered 35 percent of the time.

Certain diseases or conditions are more amenable to practice guidelines and usually get included first (Exhibit 3–6). By a wide margin, the two most likely subjects of guidelines are back pain and asthma. They are addressed by two-thirds of the groups who use guidelines.

Practice guidelines serve no purpose unless they produce positive effects. About half of the groups using guidelines claim that they have

Exhibit 3–5 Use of Medical Practice Guidelines by Group Practices, by Type of Guideline (type of practitioner covered)

Primary Care Only	10%
Specialty Care Only	20%
Nonphysician Professional Care Only	5%
Primary and Specialty Care	35%
Primary and Nonphysician Professional Care	15%
Specialty and Nonphysician Professional Care	—
All Three Types of Practitioner	15%

Source: Adapted with permission from *Medical Group Practice Digest*, p. 30, © 1996, Hoechst Marion Roussel.

Exhibit 3–6 Use of Medical Practice Guidelines by Group Practices, by Area of Guidelines (disease or condition)

Back Pain	63.2%
Asthma	63.2%
Diabetes	47.4%
Immunization	42.1%
Respiratory Infections	42.1%
GI Disorders	36.8%
Obstetrics/Gynecology	36.8%
Hypertension	31.6%
Other*	31.6%

*"Other" includes allergies, urinary tract infections, cholesterol evaluations, congestive heart failure, and multiple surgical diagnoses.

Source: Adapted with permission from *Medical Group Practice Digest*, p. 30, © 1996, Hoechst Marion Roussel.

helped identify areas for quality improvement and reduce variations in practice patterns (Exhibit 3–7).

Two-thirds of these practice guidelines were developed by the medical group using them (Exhibit 3–8). The second most common source was medical specialty societies.

Writing practice guidelines and putting them in place is one thing, getting physicians to follow them is another. Only one-third of the groups with guidelines reported that their physicians complied with them "frequently" (70 percent to 100 percent of the time) (Exhibit 3–9). The physicians in most of the other groups complied only "occasionally" (30 percent to 69 percent of the time).

Physician groups have adopted a number of other quality assurance measures. Five of them are summarized in the following table (Table 3–19). Far and away the most popular are patient satisfaction surveys, used by three-quarters of all groups. About one-third each have established a drug formulary, conducted outcomes studies, and begun benchmarking. Accreditation hovers

Exhibit 3–7 Use of Medical Practice Guidelines by Group Practices, by Positive Effects Produced

Identified areas for quality improvement	52.6%
Reduced variations in practice patterns	47.4%
Improved pharmaceutical therapy	21.1%
Reduced use of diagnostic tests	21.1%
Improved patient outcomes	21.1%
Unknown	21.1%
No effect on practice patterns	10.5%

Source: Adapted with permission from *Medical Group Practice Digest*, p. 31, © 1996, Hoechst Marion Roussel.

Exhibit 3–9 Use of Medical Practice Guidelines by Group Practices, by Frequency of Compliance with Guidelines

Frequently (70–100% of the time)	33.3%
Occasionally (30–69% of the time)	58.3%
Seldom (0–29% of the time)	8.3%

Source: Adapted with permission from *Medical Group Practice Digest*, p. 31, © 1996, Hoechst Marion Roussel.

around 15 percent until a group reaches more than 100 physicians, when the percentage relying on it jumps to 40 percent.

As a general rule, the likelihood that a group will pursue any of these initiatives increases as the size of the group increases. Larger groups are more likely to have the necessary resources. Once again, multispecialty groups implement these measures much more often than single specialty groups—with the exception of outcomes studies where the two group types are almost the same.

Exhibit 3–8 Use of Medical Practice Guidelines by Group Practices, by Primary Source of Guidelines

Own Medical Group	66.7%
Specialty Society	26.7%
Government	6.7%

Source: Adapted with permission from *Medical Group Practice Digest*, p. 30, © 1996, Hoechst Marion Roussel.

Internal review mechanisms are traditional devices for monitoring quality, and they continue to be popular in the age of managed care. Over three-quarters of all group practices employ a formal internal peer review process (Table 3–20). A little less than half maintain a formal medical practice review committee.

Some of the same patterns persist here as with other clinical management procedures—larger groups are more likely to implement internal review mechanisms, and they seem less necessary to single specialty groups than to multispecialty groups. As expected, the procedures show up more often in groups with higher levels of managed care involvement.

The following table presents more detailed information on the use of drug formularies by group practices (Table 3–21). About half the groups covered by these data use some kind of formulary. An open formulary is the most popular.

In addition to formularies, several other control methods help ensure only the appropriate utilization of drugs (Exhibit 3–10). A regular drug utilization review is the most common approach. In nearly 70 percent of the cases, the drug utilization controls are applied to the group practice by an HMO with which it contracts. The control authority is located within the group half of the time.

Another method groups use to reduce the costs of care delivery without impairing quality is to employ midlevel providers (MLPs) under the supervision of physicians (Table 3–22). "Mid-level providers" include physician assistants and nurse practitioners.

The percentage of multispecialty groups that use MLPs is increasing steadily. Virtually 100 percent of such groups with 76 or more physicians rely on MLPs. The likelihood that a group will use MLPs increases both with the size of the group and the degree of its involvement with managed care.

The median MLP staff of physician groups is in the range of 0.15 to 0.20 per FTE physician, rising to 0.27 MLPs per doctor in the very largest groups.

The aggressive use of MLPs is not restricted to multispecialty groups; single specialty groups have become part of the trend. MLP usage seems to be the highest in the following subspecialties (Exhibit 3–11).

A physician in a multispecialty or single specialty group might want to compare the number of MLPs in her group with these figures.

In maximizing net income under managed care, groups must be just as concerned with expenses as they are with revenues. As managed care involvement grows, some of the utilization control mechanisms might be expected to reduce certain operating expenses. At the same time, the cost of implementing those mechanisms, along with quality control measures and other reporting systems, would increase expenses.

In fact, median nonprovider expenses per FTE physician clearly increase as a multispecialty group's involvement in managed care grows (Exhibit 3–12). Expenses take a big leap when managed care revenues exceed 50 percent of the group's total. Per physician expenses also increased far more from 1994 to 1995 for heavily managed care groups than for any others. It appears that the costs of competing for managed care contracts and performing successfully under them are not insignificant.

To understand what cost items are included within "nonprovider expenses" and in what proportions, consult Exhibit 3–13. In a labor-intensive enterprise like health care delivery, it is not surprising that support staff compensation and benefits consume over half the expense budget.

Table 3–19 Quality Assurance Activities of Group Practices, by Group Size and Specialty Composition

	Patient Satisfaction Studies (%)	Drug Formulary (%)	Outcomes Studies (%)	Bench-marking (%)	Accredi-tation (%)
Group Size					
10 or fewer	72.6	34.1	28.0	21.0	15.9
11–25	76.9	29.7	31.2	30.6	8.1
26–50	91.5	42.0	39.7	50.0	18.8
51–100	94.6	48.6	47.2	50.0	18.2
101 or more	88.0	48.0	58.3	58.3	39.1
Specialty Composition					
Single Specialty	66.3	29.8	31.1	19.8	13.6
Multispecialty	82.7	38.3	33.5	35.4	16.4
All Groups	75.6	34.2	32.3	28.3	16.0

Source: Adapted with permission from *Medical Group Practice Digest*, p. 14, © 1997, Hoechst Marion Roussel.

Table 3–20 Use of Internal Peer Review Mechanisms by Group Size, Specialty Composition, Managed Care Involvement, and Ownership

	Formalized Internal Peer/ Medical Review Process (%)	Formalized Medical Practice Review Committee (%)
Group Size (# of FTE physicians)		
25 or fewer	50.0	12.5
26–100	71.4	50.0
101–160	85.7	42.9
161 or more	100.0	87.5
Specialty Composition		
Single Specialty	25.0	—
Multispecialty with Primary Care	84.0	54.2
Managed Care Involvement		
50% or Less Revenue	68.8	33.3
More Than 50% Revenue	84.6	61.5
Ownership		
Group Physicians	72.7	42.9
Physician Practice Management Company	66.7	33.3
Other*	100.0	80.0
All Groups	76.7	48.3

*"Other" includes ownership by a single physician and by an IDS.

Source: Adapted with permission from *Medical Group Practice Digest*, p. 32, © 1996, Hoechst Marion Roussel.

The employment of support staff is as important to managed care success as midlevel providers. Multispecialty groups use an average of four to six support persons per FTE physician (Table 3–23). The numbers increased from 1994 to 1995. They are higher for larger groups and for groups that receive more of their revenues from managed care. These are all predictable trends.

In addition to these operational changes in the way they practice medicine, some physicians have been making strategic adjustments as well.

In the three years prior to a recent survey,* 39 percent of physicians had increased the number

---

*In 1995, researchers from Harvard University and Louis Harris and Associates, Inc., funded by The Pew Charitable Trusts, conducted five surveys. They contacted 2,003 physicians and the strategic planning and staffing officials in 502 hospitals and health systems, 152 HMOs, 100 PPOs, and 151 medical group practices by phone about their perceptions of medical practice in the age of managed care.

Table 3–21 Use of Drug Formularies by Group Practices by Group Size, Specialty Composition, Managed Care Involvement, and Ownership

		Those Groups Using Formularies (%)		
	% Using Formularies	Open Formularies	Closed Formularies	Both Open and Closed
Group Size (# of FTE physicians)				
25 or fewer	37.5	100.0	—	—
26–100	42.9	66.7	—	33.3
101–160	85.7	50.0	16.7	33.3
161 or more	50.0	75.0	25.0	—
Specialty Composition				
Single Specialty	25.0	—	—	—
Multispecialty with Primary Care	60.0	66.7	13.3	20.0
Managed Care Involvement				
50% or Less Revenue	50.0	87.5	12.5	—
More Than 50% Revenue	61.5	50.0	12.5	37.5
Ownership				
Group Physicians	40.9	66.7	11.1	22.2
Physician Practice Management Company	100.0	66.7	33.3	—
Other*	80.0	75.0	—	25.0
All Groups	53.3	68.8	12.5	18.8

*"Other" includes ownership by a single physician and by an IDS.

Source: Adapted with permission from *Medical Group Practice Digest*, p. 36, © 1996, Hoechst Marion Roussel.

of other physicians they practice with, and 24 percent increased the number of nonphysician (midlevel) providers. In the three years after the survey, 40 percent of the physicians planned to increase the number of other doctors they work with.

In the last three years, 14 percent of the physicians had changed the geographic location of their practices. In the next three years, 12 percent were considering doing that.

In the past three years, 11 percent of physicians had changed to a salaried or capitated practice setting. In the coming three years, another 11 percent expected to make such changes.

In the previous three years, 5 percent of the doctors surveyed had sold their practices to larger organizations. A further 13 percent were considering selling during the next three years.

In the coming three years, 14 percent of the physicians were thinking about leaving their clinical practices to go into administration, teaching, or research. An additional 25 percent were considering retiring or abandoning their practices for other undescribed pursuits.

Because of the demand of MCOs for primary care physicians and the alleged surplus of specialist physicians, arguments have been made that the specialists should try to shift to primary care

Exhibit 3–10 Methods and Sources of Drug Utilization Controls in Group Practices

Methods of Control	
Drug Utilization Review	42.3%
Quality Assurance	30.8%
Capitation	26.9%
Financial Withholds	26.9%
Treatment Protocols	26.9%
None	23.1%
Sources of Control	
HMO	68.8%
In-House Control	50.0%
Pharmacy Business Management Company	6.3%

Source: Adapted with permission from *Medical Group Practice Digest*, p. 37, © 1996, Hoechst Marion Roussel.

medicine. So far, only 6 percent of medical specialists and surgeons have said they were willing to get additional training to be able to practice primary care. Sixty percent of HMOs and 31 percent of hospitals already operate primary care residency training programs. Now, 23 percent of the HMOs and 7 percent of the hospitals have also developed programs to retrain specialists to deliver primary care.

With all these changes in the traditional ways of practicing medicine, one might expect that current physicians would be reluctant to recommend a medical career. This is not entirely the case.

Fifty-nine percent would recommend medicine as a career to a qualified college student, and 67 percent would recommend their particular specialty to a qualified medical student. Seventy-three percent of primary care physicians would recommend their specialty. Ninety percent of institutional leaders, who do the hiring of many physicians, agree on the value of training in primary care. Sixty-four percent of medical specialists and 60 percent of surgeons would recommend their respective specialties. About 50 percent of institutional leaders share the same view.

Perhaps the most deliberate and ambitious physician response to the inroads of managed care, and the one advocated by this book, is to integrate the practice with other provider organizations. The following table displays some information on the percentages of group practices that have implemented certain integration strategies (Table 3–24). Because the survey underlying the table is based on a rather small sample, it would not be a good idea to rely too heavily on the specific numbers. However, this does represent a good listing of the integration strategies available to physicians and their groups.

Many group practices that have not integrated plan to do so in the near future (Exhibit 3–14). The most popular option with the groups in this survey was a joint venture with a hospital and the development of an HMO entity.

LEADING TRENDS

- Over three-quarters of doctors believe that it has become harder to practice medicine as a result of managed care. The only thing that has increased is the time they spend on paperwork and administration.
- Managed care has affected the referral patterns of nearly half of all physicians to a "great extent."
- The positive effects of managed care (e.g., use of clinical information technology, clinical protocols, broader responsibility for patient care) are much more often felt in multispecialty groups.
- About one-fifth of doctors have been either denied a managed care contract or dropped from an MCO's provider panel.
- There is solid evidence that managed care has reduced the average length of hospital stays and hospital charges per admission,

Table 3–22 Use of Midlevel Providers (MLP)* by Multispecialty Groups, by Group Size and Managed Care Involvement

	Median MLP Staff per FTE Physician	% of Groups with MLPs
Group Size (# of FTE Physicians)		
10 or fewer	0.31 (0.25)	57.1 (59.0)
11–25	0.16 (0.11)	71.0 (67.4)
26–50	0.14 (0.11)	80.2 (79.7)
51–75	0.19 (0.14)	93.3 (100.0)
76–150	0.16 (0.22)	97.5 (89.7)
151 or more	0.27 (0.26)	100.0 (93.3)
Managed Care Involvement		
No MC Revenue	0.18 (0.16)	68.3 (70.0)
1–10% MC Revenue	0.17 (0.14)	75.2 (83.6)
11–50% MC Revenue	0.19 (0.17)	85.3 (72.4)
51–100% MC Revenue	0.21 (0.16)	90.0 (76.7)

*Midlevel providers are specially trained and licensed nonphysician providers who can provide medical care and billable services. They include audiologists, certified registered nurse anesthetists, dietitians/nutritionists, midwives, nurse practitioners, occupational therapists, optometrists, physical therapists, physician assistants, podiatrists, psychologists, social workers, speech therapists, and surgeon assistants.

Note: Figures in parentheses are from 1994.

Source: Adapted with permission from *Medical Group Practice Digest*, p. 21, © 1996, Hoechst Marion Roussel.

Exhibit 3–11 Use of Midlevel Providers (MLP) by Select Single Specialty Groups Median Staffing per FTE Physician

Cardiology	0.26 (0.22)
Family Practice	0.25 (0.25)
Internal Medicine	0.18 (0.15)
Ob/Gyn	0.33 (0.26)
Pediatrics	0.19 (0.21)

Note: Figures in parentheses are from 1994.

Source: Adapted with permission from *Medical Group Practice Digest*, p. 21, © 1997, Hoechst Marion Roussel.

while increasing the volume of outpatient services delivered per 1,000 covered lives.

- Over half of all physician groups are using treatment protocols.
- By using medical practice guidelines (i.e., treatment protocols), around half of group practices claim to have identified areas for quality improvement and reduced variations in practice patterns.
- Three-quarters of all groups rely on patient satisfaction studies to maintain quality. At least one-third are also using drug formularies, outcome studies, and benchmarking.
- Three-quarters of the groups operate a formal internal peer review process, while one-half have created a medical practice review committee.

Exhibit 3–12 Median Nonprovider Expenses per FTE Physician in Multispecialty Groups in 1995 by Degree of Managed Care Involvement

No Managed Care Revenue	$236,444 ($228,569)
10% or Less Managed Care Revenue	$233,599 ($227,751)
11% to 50% Managed Care Revenue	$260,270 ($254,992)
51% to 100% Managed Care Revenue	$353,301 ($282,538)

Note: Figures in parentheses are from 1994.

Source: Adapted with permission from *Medical Group Practice Digest*, p. 18, © 1997, Hoechst Marion Roussel.

Exhibit 3–13 Percentage Breakout of Median Nonprovider Expenses per FTE Physician in Multispecialty Groups in 1995 by Expense Category

Support Staff Compensation	43.4
Building and Occupancy	11.4
Support Staff Benefits	10.2
Medical and Surgical Supplies	6.9
Other Nonprovider Expenses	6.2
Laboratory	5.0
Insurance Premiums	3.3
Administrative Supplies and Services	3.2
Information Services	3.1
Ambulatory Surgery Center	2.8
Furniture and Equipment	2.6
Radiology and Imaging	1.9

Source: Adapted with permission from *Medical Group Practice Digest*, p. 19, © 1997, Hoechst Marion Roussel.

Table 3–23 Use of Support Staff by Multispecialty Groups Median Staffing per FTE Physician, by Group Size and Managed Care Involvement

	Median Support Staff per FTE Physician
Group Size (# of FTE Physicians)	
10 or fewer	4.02 (4.50)
11–25	4.62 (4.62)
26–50	4.73 (4.70)
51–75	5.02 (4.95)
76–150	5.17 (5.11)
151 or more	4.69 (4.60)
Managed Care (MC) Involvement	
No MC Revenue	4.60 (4.73)
1–10% MC Revenue	4.25 (4.44)
11–50% MC Revenue	4.70 (4.76)
51–100% MC Revenue	5.85 (4.99)
All Groups	4.63 (4.75)

Note: Figures in parentheses are from 1994.

Source: Adapted with permission from *Medical Group Practice Digest*, p. 22–23, © 1997, Hoechst Marion Roussel.

Exhibit 3–14 Future Integration Plans of Group Practices (Within 2 Years)

	% of Groups
Joint Venture with a Hospital	57.9
Practice Will Own HMO	42.1
Management Company Will Own Practice	26.3
Plan To Participate in "Clinic without Walls"	15.8
Other Planned Arrangements	26.3

Source: Adapted with permission from *Medical Group Practice Digest*, p. 29, © 1996, Hoechst Marion Roussel.

Table 3–24 Forms of System Integration Adopted by Group Practices

Integration Forms	Percentage of Managed Care Revenues		Multi-specialty with PC Doctors
	50% or less	51–100%	
Practice is a hospital or a department within a hospital	16.7	—	5.0
Hospital owns the practice	16.7	—	10.0
Practice owns the hospital	—	—	—
Practice and hospital have joint ventured	8.3	41.7	25.0
Practice owns HMO	35.7	7.7	25.0
Hospital-owned MSO provides management services for a fee	8.3	8.3	10.0
Physicians are hospital employees through a PHO	—	—	—
Hospital and practice participate in risk-bearing PHO	25.0	33.3	20.0
Hospital and practice participate in non–risk-bearing PHO	41.7	25.0	30.0
Practice participates in a "clinic without walls"	—	—	—
Practice physicians are employees of a hospital-owned medical foundation	—	8.3	5.0
Practice and hospital are subsidiaries of a management company	8.3	8.3	15.0
Other arrangement	41.7	33.3	40.0

PC = primary care, MSO = management services organization, PHO = physician–hospital organization

Source: Adapted with permission from *Medical Group Practice Digest*, p. 29, © 1996, Hoechst Marion Roussel.

- The percentage of multispecialty groups employing midlevel providers is greater for larger groups and for those with a larger share of managed care revenues. The number of MLP staff per physician is also greater for the same groups. For nearly all groups, these figures are increasing over time.

- Nearly half of all physicians have increased the number of physicians they are practicing with or have plans to do so.
- About half of group practices intend to joint venture with a hospital or offer an HMO product within the next two years.

## CHAPTER 4

Industry Trends That Are Forcing Physicians To Rethink Their Long-Term Strategies

Physician and Patient Attitudes toward the New Health Care System

INTRODUCTION

This final data chapter reviews the attitudes of both physicians and patients toward the new health care system that is taking shape.

Once a person has experienced the rapidly evolving U.S. health care system, as a provider or recipient of services, it is hard not to have some strong views on how well it is working. These opinions can be important to physicians. They may indicate the attitudes of professional colleagues who are going through the same experiences. The attitudes of American citizens on the health care system can be powerful forces in shaping that system. One example is the spate of remedial legislation in response to public criticisms of physician gag rules and drive-through pregnancies.

The opinions of physicians about the health care system have waxed and waned over the years. Currently, opinions are not very positive (Table 4–1). Two-thirds of physicians believe that the system needs at least fundamental change. Bear in mind that the exact nature of the change desired by each physician may vary considerably.

A 1995 survey looked at physician satisfaction levels in different states, classified by their degrees of health maintenance organization (HMO) penetration (Table 4–2). The percentage of physicians who felt that the health care system had become worse in the past year increased as HMO penetration increased. It went from 47 per-

cent in states with low penetration to 60 percent in states where HMOs had the greatest presence. The same trend showed up when physicians were asked about their satisfaction with their current practice. As the level of HMO penetration increased, so did the level of dissatisfaction. In fact, it doubled from low- to high-penetration states.

A more recent, more detailed survey on physician satisfaction with medical practice produced less conclusive results (Table 4–3). Dissatisfaction levels do seem to creep up as a medical group's involvement in managed care rises. Yet, when 75 percent or more of a group's patients are members of a group or staff model HMO, the

---

Table 4–1 Physician Satisfaction with the U.S. Health Care System over the Years

	Needs at least fundamental change (%)	Works well overall (%)
1984	51	49
1990	69	31
1992	77	24
1994	57	42
1997	67	32

Courtesy of Louis Harris & Associates, Inc., New York, New York.

Table 4–2 Physician Satisfaction with Health Care System and Current Medical Practice, by Degree of HMO Penetration

	All Physicians (%)	High HMO Penetration States (%)	Medium HMO Penetration States (%)	Low HMO Penetration States (%)
Health Care System in Past Year Is:				
Better	8	9	8	9
Worse	55	60	56	47
Same	36	31	35	43
	100	100	100	100
Dissatisfied with Current Practice	23	27	24	13

Source: Adapted with permission from *Health Affairs,* Vol. 16, No. 5, p. 142, Copyright © 1997, The People–to–People Health Foundation, Inc., All Rights Reserved.

most tightly regimented forms, the dissatisfaction ratings plummet to half of what they are for all other groups—even those with no managed care at all. It would appear that those kinds of HMOs find ways to keep their physicians quite happy.

Physicians' levels of satisfaction with their profession (which may be interpreted differently from the "practice of medicine") also vary a bit by specialty (Figure 4–1). The most unhappy are ob/gyns and otolaryngologists. Satisfaction is

Table 4–3 Physician Satisfaction with the Practice of Medicine, by Managed Care Involvement

	All Practicing Physicians (%)	% of Practice in Managed Care				75+% of Patients in Group/Staff Model HMOs
		None (0%)	Light (1–10%)	Moderate (11–49%)	Heavy (50+%)	
Very Satisfied	24	35	31	20	20	36
Somewhat Satisfied	41	30	37	43	44	46
Total Satisfied	**64**	**65**	**68**	**63**	**64**	**82**
Somewhat Dissatisfied	26	23	23	28	28	16
Very Dissatisfied	9	12	9	9	8	2
Total Dissatisfied	**35**	**35**	**32**	**37**	**36**	**18**

Courtesy of Louis Harris & Associates, Inc., New York, New York.

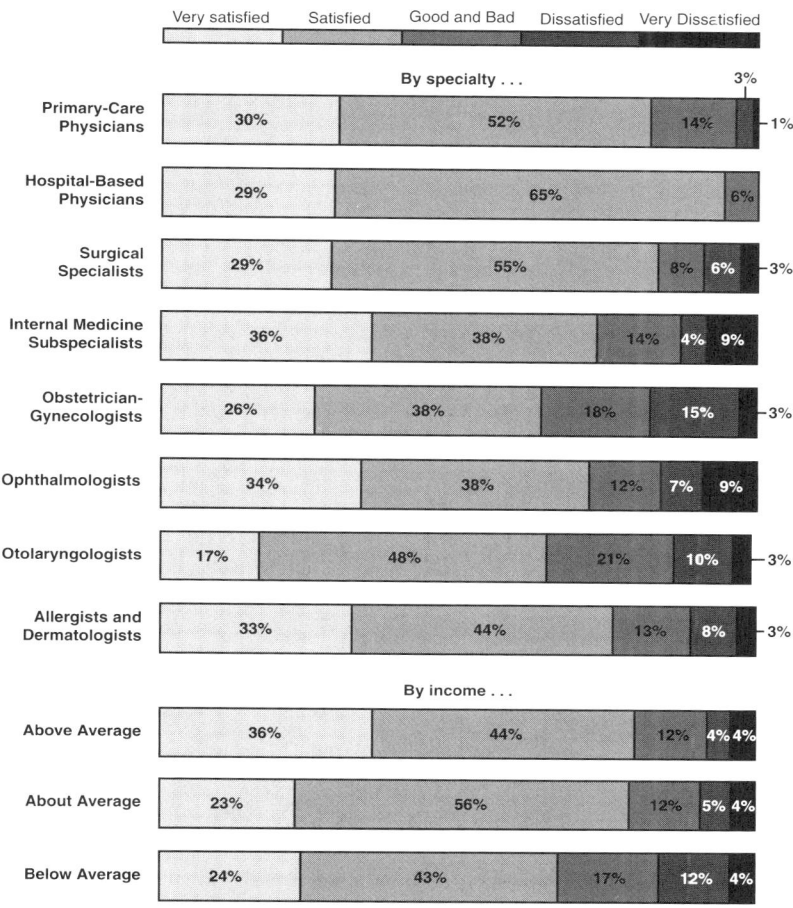

Figure 4–1 Doctors' Level of Satisfaction with Their Profession. *Source:* Copyright © 1997 by Medical Economics Publishing. Reprinted by permission from *MEDICAL ECONOMICS Magazine.*

highest for hospital-based surgical specialists, internal medicine specialists, and primary care physicians. The overall levels of professional satisfaction are quite substantial for all specialties. They range from 65 percent of otolaryngologists who are either "very satisfied" or "satisfied" to 94 percent of the hospital-based surgical specialists who feel the same way.

There is a dramatic difference in satisfaction levels of physicians in different practice settings (Exhibit 4–1). Solo practitioners are four or five times more likely to be "very dissatisfied" with

Exhibit 4–1 Physician Satisfaction with Current Practice Situation, by Practice Type

	Very Dissatisfied
Single Specialty Group	4%
Multispecialty Group	5%
Solo Practice	21%

Courtesy of Louis Harris & Associates, Inc., New York, New York.

Table 4–4 Physician Satisfaction (%) with Current Practice Situation, by Years in Practice

		Number of Years in Practice			
	Total	1–9	10–19	20–29	30+
Very Satisfied	22	30	32	17	10
Somewhat Satisfied	50	60	50	53	44
Somewhat Dissatisfied	18	10	15	16	26
Very Dissatisfied	10	—	4	14	19

Courtesy of Louis Harris & Associates, Inc., New York, New York.

their current practice situation than their colleagues in single- and multispecialty group practices. These findings reinforce the view that solo practice is no longer a viable practice model.

The common wisdom is that older physicians are having a harder time adjusting to managed care. This is confirmed by data that demonstrate a direct relationship between the number of years a physician has been practicing medicine and his dissatisfaction with his current practice situation (Table 4–4). Yet, even 54 percent of those who have been practicing for 30 years or more are "very satisfied" or "somewhat satisfied."

There is a reasonable concern among many physicians that their personal incomes will suffer as a result of MCO pressures constantly to reduce costs. Data on their expectations about future earnings reflect this concern (Table 4–5). Those most hopeful, expecting to actually earn more in the future, are more likely (24 percent) to belong to a multispecialty group practice. Single specialty group physicians who feel the same are close behind (22 percent), but half again as many of them (46 percent versus 31 percent) expect to earn less. Once again, the solo practitioners are the most pessimistic.

Physicians have been very specific about the problems they have experienced while practicing under managed care (Table 4–6). The biggest gripes by single specialty and multispecialty group doctors are over the "continuity of rela-

tions" with other providers and the "limitations on other referrals" to physicians (about 25 percent each). The extent of unhappiness with all these issues is much higher with solo practice physicians. Note that a good 75 to 80 percent of group doctors do not express concern with these problems.

The next set of data (Table 4–7) provides more detailed feedback on the problems physicians are having with the requirements managed care organizations (MCOs) impose upon them. In particular, they relate the incidence of physician problems to the degree of HMO penetration. A significant proportion of physicians in this survey, well over half in some cases, complained of practice difficulties with managed care demands and procedures. Upset with many of these prob-

Table 4–5 Physicians' Future Earning Expectations, by Practice Type

	Expect To Earn More (%)	Expect To Earn Less (%)
Solo Practice	14	52
Single Specialty Group	22	46
Multispecialty Group	24	31

Courtesy of Louis Harris & Associates, Inc., New York, New York.

Table 4–6 Physician Practice Problems with Managed Care, by Practice Type

	Solo Practice (%)	Single Specialty (%)	Multispecialty (%)
Continuity of Relations	41	21	25
Lack of Coordination with Other Doctors	24	15	13
Limitations on Other Referrals	35	26	24
External Review	29	22	18

Courtesy of Louis Harris & Associates, Inc., New York, New York.

Table 4–7 Physician Practice Problems with Health Care System Requirements by Degree of HMO Penetration in State

Serious Problem in Practice With:	All Physicians	Degree of HMO Penetration (%)		
		High	Medium	Low
Movement of patients in and out of your practice because of changes in insurance coverage	62	67	65	48
Administrative paperwork requirements for the referral of patients to specialists	56	59	59	42
Limitations on referring patients to specialists of your choice	53	55	57	33
Limitations on hospital length-of-stay for your patients	48	44	49	49
Patients who should have been referred for medical attention sooner	42	44	43	37
Limitations on deciding if patients are admitted to the hospital	41	35	43	36
Limitations on referring patients to appropriate special- ists	40	42	27	26
Limitations on ordering diagnostic tests and procedures you think are best for your patients	39	41	42	27
Financial incentives to do less than what you think is best for your patients	38	39	40	31
Pressure to see a greater number of patients than you think is appropriate	38	37	40	28
Limitations on prescribing drugs you think are best for your patients	31	38	30	28

Source: Adapted with permission from *Health Affairs,* Vol. 16, No. 5, p. 142, Copyright © 1997, The People–to–People Health Foundation, Inc., All Rights Reserved.

lems seems to jump when an area goes from low to medium penetration. In no case did it increase steadily from low to medium to high. Some of the problems actually became less troubling when HMO penetration grew from medium to high. If nothing else, this is an excellent listing of the kinds of challenges physicians can expect to encounter when they deal with MCOs.

In the battle for the affections of U.S. consumers, if such a battle is really going on, physicians are winning handily. Over 80 percent of consumers believe that medical doctors do the best job of serving their interests. Only about 50 percent feel the same way about health insurers and managed care companies.[1]

On the whole, about 60 percent of HMO members are "highly satisfied" with the care and service they are receiving (Exhibit 4–2). These feelings vary from city to city, with Boston area HMOs scoring the highest. But, the range is fairly narrow.

Doctors polled by the American Society of Internal Medicine gave some very low grades to a group of five selected HMOs. With one minor exception (patient choice at AvMed), none received a passing score for any of the key attributes measured. The two-thirds of physicians who would not recommend the CIGNA HMO was the best showing of any of these five HMOs.[2] These extremely negative findings are a bit at

Exhibit 4–2 Percentage of HMO Members Who Were Highly Satisfied

Boston	71%
Denver	67%
New York City	63%
Milwaukee	62%
Detroit	61%
Philadelphia	60%
Portland, OR	60%
Arizona	58%
North Carolina	58%
Dallas/Fort Worth	56%
NATIONAL AVERAGE	60%

Source: Adapted with permission from Professional Beat section, Medical Economics, Vol. 74, No. 5, p. 57, Medical Economics Publishing Company, Inc.

odds with some other studies and probably should not be overemphasized.

One of the many controversies over the way health care is delivered in the United States concerns its growing commercialization. A recent survey sought public opinions on the qualities of not-for-profit (NFP) and for-profit (FP) hospitals and health plans (Table 4–8). Sixty percent of the

Table 4–8 Public Opinion of For-Profit (FP) and Not-For-Profit (NFP) Hospitals and Health Plans

	Hospitals (%)		Health Plans (%)	
	NFP	FP	NFP	FP
Are more helpful to the community	61	23	60	24
Cost you less	57	18	58	21
Are more responsive to customers	40	41	41	40
Provide better quality care	37	42	37	39
Are more efficient	31	48	35	44

Source: This table was reprinted with permission of the Henry J. Kaiser Family Foundation of Menlo Park, California. The Kaiser Family Foundation is an independent health care philanthropy and is not associated with Kaiser Permanente or Kaiser Industries.

respondents feel that NFP versions of both hospitals and health plans "are more helpful to the community" and cost them less. Whether consumers actually seek out this information and allow it to affect their choice of health care institution is another question. On the other hand, just under 50 percent believe that FP entities "are more efficient" in delivering care. It is a standoff between NFPs and FPs regarding "responsiveness to customers" and "quality of care." The controversy is sure to continue.

It is a popular belief that there are too many specialist physicians and not enough primary care physicians. Most physicians do not share this view (Table 4–9). Between 30 percent and 40 percent of all physicians perceive that the supply of all practicing physicians in their community exceeds the demand. About 50 percent believe that supply and demand is pretty well balanced. Hospitals and health systems have the most contrary positions on physician supply—only 23 percent think there is an excess and a surprising 42 percent feel that a shortage exists. It is the MCOs that believe most strongly that the supply of physicians is too large (55 percent of HMOs and 48 percent of preferred provider organizations (PPOs).

Physicians do not agree with the view of many experts that there is an oversupply of physicians (Table 4–10). The proportion of physicians in this survey who perceived an oversupply is the same as the proportion in a 1988 American Medical Association (AMA) survey of physicians and 10 percent lower than the proportion in a 1986 AMA survey. Thus, it is not surprising that there is little interest in retraining medical and surgical specialists to primary care practice.

Table 4–11 compares physician perceptions of over- and undersupply by the degree of HMO penetration in the areas where they practice. The pattern of results is exactly what one would predict. In all specialty categories, the percentage of physicians who saw an oversupply of physicians increased as the penetration level increased. The more efficient use of physicians by HMOs rendered more and more of the doctors redundant.

There are significant variations in the perceptions of physician supply in different specialties (Table 4–11). The greatest sense of undersupply is among family practice doctors. Oversupply is seen most often in gastroenterologists, cardiologists, general surgeons, and cardiovascular surgeons.

Physicians just entering the medical profession are generally the best informed about the changes sweeping the health care system and the problems they will face in different practice settings. It is interesting to examine their preferences for work environment and reimbursement method (Table 4–12).

Multispecialty group practices have surged over the last two years to become the most popular (32.7 percent) practice destination for senior medical residents. The preference for single specialty group settings has faded from 39.0 percent to 29.4 percent. Partnerships with other physicians became slightly more appealing. Rather small fractions of residents want to work for an HMO or a hospital. These trends reflect some wisdom on the part of the residents—multispecialty group practices are one of the best ways for physicians to engage with managed care without completely sacrificing their autonomy and control.

During the same two years, the percentage of residents who preferred to receive a salary or salary bonus climbed from 55 percent to 86 percent. Only 11 percent now want an income guarantee, down from 41 percent in 1995. Some radical shifts in attitude toward managed care and compensation are going on among the newest members of the medical profession.

LEADING TRENDS

- Two-thirds of all physicians believe that the U.S. health care system needs fundamental change.
- About one-fourth of physicians are dissatisfied with their current medical practice. The "dissatisfied" percentage is twice as high in states with high HMO penetration than in low penetration states. The "dissatisfied"

Table 4–9 Physician and Marketplace Perceptions of Physician Supply

	Percent Reporting the Supply of All Practicing Physicians in Their Community Is:		
	Greater Than Demand	Less Than Demand	About Right
All Physicians	36	14	49
Primary Care Physicians	31	17	52
Surgeons	39	12	48
Medical Specialists	41	12	46
Hospitals/Health Systems	23	42	34
Group Practices	42	15	43
HMOs	55	13	32
PPOs	48	11	41

Source: Adapted with permission from *Health Affairs,* Vol. 16, No. 5, p. 143, Copyright © 1997, The People–to–People Health Foundation, Inc., All Rights Reserved.

Table 4–10 Physician Perceptions of Physician Supply, by Physician Specialty and Degree of HMO Penetration in State

	Percent Reporting the Supply of Practicing Physicians in Their Community Is:		
	Greater Than Demand	Less Than Demand	About Right
All Physicians			
High HMO States	52	8	40
Medium HMO States	35	13	51
Low HMO States	25	22	53
Primary Care Physicians			
High HMO States	48	12	40
Medium HMO States	29	17	53
Low HMO States	21	21	59
Medical Specialists			
High HMO States	60	4	36
Medium HMO States	39	10	50
Low HMO States	26	29	44
Surgeons			
High HMO States	51	7	42
Medium HMO States	39	11	49
Low HMO States	29	21	51

Source: Adapted with permission from *Health Affairs,* Vol. 16, No. 5, p. 144, Copyright © 1997, The People–to–People Health Foundation, Inc., All Rights Reserved.

Table 4–11 Perceptions of Physician Supply in Particular Specialties

	Perception of Physician Supply by: (more or less than demand)									
	Physicians in Specialty (%)		Group Practices (%)		Hospitals and Health Systems (%)		HMOs (%)		PPOs (%)	
	More	Less	More	Less	More	Less	More	Less	More	Less
Primary Care										
Family Practice	8	48	7	54	6	65	5	60	8	54
General Internal Medicine	20	28	9	38	10	41	13	33	15	34
Pediatrics	19	21	7	31	8	37	11	49	5	40
Medical Specialists										
Hematology/Oncology	22	6	18	15	9	24	26	14	25	20
Gastroenterology	55	0	24	8	16	12	45	3	37	6
Cardiology	71	3	32	11	25	15	65	4	54	5
Surgeons										
Cardiovascular Surgery	55	0	32	10	18	15	56	11	51	11
Neurologic Surgery	—	—	19	17	12	27	31	21	34	19
General Surgery	33	14	32	5	24	17	63	2	51	3
Ob/Gyn	33	10	19	15	11	35	34	22	27	26

Source: Adapted with permission from *Health Affairs,* Vol. 16, No. 5, p. 145, Copyright © 1997, The People–to–People Health Foundation, Inc., All Rights Reserved.

Table 4–12 Kind of Practice Sought by Senior Residents

	1995 (%)	1997 (%)
Multispecialty	14.0	32.7
Single specialty	39.0	29.4
Partnership	9.0	12.7
Outpatient clinic	—	6.0
HMO	7.8	5.3
Association[*]	3.9	5.3
Hospital employment	9.0	4.0
Other[**]	11.6	2.6

[*]Physicians share office and staff, but not finances.

[**]Academic, locum tenens, urgent care, and no preference.

Source: Adapted with permission from *Hospitals and Health Networks,* © 1997, American Hospital Publishing, Inc.

percentage is four times as high among solo practice doctors than those in group practice.

- Physicians' expectations for future earnings are more optimistic in multispecialty groups than in single specialty groups or solo practices.
- The biggest practice problems physicians have with health plan requirements are the movement of patients in and out because of changes in insurance coverage, paperwork requirements connected with referrals, and limitations on physician choice in making referrals.
- Americans believe that physicians do a much better job of serving consumers than managed care companies.
- Physicians are more likely than hospitals and health systems to believe that there are too many doctors practicing in their communities.

- Senior residents are showing a steadily increasing interest in practice with multi-specialty groups, as opposed to single specialty groups and hospital employment.

REFERENCES

1. L. Light, "Who Does the Best Job Serving the Consumer?" *Business Week*, no. 3523 (1997): 6.

2. "Rating HMOs," *Medical Economics*, 10 March 1997.

## CHAPTER 5

A Step-by-Step Strategy To Take You from Solo Practice to an Integrated Delivery System

INTRODUCTION

You bought this book because you are apprehensive about the changes occurring in the U.S. health care system and the role of your practice within it. The first four chapters were intended to document the nature and scope of that change. You are seeking guidance on new strategic moves you might make to position your practice better for the future. You are wondering about what kinds of adjustments you will have to make in your style of practice, in the management of your practice, and in the structure of your practice.

This chapter first explains why physicians and group practices need to adopt formal long-term strategies for the development and evolution of their practices. It provides an example of what such a strategic plan should look like. Finally, it summarizes the overall, beginning-to-end strategy recommended. This is an outline of the 11 steps described in greater depth in the remainder of the book. It includes several other related strategic and operational recommendations.

It is important to understand that these 11 steps, and some of their more numerous variants, need not be followed in linear fashion. Frequently, it will make sense to leap ahead a step or two in response to a unique opportunity or competitive pressures. At certain points in a good strategy, there may be two or more structural options to choose from. The goal of this book is to guide the

physician through this complex maze of organizational possibilities.

The intended result of this chapter is that the reader-physician accepts the need to do formal long-range planning for his career and medical practice, learns the basic outlines and benefits of such planning, and understands the progression of steps his practice must move through.

WHO SHOULD READ THIS CHAPTER

If you read only one chapter in this book, it should be this one.

Of course, if you already have a specific need for advice on managed care contracting, practicing under capitation, joining a management services organization, or another of the key strategic steps, you could go directly to the appropriate chapter. However, this chapter puts it all in context.

A GENERIC STRATEGIC PLANNING FRAMEWORK FOR SOLO OR GROUP PHYSICIAN PRACTICES

There is a saying in business management circles, "If you don't know where you are going, you'll never know when you get there." It could be added that, "You'll probably never get there at all."

It is essential for any business operation such as a medical practice—large or small—to put down on paper what you intend to achieve in the future and how you intend to achieve it. This is the process of planning. Its key elements are

- the ultimate achievements you desire
- the intermediate steps necessary to reach the final goals
- the interrelationships and dependencies among all the goals and steps
- the resources that will be necessary to implement them
- a timetable for reaching each step and each final goal
- an analysis of the environment in which these actions will take place
- an analysis of the barriers that may arise to implementation of the plan

Because planning involves trying to predict or shape the future, it often makes sense to lay out one or more alternative plans in case the primary plan becomes unworkable.

Businesses around the world have practiced formalized strategic planning for decades. Their experience has produced a well-tested framework for the process. It goes this way.

At the highest level of abstraction, an organization prepares a *Mission Statement*. This is a description of the most fundamental reasons that the organization was created and continues to operate. It may also be viewed as the ultimate purpose or goal of the organization. The mission statement is intended to guide the organization for 10 or 20 years, or longer.

The best mission statement is expressed in one sentence. You will see many that go on for several paragraphs. The mission statement should be memorable, literally. Owners and employees of the organization should be able recite it from memory. They should be able to grasp its simple meaning and incorporate it into all their work for the organization. Frequently, the mission statement is placed on bulletin boards, in waiting rooms, on company stationery, on company vehicles, and woven into the company logo. The essence of the organization is reflected in the mission statement and the essence of the mission

statement is reflected throughout the organization.

Because owners and managers often want to say more than will fit into a single sentence, the mission statement sometimes includes a set of basic values important to them.

With the mission statement as a foundation or guiding light, the directors of the organization prepare a *Strategic Plan*. This plan is a list of goals or objectives that, if achieved, will carry out the organization's mission. (Note: Do not be confused by terminology; just make sure you understand each phase of the strategic planning process regardless of what it may be called.)

There are two critical features of any goal or objective. First, it must be measurable. That is, it is stated in such terms that there can be no disagreement about whether it has been achieved or not. For example, the goal, "Reduce utilization rates" is not nearly as useful as "Reduce primary care utilization rates by 14 percent, specialty referrals by 17 percent, and hospital utilization by 9 percent." Second, there must be a specific time deadline for its completion.

It normally is not practical to project a strategic plan beyond five years or so. At that distance, circumstances are so unpredictable and speculative that any goals set are likely to become unrealistic. As it is, there is a good chance that goals in the later years of the strategic plan itself will be adjusted.

Keep the number of strategic goals under 10. Six or seven is a good, workable figure. Some organizations tend to prepare a long laundry list of everything they would like to accomplish in the next five years. A shorter list is better because it focuses the energies of the organization.

The next element in the planning process, as it comes increasingly closer to the present, is an *Annual Operating Plan*. This is a much more detailed description of what the organization will do over the coming year to move toward achievement of its strategic goals. Because it is much shorter term, it is less speculative and more amenable to clear definition. At the very least, this aspect of the planning process will include a more extensive list (perhaps running two or three pages) of objectives, a list of tasks designed to achieve those objectives, and a budget showing the expenditures necessary to support those tasks.

Keep in mind that no part of the strategic planning process is immutable. Nothing is set in concrete. Just because the board of directors chose three years ago to pursue a particular strategic goal does not mean that the organization must follow through even when circumstances make achievement of the goal impossible or inadvisable. View planning as a continual "process," not a series of discrete, mandatory documents or programs.

Indeed, the planning process typically is carried out in a routine annual procedure. The board of directors and top executives go away on a one-day planning retreat. They reexamine the mission statement. Unless the political, economic, and competitive environment has changed radically, it is left unchanged. The board renews its commitment to it.

The directors then look very closely at the strategic goals. They note those which have been achieved and ask for explanations why others have not been achieved. If the assumptions upon which some remaining goals are based have changed, those goals may be adjusted or eliminated. Then, the directors may add new strategic goals to carry the organization another year into the future.

The strategic plan is really a rolling plan. Annually, the current year is dropped off and a new fifth year added to the far end of the plan.

The strategic plan that comes out of that retreat is communicated to the executives. They digest it and submit to the directors an *Annual Operating Plan* that they propose to follow during the coming year in pursuit of the strategic goals.

After it has been conducted for two or three years, the planning process becomes fairly intuitive and easy to execute. It requires a healthy amount of preparation by directors and managers. The game plan that guides all the organization's activities is more than worth that effort.

Some variation of this planning process should be carried out by every physician practice, from a solo practice to a large integrated multispecialty

group practice. It will take some time, but it will save you even more time.

PRIMARY DOCUMENTS FOR STRATEGIC PLANNING BY A SOLO OR GROUP PRACTICE

There are several documents that play key roles in the strategic planning process.

The first is the *Articles of Incorporation* or *Partnership Agreement* for the practice organization. These were the original legal documents that brought your organization into existence as a legal entity. Most of the language in them is what lawyers call "boilerplate," standard provisions that appear in all documents of this sort.

However, they include a couple sections that bear on strategic planning: the statements of the organization's purposes and its powers. Good lawyers draft these sections broadly, to give the organization wide latitude in what it does and how it may do it. They are worth checking, however. They will give some guidance on the original motives of the founders of the organization. The language also will reveal any restrictions on the kinds of authority one can exercise in pursuing the organization's mission. If the documents do not address the organization's current needs, they can be amended.

The *Mission Statement* is the internal document that describes the essence of why the organization exists. Exhibit 5–1 is an example of a mission statement for a small group practice.

Exhibit 5–2 is a set of *Strategic Goals* that might issue from such a mission statement.

The fourth key planning document is the *Annual Operating Plan*. It usually is too voluminous to present an example here. This plan is prepared by the administrative head of the organization (general manager, president, chief executive officer (CEO), managing partner) as a manifestation of the directors' strategic goals. The directors review the plan, make appropriate changes, approve it, and return it to the general manager. The plan is the blueprint for everything the general manager does during the coming year

Exhibit 5–1 The Riverside Primary Care Associates P.C. Mission Statement

To maintain the health of a dedicated community of patients, within the framework of an integrated community of providers delivering a full continuum of health care services. In pursuit of that mission, our values are to

1. Maintain health through patient education and illness prevention.
2. Practice cost-effective medicine and be able to prove it.
3. Practice efficacious medicine and be able to prove it.
4. Satisfy our patients and be able to prove it.

5. Produce rewards for ourselves and our employees commensurate with our experience, training, and abilities.
6. Ensure that clinical medical decisions are always made by physicians or their agents.
7. Deliver medical services in an environment that is nurturing, caring, and respectful for patients and employees.
8. Practice medicine in organizations in which physicians have significant ownership and governance roles.
9. Constantly grow and adapt to responsible changes in the health care system.
10. Affiliate with organizations that, to the fullest extent possible, share these values.

and the standard against which her performance is measured. The most important pieces of the plan are these.

- brief statements of operational objectives that the general manager will pursue during the year, accompanied by her reasons for choosing them (the rationales frequently will refer to particular strategic goals that an operational objective will serve)
- operating budget for the coming year, with relatively detailed revenue and expense breakdowns
- cash flow projections for the coming year
- projected balance sheet for the end of the coming year
- projections for other key financial and practice indicators (e.g., utilization rates, shares of revenues from various payers)

A *Business Plan* is another planning document that would be strongly advisable if you are creating an entirely new organization or taking your current practice in a dramatically new direction. The best examples of such plans are those submitted by entrepreneurs to venture capitalists

from whom they are seeking capital. In fact, this may be one of the uses to which you put your business plan.

Business plans typically are 50 to 100 pages long. There are several good books and computer software programs that will guide you in preparing one. They take a lot of work if done well. The result is a bible for running your practice for at least the next two years. A comprehensive business plan includes the following sections:

- a description of products and services to be offered
- an evaluation of the market to be served
- an assessment of the organization's competitors
- an explanation of what distinguishes those products and services in that market
- an analysis of the legal, political, social, and economic environment in which the organization will operate
- an organizational SWOT (strengths, weaknesses, opportunities, threats) analysis
- a description of initial marketing activities
- a listing and description of leading revenue sources, particularly health care payers

Exhibit 5–2 The Riverside Primary Care Associates P.C. Strategic Goals: 1995 to 2000

1. Increase the number of primary care physicians in the group to at least 14 by the end of year 1996 and at least 20 by the end of year 1998.
2. Add at least 8 specialist physicians to the group by the end of year 1996 and 4 more by the end of year 1998.
3. Explore the pros and cons of joining an independent practice association and, if the move proves advisable, do so by the end of year 1996.
4. Explore the pros and cons of forming a joint venture or affiliation with one of the two largest community hospitals in town and, if the move proves advisable, do so by the end of year 1997.
5. Hire a full-time general manager to direct the business affairs of the group by the end of the year 1997.
6. Increase the group's proportion of total revenues coming from capitation fees to the following percentages by the end of the following years:

1996	29%
1997	35%
1998	50%
1999	70%
2000	85%

7. Institute a computerized management information system that generates data on utilization rates by physician, patient, and payer and on practice costs by CPT code. Have this system up and running by the end of year 1998.
8. Establish a task force within the group to plot a strategic course that will take the group into an integrated delivery system by the end of the year 2000.

- a description of and an implementation schedule for management systems key to the organization's success (cost tracking, utilization management, outcomes measurement, patient satisfaction measurement, electronic communication links with stakeholders)
- an outline of key planned events during the first three to five years of the organization's life
- a description of the organization's management team and their qualifications
- a cash flow projection for three years—monthly for the first year, quarterly thereafter
- an income statement projection for five years, on a quarterly basis
- a balance sheet projection for five years, on a quarterly basis
- a projection of other key performance indicators

If you can gather information this thorough and detailed, you will be in excellent shape to create a successful new venture and to attract investment capital to it.

ESSENTIAL STEPS IN A GRAND STRATEGY FOR PHYSICIAN PROSPERITY IN THE NEW HEALTH CARE SYSTEM

The following are recommendations for principal components of a strategy that will enable any physician practice to thrive and prosper in the new health care system now emerging in the United States. The strategy cannot be pursued all at once. As a practical matter, many of its steps must be followed sequentially. On the other hand, your resources, entrepreneurial skills, and aggressiveness may permit you to skip over some steps. Certain strategic moves are really ongoing processes—such as continually improving your ability to deliver cost-effective medicine. You may also choose to design your own unique strategy, using this as a model or framework.

Enter into More Contracts with Managed Care Organizations (MCOs)

Managed care has represented the future of health care delivery for at least a decade. Enter into more contracts with MCOs to provide health care to their member-patients. Do not do this recklessly. Do not look only for an acceptable reimbursement rate and then sign every contract offered you. Read and evaluate each one thoroughly, concentrating on the most problematic provisions. Read Chapter 8, "Step Two: How To Analyze and Evaluate a Managed Care Contract," for more guidance on this task.

Gain the experience of *negotiating an agreement* that influences the flow of revenues to your practice and income to you. You will participate in more negotiations like that in the future, and you had better become adept at it. Read Chapter 9, "Strategies for Negotiating with a Managed Care Organization," to learn more about negotiating.

Gain the experience of thinking, perhaps for the first time, of *your practice as a business organization* that must make rational, thoughtful decisions and plan for a radically different future.

Gain the experience of *working with another organization* in deciding how your practice will be structured and how patients will be treated. Depending on the MCO you contract with, normally it will not dictate directly to you. However, the incentives will be powerful persuaders to reexamine all your assumptions and habits about medical practice. Look for MCOs and MCO contracts that will foster a partnership relationship between you—so that you do not feel threatened or imposed upon.

Gain the experience of *practicing under reimbursement schemes* designed to make you more cost and quality conscious. The MCO may propose reimbursement on a discounted fee-for-service basis, add a utilization management requirement, subject you to risk pool withholding, or wish to share risk with you through capitation

rates. All of these methodologies may have a role in the emerging health care system. You would do well to understand them. Practicing under such contracts, before they are a dominant source of your revenues, is a good way to learn. Read Chapter 25, "The Kinds of Physician Reimbursement Systems You Can Expect under Managed Care," for more information on physician reimbursement.

More important, all of these reimbursement systems point physicians in the same direction—practicing cost-effective medicine. The incentives of these schemes will compel you to become proficient at such practice or suffer loss of patients and income.

Gain the experience of *learning new methods for practicing* cost-effective medicine. This is the most important skill for a physician to learn now to assure his future survival. For many doctors, it means reprogramming impulses and habits instilled in medical school. It does not come easily, even when approached with enthusiasm. You cannot start too soon. Read Chapter 6, "A Physician's Life under Managed Care," and Chapter 7, "Step One: Preparing Your Practice for Operation under Managed Care," to learn more about medical practice under managed care.

Develop Competence at Practicing under Capitation

Current evidence suggests that capitated contracts will become the reimbursement method of choice within the next 5 to 10 years. Begin now to learn the terms of such contracts and their pluses and minuses for your practice. Even more important, start training in the necessary, new ways of practicing medicine and organizing your practice. Read Chapter 20, "Negotiating and Practicing under a Capitation Contract," for more details on evaluating capitation contracts and practicing medicine under them.

Grow Accustomed to Being "At Risk" for the Cost of Medical Services Provided to Your Patients

One of the scariest and most revolutionary aspects of the new health care system is the new kind of risks to which it exposes physicians. In the good, old days of fee-for-service medicine, the primary risk faced by physicians was the possibility of a malpractice lawsuit. The only response was to practice as carefully as possible and set aside a big chunk of revenues for professional liability insurance premiums.

Rapid changes in the industry have multiplied physician risks. The ones to know about and adjust to are

- Risk of business failure. Competition and the demands of managed care require that medical practices be managed in a professional, businesslike manner. Poorly run practices will fail.
- Risk of contracting with the wrong MCO (unethical, financially unstable).
- Risk of not contracting with the right MCO.
- Risk of forming or joining a new entity that proves to be competitively nonviable.
- Risk of having specialist skills no longer needed in such great numbers.
- Risk of lacking primary care skills now in greater demand.

However, when MCO executives talk about "risk-sharing" with providers, they really are referring to two primary risks. First, there is a risk that the patients for whom you have assumed responsibility will be sicker and require more medical services than the actuarial projections called for. Since your capitation rate or discounted fee schedule was based on those projections, you will not have enough money to pay for the services. Still, there are mechanisms for reducing that risk, such as stop-loss insurance. Second, there is the risk that you simply are unable to practice medicine cost-effectively enough to stay within the capitation rate. Again, you will lose money. The remedy is not as easy. Through consultation, continuing education, and practice you must develop a new practice style that meets managed care requirements.

The challenge of managing risk is discussed more thoroughly in Chapter 26, "Managing Risk in the Practice of Medicine."

Think in Terms of Managing the Demand of Patients for Health Care Services

There are two ways to lower costs under a managed care arrangement. One is to restore a sick patient to health with fewer or lower cost medical services. The other is to keep the patient from getting sick in the first place.

After improving the cost-effectiveness of your clinical decision making, work with your patients to help them stay healthier. This does not mean persuading them to stay away when they truly need a doctor's attention. It means

- conducting formal patient education on these issues
- explaining to patients how "managed" health care works, and how they can use it to greatest advantage
- encouraging patients to seek your help early in the course of a disease rather than later
- encouraging patients to obtain regular checkups and tests
- giving patients specific recommendations on creating a healthier lifestyle
- offering patients programs for improving their lifestyle (e.g., stress reduction, weight loss, smoking cessation, food nutrition, child rearing)
- teaching patients how to treat minor ailments themselves, at home, without seeking physician assistance on every occasion

Remember, "health maintenance organizations" originally received their name because of the expectation that they would offer services to maintain the health of their members, rather than simply restore it after it had deteriorated. These MCOs are just now beginning to act on that early promise. You can benefit by joining with them in the effort.

Get Out of Management or Get Out of Medicine

If you believe that you are competent in practice management and enjoy those challenges, get an MBA and build a career as a manager, then executive, of health care delivery organizations. If you still prefer the stimulation of diagnosing and treating illness and interacting with patients, concentrate on being a clinical practitioner. Do not try to do both simultaneously.

It used to be possible. Even now, there are large numbers of physicians managing large clinical departments and entire hospitals, while carrying on active medical practices. In the past, cost-based reimbursement allowed some leeway for misjudgments by nonprofessional physician managers. The margins for error have disappeared.

Competitive pressures require that health care managers and executives have professional management skills. They also must work 40, 50, and 60 hours a week at managing. It requires their full attention. The transformation of physician practice styles to accommodate managed care also is a full-time job.

Many physicians have developed into excellent managers. More than ever, the medical profession right now needs to have representatives with an understanding of clinical issues, with medical training, in the executive suites of the large and growing MCOs and other provider organizations. If you can be one of those people, get the necessary training and make a career of it. Otherwise, you short-change yourself, the organization, and the profession.

> **Note:** Management is not the same as ownership or even control. You can own shares of stock in a corporation or have a financial partnership interest without being the CEO of the organization. Ownership usually allows you to vote for the board of directors, who select the CEO. You also can be one of the directors on that board. The time commitment and required business knowledge is much less than what you will expect of the CEO you choose. As an owner or director, you will influence and control the broad strategic policy issues that shape the organization. They are more powerful positions than the CEO's.

Form or Join Groups with Increasingly Larger Numbers of Physicians

Move aggressively to form larger and larger aggregations of physicians organized legitimately into larger and larger physician-controlled integrated delivery entities serving larger and larger geographic areas. One of the reasons that physicians are losing influence in the shift to managed care is the ability of much larger, better capitalized, more professionally managed MCOs to overwhelm and outnumber solo or group practices of just a few physicians. These small physician clusters lack the experience, expertise, resources, bargaining power, or time to stand up to determined managed care entities.

The answer is collaboration and consolidation. Prescient physicians began moving in this direction 5 and 10 years ago. You must start now!

You cannot get to where you need to be overnight. It is an unavoidable fact that time must pass in order to gain experience, acquire expertise, and amass capital and other resources. It is a process of several steps that must be followed more or less in sequence. A solo practitioner first becomes part of a small, single specialty group practice. That group grows, adds physicians and services, accumulates capital, and evolves (through merger or acquisition) into a large, multispecialty group practice. This group continues to expand and grow in competence, perhaps emerging eventually as a fully integrated system. At a certain point, the group achieves a critical mass of providers and resources, permitting it to bargain and compete on equal terms with MCOs and employers.

The purpose of this grand strategy is to move you along this growth path as quickly and efficiently as possible. Remember, the key is in size and numbers. Get bigger and wiser as fast as you can. (There are serious legal implications in the ways that physicians choose to collaborate with each other. Read more about these in Chapter 28, "Collaborating with Other Physicians without Legal Risk.")

The following are some of the key strategic steps or changes you should implement as part of that strategy.

Form or Join a Small, Single Specialty Group Practice

If you currently are a solo practitioner, this is your best first move. The same thing is true for two or more physicians sharing a medical suite but not really functioning as a cooperative group. Begin sharing ideas and experiences on your clinical and practice management problems. Legally reorganize yourselves into a partnership or professional corporation. Start thinking in terms of how "we" rather than "I" can plan for the future. Get used to compromising some of your personal desires in the interests of the common good of the group. Learn what it is like to take a team approach to at least part of your practice duties. Get serious about the need to change and start planning for it. Chapter 10, "Step Three: Forming or Joining a Small, Single Specialty Group Practice," examines this step more closely.

Participate in a Preferred Provider Organization (PPO)

A PPO is run by an insurance company, private broker, or physicians to obtain fee-discounted indemnity contracts for participating providers. Reimbursement is on a discounted fee-for-service basis. You and other physicians, as well as selected hospitals, will be the "preferred providers" for members who pay lower premiums, co-payments, or deductibles when receiving medical services from you.

There are three possible reasons for becoming part of a PPO. One is for the additional patients and revenues that will be steered your way. The second reason is the pressure you will feel from the fee discounts to practice more cost-effectively. The last reason for hooking up with a PPO is simply for the sake of getting yourself moving, taking some action, and having the tenuous feeling of being part of a greater whole.

Just be aware that PPO participation leads nowhere. Discounted fee-for-service is a waning form of reimbursement. PPO providers do not integrate their practices, share risks, jointly manage utilization, or take any of the other strategic initiatives required of them.

Participating in a PPO is better than doing nothing, but joining an independent practice association (IPA) is a superior alternative.

Join an Independent Practice Association

An IPA is a physician-run organization that obtains managed care contracts for its membership composed of solo physicians and group practices. Physician members remain in their individual practices, continue to see fee-for-service patients, can belong to more than one IPA, and may be able contract directly with non-IPA managed care plans.

This is an excellent option for a small group practice that has been together at least six months to a year. It is a small, positive, nonthreatening step toward the managed care future of medical practice. Many IPAs have negotiated risk-sharing capitated contracts, instituted utilization management controls, and become more selective in accepting physicians as members.

An IPA is an excellent training ground for all the skills and knowledge you will need as you progress through your long-term practice strategy. If you remain in an IPA for longer than two years without integrating and consolidating further, you are wasting time. Learn more about how IPAs operate in Chapter 11, "Step Four: Joining an Independent Practice Association."

Form a "Group Practice without Walls" (GPWW)

The natural next strategic step beyond an IPA goes under several names: "clinic without walls," "group practice without walls," or "partially integrated medical group." The GPWW is a single legal entity resulting from the merger or acquisition of several smaller practices. Some operational aspects of the practices are integrated, while others remain under the control of each practice. The practices usually stay at their separate locations. The best GPWWs are no more than a transitional phase on the way to a fully integrated multispecialty group practice.

The GPWW should be in constant ferment as it explores and adopts new forms of collaboration and integration. It can be a stressful time; after all, you are forcing the transformation of the practice of medicine.

Do not stay in this model for longer than two years. You will find more information about GPWWs in Chapter 12, "Participating in a Group Practice without Walls."

Grow into a Large, Fully Integrated, Multispecialty Group Practice

This should be the five-year strategic goal for your practice.

It represents the zenith of physician collaboration. Strategic development beyond this point requires affiliation with other nonphysician providers. Indeed, it is conceivable that a multispecialty group practice could become large and well organized enough to thrive indefinitely through well-negotiated contracts with integrated delivery systems (IDSs) and MCOs. Much greater detail about forming, selecting, and managing fully integrated, multispecialty group practices is available in Chapter 13, "Step Five: Growing into a Larger, Multispecialty Group Practice."

Be Careful of the Ways You Collaborate with Other Physicians

In the course of forming, acquiring, and merging with group practices, you must talk and plan together with other physicians. Most of the conversations will seem perfectly natural to you. Be alert to the serious legal implications of whom you talk to and what you talk about.

The primary hazard is an unknowing violation of federal or state antitrust laws. You may be accused of price fixing, restraint of trade, and, occasionally, monopolistic behavior. These legal problems arise most often in a few specific situations. The physician network you have formed to negotiate for managed care contracts is a sham for illegal agreements among independent physicians to set prices. The IDS you helped found has contracted with such a large percentage of key physicians in the area that other systems or MCOs are prevented from entering the market. Due to the attempts to select only the most cost-effective practitioners for an integrated physician-hospital organization, excluded physicians claim to be deprived of the opportunity to earn a livelihood.

There are clear-cut ways to avoid these legal risks. The best course is to move as quickly as possible to thoroughly integrate your group of physicians and share risks among yourselves. Chapter 28, "Collaborating with Other Physicians without Legal Risk," provides a lot more information on how to collaborate safely.

Concentrate on Bringing Primary Care Physicians into the Group and Giving Them Considerable Clinical and Managerial Decision-Making Authority

Whether you call them "gatekeepers" or "portals of entry," primary care physicians are assuming a dominant role in the new health care system. They increasingly have primary responsibility and authority for deciding which, of all available medical services, each patient will receive. The initial diagnosis, the tests, the specialist referrals, many hospital admissions, and many drug prescriptions are all in their hands. In making those decisions, they also directly influence which costs will be incurred. Their growing power cannot be overestimated.

You must take this new status of primary care physicians into account in planning your future practice strategies.

If your goal is, as it should be, to become a large multispecialty group practice, *you must develop an appropriate proportion of primary care physicians on your panel or staff.* The exact percentage depends a lot on the type of patient population you are serving. In many cases, 50 percent primary care doctors is not too high. For many group practices that have been formed or are led by specialist physicians, this requirement means hiring a substantial number of primary physicians.

Because they traditionally received comparatively low compensation and are now in such great demand, it probably will be necessary to *offer significantly higher salaries or income guarantees to your primary care doctors*. Initially, this may require that the specialty physicians accept less income than they are used to. The proper primary care-to-specialist ratio will ensure that, in the end, everyone prospers.

You will have to *assign to the primary care physicians the preeminent clinical decision-making authority* that managed care demands. Concomitantly, patients must be denied direct access to specialty care physicians. This may be a discomforting adjustment for some specialists. It is unavoidable.

It also is necessary to make a special effort to *give primary care doctors a major role in the governance* of the group practice, physician network, or delivery system. Some commentators insist that they have a controlling representation on the board of directors. This dominant position does two things: one, it ensures that the organization will give proper emphasis to the gatekeeper responsibility of primary care doctors, and two, it demonstrates to MCOs with whom you might contract that your group is firmly committed to managing the care it delivers.

Begin Amassing the Investment Capital Required To Expand the Practice, Install New Information Systems, and Support the Formation of New Ventures and Organizations

Most of the strategic initiatives we are discussing cost money, some of them a great deal of money. There are organizational start-up costs, working capital costs for growing organizations, and capital equipment costs for new information systems. Exhibit 5–3 shows some very rough estimates for starting certain popular entities. The

estimates probably should be doubled for projects begun in 1999.

This money can come from three general sources. One is traditional financing institutions—venture capital firms and other investment capital sources, banks, and other loan capital sources. A second is the larger organizations (hospitals, insurance companies, MCOs) with whom you might partner. The third is the revenues generated by the practice entity itself.

Arranging financing for your strategic moves is discussed in greater detail in Chapter 27, "Financing Strategies To Support Your Integration Plans." There are two issues to keep in mind immediately. When one of your strategic partners agrees to invest significant amounts of capital in a new venture, it will want something in return—a significant control interest in that venture. There is always a trade-off between money and control with investors. Be prepared for it.

Physicians historically have not included capital accumulation as a line item in their practice budgets. At the end of each fiscal year, they generally withdraw any revenues left after expenses as personal income. Now is the time to begin budgeting for future capital purchases and invest-

---

Exhibit 5–3 Rough Estimates for Capital Necessary To Start Popular Entities

IPAs	$1.2 million
Physician-hospital organizations	$2.2 million
Staff-model physician organizations	$7.8 million
Management services organizations	$9.6 million
Free-standing medical groups	$19.7 million
Foundation-model medical groups	20 million

Source: Data from Assessing Healthcare Market Trends and Capital Needs: 1996–2000, *Healthcare Financial Management,* © 1995.

ments. Set aside a significant share of the money you might otherwise keep for yourself in a special strategic nest egg. Insist that your physician partners do the same.

Install a Computerized Information System That Tracks Costs by CPT Code, Physician, and Payer

In order to know which administrative and clinical expenses you can cut without impairing quality of care, you must be able to associate individual expense items with particular services (designated by CPT code), physicians, and patients. This will permit you to identify unnecessary or cost-ineffective services, as well as more cost-effective alternatives. The data will reveal the physicians who tend to practice less cost-effective medicine; they will identify those who are more efficient and may serve as role models for the rest. Some patients will emerge as consumers of more costly care. They may require more intensive case management.

The system that gathers this information will be an offshoot of the accounting system and must be computerized to handle the volume and complexity of data. From these data, you will learn surprising things about where the money goes in your practice. The data will empower you to take control of your practice expenditures to a degree you might not imagine.

A system like this is essential for competing successfully in the managed care marketplace. Many MCOs will ask for evidence that you operate such a system.

Install a Computerized Information System That Records Utilization Rates by Physician, Patient, and Payer

Managed and reduced utilization of services and resources is the keystone of successful practice under capitation. Your practice organization cannot carry out this task without a computerized system for tracking actual utilization rates. It will tell you which physicians are excessive utilizers and require further training. It will tell you which patients are heavy consumers of medical services and require closer case management. It will tell you when utilization rates are particularly high for members of certain payers. This may suggest unique demographics of that payer's members that deserve risk adjustment in the capitation rate.

A system like this is essential for competing successfully in the managed care marketplace. Many MCOs will ask for evidence that you operate such a system.

Install an Electronic Communication System That Links Your Practice with Its Key Stakeholders (MCOs, Insurance Companies, Employers, Referring Physicians, Specialist Physicians, Hospitals, and Other Providers)

In adding computerized systems, this communication module probably has secondary priority to the utilization management capability described above. However, its early implementation will give your practice a clear competitive advantage over more hesitant physician groups. Your high-tech efficiency will impress all that deal with you, particularly MCOs, insurance companies, and payers. Physician members at separate locations will be able to share key patient information. Physicians and their hospitals can more easily exchange medical records, test results, and patient status information. Billing submissions and any subsequent disputes will be handled more expeditiously, resulting in prompter payments to the group. You will be able to meet a payer's reporting requirements more smoothly with this capability. The overall result of these gains will be lower operating costs and increased revenues.

As you install the other more necessary computer-based systems, you will reach a level of electronic automation that will permit you to add this communication capacity with relatively little additional expense. When the opportunity arrives, do it.

Install an Electronic Information System That Accumulates Data on the Clinical Outcomes of Your Medical Decisions

You can expect more and more MCOs with which you contract to require regular reporting on the quality of care that you provide to their members. They do this to ensure that a proper balance is maintained with cost control and utilization management efforts. Quality of care means evidence of the outcomes produced by various therapies and treatments.

Besides assuring your MCO contractors of the efficacy of your clinical decision making, outcomes data are a useful tool for fine tuning the manipulation of utilization rates. They also can be powerful persuaders in contract negotiations with MCOs.

A regular system for gathering and analyzing these data will be a mandatory feature of every practice organization in the new health care system. It will be a complex and expensive undertaking, and can be placed lower on your list of capital projects. However, begin now creating the structure for this kind of data-gathering and steadily increase the volume of outcomes measured.

Institute a Regular Procedure for Measuring the Satisfaction of Patients

You and your MCO partners will look at quality of care from two perspectives. One is the actual results or outcomes produced. The other is the patient's perception of that quality, her satisfaction with the entire clinical treatment experience. The MCO will want to know this information and expect you to collect it.

Establish a routine procedure for obtaining detailed feedback on patients' satisfaction with every phase of their encounter with your practice—first contact after enrolling; making appointments; interactions with phone operator, receptionist, ancillary personnel, and physician; treatment procedures; treatment results; and co-payment and deductible billing. Satisfaction survey forms may be given to patients during each

visit or sent to their homes at regular intervals. Periodic focus groups of patients will provide more personalized information and permit deeper probing into the real causes behind patient upsets.

These data need to be gathered, compiled, digested, reported, and disseminated to people who care about them. The organization must be prepared to acknowledge problems brought to its attention and take immediate, appropriate action.

MCOs will gravitate toward delivery organizations that are this attentive to their patients.

Study and Consider Using Practice Guidelines, Clinical Pathways, or Practice Protocols in Your Medical Decision Making

The outcomes data that you gather will lead to general conclusions about which therapies are the most efficacious, cost-effective responses to which diagnoses. When these conclusions are codified, they become practice guidelines or clinical pathways. Such guidelines may be developed informally within your organization or you may adopt the more formal, scientifically researched precepts emerging from various specialist societies.

Use of practice guidelines offers several benefits. By applying proven standard treatments and procedures in appropriate situations, a physician reduces the expense of diagnostic time and tests spent figuring out the treatment each time that situation presents itself. Furthermore, guidelines that have been thoroughly tested are more likely to produce optimal outcomes. An organization's familiarity with practice guidelines also is appealing to prospective MCO partners.

Enter into Strategic Partnerships, Affiliations, or Mergers with Other Provider Organizations

After gathering a critical mass of physicians into a highly integrated, physician-controlled organization, the second major phase in the competitive strategy is building alliances and affiliations with the other necessary entities in a full-service health care delivery system. The other parties will include hospitals, ambulatory or emergency care facilities, long-term care institutions, certain single specialty group practices, ancillary provider groups, and testing laboratories.

The affiliation can take several forms. One organization can purchase or sell out to another organization. Two or more organizations can jointly own and control another organization. Two organizations can enter into a contract to sell or exchange services between themselves. Two organizations can use a contract to form a more substantial joint venture operation. Two or more organizations can simply merge with each other, both disappearing, creating a new third organization.

Focus on the types of relationships you want with other people and organizations and the flow of money, goods, and services you wish to take place. The law is flexible enough to define and create the necessary organizations and linkages. There are a few inhibitions, like antitrust and anti–self-referral laws, but generally a good lawyer can enable what your mind can imagine.

Sell Your Practice to a Hospital or MCO. Selling your practice is probably not what you had in mind when you picked up this book. Nonetheless, it could be just the right decision under the appropriate circumstances.

Physicians typically sell their practices to a management services organization (MSO), a physician practice management company (PPMC), an insurance company, an MCO, or a hospital. The MCO or the hospital then negotiates a compensation agreement with the physician that does not violate the physician self-referral laws, but does sufficiently bind the physician to the purchaser so that he wants to refer his patients to them.

From the physician's point of view, a practice sale makes sense for two reasons. The physician has grown weary of managing the business side of a medical practice, particularly in the face of multiple MCO payers and their more complex practice requirements. She is content to sell out to a larger, competitively well-placed organization, turn over practice administrative responsibilities, and accept a steady salary as an employee for the rest of her career. Many physicians are making exactly this decision right now. The strategy begins and ends with this one choice.

A very different rationale is involved when a physician sells his practice to a physician-run organization with ambitious strategic plans for integration and growth. He reaps several benefits from the transaction. He may immediately receive a shareholder interest in the organization, as well as a role in its governance. He enjoys the comfort of knowing that key managerial and clinical practice decisions will be made with the physician's interests in mind. He has placed himself in an environment where it will be easier to acquire necessary new practice skills. The physician's career is now aligned with a professionally managed organization with a clear strategic mission. He is well placed for the future.

Chapter 18, "Step Nine: Selling Your Practice to a Hospital, Managed Care Organization, or Physician Practice Management Company," explains a lot more about how to plan and carry out the sale of your practice—or the purchase of another physician's practice.

Contract with a Management Services Organization (MSO). A sale of a physician's practice to an MSO is normally a statement that he simply does not want to think anymore about the management or strategic planning of his practice. An MSO typically is founded by a hospital or profit-driven entrepreneurs, though it sometimes is the result of a joint venture between a hospital and physicians.

Bear in the mind the following questions when contemplating a deal with an MSO:

- What is the range of practice management services it will provide to you?
- What price will it pay in purchasing your practice assets?
- What price could you get if you sold the assets on the open market?
- At what rate will it lease the assets back to you?

- What is the financial history and strength of the MSO?
- Are you confident that it, and your practice assets, will still be around in five years?
- What plans does the MSO have for reconfiguring the practices that it owns and services?
- Is there any potential for payer contracting and integration initiatives to occur through the MSO?
- Could the MSO evolve into a physician-hospital organization (PHO)?

Sale and leaseback with an MSO is not a strategic end point. It solves some immediate cash flow and practice management problems. It normally does nothing about consolidating your practice with other physicians, advancing the operational integration of your practice, negotiating payer contracts, or striking up the strategic alliances essential to future success. It can move in those directions and then become a different kind of organization. Before you sell out to an MSO, get clear on whether you can rely on it for strategic leadership.

For more information on MSOs and PPMCs, refer to Chapter 16, "Step Seven: Partnering with a Management Services Organization or Physician Practice Management Company."

Form or Join a Physician-Hospital Organization (PHO). Joining in the creation of a PHO is one of the most popular first strategic affiliations for physicians with a nonphysician provider. A hospital is an obvious key component if one is building a full-service delivery system. Your strong, integrated physician group should have an affiliation with a good hospital no later than two or three years after reading this book.

Be alert to the pitfalls in forming one of these organizations. If the hospital contributes most of the capital, it is likely to end up controlling the organization. It may then steer the PHO in directions more beneficial to the hospital than the doctors. From a competitive standpoint, if there are several hospitals in town, the one forming the PHO may not be the best affiliation partner for your practice. The hospital may pursue the PHO option as a last effort to shore up its deteriorating financial condition. Your PHO partner may declare bankruptcy in a few years. Formation of a PHO is not an end in itself. The organization needs to have a strategy for moving toward further integration and developing cost-effective delivery skills among all its providers. PHOs sometimes are simple combinations of a hospital and its medical staff. As the organization accepts more and more capitation contracts, it must winnow out those physicians incapable of practicing cost-effective medicine.

The PHO is an excellent first-stage mechanism for building the necessary strategic alliances with nonphysician providers. Turn to Chapter 15, "Step Six: Forming a PHO—An Affiliation between Your Group Practice and a Hospital," for more detailed advice on forming and managing a PHO.

Be Very Selective in the Provider Partners You Choose To Affiliate or Merge with. Physicians and hospitals are not interchangeable. Some are better than others are. Choose them for their suitability as strategic partners.

Seek physicians who satisfy these criteria.

- They understand the inevitability of managed care and are willing to embrace its basic tenets.
- The are flexible enough to learn and apply the new practice skills necessary to succeed under managed care.
- They are willing to assume risk in a capitated environment.
- They have demonstrated the ability to practice cost-effective medicine, where possible.
- They possess reputations for delivering only good quality care.
- Their practice locations are distributed appropriately throughout the targeted market.
- They are willing to contribute capital to new strategic ventures within the limits of their personal finances.

- They have a commitment to work as part of a team toward the good of the entire organization.
- They accept the value of professional management of the organization, even if that means nonphysician managers.
- They accept the leadership role for primary care physicians in the process of clinical decision making and resource allocation.
- They have the determination to create physician-controlled organizations for influential roles within the health care industry.

Seek hospitals that satisfy these criteria.

- They understand the inevitability of managed care and are willing to embrace its basic tenets.
- They are flexible enough to learn and apply the new delivery management skills necessary to succeed under managed care.
- They are currently in strong financial condition.
- They recognize that physicians must play a dominant role in the health care delivery system and in the PHO.
- They accept the leadership role for primary care physicians in the process of clinical decision making and resource allocation.
- They possess a reputation for delivery good quality care.
- They are willing to assume risk in a capitated environment.
- They have a full appreciation of the internal systems necessary to support high-quality, cost-effective health care delivery.
- They accept the value of professional management of the organization.

Use these criteria and others that seem relevant to you in making all affiliation decisions. Prepare a list before the choices have to be made and apply it rigorously. The success or failure of your strategic plans will turn on the quality of the people and organizations that join you in those plans.

Chapter 24, "Choosing the Best Strategic Partners for Your Group Practice, Physician Hospital Affiliation, or Integrated Delivery System," looks at the selection of strategic partners in greater depth.

Increase the Level of Integration and Risk-Sharing in Your Provider Network or Group

The most successful provider organizations are the ones moving most rapidly to integrate and assume risk.

The term "integration" has at least three meanings in the health care delivery context. When physicians begin to form alliances with each other (through mergers, acquisitions, or contracts) instead of operating as wholly autonomous medical practices, they are combining their resources and aligning their strategies in order to wield greater influence with insurance companies, MCOs, and other payers. This is called "horizontal integration." When a physician group forms strategic partnerships with other entities in the health care delivery chain (hospitals, specialist groups, long-term care facilities, MCOs, employers), they are carrying out "vertical integration." These are forms of structural integration.

However, the current usage of the term usually refers to the internal, operational melding of physician interests and actions within the group. This kind of integration occurs in a multitude of ways.

- measuring and comparing utilization rates of all physicians and working together to reduce excessive rates
- accepting responsibility, as a group of physicians, for an entire community of covered lives (rather than as individual physicians for individual patients)
- agreeing on and operating under a common vision and set of strategic goals
- consolidating within the group all contract negotiation and execution for all providers in the group
- measuring patient satisfaction with group encounters and assuming joint responsibility for remedying dissatisfaction
- managing every aspect of the group, including individual physician practices, under a single operating budget

- creating and coordinating compatible operating systems in the areas of accounting, billing, collections, data processing, communications, information systems, utilization management, outcomes measurement, quality assurance, and medical records
- combining capital contributions to create new organizations, purchase equipment, and support growth that benefits the entire group
- sharing the financial risk of excessive utilization by certain physicians or unanticipated high demand for services by certain patients
- sacrificing some individual physician interests for the good of the entire group
- cooperating as a team of physicians to resolve problems that confront the group
- delegating governance of the group's affairs to an elected board of directors
- delegating management of the group's operations to professional managers chosen by the board of directors

This is the direction in which your group must move. The sooner you can develop these "team" attitudes and implement these integration measures, the more competitive you will become in winning managed care contracts and larger populations of covered lives.

Increasing the level of integration in a provider organization is explained further in Chapter 19, "Step Ten: Increasing the Level of Integration in Your Provider Organization."

Create or Join a Fully Integrated, Full-Service Delivery System

This is the second of three possible end points in your practice development strategy. The first is the fully integrated, multispecialty group practice. The third is the complete delivery and financing system.

An integrated delivery system is a single legal entity that operates an entire health care delivery system. It consists of a group of affiliated organizations through which physicians, hospitals, and other providers combine their resources, energies, risks, and rewards in order to deliver comprehensive health care services to an identified community. A payer can contract with a single IDS to meet all the health care needs of its members.

If you do not choose to take the initiative to build your own IDS, you will inevitably become one of the affiliated components of an IDS. The IDS is the natural next evolutionary step after a large integrated full-service multispecialty group practice has entered into a solid joint venture with one or more hospitals. A well-integrated PHO comprises 75 percent of an IDS. Only the addition of some additional provider organizations and ancillary facilities and the further unification and consolidation of systems stands between a PHO and an IDS. The challenges in forming and operating an IDS are explored in more detail in Chapter 21, "Step Eleven: the Final Step–Evolving into a Regionwide Vertically Integrated Delivery System."

Consider your strategic future this way. Either build a multispecialty group practice so dominant that it can prevail in contract negotiations with an IDS or MCO or develop an IDS that deals directly with insurance companies and large MCOs.

Take Over the Financing of the Health Care Provided by the System

When you add a financing or insurance component to an IDS, the result is an MCO. This is the ultimate destination for any practice growth strategy. Beyond this stage, progress is measured in terms of more providers serving more covered lives in more markets. The nature of the organization does not really change. The size simply continues to increase.

Development of a full-blown MCO is a plausible strategic step only for the most ambitious physician or physician group. The cost is immense, well exceeding $100 million. The challenges and complexities of assembling the necessary people, organizations, and resources are considerable. This does not make sense as a high priority long-term goal for most physician groups right now.

However, events in the health care industry are moving at a pace no one would have predicted 10 years ago. It is possible that, by the year 2005, your group will be in such a strong financial and competitive position (perhaps having evolved into an IDS) that the assumption of full financial risk will seem within your reach. Keep it in the back of your mind.

RESOURCE LIST

J. Blair and M. Fottler, *Strategic Leadership for Medical Groups* (San Francisco: Jossey-Bass, Publishers, 1998).

S. Hillestad and E. Berkowitz, *Health Care Strategic Plans*, 3rd ed. (Gaithersburg, MD: Aspen Publishers, Inc., in press).

G. James, *Making Managed Care Work—Strategies for Local Market Dominance* (Winchester, IL: Healthcare Financial Management Association, 1997).

Making Sense of Managed Care—Vol. I: Building Blocks and Fundamentals (San Francisco: Jossey-Bass, Publishers, 1998).

Making Sense of Managed Care—Vol. II: Strategic Positioning (San Francisco: Jossey-Bass, Publishers, 1998).

Making Sense of Managed Care—Vol. III: Operational Issues and Practical Answers (San Francisco: Jossey-Bass, Publishers, 1998).

F. McCall-Perez, *Physician Equity Groups and Other Emerging Entities: Competitive Organizational Choices for Physicians* (Winchester, IL: Healthcare Financial Management Association, 1997).

The Physician Strategist. Setting a Strategic Direction for Your Practice (Burr Ridge, IL: McGraw-Hill Healthcare Education Group, 1996).

Strategic Choices for Medical Groups: Navigating Your Strategic Web, book #5069. Medical Group Management Association, 1998.

Strategic Planning, Super Search Packet #0992. Medical Group Management Association.

I. Studin, *Strategic Healthcare Management: Applying the Lessons of Today's Top Management Experts to the Business of Managed Care* (Winchester, IL: Healthcare Financial Management Association, 1995).

CHAPTER 6

A Physician's Life under Managed Care

INTRODUCTION

Most physicians do not have to be told that the life of a practicing physician is dramatically different now than what it was 20 years ago—due largely to the spread of managed care. A lot of what they have heard has been negative. At best, there is often a lot of confusion and worry about what it will be like to practice medicine in an intensely managed care environment.

This chapter describes all the facets of a physician's professional life in the practice settings typical of the late 1990s. Its goal is to leave physician-readers with a more realistic and perhaps more inviting sense of what her work life might be to help her make better informed decisions about practicing in a managed care setting.

The chapter starts with a brief look at the kinds of organizations for which a physician is likely to work. It focuses on the practice setting where he will spend most of his working day. The physician will learn about a typical practice schedule, the work hours, flexibility in setting them, and off-hours availability. She will become familiar with the gamut of practice controls likely to be imposed on her—passively or actively. This includes utilization management (UM), clinical guidelines, practice profiles, patient satisfaction surveys, and clinical outcomes measurements.

After reading the chapter, the physician will better understand

- how he is likely to fit into a "gatekeeper" system (depending on his specialty)
- what kinds of information he is likely to receive and give to a managed care organization (MCO) to support the care management process
- what techniques are available for managing the demand for his services

The chapter also includes material on the administrative duties a physician may be asked to assume and the growing importance placed on the interpersonal skills of physicians. Finally, there is some discussion of the further career opportunities available through managed care.

WHO SHOULD READ THIS CHAPTER

There are probably quite a few physicians who already have enough experience working under managed care contracts or for a large, capitated multispecialty group practice to have a pretty good idea of what professional life in managed care is like. Those physicians may want to skip this chapter and go directly to the chapters that discuss the strategic alternatives that intrigue or puzzle them.

A great many other physicians still do not have enough exposure to managed care to even begin thinking positively about which strategic options they want to consider. Nothing can take the place of day-to-day practice in a managed care environment to learn its impact on the practice of medicine. This chapter attempts to provide a balanced introduction to the real-life world of managed care. With this foundation, a physician may feel better prepared to choose where she would like to locate herself in the health care delivery infrastructure and what role she wants to play in shaping it.

Even those physicians with some working experience in managed care could have something to gain from reading this chapter. Not all managed care practice settings (arm's length contract, MCO employee, group practice partner) have adopted care management principles in the same way and to the same extent. This chapter describes a typical or optimal practice situation. It could be valuable to compare this model with what a physician is currently experiencing.

Those readers in positions of influence (management or governance, usually) in physician-run organizations might simply want to follow the concepts laid out in this chapter.

KINDS OF ORGANIZATIONS FOR WHICH YOU WILL WORK

Broadly speaking, there are three types of managed care-oriented organizational structures in which a physician can expect to work.

Solo or Small Group Practice under Contract with an MCO

It may come as a surprise to know that thousands of physicians are still in solo or small group practices. Among medical group management association (MGMA) physician members, roughly 25,000 are in groups of 10 physicians or less. This represents about 14.5 percent of all MGMA physicians,[1] comprising a few distinct groups.

- A few of them are located in areas not yet penetrated at all by managed care. They are practicing pretty much the old-fashioned way, filing claims for reimbursement under their patients' indemnity insurance policies.

- A great many others have contracts with one or more MCOs to provide services on a variety of terms. These contracts may be with either health maintenance organizations (HMOs) or preferred provider organizations (PPOs). Of MGMA groups with 10 physicians or less, the following percentages have contracts with these kinds of MCOs: PPO (76.5 percent), independent practice association (IPA)-HMO (32.9 percent), network HMO (32.9 percent), group HMO (23.5 percent), and staff HMO (7.1 percent).[2] The physicians may be reimbursed on the basis of discounted fee schedules, capitation, or other risk-sharing formulas. In 1995, 60.6 percent of MGMA groups with 10 physicians or less derived revenue from at-risk managed care contracts.[3] Under these contracts, the physicians may be subject to UM, quality assurance, and other practice management requirements.

- Another group of physicians is composed of members of loosely structured IPAs or physician-hospital organizations (PHOs) that negotiate managed care contracts on their behalf. Their compensation may come in the form of discounted fee-for-service (FFS), capitation, or other at-risk arrangements.

What is unique about all these scenarios is that the physicians remain legally and physically independent. In the less competitive markets, there may be relatively little pressure to reduce utilization or to watch quality any more closely than in the past. The physicians are not yet practicing under some of the more onerous care management programs.

What is also inevitable about these physicians and small groups is that they will develop the ability to manage both cost and quality, they will learn to satisfy patients, they will meet MCO reporting requirements, and they will follow rules prescribed by the MCO. They will do this independently or, if that setting does not provide adequate resources, they will become part of a larger, better-financed entity, such as a multispecialty group practice, a management services organization (MSO), a more highly integrated PHO, or another form of physician-run organization.

Member or Employee of a Large Group Practice or Other Provider Organization That Has Contracts with MCOs

The movement among physicians is toward participation, in some form, in larger delivery organizations, such as a large integrated multi-specialty group practice, a network sponsored by a physician practice management company, a more integrated PHO, a more integrated IPA, or a full-blown integrated delivery system (IDS). They can have different relationships with each of those entities. Basically, a physician may have an arm's length contract with an organization, may be an employee of that organization, may be a shareholder (if it is a for-profit corporation), or may be a partner (if it is a partnership).

The organization in which the physician participates then turns around and contracts with an MCO to provide medical services to its enrollees through the organization's providers. The key distinction of these scenarios is that the physician is part of a separate and substantial organization that negotiates with the MCOs. Because of its greater size, the organization carries more weight in the negotiations with an MCO. It can achieve better results. Its greater size also gives it the resources to purchase and implement the sophisticated care management and information systems necessary to satisfy the MCOs and to compete with other delivery organizations. Because it is a separate legal entity, it presents the opportunity for physicians to own and run it. This can be the vehicle by which physicians reclaim their authority over clinical decision making and earn an equal place at the bargaining table with MCOs.

Direct Employee of an MCO

There is one kind of MCO that is likely to directly employ the physicians it needs. The physicians in a staff-model HMO are either employees of a specially formed professional group practice that is an integral part of the HMO or are salaried employees of the HMO itself. In 1996, the 46 staff-model HMOs then operating used 52,670 physicians. Most of those physicians were employed, but a significant number had contractual relationships with the HMO.[4] They are as far removed from the traditional solo practitioner as they are ever likely to be. The HMO tells them where to practice and what hours to work. As long as they remain in the HMO's employment, they abide by its requirements concerning resource utilization, quality control, clinical outcomes and protocols, patient satisfaction, administrative duties, and collaboration in teams. Once a physician has made it through two or three years of employment by an HMO, she can be rather confident that she is meeting the HMO's requirements for a modern managed care physician. She has achieved the health care equivalent of tenure.

WHAT YOUR PRACTICE SETTING WILL LOOK LIKE

Physicians who do not yet have relations with an MCO or who are participants in an early-stage, loosely combined IPA or PHO are practicing just where they have been all along. If they are seeing patients in a medical office building, in a suite in a strip mall, or in an office carved out of their personal residences, that is where they are staying. As managed care becomes more prevalent in their areas, these physicians will come under pressure to relocate.

Once physicians become more involved with managed care, particularly after they join larger provider organizations, relocation may become necessary for several reasons.

- The overhead expense of maintaining their separate locations may become unacceptable.
- The size of their current locations may restrict their ability to see the volume of patients or provide the range of services required by the organization.

- The organization may feel unable to carry out its care management and information-gathering procedures without its physicians practicing in a central location.
- The physicians' current location may not be as accessible to the organization's patients as it could be.

The relocation may take different forms. A lot will depend on the organization's strategic vision for the kind of system that it wants to build. A physician may be asked to move her solo practice to an area of the city where more of the organization's patients are concentrated. To meet the basic ambulatory medical needs of a community or neighborhood, the organization may set up a modest clinic staffed with primary care specialists (e.g., family practitioner, pediatrician, obstetrician/gynecologist). Each specialist will come from another location to this clinic. The doctors will be supported by some administrative and ancillary personnel. If or when there is a large enough concentration of covered lives in an area, the organization may choose to establish a much larger multispecialty clinic that offers a more comprehensive range of services.

Some provider organizations, particularly those in rural or lightly populated areas, automatically pull all their physicians into a large, central clinic facility (perhaps located close to one of the only hospitals in the area) where the clinical and financial features of their practices can be more tightly integrated. In fact, as health care providers gain more experience in organizing themselves, some physicians may find themselves first relocated to a central facility. Then, as it becomes clear that enrollees prefer more convenient primary care access, they may be sent back out to a strategically located satellite clinic.

One thing a managed care physician can count on is that he will be practicing in an organization, and often a facility, with a larger number of other physicians than he may be used to. He will not be the only professional of concern in the organization (as in a solo practice), nor will he be among just a few rather familiar colleagues (as in a small group practice). He will work among a great many other physicians, many of whom are relatively unknown to him. He will be expected to work for the common welfare of the entire organization, rather than exclusively for his own benefit. As a result, he will ultimately do better than if he focused on his own needs.

HOW YOU WILL BE COMPENSATED

There used to be one simple, universal method for reimbursing physicians. After performing whatever services she felt clinically necessary, without thinking for a second about the attendant costs, the physician sent a claim for her fee for that service (usually pretty similar to the fees of other area physicians for the same service) to the patient's insurance company. The insurance company paid the claim in full, also without asking many questions. If the patient did not have medical insurance, he might pay the physician's fee out of his own pocket. If the patient also had a low income, the physician might forgive the fee. There was little contentiousness over the amount of the claim or the need for the service that it covered.

All that has changed. There is a multitude of ways that a physician can now expect to be compensated for work.

Traditional FFS

There may be a few physicians who still have the luxury of having their claims paid automatically under an insurance indemnity policy. However, most paid on this basis actually fall in the following two categories:

Discounted FFS

When it became apparent that traditional FFS served as an incentive for physicians to perform more services, driving up health care costs, the MCOs began negotiating for discounts from the physician's usual and customary fee schedule. In return for accepting 10 to 20 percent less than her normal charges, the physician gained access to a new, large pool of patients.

FFS or Discounted FFS Plus Basic UM

Even with discounted FFS, physicians could make up the lost income by performing proportionately more services. The MCOs adjusted again by instituting the first crude UM procedures. These require that, before performing certain services or even admitting a patient to a hospital, the physician obtain the consent of the MCO. The consent often is obtained by placing a call to a UM person (usually a trained nonphysician practitioner employed by the MCO or by a UM company under contract with the MCO). On the basis of the patient's condition and diagnosis, and after consulting a book of guidelines and protocols, the person states that the MCO will or will not pay for the services prescribed by the physician.

That leaves the physician with four choices. She can take advantage of the appeal procedure that is part of a good UM program. She can perform the service and absorb the cost herself. (This does not work, of course, if the prescription is for a service to be performed by others.) She can tell the patient that he must pay for the service out of his own pocket. Or, she can change her original prescription and not perform the service.

This reimbursement method is quite common in the more loosely structured physician networks, such as IPAs and PHOs. The lack of integration makes it hard to impose UM measures that rely on clinical protocols, sharing of comparative data, a healthy dose of peer review, and not a little peer pressure. Because the physicians are usually still legally independent at this point, they are not likely to want to work for the greater good of the entire organization, as is the case under many capitation and risk-sharing schemes.

Capitation

Capitation can occur at two levels. The entire physician group or organization can be capitated, and then compensate its member physicians through any one of these methods here. It is also possible to capitate individual physicians. Under such capitation, each physician receives a fixed amount of money per month to provide a defined package of services (within the physician's specialty and range of ability) to each of a large number of patient-members. For this method to work, the physician must be responsible for a large enough pool of patients so that actuarial probabilities will come into play. A very few of the patients will be extremely ill, requiring services that cost far more than the per member–per month (PMPM) capitation fee. Most of the remaining members will not be sick at all and will not require any services, allowing their capitation fees to be applied toward the very sick patients. A significant minority of members will be sick enough to need some services, but the cost will not exceed the capitation fee. A lot depends on the amount of the capitation fee, the size of the physician's assigned pool of members, and the accuracy of the actuarial projections of the incidence of sickness among those members. It will have a direct impact on how much net income the physician receives.

The common wisdom has been that the best candidates for capitation are physicians in the primary care specialties. They are the participants in any physician group likely to see the greatest number of patients. However, where the group or organization is large enough, even narrow subspecialists may be tied to a large enough member pool to warrant paying them on a capitated basis. Several MCOs and physician organizations are doing exactly that.

Salary

If FFS payment was criticized for encouraging physicians to provide too many services, capitation has seemed like an incentive to perform fewer services than the patient really needs. Some delivery organizations have turned to paying their physicians a salary as a sort of neutral middle ground between FFS and capitation. The thought is that the physician knows exactly how much income he is going to receive and can concentrate on providing the best medical care without feeling financial pressure to do too much or too little. In practice, some organizations have found that, with no monetary incentives at all, some physicians do the least necessary to get by. Their productivity is not good.

Salary or Capitation Plus Risk Sharing

Under this arrangement, a single physician or group of physicians receives a guaranteed income base (via salary or capitation) that represents 70 to 90 percent of their potential total income. The remaining 10 to 30 percent is put into a risk pool or a risk withhold, to be paid out to the physicians only if their utilization of resources does not exceed a certain level. The formulas by which the pools or withholds are calculated and their funds allocated can be quite complex.

Salary Plus Incentives Bonuses

This method of physician compensation is the latest and, arguably, the most sophisticated yet. Physicians are paid a salary that is more or less competitive with what others in the area are earning. At the end of the year, they may also receive bonuses, depending on their achievement of predetermined goals in the areas of productivity (i.e., number of patients seen, not services performed), resource utilization, cost reduction, quality standards, compliance with organization-mandated clinical protocols and other administrative procedures, patient satisfaction, interpersonal relations with ancillary staff and other physicians, participation in multidisciplinary teams, and assumption of managerial responsibilities. Few organizations are currently paying their physicians for their performance in all these areas, but this method is an indication of where physician compensation is headed.

The compensation methods involving capitation, salaries, risk withholds, and bonuses are typically employed by organizations that are much more tightly integrated. In many cases, physicians are employees of the organization.

Delivery organizations continue to experiment with physician compensation methodologies. Though the current "mode" seems to be capitating primary care physicians (PCPs) and paying

specialists a discounted FFS, a few places are trying the very opposite—using capitation fees with the specialists and paying salaries to the primary care doctors. The quest for a compensation mechanism that encourages the desirable behavior in physicians while aligning their goals with those of the entire organization will continue.

DIFFERENCES IN CLINICAL ROLES OF PRIMARY CARE AND SPECIALIST PHYSICIANS

The real-life clinical roles of physicians in different specialties have always varied tremendously. The setting and tempo of the daily work routine are dramatically different among family practitioners, orthopedic surgeons, and cardiologists. In managed care environments, these roles have become more formally defined, divided, and regimented. Historically, patients tended to visit primary doctors first to determine the nature of their ailments. If the primary doctor could diagnose and treat the problem, that was the end of it. If the problem was beyond his training and abilities, he referred the patient to a specialist.

In the majority of MCOs and their provider organizations, this triage function of the PCP has been codified into the so-called gatekeeper. When they first join the MCO, members are required to choose a personal physician from among the available gatekeepers. Whenever she feels she needs medical care, the patient is expected to arrange a visit with that particular physician. Only after seeing the gatekeeper and getting a referral to a specialist may the patient proceed to see a specialist.

Gatekeepers frequently receive training from the MCO in carrying out their duties. It is a challenging position to be in. They must determine, in a minimal amount of time—remember, productivity and throughput are important—the nature of the patient's ailment and whether the patient requires or deserves access to the remainder of the MCOs provider network. They are directly in the middle of the opposing forces in managed care—the desire to keep costs as low as possible while keeping quality as high as possible.

In the good MCOs, the primary care physician role goes beyond opening and closing a gate. She may function as the coach of a multispecialty, multidisciplinary team through which she coordinates the care required by each patient. She directs access, rather than preventing it. She may also be expected, with the appropriate education and training, to personally treat a much wider range of patient conditions than PCPs traditionally have done. Some have suggested that a so-called superdoctor might be able to provide over 90 percent of the care a patient will ever need. Still, the PCP knows when to refer to a specialist. Conceived this way, the gatekeeper role becomes more appealing.

Some other new practitioner roles are also being carved out, with effects for physicians. A few MCOs have begun experimenting with gatekeepers for the gatekeepers. They are using non-physician providers, particularly nurse practitioners, to carry out certain tasks performed previously by physicians. Members of certain health plans can choose a nurse as their principal primary care provider. Those nurses are reimbursed at the same rates as are PCPs. They work with physician partners, to whom they refer patients when they need a specialist, when there is an emergency, or when the patient's problem exceeds their abilities. The nurses are given the authority to admit patients to the hospital and to write prescriptions. In the states where they are licensed, nurse practitioners usually are permitted to

- diagnose illnesses
- perform physical examinations
- order and interpret laboratory tests
- design and carry out treatment plans, suture wounds
- provide preventive health services

There is an expectation that the nursing skills of these practitioners may better enable them to handle the health education and disease prevention functions for which physicians no longer have the time and yet which are becoming essential in managed care.

Primary care physicians and even some specialists, who spend the bulk of their practice engaging with patients on an outpatient basis while periodically rounding on their hospitalized patients, are being encouraged to focus entirely on the outpatient segment. As one physician put it, "It's very difficult to be a gatekeeper when you have two gates to keep." After the PCP has decided to admit a patient, that patient's care is turned over to a full-time, specially trained, hospital-based physician who is coming to be called a *hospitalist*. Some MCOs and group practices are requiring the transfer of clinical responsibility; others are leaving it at the discretion of the PCP gatekeeper. In one group practice where the use of a hospitalist was voluntary, 75 of the 160 physicians turned over all of their hospitalized patients and another 60 trusted the care of some of their patients to the hospitalists.[5]

Some of the advantages claimed for this new category of practitioner are

- no wasted time shuttling between the hospital and the outpatient office
- no need to juggle the demands of an outpatient practice with urgent calls from the hospital
- ability to receive results of crucial tests more quickly for immediate action
- ability to catch promptly a redundant test or marginally indicated procedure proposed by a consultant
- more time to spend with patients and their families
- more time to spend on patient education
- better ability to consider each patient's treatment preferences
- more familiarity with the internal workings of the hospital
- more knowledge about the hospital's inpatient protocols
- better knowledge of the qualifications of the specialists on the medical staff
- greater experience with hospital medicine as a result of rounding on many more patients each year

The early results from plans and groups that have been using hospitalists for a year or more are that they can cut hospital stays by one-half to one full day and reduce total costs per stay by 10 to 20 percent.

The professional lives of specialists have changed under managed care, as well. In fact, it may be going through two opposing phases. Under the original gatekeeper system, which still exists at most MCOs, the specialist is quite dependent on referrals from the gatekeepers. Because the gatekeepers have incentives to minimize such referrals and because many specialists are paid a discounted FFS, the volume of patients seen and income earned by the specialists drops. As the MCOs overall utilization of specialists declines, it usually concludes that it needs to have fewer physicians—specialists, in particular—on its provider panels. Some specialists currently under contract with the MCO are dropped and are likely to have great difficulty contracting with another plan. Other specialists who decide too late to join the managed care game will never get a chance at a contract.

There are two other trends pushing patients toward specialists rather than away from them. They both stem from concern that tightly closed panels limit patient choice of physicians too much. Health plans with point-of-service (POS) options allow members to decide whether they will use a panel physician or a nonpanel physician at the time that they need medical care. If they choose a nonplan physician, the members must pay more out-of-pocket, in the form of higher copayments or deductibles. However, the nonplan physician may be just the specialist that the health plan would not allow them to see.

Several MCOs have begun experimenting with allowing members to make appointments directly with specialists, without first obtaining a referral from a PCP gatekeeper. The motive for this radical procedural shift is also concern for patient choice of physicians. The change can take different forms. Once a patient has seen the specialist at least once, perhaps in connection with a chronic illness, she will be authorized to return to that specialist at her discretion for further treatment of that illness. Alternatively, the gatekeeper may give the patient initial authority to contact a specialist a fixed number of times, five, for example, at her discretion and without getting further permission from the gatekeeper. Only the most daring MCOs are willing to let patients make their own decisions in all cases about whether their condition warrants seeing a specialist and which one to see. Prior experience indicates that it is usually more expensive to allow patient judgments to supersede those of a trained gatekeeper physician. Time will tell whether patients are willing to pay for this degree of freedom of physician choice.

HOW UM PROCEDURES WILL BE APPLIED TO YOU

Utilization management has been the heart of managed care. Approximately 80 percent of the costs incurred for health care services are the result of decisions made by physicians. These are decisions to directly provide services and perform procedures, to refer the patient to another physician, to order a variety of ancillary services, to hospitalize the patient, to prescribe medications, and to obtain tests. Managed care's original mandate is to control costs, and the primary method for achieving this is to control physician decisions on the utilization of resources.

MCOs employ a variety of UM techniques, some of which are applicable to only certain types of resources. These are the most common techniques.

Utilization Review

The first form of UM employed by MCOs was utilization review by a third party, usually prior to performing certain procedures or to hospitalizing a patient (prospective), or while the patient is in the hospital (concurrent). Variations of this approach can still be found in many MCOs. The review process may be handled by the MCO's employees or by a third-party utilization review organization. Several states require that third-party review entities obtain licenses from them.

The actual reviewers typically are trained registered nurses. The process should always include a reliable appeals procedure (first one doctor, then a panel of doctors, in the appropriate specialty).

Provider Education

The best provider organizations combine other UM techniques with programs of education in the most cost-effective treatment methods. This may come through peer mentoring or consultation, formal in-house workshops, or by sending physicians to outside continuing medical education (CME) events on this topic. Do not expect to see provider education as the sole means of controlling utilization. Evidence has shown that it must be backed up by comparative physician-specific utilization data, visible support of clinical authority figures, and appropriate economic rewards and incentives.

Physician Profiling

The MCO or group practice tracks a variety of utilization data for each physician to build up a profile of that physician's practice style (how much of each kind of resource the physician typically uses) across multiple patients. The goal is to use these data on past physician practices to influence their current behavior. The following are the data categories most often used.

Inpatient Utilization Data

hospital days per 1,000 patients
average length of hospital stay
average per diem cost during hospital stay
average cost per case (per admission)

Outpatient Utilization Data

primary care encounter data

- patients seen per day
- visits per member per year
- intervals between visits for same patient

lab referrals per patient visit

X-ray referrals per patient visit
medication prescriptions

- prescriptions per visit or per member per year
- average cost per prescription
- percentage of prescriptions that are generic
- percentage of prescriptions within the formulary

specialist referrals

- referral rate per 100 primary care visits or per 1,000 members per year
- comparison to referral rate of comparable physicians
- initial referrals as a percentage of total referral visits
- cost per referral (by PCP, specialty, and plan average)
- number of visits and their costs (by specialty)

As important as the existence and thoroughness of physician profiles is, the way the information is used is even more significant. Some organizations simply pass the information on to each physician, usually with comparative figures for other similarly situated physicians within or without the group, and leave it to her individual conscience to decide what adjustments to make.

The physician members of a peer review committee may sit down with physicians who appear to be utilizing resources to excess to explore possible causes and agree on corrective measures to be taken. The organization may steer an outlier physician who has trouble managing utilization on his own to an appropriate outside CME workshop or, if the organization is large enough, have one conducted in-house. It may leave it to the physician's discretion whether to attend or, in more serious cases identified by the peer review committee, may require that he attend.

After exhausting all attempts to correct excessive utilization, the organization may choose to dismiss the physician from the group or provider panel. It can be expected that a physician-run organization would do this only as a last resort, that it would try much harder than a totally profit-driven organization to correct a physician's unacceptable behavior before dismissing him.

Capitation Compensation

By putting the physician at risk for excessive utilization and permitting her to retain the savings from reduced utilization, the monetary incentive of capitation payments (coupled with reasonable quality standards) can be a strong motivator to self-control utilization. This risk-sharing approach can take other forms, too, such as risk pools or withholds. Even under a capitation arrangement, physicians need utilization data to know how close they are to benchmarks or group norms.

Other Monetary Incentives

Other, more traditional monetary incentives may be used to encourage desired physician practice behavior. A certain portion of a physician's pay may be made conditional on his achievement of predetermined goals for utilization, as well as on other areas. Bonuses can be awarded for similar reasons.

Practice Guidelines

The publication and enforcement of practice guidelines may have the partial intent of pushing physicians to utilize the ideal volume of resources—and not a bit more. The guidelines offer model diagnostic and therapeutic modalities for patients with narrowly defined diseases or symptoms. Unless the treating physician can point to something exceptional in the patient's condition, she is expected to follow the guidelines in her clinical decision. As with the physician profile data, the guidelines may be used passively (let the physicians see them and choose how to respond) or actively (strongly urge, incent, or coerce the physicians to follow them).

Gatekeepers

The current UM strategy of choice is using PCPs as exclusive portals of entry, or "gatekeep-ers," to the full range of an organization's services and resources. Without the gatekeeper's authorization, the patient may not have access to those resources. Generally, physicians affiliated with a gatekeeper organization will be either filling the gatekeeper role (if they are trained in certain primary care specialties) or will see patients only when the gatekeeper concludes it is necessary (if they are specialists typically on the receiving end of referrals). The implications are dramatic. The PCPs are the primary managers of utilization; they must make the hard decisions about which resources will be applied to each patient's case; they often have powerful incentives (in the form of individual capitation compensation) to minimize utilization; and, ultimately, they decide when their specialist colleagues will see patients. The specialists must know that their group or managed care contract partners want to use their services as little as possible. This means that the UM system is designed to minimize their income.

KINDS OF INFORMATION YOU WILL GIVE AND RECEIVE

The cost-effective delivery of quality health care becomes more and more dependent on the gathering, analysis, dissemination, and utilization of information. Much of that information flows to and from physicians. Both MCOs and physician organizations under contract with MCOs require their participating physicians to furnish them with certain data about their practice operations. If a physician is a member of a large integrated group practice, these data will be collected for her, and about her, by the management of the group practice. They will pass on to MCO partners any of the information they need to see. If the physician is a solo or small group practitioner and has contracted directly with the MCOs or is a member of a largely unintegrated IPA or PHO with MCO contracts, she will have the responsibility of gathering the data and presenting them in the proper format for the MCOs.

These are typical examples of the kinds of data that the physician organization and, ultimately, the payer (MCO or insurance company) will want to see.

Start with the list of items just above, typically found in a physician profile. These relate primarily to the physician's clinical practice behaviors.

Claims data will be of interest where the physician is paid on a fee-for-service basis. In fact, some MCOs even require their capitated physicians to file shadow claims to track their practice activity. The claims data may be reviewed to determine whether

- the diagnosis was appropriate to the patient
- the treatment was appropriate to the diagnosis
- the treatment provided was appropriate to the patient's age, sex, and medical history
- the maximum number of acceptable treatments was exceeded
- the conditions of coverage were met
- the treatment or diagnosis typically involves coordination of benefit issues

Data may be sought from the member services office on

- the number and nature of patient complaints against the physician
- patient-initiated transfers away from assignment to the physician
- other administrative problems there may have been with the physician

Increasingly, physicians are being evaluated on their performance of certain nonclinical responsibilities. This can require the collection of data on

- productivity (measured by number of visits per week or hours worked or office visits per member per year, efficient use of time)
- medical charting (charts evaluated for legibility, timeliness, thoroughness, and compliance with charting systems in effect)
- dependability (arriving on time for work, sticking to a schedule, compliance with general administrative and procedural rules)
- after-hours call duty (responsiveness, appropriate use of emergency medical resources,

proper documentation, ensurance of continuity of care through follow-ups or transfer of care to another appropriate physician)
- medical knowledge (level of medical knowledge, demonstration of technical skills, evidence of proper medical judgment, awareness of limitations in skills and knowledge, appropriate use of CME opportunities)
- management of patient care (logical and efficient plans for diagnosis and treatment, proper discharge planning, appropriate follow-up intervals)
- management of outside resources (appropriateness, cost-effective use, and maintenance of continuity with regard to consultants and ancillary services—both diagnostic and therapeutic—referrals per member per year, total referral costs per member per year)
- cooperation with precertification and authorization requirements (percentage of admissions precertified, percentage of referrals preauthorized)
- use of plan providers (percentage of use of other providers participating in the plan, rather than nonparticipating providers)
- cooperation with quality management programs and procedures (participation in peer review, responsiveness to quality warnings, compliance with protocols)
- patient relations (ability to communicate effectively with patients, quality of patient relations, level of member satisfaction)
- staff relations (ability to communicate and cooperate with other members of the medical staff or provider panel and with support staff)
- attitude and leadership (enthusiasm, interest, commitment, flexibility, responsiveness, ability to train others, to motivate and to lead, decision skills in nonclinical matters)
- participation (in group or plan committees and meetings, including attendance, contribution, and initiative in taking responsibility)

The other side of this arrangement is that the physicians should have access to the data that the MCO is using to evaluate their performance.

These are data that may bear on their compensation or potentially lead to their deselection. Some of the data may come from the physicians themselves, in the reports they send to the MCO. Others may be gathered separately by the MCO—for instance, patient satisfaction survey results, comparative claims or utilization data, and tabulation of clinical outcomes or compliance with practice guidelines.

Physicians require this information to make adjustments in their practice style necessary to satisfy the MCO's performance criteria. Guaranteed access to the information should be written into the contract between the physician and the MCO.

PROGRAMS TO MEASURE AND IMPROVE THE QUALITY OF CARE THAT A PHYSICIAN PROVIDES

To balance aggressive cost-cutting initiatives, wise provider organizations and MCOs have instituted a variety of measures to maintain and elevate levels of quality of care. They expect cooperation and compliance from participating physicians. Look for measures like these when practicing in a managed care setting:

Continuous Quality Improvement (CQI) Techniques

For over 20 years, many provider organizations have been engaged in efforts to apply to health care delivery the CQI techniques developed by J. Edwards Deming in his groundbreaking work with Japanese industry. By definition, this is work that will go on continuously. Physicians can expect to be drawn into multidisciplinary teams whose short- or long-term assignments will be to redesign or reengineer processes and systems of all sorts. The processes may initially deal with administrative and procedural issues, but eventually the teams usually find themselves looking at clinical processes. The goal always is to improve the qualitative or quantitative output of the process. Besides frequently participating on these teams, physicians must be prepared to carry out the process changes they recommend. They also

will be asked to attend workshops explaining basic CQI principles.

Reduction of Clinical Variation and Practice Outliers

When provider groups decide to get serious about quality, their first aim often is to reduce the variation in treatment of identical conditions or diagnoses. Physicians can expect to have risk-adjusted data gathered on their treatment decisions, to have those data compared with comparable data from other physicians, and to receive attention from the group when their treatment patterns appear to be too far outside the norm. That attention will take the form of respectful questioning about the reasons for the treatment deviations, suggestions for adjustments in the physician's treatment decision making, recommendations that the physician attend appropriate clinical practice improvement workshops, mentoring by another group physician in the same specialty, and other corrective measures.

Development and Implementation of Clinical Guidelines

As CQI teams begin to explore clinical quality issues and to wrestle with the matter of treatment variation, they inevitably want to reshape some of the clinical processes involved. The natural next step is the development and implementation of clinical guidelines. Whether referred to as *guidelines, protocols*, or *pathways*, these are a kind of flowchart of the care and treatment steps that should be provided to a typical patient across a general diagnosis within a specified period of time. Physicians can be affected by clinical guidelines in two ways.

1. They may be asked to help in their development by the organization.
2. Once the guidelines are developed, they will be expected to follow them as closely as possible.

Some provider organizations have chosen to acquire their guidelines from outside sources, such as medical specialty boards. Though this saves the effort of preparing them in-house, such guidelines may be too general for practical application and may not take into account the resources available in a particular market area.

Clinical guidelines are developed or acquired for the most common illnesses or procedures. Physicians dealing with these diagnoses can expect to encounter guidelines for

- breast cancer detection and early treatment
- lower back pain
- specialty treatment of depression
- stroke
- hysterectomy
- diabetes
- knee care
- asthma in children
- viral upper respiratory infection in children
- vaginal birth after Caesarean
- urinary tract infections in women
- hypertension diagnosis in stable coronary artery disease
- acute myocardial infarction
- degenerative joint disease
- glaucoma

Measuring the Quality of Your Work with Clinical Outcomes

In reengineering processes and developing guidelines, provider organizations and health plans have been forced to consider exactly what they want those processes and guidelines to achieve. The answer is normally stated in terms of some quality benefit to the patient. For physicians, quality is usually a function of clinical outcomes, diagnostic acumen, and surgical technique. Patients have a much broader definition of quality of care, including matters like the food served in the hospital and the physician's bedside manner.

Increasingly, physicians can expect to have their practice decisions evaluated for the clinical outcomes they produce—a reduction in disease rates, symptom burden, or prevention of illness. This is still a rudimentary science; a great deal of

research is in progress, and it is proving difficult to define accurate and reliable measures of outcomes that correlate with a physician's treatment decisions. As outcomes measures are perfected, they first are used to determine optimal pathways or guidelines for treatment, eventually to be codified as clinical protocols. However, it is a small leap from there to using the outcomes data to rate an individual physician's performance and to determine part of his compensation.

Already, several MCOs are offering financial incentives or bonuses to participating physicians for their satisfaction of less sophisticated quality criteria. At Aetna U.S. Healthcare, physicians can earn a performance incentive equal to 10.5 percent of their base capitation by doing well on three measures of quality of care

- member satisfaction, as measured by patient surveys and the rate at which patients transfer out of one practice and into another
- chart reviews, conducted twice a year
- patient-care management, measured by the physician's cooperation and participation in health plan initiatives like pharmacy selection profiles, disease management programs, and diagnostic test selection

At the BlueChoice HMO in St. Louis, physician groups gain an immediate 12.5 percent jump in their capitation rates just for participating in the quality incentive program. Then they can earn an additional 8 percent in bonuses by meeting certain quality standards. The potential bonus is split evenly between

- scores on patient satisfaction surveys
- meeting HEDIS performance standards in the areas of cholesterol, breast cancer, diabetic retinal screening, asthma treatment for adults and children, prenatal care, and childhood immunization[6]

USING HEDIS VARIABLES AS PERFORMANCE CRITERIA

It is worth noting that the standard by which MCOs are being measured by their primary customers (employers and Health Care Financing Administration/Medicare) is becoming accreditation by the National Committee for Quality Assurance (NCQA) and the MCOs performance on NCQA's Health Plan Employer Data and Information Set (HEDIS). Many of the HEDIS measures concern the performance of the providers under contract with the MCO. Physicians should reasonably expect that MCOs, to boost their HEDIS scores, will begin to begin to use HEDIS measures as a basis for evaluating their providers. It would be a good idea to become familiar with them.

The HEDIS data set is in its 3.0 iteration. The NCQA has proposed a new version to take effect in 1999. It will include 53 measures (see Exhibit 6–1).

PARTICIPATION IN MULTIDISCIPLINARY TEAMS

Administrative and clinical processes are carried out by health care personnel in a variety of disciplines. Reengineering those processes, as with most CQI initiatives, requires the participation of representatives of all those disciplines, collaborating on more or less equal terms. This need has been addressed by the development of multidisciplinary teams.

The teams may be organized on an ad hoc basis to respond to a crisis or identified problem, or to implement a short-term quality improvement project. They may operate continuously to monitor the activities and performance of individual departments, clinics, or projects. In a typical case, a team will include an administrative director, a head nurse, and a physician manager. While reporting to their separate superiors in administration, nursing, and the medical staff, they also will be responsible for mediating conflicts, improving quality, and adapting to change within the team domain.

It can be challenging for a physician to participate on such a team. The physician will not automatically be looked to as the leader, but he must effectively communicate the perspective of his discipline (professional medicine) while listening sensitively to the perspectives of the other disciplines. Teamwork demands new skills of all participants. As with the other members, physicians can expect to be evaluated for their cooperation with the team effort and the accomplishments of the team.

MANAGING THE DEMAND FOR YOUR SERVICES

The managed care regimen has searched constantly for new ways to reduce the costs of meeting the health care needs of enrolled patients. It has negotiated discounted fees for service with providers; has managed and reduced the utilization of resources, particularly hospitals; has shifted the treatment of an entire range of diagnoses from an inpatient to an outpatient basis; has shifted the actuarial and financial risk of nearly all clinical decisions to the providers themselves; and has studied and routinized the treatment strategies for the most common diagnoses. One of the latest managed care initiatives is to manage the actual patient demand for health care services. The least expensive health care is the health care that never is delivered at all.

Demand management takes several forms. It starts with education of patients, designed to make them more discriminating consumers of health care services. They are taught which symptoms indicate serious medical problems requiring the immediate attention of a professional, which are likely to disappear on their own, and which should simply be watched to see whether they worsen. Patient education also can include directions on when and how the patient can self-treat. This information can be communicated to patients through literature, videotapes, home visits, and classes at health care facilities and in the community. All practitioners who interact with patients may have instructional roles to play. Although it is not always the best use of their time, physicians may get involved in this educational process.

When patient symptoms indicate a need for professional advice, the expense of an actual visit to a health care facility may be further postponed

Exhibit 6–1 New HEDIS Measures

EFFECTIVENESS OF CARE

- Childhood immunization status
- Adolescent immunization status
- Advice on quitting to smokers
- Flu shots for older adults
- Breast cancer screening
- Cervical cancer screening
- Prenatal care in the first trimester
- Low-birth-weight babies
- Checkups after delivery
- Beta blocker treatment after a heart attack
- Eye exams for people with diabetes
- Cholesterol management after acute cardiovascular events
- Health of seniors
- Follow-up after hospitalization for mental illness
- Antidepressant management
- Comprehensive diabetes care

ACCESS/AVAILABILITY OF CARE

- Adults' access to preventive ambulatory health services
- Children's access to primary care providers
- Initiation of prenatal care
- Annual dental visit
- Availability of language interpretation services

SATISFACTION WITH THE EXPERIENCE OF CARE

- HEDIS Consumer Survey (commercial, Medicaid)
- Experiences with children's care survey (commercial, Medicaid)

HEALTH PLAN STABILITY

- Disenrollment
- Provider turnover
- Years in business/total membership
- Indicators of financial stability

USE OF SERVICES

- Frequency of ongoing prenatal care
- Well-child visits in the first 15 months of life
- Well-child visits in the third, fourth, fifth, and sixth years of life
- Adolescent well-care visit
- Frequency of selected procedures
- Inpatient utilization—nonacute care
- Discharge and average length of stay—maternity care
- Caesarean section and vaginal birth after a Caesarean (VBAC) rate
- Births and average lengths of stay—newborns
- Mental health utilization—percentage of members receiving inpatient, day/night, and ambulatory services
- Chemical dependency utilization—inpatient discharges and average length of stay
- Chemical dependency utilization—percentage of members receiving inpatient, day/night, and ambulatory services
- Outpatient drug utilization

COST OF CARE

- Rate trends
- High-occurrence/high-cost DRGs

HEALTH PLAN DESCRIPTIVE INFORMATION

- Board certification/residency completion
- Provider compensation
- Arrangements with public health, educational, and social service organizations
- Total enrollment
- Enrollment by payer (member years/months)
- Unduplicated count of Medicaid members
- Cultural diversity of Medicaid membership
- Weeks of pregnancy at time of enrollment in the health plan

Courtesy of National Committee for Quality Assurance, Washington, DC.

by the use of telemedicine. Under appropriate circumstances, the patient is encouraged to speak by phone with a clinician, such as a physician assistant or nurse practitioner, even a physician if absolutely necessary. It is often possible, by these means, to perform a preliminary assessment and diagnosis, and to recommend a treatment plan that does not require professional intervention. If the clinician discerns a more serious condition, a visit can be scheduled.

To minimize the future use of resources, health plans and providers organizations may offer early detection and preventive care services to patients when they do come in for visits. Not only must the services be available and prescribed for individual patients, but the health plan should provide payment coverage to encourage their use. Physicians are frequently drawn into this phase of demand management. Their performance may be assessed on the frequency with which their patients are given mammograms and Pap smear tests, for instance. A balanced program of early detection and preventive care can literally prevent certain diseases from ever developing and can catch the emergence of others so early that less expensive and less invasive procedures are sufficient to treat them.

The still-growing use of gatekeepers and physician extenders can be viewed as a mechanism for reducing the demand for physician services. There is a strong tendency in health care delivery systems to push the provision of services down to the least skilled, least expensive provider capable of competently providing them. For physicians, this means that their clinical work will be narrowed to those tasks that only they are uniquely qualified to perform. The net result may be to remove a lot of the human element from that work.

INCREASED IMPORTANCE OF INTERPERSONAL SKILLS

The physician in modern managed care settings is expected to interact effectively with those around him much more than was ever necessary in solo or small group practices of the past.

- He must collaborate with physician colleagues to manage utilization of resources and maintain or improve quality of care.
- In a system using gatekeepers, hospitalists, and physician extenders, he must work with them to assure a seamless treatment experience for the patient.
- He must work amicably and productively with ancillary personnel—both clinical and administrative—in some cases, supervising them for maximum effect.
- Given the opportunity and the desire, the physician may assume managerial responsibilities over larger numbers of people—a task that more and more requires professional training and ability.
- Besides displaying the traditional salutary "bedside manner," he will be expected to create patient satisfaction in a variety of other ways.
- If the physician is more directly involved with contracts with MCOs or other payers, he may need to maintain positive working relationships with officials of those entities.
- To a more limited extent, a managed care physician must work to please government regulators and accrediting organizations on which he is dependent for continued freedom to practice medicine.
- He must be asked to participate constructively in multidisciplinary clinical teams.

The physician's continued career success will depend on his ability to demonstrate to his superiors and the key decision makers in his organization that he possesses these skills. Increasingly, his performance and compensation will be evaluated partially on these grounds.

YOUR ASSUMPTION OF ADMINISTRATIVE DUTIES

Many physicians are turning eagerly to managed care for the chance to forget about the business of running a practice and to concentrate on what they really want to do—practice medicine. On the other hand, with the recent movement toward physician-sponsored organizations and reassertion of physician control over at least the clinical side of health care delivery have come opportunities for physicians to assume significant managerial roles in their organizations. This can range from serving on board committees for physician credentialing or compensation and sitting on peer review or performance appraisal panels to working nearly full time as a facility or department manager. One thing is certain; physicians seeking these positions usually must obtain some formal management training, in addition to their scientific medical skills. They also must expect their managerial performance to be scrutinized by their superiors (often the board of directors) and their competitors.

CAREER OPPORTUNITIES UNDER MANAGED CARE

One of the advantages of participation in larger, more professionally managed organizations is the greater variety of career opportunities they offer to physicians. The possibilities available will depend on the organizational structure, geographic location, market environment, and strategic plans of each organization. These are the most likely career paths.

- *straight clinician*—do nothing but practice medicine 8 to 10 hours a day, with no business or administrative worries, a chance to hone practice skills, to improve the quality of outcomes, and to concentrate on patient interaction
- *researcher and developer of clinical outcomes measures and practice guidelines*—in addition to seeing patients, apply rigorous scientific procedures to the study and design of measures and guidelines that enable other physicians to deliver high-quality, patient-centered care with possibilities for presentation of findings at conferences and publication of research papers
- *midlevel manager of departments, clinics, and other separate facilities*—assume significant managerial responsibility for specialty department or clinic within a larger organization; deal with issues of human resources, financial management, planning, and resource allocation with an opportunity to take some initiative in creating an environment that is supportive of physicians and patients alike; patient contact may still be possible
- *high-level executive of major business functions in provider organizations*—key executive responsibility for functions such as finance, planning, marketing, network development, or managed care relations; full-time commitment requiring specialized management training; opportunity to have major impact on a major portion of a provider entity; often viewed as step on a career path to higher level executive positions; best suited for a physician willing to forgo routine clinical involvement to balance legitimate clinical and financial concerns of the organization
- *chief executive officer of a provider-sponsored organization*—a position of leadership in the ongoing transformation of the health care system; challenging and stressful work; requires substantial management training and experience; makes major strategic and policy decisions affecting many physicians (often hundreds), support personnel, patients, and payers; success can bring great material and status rewards
- *member of the board of directors of a provider-sponsored organization*—monitor and oversee the strategic direction of the organization and the performance of the chief executive officer (CEO); deal only with highest-level issues, including relations with other organizations; ultimate responsibility for the total organization; may be combined with patient care and research; opportunity to shape a provider organization in the model you have always dreamed of

Still other variations on these career paths are available in particular organizations (academic faculty practice, staff-model HMO). The new world of managed care is capable of meeting just about any career aspiration a physician might have. To qualify, however, the physician must be prepared to acquire appropriate training and experience, to make a firm, often full-time commitment to the chosen career, to work constantly to improve her vocational capabilities, and to accept accountability for the level of her work performance.

WHAT THERE IS TO LIKE ABOUT PRACTICING MEDICINE UNDER MANAGED CARE

Physicians have a lot to dislike about the impact of managed care on their role in the delivery of health care. However, it looks like it is going to be around for a while. So it might be a good idea to focus on the more appealing attributes of managed care.

- Managed care allows a physician to concentrate on practicing clinical medicine and nothing else, if that is what he wants.
- Physicians have the opportunity to assume substantial managerial and leadership responsibilities under managed care, with accompanying rewards and recognition.

- The assertive, qualified physician can be a catalyst in redefining the health care delivery model in the United States while protecting the role of physicians within it.
- Managed care offers the opportunity to work regular, predictable hours without worry about on-call responsibilities.
- A physician under managed care can earn a comfortable income without working extraordinary hours or the nagging headaches of managing the personnel and finances of a practice.
- Physicians in integrated groups serving MCOs have the ability to engage in genuinely collegial dialogue with other physicians about the most effective and quality-conscious methods of treating patients (either informally, as the member of a peer review group, or as a team member developing clinical protocols).
- Managed care gives physicians the chance to be part of an organization that is working constantly to improve the quality of medical care it provides and supports them in doing the same.

REFERENCES

1. Medical Group Management Association Member Database, data from 1996 (1997).
2. Medical Group Management Association Member Database, data from 1996 (1997).
3. Medical Group Management Association Cost Survey: 1996 Report Based on 1995 Data (1996).
4. SMG Marketing Group (1997).
5. "Turning Over Inpatients to a 'Hospitalist,'" *Medical Economics*, 22 December, 1997.
6. "Quality Counts—Right in Your Wallet," *Medical Economics*, 27 October, 1997.

RESOURCE LIST

American Medical Association. *Managing Managed Care in the Medical Practice* (Chicago: 1996).
"HMO Coverage Battle Rages On—Quality Issues at Core of High-Profile Case," *American Medical News*, 26 February, 1996.
W. Knight, *Managed Care, What It Is and How It Works* (Gaithersburg, MD: Aspen Publishers, Inc., 1998).

P. Kongstvedt, *Essentials of Managed Care*, 2d ed. (Gaithersburg, MD: Aspen Publishers, Inc., 1997).
P. Kongstvedt, *The Managed Health Care Handbook*, 3rd ed. (Gaithersburg, MD: Aspen Publishers, Inc., 1996).
"Making Physician Networks Work: Why It's Important To Educate Physicians about Managed Care," *Health Care Strategic Management*, 1 April, 1996.

Making Sense of Managed Care—Vol. I: Building Blocks and Fundamentals (San Francisco: Jossey-Bass, Publishers, 1998).

"Managed Care Relationships from the Physician's Perspective," *Topics in Health Care Financing,* 22 December, 1993.

D. Nash, ed., "Life of the HMO Physician," in *The Physician's Guide to Managed Care* (Gaithersburg, MD: Aspen Publishers, Inc., 1994).

"Old Traditions, New Realities—Dealing with New Health Care Delivery Systems," *Hospitals & Health Networks,* 5 December, 1995.

"Pediatric Practice: How To Survive and Thrive in the Changing Health Care System—A Look at the Private Practice of the Future," *Pediatrics,* October 1995.

"Primary Care in Transition," *JAMA,* 16 November, 1994.

R. Rognehaugh, *The Managed Care Dictionary,* 2d ed. (Gaithersburg, MD: Aspen Publishers, Inc., 1998).

## CHAPTER 7

Step One: Preparing Your Practice for Operation under Managed Care

INTRODUCTION

Many physicians would have trouble adjusting if suddenly thrust into a managed care practice environment as described in the previous chapter. The changes in practice style, group culture, interactions with other physicians, and permitted use of resources are radical departures from medical practice in a solo or small group setting. The chances of success would be limited.

There are steps a physician can take to assess his readiness to compete in the managed care world. Where deficiencies are revealed, he can begin to make improvements before trying to practice managed care medicine.

This chapter highlights the areas of medical practice critical to success with managed care organizations (MCOs). It proposes and describes a formal audit of practice features to assess readiness. Then it recommends practical measures for modifying the nature of the practice and the attitude of the physician toward managed care.

The purpose of this chapter is to teach the physician-reader what abilities she needs to do well at managed care, to help her figure out whether she currently has those abilities, and to guide her in acquiring them.

WHO SHOULD READ THIS CHAPTER

Practicing medicine under managed care—in the manner described in Chapter 6—is not intuitive. Your medical school training and previous practice experience is likely to have taught you the wrong impulses for managed care: testing thoroughly before diagnosing, applying treatment in optimal quantities and at highest technology levels, and spending time informing and reassuring the patient.

It makes sense to think deliberately about what MCOs will demand of you, then to train and prepare yourself in advance for those challenges, so that you are effective and successful at the new game. Do not learn how to deliver "managed" care on the MCO's time. You may find yourself deselected before you are halfway up the learning curve.

If you plan to be moving into managed care practice for the first time in the near future, read this chapter for recommendations on steps you can take immediately (changes you can make in your practice style and in the operation of your practice) to hone the necessary skills.

If you have experience contracting with MCOs, you have had a taste of the managed care life. However, you probably have not been subjected to the full press of risk-sharing and utilization management that will be your future. There are several further adjustments you must make in the way you deliver medicine; this chapter will lay them out for you.

You may be able to skip this chapter if you have practiced for a year or two under a capitated agreement, particularly in a larger group practice setting. Still, there may be some additional lessons you can learn here. Except for the managed care hot spots, such as Southern California and Minnesota, very few physicians have spent enough time at this new kind of medicine to be fully adept at it. Read the chapter!

ACTION STEPS IN PREPARING FOR MANAGED CARE

1. Start with a New Perspective

You probably began reading this book with the attitude that it could enhance and secure your professional well-being. Fine. However, the key to practice success is also viewing your practice from a marketing perspective.

If you were an MCO, would you want to contract for medical services from a physician like you? Do you provide the type of services required by the MCO's plan for "one-stop shopping" health care? Are the services of a quality and at a cost commensurate with the health care package being marketed by the MCO to payers and patients? Can you participate effectively in the MCO's utilization management and quality assurance programs? Are you flexible enough to adjust as the MCO changes its provider relations in the future (perhaps incorporating practice guidelines) to adapt to evolving market conditions?

If you were a payer, would you want to pay limited monies for the medical services that you deliver? Are your services worth the money you would be paid? Do you have the skills to constantly improve the cost-effectiveness of your practice style? Do your services result in the outcomes that the payer wishes to offer to its customer/patients?

If you were a patient, would you want to be treated by a physician like you? Does medical care at your hands produce outcomes acceptable to the kinds of patients you will be treating in the future? Do you know and understand what kinds of patients will be steered your way by the MCO and payer? Apart from actual outcomes, how sat-

isfied are patients with a treatment experience in your practice?

There are two basic characteristics of medical care: *quality* and *cost*. A third characteristic is *value*—a combination of the first two.

Some would say that the traditional American attitude toward its medical care has been: "Provide the absolute highest quality care, regardless of the cost." Today, others would say that MCOs are demanding that physicians "provide the absolute lowest cost care, regardless of the effect on quality."

In the late 1980s, managed care did tend to stress cost containment. However, the age of unrestrained discounting is almost over.

In the 1990s, if you come upon an MCO that genuinely demands the latter brand of care from you, avoid it! You probably are unwilling to practice that kind of medicine at all. More important, an MCO that offers that kind of product will not survive long in the marketplace. Fortunately, the majority of MCOs you will encounter are after something else—good quality care at a reasonable cost.

2. Put Your Practice under a Microscope

Gather data that will permit you to evaluate the following practice characteristics:

- patient demographics
- medical services required
- payer mix
- referral source mix
- referral source satisfaction
- patient satisfaction
- treatment outcomes

Patient Demographics

From your medical records, compile aggregate figures on the age, sex, and place of residence (by ZIP code) of all your patients. Similar historical information will reveal possible trends in these characteristics. These data will help you assess contract or affiliation opportunities with MCOs and integrated delivery systems (IDSs).

If you have been treating patients of particular ages or sex, you may not be interested in or capable of handling a dramatically different patient population offered by an MCO. If you discover that your patients traditionally have come certain geographic distances from certain communities, an MCO's members living in other communities or at greater distances may be unwilling to frequent your practice. The result will be an attractive contract that produces few patients who select you for their care.

Medical Services Required

Examine your billing records to prepare a profile of the medical services typically provided to your existing patients. This could be nothing more than a list of the ten most frequently billed codes. You may be surprised by what you find. This information will tell you a lot about the nature of your practice (the kinds of patients you are seeing, the problems they present, and the therapies you most commonly deliver). It also becomes the basis of comparison with what will be expected of you under each managed care contract. A large difference between those expectations and your current practice may cause you to reconsider entering into the contract.

Payer Mix

Billing records should also reveal to you the percentage of patients and revenues coming from each payer and type of payer. The trends are just as important as the absolute figures. If many or most of your patients are covered by indemnity policies when managed care already has made inroads into your market, you are behind the competitive curve. If many or most of your patients are employees of a single employer or of a very few employers, you may be left in the lurch if that employer switches to an MCO with which you do not have a contract. The best situation is a growing percentage of patients and revenues from managed care sources, coupled with contracts with most of the larger employers in the area. Of course, what is appropriate depends on

the economic and competitive conditions, as well as on the intensity of managed care activity in your area.

Referral Source Mix

If you practice in a specialty that relies extensively on referrals for patients, you must be concerned with the sources of those referrals. Your medical records should document how each patient came to you. If not, set up a simple system right now to begin gathering this information. Your patients will be either self-referred or directed to you by other patients, other physicians, a physician referral service—hospital or preferred provider organization (PPO)-based— or an MCO with which you have a contract. The incursion and expansion of MCOs into your market area can disrupt established referral patterns. Primary care sources may be restricted by their MCOs to a select group of specialists—cutting you out. Or, as a primary care physician, you may be prevented from continuing to refer to specialists who are long-time colleagues and friends. If you are aware of your current referral sources, you can better understand how they may change under a particular managed care contract.

Referral Source Satisfaction

Even if the managed care plan does not try to influence your referral patterns, you should make sure that your sources are happy with your handling of their patients. In times of high competitive stress and pressure from MCOs to minimize utilization while employing the most cost-effective resources, you cannot afford to be complacent about their satisfaction. Begin immediately contacting your major referral sources and soliciting their feedback on every aspect of their referral relationship with you. At the same time, establish a regular procedure for surveying referral source satisfaction.

Patient Satisfaction

You probably believe that your patients are more than pleased with the health care they receive from you. You are probably right. However, in the off-chance that they do have some gripes about your practice, it is preferable to learn about yourself before entering into managed care contracts than to have the MCO discover the problems later, through its own member surveys. It is time to institute regular surveys of all your patients to gauge their levels of satisfaction. When problems are revealed, act promptly to correct them and advise the complaining patient of the remedy. If the surveys confirm your patients' contentment, you have documentary evidence to show to MCOs. They will be interested—before and after they enter into a contract with you.

Treatment Outcomes

You are not likely to have scientific data demonstrating the efficacy of your clinical decisions, as measured in the outcomes realized by patients. Do assemble whatever facts you do have that tend to demonstrate the quality of your care. This will be found largely in patient medical records but may also be reflected in your levels of clinical privileges at local hospitals, statements about your general reputation, testimonials from referring physicians, and so forth. You ought to begin planning the implementation of a formal system for assessing the outcomes of your practice methods. This is a complex task; outcomes research at major teaching hospitals has been going on for only five years or so. It will take your group a significant amount of time and money. Eventually, when you are operating fully under managed care and capitation, systems like this will be mandatory. The sooner you get started, the better.

3. Educate Yourself and Your Colleagues about Managed Care and the Business of Medical Care Delivery

You need to acquire further knowledge in two broad areas to prosper in the American health care system of the twenty-first century. You first must understand how that system works, who the key players are, how the money flows among them, and what determinants of success are. You

have to fully grasp the nuances of medical practice under the managed care concept. Your second area of new learning concerns the basic business functions that underpin a modern, well-managed medical practice.

These are some specific topics you might concentrate on:

- economics of the U.S. health care system
- practicing medicine under capitation
- assessing outcomes of care
- clinical practice guidelines in the outpatient setting
- basic management of service businesses
- creating a vision and strategic planning
- basic business accounting (cash and accrual methods)
- basic financial management
- sources and terms of investment capital for health care providers
- basic marketing, advertising, and promotion
- people management skills for health care practitioners
- teambuilding among physicians

Look for courses on these topics in several places. The most common sponsors of seminars/workshops running one or more days, as well as courses spread over several weeks, are professional medical societies, group practice trade associations and publications, independent seminar companies, and college and university professional development programs, night schools, and extension programs. Education courses for physicians and group managers on these topics are "hot" right now. Contact these organizations, get on their mailing lists, and pick the courses that excite your interest. Stress physician-focused courses in health care economics and accounting of financial management.

Research the health care market in your area. (Read Chapter 14, "Assessing the Market for Managed Care/Integration Opportunities" for more information.) Familiarize yourself with the key players and their strategic plans and motives.

Strongly encourage every member of your group to participate in this education effort. It is important that every physician member have a solid foundation of knowledge upon which to base the business and practice decisions he will have to make in the future. This also is a good activity to pursue if you are currently unwilling or unable to take overt action to move your practice strategically.

Learning requires no commitments. When you are ready to move, you will be able to make prompt, informed decisions.

4. Know and Keep Constantly in Mind the Professional, Financial, and Personal Goals of Each of Your Group Members

Meld them into your organizational goals. Work consistently to keep each other contented. These goals are the reasons that each of you is practicing medicine, the reasons that you have come together in a group, and the reasons that you are planning new strategic initiatives. All this effort is pointless if it does not serve the goals. If the group activities stray too far from each member's goals, the risk is alienation, disruption, and eventual dissolution.

Early in the new planning and growth process you are embarking upon, meet as a group, away from work and office, perhaps on a Saturday retreat, to get clear on everyone's goals. Write them down. Consult them closely as you develop a vision and a strategic plan for the group. Revisit the goals annually and whenever a significant new strategic move is contemplated. Pay serious attention to complaints and upsets from any of your partners. Resolve them promptly and thoroughly or they will fester and corrode the organization.

5. Make Sure That the Goals of all the Physicians in Your Group Are in Alignment, in Terms of Culture, Cost Emphasis, Quality Emphasis, Physician Control and Autonomy, and Strategic Ambition

"Alignment" does not require "agreement." It means that each physician's goals for what he or she wants to achieve through the organization are compatible with those of everyone else in the group. They can coexist.

In the excitement of creating a new organization, acquiring new skills, or securing new managed care contracts, the physicians may not take the time to check that they all want approximately the same things from their common venture—not only now, but also in the future. These unexplored personal agendas can sabotage the long-range strategic plan. If alignment cannot be achieved, some group members may have to leave.

6. Begin Developing a Critical Mass of Physicians with the Intention of Creating a Significant Market Presence

As in almost every field of human endeavor, numbers and size make a difference. Larger groups are more powerful competitors—for several reasons. You will have more resources to start with, and your revenue-earning potential will command even greater additional resources. Bankers and investors feel more comfortable financing the operations of larger, more established entities. You will have greater appeal when recruiting new physicians. Your larger size will support more sophisticated practice management systems. Your greater size takes up more space in the community consciousness and in the media, attracting even more business. A larger group of physicians can handle a larger population of patients; under a risk-sharing contract, this allows you to spread the risk over more covered lives.

You will have greater leverage in negotiations with MCOs, insurance companies, employers, other payers, and any other parties. Hospitals listen more closely to large groups of doctors. MCOs are more willing to negotiate contract terms with more sizable physician-hospital networks. Employers are more interested in contracting directly with full-service, broad geographic coverage delivery systems. Most MCOs actually prefer to deal with larger, and presumably more businesslike, physician groups. (Note: A few MCOs are threatened by bigger, stronger groups and prefer to go after smaller, weaker practices. You do not want to work with them, anyway.) Remember also that every physician who is part of your group is not part of another group that might compete against you.

Building a "critical mass" simply means steadily and systematically expanding the size of your group or organization, particularly in terms of numbers of physicians, specialties covered, affiliated hospitals, ancillary personnel, and points of presence. Hire new physicians, acquire the practices of established physicians, bring in physicians in new specialties, establish partnerships of various sorts with hospitals, set up clinics and other satellite facilities, and invest in ancillary service facilities. What constitutes a critical mass will vary. The number may be 20 physicians in one town and 200 in a nearby city.

Picture physician groups as many drops of water on a flat surface. When one runs into another, they become a new, larger drop, in a much stronger position to absorb still other drops. The smaller drops seem almost drawn to the larger ones. Eventually, one drop becomes so large that it is really a substantial pool of water that dominates the area.

7. Build an Internal Governance Structure That Is Flexible and Responsive Enough To Carry Your Group through the Changes and Decisions Required over the Next 5 to 10 Years

The chances are that you and your partners have governed your small group practice in a pretty informal way. In fact, some well-established multispecialty groups have rather loose, impromptu governance mechanisms. These work fine under conditions of low competitive pressure and few challenging decisions.

In the next few years, your practice will be subjected to severe competitive forces. You and your colleagues will be called upon to make strategic and tactical decisions that will determine your professional futures. The decisions will entail new relationships with unfamiliar people and organizations, a reshaping and resizing of your organization, the expenditure of large sums of money, and the acceptance of high risk. Frequently, the decisions will have to be made on short notice. They will involve controversial issues that threaten to alienate some of your colleagues.

Your group needs a governance structure that is up to these challenges. Now is the time, before the pressure builds, to institute a mechanism that produces wise decisions, based on thorough background analysis and full awareness of every partner's wishes. Some important principles of good governance are

- adequate representation on the governing body for key constituencies within the group
- willingness of group members to abide by decisions of the governing body (or leave the group)
- commitment to gathering full background information before making decisions
- formal procedure for soliciting the views of all group members before making major strategic decisions
- established procedure for submitting proposals and voting on decisions in a timely fashion
- explanation of the levels of majority necessary to make decisions of different levels of importance
- formal procedure for reporting all decisions of the governing body to the full membership of the group

Think deliberately about these elements of governance structure.

- which governing bodies (i.e., board of directors, executive committee, various subcommittees) will make which decisions
- how the members of those bodies will be chosen
- how often the bodies will meet
- the decision-making processes they will follow (i.e., unanimous vote, majority vote, supermajority vote on select issues)

- how much authority to delegate to individuals, particularly managers (both physician and nonphysician)

Keep in mind that the structure will have to evolve as the organization grows, assimilates new constituencies, enters into new external relationships, and faces new challenges. Chapter 22, "Creating an Effective Governance Structure for an Affiliated or Integrated Physician Group," provides more detail on designing an effective governance structure for integrated physician groups.

8. Identify and Develop Physician Leaders within Your Group Who Have the Necessary Business Acumen, Professional Reputation, and Strategic Wisdom

To plan and carry out managed care strategies and tactics requires the ability to envision a bold new future for the group or organization and to mobilize all its members to create that future. Some leaders are born, but they also can be made. This involves identifying those physicians most qualified and interested in moving into leadership positions. Design systematic custom-tailored programs to build their leadership skills through education and experience. Provide them with in-house and outside opportunities to study leadership and management in formal settings. Give them increasingly responsible leadership assignments within the organization. Do not hesitate to remove from positions of authority those who do not demonstrate the necessary leadership qualities. If you do not, the entire organization will pay the price.

9. Develop Skills in Working Collegially among the Physician Members of Your Group

Aim to grow comfortable in collaborating on both business and clinical matters. The new paradigm in practice management places the well-being of the group above the parochial interests of individual members. MCOs are looking for groups of physicians who act as a unit, support

and critique each other's clinical practices, stand by the decisions of the group, and—together—share the risks of treating an entire population of covered lives. It will take deliberate action to create such a collegial work atmosphere.

Attend and learn from one of the many workshops on team building. Implement a governance structure that requires and rewards group decision making that is as consensual as possible. Establish procedures and routines for joint activities among group members: peer review, utilization management, strategic planning, continuing education, and other opportunities that present themselves. When discussing the group with your partners or others outside the group, speak of "we" rather than "I." Constantly tend to the needs of each other in the group. Establish procedures for dealing with the problems, complaints, and upsets that some group members will have with changes in structure and culture as the group evolves.

This change in the working relationships among physicians is a radical departure and will take time. Be dedicated and persistent. It is essential to the long-term health of the group.

10. Develop a Staff of Individuals Who Understand and Adjust to Their New Roles in Managed Care

The same adjustment in attitude and knowledge regarding managed care required of physicians must be carried out with the group's support staff. Give your staff the same kinds of training in managed care concepts and alternatives that you are receiving. Help them to understand how managed care contracts, new affiliations for the group, and perhaps even a new group structure will affect the way the organization functions. Teach them what their new roles will involve as the group changes. Keep them up to date on your managed care plans and strategies. Arrange for additional training in the new skills they will need. Generate in your staff a sense of enthusiasm and optimism for the new practice paradigm.

Hire new staff people with prior experience in managed care environments. Begin creating and filling new staff positions to perform uniquely managed care tasks, such as

- obtaining MCO-required prior authorizations
- checking patient eligibility
- gathering and analyzing utilization data
- tracking costs by procedure
- measuring and managing patient satisfaction
- assessing and enhancing clinical outcomes
- developing practice guidelines and clinical pathways

People in these job categories will be essential to the smooth operation of the group under managed care and capitation.

Generally upgrade the competence of all your support staff. A professionally-managed practice employs fully trained, well-motivated, industry-knowledgeable, competition-aware people.

11. Develop an Outwardly Focused Orientation Supported by Externally Focused Systems

Gone are the days when you could just deliver good quality care and count on enough new patients showing up. In the new competitive health care industry of the 1990s, you must reach out aggressively to attract not only patients, but MCOs, insurance companies, employers, other payers, referral sources, and prospective strategic partners. This is addressed through these functions.

- market research (to find out what your competitors are doing, what your customers want, and how your practice is perceived by the public)
- marketing (to broadcast your existence, your capabilities, and your services to the public)
- public relations (through more subtle means, to create a favorable impression of your practice in the eyes of both stakeholders and the public)
- outreach (through mailings, workshops, health fairs, and the like, to make a noncommercial connection with the community)
- patient relations (through mailings, phone calls, and direct conversations, to maintain a supportive relationship that continues beyond their specific medical episodes)

Within those functions, here are a few of the initiatives you should consider taking.

- Get very clear on what the strengths or advantages of your group are and what distinguishes you from other similar groups.
- Start to define and pay attention to who your competition is. (Note: If an MCO comes into town and is thinking about contracting with your group, what alternative groups might they contract with?)
- Define all your stakeholders, find out what they want, and adopt some kind of conscious strategy for each one.
- Assertively contact MCOs and employers with which you might contract and ask them, "What can we do to support you and help you succeed?"
- Take a course in basic principles of marketing for health care providers.
- Explore the form and content of marketing that you might do for your organization.
- Take steps to project the perception to the community that you are meeting its needs.

> **Note:** Think seriously about hiring a public relations firm for the purpose of placing the positive attributes of your practice more noticeably in the public eye. This is not a form of lying; it is not even advertising. It is simply a matter of finding forums and venues (media appearances, speaking engagements, article publications) in which the abilities of your physicians and the unique qualities of your practice can be presented to the community. If a new MCO moves into the area and finds everyone talking about your group, they will think you are special and will be more inclined to seek a contract with you.

12. Prepare Yourself To Be the Kind of Physician That MCOs Want

There are certain characteristics that MCOs find appealing in the physicians who will join their provider panels. They are indicators that the MCO's members will be well served, the members' employers or other premium payers will be content with value received, and the MCO will prosper financially.

Create the ability to "show and tell" MCOs what they want to know about your group: what is good and attractive about the group, what abilities and systems you have, what your attitude is, what your record and reputation are, and what you can do for them and their customers.

This ability to demonstrate—to prove the existence of—certain features of your practice is valuable in persuading an MCO to contract with you initially, and mandatory if you wish to maintain the contract. Here are some of the attributes that MCOs are looking for in their physician groups.

- evidence that your practice delivers high-quality care
- evidence that your practice delivers cost-effective care
- evidence that patients are happy with the care they receive from you
- comparisons of your practice's costs, utilization rates, quality measures, and patient satisfaction with regional or national averages
- systems in place to measure and manage quality
- systems in place to measure patient satisfaction and correct problems
- systems in place to measure and control costs
- systems in place to measure and manage utilization
- procedures for rigorously credentialing and monitoring all of your physicians

Show quality commitment through

- strict criteria for adding new physicians
- good recordkeeping
- benchmark of your quality data with local, state, or national standards
- quality assurance programs
- assessment and surveys of patients on a regular basis

Some of the more subjective characteristics sought after by good MCOs are

- good skills in communicating with each other, with staff, with patients, with other practitioners, and with the MCO
- enthusiastic knowledge and embrace of the managed care concept
- willingness to change and adapt to constantly evolving conditions in health care delivery
- appreciation of the goals and needs of MCOs
- personal commitment to quality of care
- geographic coverage, physical and personal accessibility, hours coverage
- willingness to go "the extra mile" in servicing the MCO's enrollees

It is not enough to tell a prospective MCO partner that your group possesses these qualities. You must show them. Be able to present the following kinds of documentation:

- procedural manuals for your data-gathering systems
- output reports from those systems (specifically, reports on utilization rates, clinical outcomes, costs by procedure)
- results of patient satisfaction surveys
- staff job descriptions indicating responsibility for managed care–related issues
- written case studies
- written testimonials from patients, colleagues, referral sources, payers, and other relevant stakeholders
- TV appearance videotapes, published articles, announcements of speaking engagements

This sort of evidence will help you to secure a first contract with the MCO. There is likely to be language in that contract requiring your group to gather and report back to the MCO data on the critical parameters mentioned above. The contract may also mandate the implementation of certain tracking and monitoring systems. The key to success under managed care is delivering high-value medical care and having the information to prove it.

13. Go After Managed Care Business

Do not wait for MCOs to approach you. Identify the most attractive managed care companies and opportunities, and aggressively pursue them. In an industry where most physicians wait passively for an MCO to come knocking, then sign anything thrust at them or become very anxious wondering whether to sign at all, a group of physicians that takes the initiative in approaching MCOs will stand out. They will get and keep contracts with the MCOs they want.

How does a physician group take a more assertive stance with MCOs? The first step is to get your practice in order. You should be well on your way to installing the tracking and control systems that are prerequisites to successful managed care participation. Then seek out and negotiate a few small MCO contracts, representing 10 percent or 15 percent of your revenues. Two to four contracts would be a good start. Through them, gain experience working with MCOs and practicing under a managed care regimen. Learn the new clinical and management skills called for. Make mistakes and grow from them. You may do so poorly initially that you actually lose one of the contracts. Try to maintain your relationships with the more physician-friendly MCOs.

After perhaps a couple of years, when your competence and confidence have improved, shift into high gear. If you have a choice, identify the largest, strongest, and best MCOs in the area. It may be one of those with which you already have a contract. Look for the following qualities:

- is financially sound and well capitalized
- acknowledges physician dominance in clinical decision making
- has a reputation for building collaborative partnerships with physician groups
- offers products with a balanced mix of quality and cost
- is committed to continual innovation and improvement
- has "good chemistry" between you and the MCOs you must work with

Then execute contracts with as many of largest, strongest, best MCOs as you can handle and as meet your criteria (Exhibit 7–1).

At some point, one of your MCO partners may begin to emerge as a market leader. Perhaps this will coincide with the development of a stronger, closer working relationship between your group and the MCO. The operating links between the two entities may increase. The MCO may account for a growing share of the group's revenues. More and more, your group and the MCO may see your futures as intertwined. It may then seem appropriate to drop the contracts with the other MCOs and concentrate on building your partnership with the one.

Take this same proactive approach with other prospective strategic partners. It works with employers with whom you might want to direct contract and other providers with whom you might want to collaborate in building an integrated delivery system.

Exhibit 7–1 Rule of Thumb about the Number and Size of Managed Care Contracts

- The portion of a provider's patient base that is closely bound to one contract or payer is not too significant.
- The more a provider relies on a particular contract as a source of revenue, the less power that provider may have at contract renegotiation time.
- Some suggest that a practice should provide services to only a specified number of MCO contracts at one time.
- The critical issue is not so much the number of contracts, but the administrative burden they place on the practice and its ability to bear them.
- An administrative and fiscal nightmare will result if the practice is not organized to function under or comply with the contract's requirements.
- At some point, even in a well-run practice, administrative costs of multiple contract administration may exceed the revenue from the additional contracts (patients). Thorough practice analysis helps the practice recognize when that point is reached.

14. Plan Future Capital Financing Needs and Start Accumulating Growth Capital

One of the primary prerequisites to bold managed care strategies for physicians is sufficient capital. Lack of adequate start-up financing is one of the main reasons new businesses fail. Ironically, one thing physicians have never done well is accumulate capital for reinvestment in their practices.

Avoid this problem and prepare for the future by doing two things now. Look ahead to anticipate the amounts of investment capital you will need in the coming years to move your practice in the directions you want to go. This simply means preparing detailed annual operating budgets and multiyear capital spending budgets, and measuring your actual performance against them. A further prerequisite to such budgets is a solid long-range strategic plan. The second step is to begin setting aside the capital you will use to support those budgets. This requires that you do not take out of the practice at the end of the year all of the money that is left after paying your expenses. Reinvest it in the practice. Place it in a relatively safe investment instrument where it can increase in value. Then it will be available when needed to acquire the information systems, physician practices, or other resources that underlie your strategic plan. This accumulated capital, or "retained earnings," will not meet all of your capital needs. Eventually, it will be necessary to borrow money and to sell shares in corporate entities you have created.

15. Start Building an Entire Array of Management Information Systems (MIS) Modules That Will Empower You To Develop, Measure, and Demonstrate the Competencies Demanded by Managed Care and MCOs

One of the leading applications of your investment capital will be the MIS needed to practice the high-quality, low-cost medicine that MCOs are looking for. This includes the hardware, the software, and the personnel. Some of the key pieces of such systems are the following:

- market-based performance measurements using external data resources
- financial reports: monthly income statement, balance sheet, payer mixes, aged accounts receivable by payer, percentage of reimbursement from each payer, gross and net collections—monitor the changes over time, the trends; line item posting of expenditures; reporting by procedure for reimbursement from each payer
- tracking of referrals, preauthorizations, and eligibility ratings
- tracking of performance of each contract
- measurements of productivity, resource utilization, outcomes
- automated medical records
- electronic interface capabilities
- electronic communication links with payers, affiliated providers, and, eventually, patients
- benchmarking

16. Implement Managed Care–Friendly Systems—Utilization Review, Physician Credentialing, and Monitoring

In addition to the tangible MIS system, there is a variety of systematic procedures and policies that facilitates care management and that MCOs expect to see. They include

- review of the utilization of resources by individual physicians
- credentialing and recredentialing of physicians for their ability to deliver quality medical care efficiently
- continual monitoring of the clinical quality of care by individual physicians
- continual assessment of patient satisfaction with their physician encounters
- development of standard protocols for the most common procedures

Move with all deliberate speed to introduce these systems. It may involve familiarizing yourself with the best approaches, choosing one that fits your group or practice, creating the necessary policies and forms, and training all personnel in its implementation. In some cases, it may make sense to purchase a proprietary system package from a vendor or other provider group. It will require the expenditure of time and money. Do not try to implement everything at once. Set priorities; follow a plan and budget.

17. Develop the Additional Infrastructure Components Necessary for Delivering Managed Care

The several care management systems are the major structural additions most physician practices must make to adapt to demands of MCOs. A few other changes are usually called for. Give greater emphasis to the role of primary care physicians. Rely on their medical skills as much as possible, until they reasonably determine that a specialist referral is necessary. Gradually move toward implementation of a "gatekeeper" system. Within the limits of the law and clinical common sense, hire and use lower-cost physician extenders (nurse practitioners, physician assistants) as aggressively as possible. Adopt or create drug formularies for use by all physicians. Pay close attention to the accessibility and availability of your services. Consider the physical location, and open satellite clinics if it makes market sense. Adjust office hours to patient needs.

18. Install a Productivity-Based Physician Compensation Plan

Regardless of how the group is being reimbursed, set up a method for compensating individual physicians that rewards desirable behavior. There are a few steps to this process.

a. Decide on what physician-controllable variables you want to encourage (patient satisfaction, clinical outcomes, resource utilization, supervisory effectiveness).
b. Establish mechanisms for measuring the performance of those variables by each physician.
c. Tie each physician's performance levels to at least some part of her compensation. For example, make a percentage of compensa-

tion contingent on meeting certain performance goals or pay out bonuses for achievement of the goals.

Money is a powerful motivator. Make sure that your monetary incentives stimulate the kinds of physician action that are good for the whole group.

19. Commit Yourselves to Assuming Risk on Several Levels

Traditional medical practice was a no-brainer, no-lose situation. You could set up practice in a convenient location and pretty much count on doing well financially for the rest of your career. If you had solid practice skills, there were few risks in practicing medicine. That is no longer true.

To succeed in a competitive managed care environment, both individuals physicians and the groups to which they belong must be prepared to take serious risks. If they do not, if they try to avoid risky decisions and transactions and relationships, if they try to play it safe, they will lose out. Attractive opportunities will pass them by because of their conservative stance.

These are some of the risks you may have to consider.

• the risk of losing the money that you invest in a new provider organization that fails
• the risk that you sell your practice to a hospital that proves incapable of managing it effectively
• the risk that you sell your practice to a physician practice management company (PPMC) whose managerial style is too heavy-handed, disrespectful of physician clinical prerogatives, or simply headed in directions you cannot support
• the risk that you sell your practice to a PPMC that lacks the wisdom or resources to compete and fails
• the risk that you acquire poorly designed, poorly installed, and poorly supported systems from the wrong vendors, leaving you incapable of managing care effectively

- the risk of contracting with certain MCOs that fail to attract large numbers of enrollees and the risk of not contracting with other MCOs that have greater market success
- the risk of contracting with the only MCO in town, only to find it an incompatible strategic partner
- the risk of agreeing to a reimbursement fee schedule or capitation rate that your group is unable to live within because of inadequate cost controls or an unpredictable incidence of catastrophic patient illnesses
- the risk of doing nothing and discovering too late that no provider organizations or delivery systems are interested in you

Except for the last one, these are all risks that you or your group may reasonably choose to accept after careful analysis and weighing of options. Business leaders and owners have made risky choices such as these for decades. The delivery of health care is now a business, and you must make similar choices. You might as well become skilled at it.

20. Get in before You Have Too Many Competitors—Those Who Take the Early Risks Will Be the Winners in the End

When the affiliation and consolidation process is completed in each market area, some physicians will be associated with the best provider networks and MCOs in town; other physicians will settle for a connection with the less attractive organizations; still others will end up on the very fringes of the delivery infrastructure; and a few will be left out entirely and will have to leave either the market or the practice of medicine. Some physicians will be in positions of ownership or management in their organizations with a lot of control over their careers and work lives. Most will be employees or small partners with little influence.

As a general rule, the sooner you take action—of almost any sort—the better your market posi-

tion will be five years from now and for the rest of your professional life. You will beat your competitors to the best provider networks, specialist affiliations, hospital partnerships, managed care contracts, and patient-member pools. In some markets, through the formation of independent practice associations (IPAs) or the mandate of patient choice, it may seem like every physician will be able to have a working relationship with every delivery system and MCO in town. In the long run, however, as those entities compete with each other, they must be more selective in the physicians with which they choose to affiliate. They will let go all but the best, most efficient practitioners.

In some markets, such as Southern California, it is nearly too late for physicians to make their first moves into the managed care arena. All the networks have been formed, all the provider panels filled. In most other markets, even those heavily penetrated by managed care, such as Massachusetts and Minnesota, there still are opportunities for late-blooming physicians to get a good seat at the table. There also are some slower-developing markets where aggressive physician groups can steal a march on the rest of their competitors. Wherever you are practicing, act now! If you are not taking any managed care initiatives, just do something. If you already trying to adapt to the new managed care paradigm, work harder at it. Become more aggressive, move faster, invest more money, and take more risks. It will pay off for you in the future.

21. Set a Goal and Attitude of Not Just Accepting, but Actually Embracing Managed Care

It may seem like a subtle distinction, but the physicians who display open enthusiasm for managed care are likely to be more successful than the ones whose managed care efforts are reluctant or halfhearted. Your attitude will influence the eagerness and commitment behind any action you take. Those you deal with, especially the MCOs and other payers, will notice it.

22. Acquire the Tools for Working Collegially

Physicians coming from a solo and small group practice tradition often lack experience in working together toward common goals. Such collaboration is essential to managed care success, whether in assembling a new integrated physician organization or simply creating a patient treatment plan with several involved physicians. It may take some concentrated effort to learn how to do this.

Start by forming work groups or task forces to attack small discrete problems. Pay a lot of attention to the interaction and process that occurs among the physicians. Critique your effectiveness. Bring in consultants or facilitators to help you acquire new team skills. Attend workshops or conduct retreats focused on building more productive physician interplay.

23. Collect and Analyze Data on Every Aspect of Your Practice Concerning Cost, Quality, and Patient Satisfaction

Use the data to control these critical factors and show them to payers to prove that you are an efficient provider of quality medical care. Track specialist referrals, return visits, drug prescriptions, and lab tests by physician. Correlate clinical outcomes and patient satisfaction with each physician's performance. Track the performance of each contract. Compare resources expended to income received. Analyze the service demands, resource utilization, and epidemiology of the group's patients by payer and by demographic classification. The primary purpose of the MIS and other systems mentioned earlier is exactly this data gathering and control.

24. Start Doing Benchmarking

Constantly compare your group to the norms or to the best in the industry. The term *benchmarking* is interpreted in several ways. In one of the better versions, it means identifying and adopting the best policies, procedures, and practices for each aspect of your group's operations. For instance, copy the excellent claims processing system of group A, the attractive waiting room décor of group B, the efficient phone system of group C, and the economic drug inventory management program of group D. You end up being better than any one of those groups because you have taken the best of each. There is no need to restrict your search for best practices to physician practices or the health care industry. One hospital that wished to improve the way that patients first were registered for a period of hospitalization studied the way that Four Seasons Hotels operated their front desks.

25. Determine and Prepare To Promote Your Strengths

Identify those practice attributes that give you a competitive edge. These could be a unique patient service, an accessible location or office hours, convenient on-site ancillary services, hospital or health plan affiliations, or a combination of physician specialties. It is important to be coldly objective about this. Be ready with facts to back up a claim of market superiority. Do not believe that you offer "high-quality medical care" unless you have been able to compare your work to what other physicians are doing.

Promote these strengths and positive characteristics to all relevant stakeholders—current patients, prospective patients, current and prospective strategic partners, referral sources, affiliated providers, MCOs and other payers, employers, regulators, politicians, community leaders, business leaders, and members of the public. Use the tools mentioned in the action step above on "externally focused systems." Do as much or as little as you feel comfortable doing. Your competitors will be doing the same.

26. Determine Your Weaknesses and Prepare To Correct Them

This is the corollary of the previous step. It may be a little harder to think honestly about what is wrong with your practice and the way you practice medicine. If you do not expose these inadequacies and move to correct them, you can be sure that someone else will discover them. It may be an MCO you have contracted with, a patient you have treated, an affiliated provider or referral source, a government regulator, or a competitor.

Possible weaknesses might be insufficient training in a procedure increasingly required by patients, poorly trained office staff, inability to track costs of providing particular services, an obsolete computer system, unfamiliarity with techniques of care management, unattractive office décor, or excessive operating costs. The practice audit suggested below is a more comprehensive way of examining these shortcomings.

The next step is to formulate an extended plan for correcting these weaknesses. Try this approach.

1. For each area of weakness, describe in detail the actions necessary to correct. eliminate, or defuse it.
2. Estimate the cost and length of time necessary to implement those actions.
3. Keeping in mind the available resources (money, staff, management time) and market pressures, set priorities for improvement among the weaknesses.
4. Begin to incorporate the highest priority corrective actions into the practice's operating and strategic plans. Be sure to set completion dates and measurable standards for determining when the problem has been resolved.

27. Carefully Review Every Managed Care Contract You Sign

Over the life of your practice, you are likely to be offered many such contracts. It is to your advantage to learn how to rigorously evaluate their language. The recommendations in Chapter 8, "Step Two: How To Analyze and Evaluate a Managed Care Contract," are a good starting point. Read a couple of the articles and books in that chapter's resource list. Consider taking a good workshop on managed care contract review for physicians. When you are getting close to

entering into a capitation contract, do the same kind of advance preparation. Chapter 20, "Negotiating and Practicing under a Capitation Contract," will give you a basic background.

KEY VARIABLES FOR SUCCESS IN MANAGED CARE

By reviewing the managed care experiences of many physicians over the last ten or so years, it is possible to describe a few fundamental prerequisites to their success.

- ability to be motivated without financial incentives
- willingness to give up complete control over all aspects of the practice—particularly those of a business nature
- ability to practice under a capitated reimbursement system
- comfort with constructive criticism from other physicians through peer review, at the least
- ability to adjust to practice guidelines or physician profiles as means of utilization review
- willingness to participate in utilization reviews or the development of practice guidelines
- willingness to perhaps earn slightly less income while working fewer, more predictable hours
- ability to practice as a member of a medical team, often including physician extenders and ancillary personnel
- willingness to delegate significant practice responsibilities to physician extenders
- if a primary care physician, ability and willingness to perform a "gatekeeper" function, balancing cost containment and quality of care
- strong interpersonal skills to facilitate more frequent interactions with colleagues and patients
- ability to handle patients
- ability to view hospitalization as a treatment of last resort

- ability to consciously manage resources, including technology, nursing services, pharmaceuticals, lab tests, and time
- willingness to read and heed profile data on the physician's practice patterns, particularly in contrast with peers
- willingness to participate on medical staff committees, most similar to those in a hospital medical staff
- willingness to give up "ownership" of individual patients and to collaborate with colleagues on their treatment
- if merely contracting with an MCO, tight enough cost accounting to determine whether the MCO affiliation is profitable
- sufficient administrative capability to meet the MCO's service and reimbursement processing requirements
- ability to practice the physician's specialty within the MCO plan's benefit limitations
- willingness to follow the MCO's referral requirements, as they may differ from current referral patterns
- ability to receive and treat what may be a very different demographic mix of patients
- if the contract is expected to produce an increase in patient load, sufficient equipment, space, personnel, and information system capability within the practice to handle it

CONDUCT AN AUDIT FOR MANAGED CARE READINESS

Using the action steps set out in this chapter, plan a systematic and objective review of your practice and yourself. It may consist of a checklist or a series of questions. The audit might rate numerically the managed care readiness of you and your practice along several key parameters. Repeat the audit at regular intervals to measure your progress in adapting to managed care.

The purpose of the audit is to evaluate the practice's and the physician's competencies and preferences for operating in a managed care setting. Use the results you get to formulate strategies for change. These will be based on the gaps or inadequacies identified in the audit. They will provide specific directions for creating within the practice

the missing managed care success factors. The physicians then may choose and implement whatever strategies they are most comfortable with.

The audit should include a review of key practice components, functions, and characteristics such as

- personnel and personnel system
- financial management system
- management information system
- resource availability
- economic climate
- organizational structure
- flexibility, including past ability to adapt to change
- medical practice environment, including competitors and market opportunities
- political environment
- provider practice patterns

The audit also should look at the practice's purposes and goals, which in turn should reflect the overall philosophy of the group and its individual members. They are the foundation from which the organization's activities evolve and are structured. Until the physicians articulate their goals and understand why their practice is organized and operated as it is, it will be hard to understand how managed care or a particular contract or affiliation will affect the practice. It may be necessary to spend some time with all the physicians discussing and drafting a clear, concise statement of the intent of their enterprise.

Carry out this audit as soon as possible, so that any necessary changes can be made at the physicians' desired pace, rather than being forced upon them by the external environment, market forces, and MCOs.

This may be the dénouement, the critical turning point, in the history of the practice and the individual providers' careers—where they must choose between sticking with their traditional attitudes and practices and adapting to the demands of managed care—the apparent future of health care delivery. For some, this may be a choice between continuing to work as a physician (with these new restrictions) and changing to another profession.

RESOURCE LIST

After the Contract: Operating the Practice under Managed Care, Super Search Packet #4905 (updated annually). Medical Group Management Association.

J. La Puma, *Managed Care Ethics: Essays on the Impact of Managed Care on Traditional Medical Ethics* (New York: Hatherleigh Press, 1998).

P. Lucash, *Medical Practice Change Management: Strategies and Techniques for the Changing Business of Healthcare* (copublished, Burr Ridge, IL: McGraw-Hill Healthcare Education Group, and Westchester IL: Healthcare Financial Management Association, 1997).

Making Sense of Managed Care—Vol. III: Operational Issues and Practical Answers (San Francisco: Jossey-Bass, 1998).

Managed Care Programs—Physician Education, Information Exchange #3802. Medical Group Management Association.

"A Road Map for Managed Care Success," *Administrative Radiology*, August 1995.

CHAPTER 8

Step Two: How To Analyze and Evaluate a Managed Care Contract

INTRODUCTION

For most physicians, the earliest manifestation of the health care revolution is the invitation to enter into a contractual relationship with a managed care organization (MCO). In the last 10 to 15 years, thousands of doctors have signed these contracts, sometimes 10 or 20 per physician. The resulting practice experiences have varied from ideal to okay to miserable. Careful research would probably show a correlation between the success of the relationship and the care with which the physician studied the contract before signing it.

Although we may be moving toward a system in which physicians are bound to a single delivery organization—perhaps through an employment agreement—managed care contracts are likely to remain a primary means of connection between physicians and one or more MCOs. It behooves the physicians to understand clearly what activities they are promising to perform for what organizations—as reflected in the contracts they sign. This is particularly true because the contract is written and enforced mainly by the MCO. It is the aim of this chapter to give physicians a framework and tools for properly examining a managed care contract before initialing it.

WHO SHOULD READ THIS CHAPTER

Certainly, if you have never executed a managed care contract before, you owe it to yourself

and to your practice to accept what this chapter has to offer. You will be much empowered when you encounter your first contract and begin your first negotiation with an MCO. The understanding of these legal documents is fundamental to every physician's interaction with the growing managed care infrastructure.

If you already are party to a few, or many, managed care contracts, you may feel seasoned enough to skip further reading on the topic. Scan this chapter anyway. You may learn something that will give you an edge in your next contract negotiation.

The physicians with the least need for the knowledge in this chapter may be the members of physician-run organizations large enough to afford full-time specialists in evaluating and negotiating managed care contracts for the entire group. If you trust their judgment and are confident that you will be with that organization for the indefinite future, move on.

What Kind of Organization Might a Physician Contract with?

The traditional model of a managed care contract results in a new legal relationship with an MCO. For individual and small group physicians, however, there is alternative. It is to contract with a provider-sponsored organization that acts as an intermediary with the MCO. Typical such organizations are independent practice associations

(IPAs), group practices without walls (GPWWs), and physician-hospital organizations (PHOs).

The contracts in each case look similar and contain many identical clauses. However, there are significant differences. Some of the more intrusive and restrictive managed care programs—periodic record audits, utilization management (UM), contract changes—will be implemented by persons controlled by and sympathetic to the interests of physicians. This alone may make your compliance with the programs more tolerable.

In addition, the contract normally is not able to define the exact managed care product or patient population you will be serving. This depends on the MCO contracts that the organization subsequently enters. Frequently, the individual physicians' contracts commit them to provide medical services through whatever MCO contracts the organization makes.

Action Plan for Entering into Managed Care Contracts

A thorough review of a proposed managed care contract has several stages, and all are important. It is best if they are approached systematically. Here is a plan of action steps for analyzing and evaluating such a contract.

1.   Conduct an audit of your practice to see how well prepared it is for meeting the demands of an MCO. Even if you did this a couple years ago and your current MCO partners seem to like you, give it another quick check. The marketplace may be changing, and the latest contracts may have greater expectations of their physician partners.
2.   Do an in-depth background check on the organization offering the contract. Unless, of course, you already have other contracts with them and know them rather well.
3.   List every provision in the contract. Number every contract provision. Then write a brief synopsis of each provision's content next to its number. The purpose is to

ensure that you have read and understand every provision, even the most mundane.
4.   Critically analyze the key contract provisions described below, as well as any others that strike you as puzzling or unacceptable. Also note any key provisions that do not seem to appear in the contract.
5.   List every provision with which you have some sort of problem. This may be because it seems confusing, inappropriate, unwelcome, or intolerable.
6.   Seek more information from the MCO about the provisions that confound you.
7.   Attempt to negotiate changes in the language of those provisions you find unacceptable. In some cases, you may wish to pursue deletion. (Read Chapter 9 to learn "Strategies for Negotiating with a Managed Care Organization.")
8.   Calculate the impact on your revenues and net income of the payments you will receive under the contract and the additional expenses you will incur in order to comply with the MCO's program requirements.
9.   Determine whether this contract with this MCO fits into your long-term strategy for your practice. Determine whether you will feel comfortable working for this particular MCO and carrying out the terms of this contract. Determine whether you can deliver care under this contract while earning the income you require.
10.   Decide whether to sign the contract.

Determining Whether Your Practice Is Ready for Managed Care

It is not a good idea to even think about signing a managed care contract until you and your practice are ready to do it successfully. Read the previous chapter on "Step One: Preparing Your Practice for Operation under Managed Care" for a detailed discussion of the how to maximize your odds of success under a managed care contract.

Briefly, the major prerequisites to a positive managed care practice experience are

- understanding managed care
- viewing private medical practice as a business
- knowing the practice's mission and operations
- developing a managed care strategy

UNDERSTANDING MANAGED CARE CONCEPTS, ORGANIZATIONS, AND RELATIONSHIPS

It is hard to have missed the discussion and debate within the medical community over managed care that has gone on during the past 10 years. Nonetheless, if you are unclear about the inner workings of a managed care system—in terms of both its financing and its impact on clinical decision making—consult the following resources:

Books

P. Boland, *Making Managed Healthcare Work— A Practical Guide to Strategies and Solutions* (Gaithersburg, MD: Aspen Publishers, Inc., 1993).

P. Kongstvedt, *The Managed Health Care Handbook*, 3rd ed. (Gaithersburg, MD: Aspen Publishers, Inc., 1996).

D.W. Lee, *Capitation: The Physician's Guide.* (Chicago: American Medical Association [AMA], 1995).

Making Sense of Managed Care—Vol. III: Operational Issues and Practical Answers (San Francisco: Jossey-Bass Publishers, 1998).

J. McCally, *Capitation for Physicians—Understanding and Negotiating Contracts to Maximize Reimbursement and Manage Financial Risk* (Burr Ridge, IL: McGraw-Hill Healthcare Education Group, 1996).

Periodicals

American Medical News, weekly newspaper of the AMA.

Medical Economics, semimonthly periodical addressing practice concerns of physicians.

Medical Group Management Journal, monthly periodical of the Medical Group Management Association (MGMA).

LOOKING AT YOUR PRIVATE PRACTICE OF MEDICINE AS A BUSINESS ENTITY

The business success of health care providers is increasingly dependent on and judged by well-established business terms, such as a product line, net profits, steady growth, market forces, operating efficiencies, customer satisfaction, and opportunities for gain and loss. It requires looking at the private practice of medicine as a commercial business venture. It can be other things—a source of personal fulfillment for the physician and a source of life-sustaining services for patients— but none of these will be possible unless the practice is a business first.

FULLY COMPREHENDING YOUR PRACTICE'S DIRECTION AND OPERATIONS

Under managed care, you will be moving your practice in new directions. Before you do that, you must fully understand its current goals, components, functions, and characteristics. Discover whether the present configuration of the practice is appropriate to the evolving health care environment and whether it puts you in a position to engage in new managed care programs. This is best accomplished through a systematic and objective practice review.

At the same time, look candidly at what you are hoping to accomplish in the long run through the conduct of a medical practice. This includes some kind of overall vision, backed up by strategic objectives and, perhaps, a set of immutable values to guide management decisions. Just creating this strategic infrastructure will be a challenge for many physicians.

FORMULATE A STRATEGY FOR THE KINDS AND TERMS OF MANAGED CARE CONTRACTS THE PRACTICE WILL SEEK

Simply waiting for MCOs to approach you and then signing every contract put in front of you is a passive, unbusinesslike way to enter into relationships that will shape your professional future. It is far better to lay out in advance a strategy or plan for selecting, negotiating, and executing managed care contracts. This means addressing these issues and answering these questions.

- What levels of financial risk and reimbursement methods are you willing to accept? Do you and your physician partners prefer discounted fee-for-service (FFS) reimbursement, or are you willing and able to take on capitation? Are you practicing in a health care delivery market where you have any choice in such matters?
- How fully and by what deadlines do you want to move into managed care (e.g., 40 percent of revenues from managed care in two years, 85 percent in five years)?
- What investments must be made in the minimum system requirements (cost accounting, UM, physician profiling, patient satisfaction, practice marketing) necessary for success under managed care? How much time will be required to accumulate the necessary capital?
- What are your preferences regarding the number of separate managed care contracts, maximum volume of patients you will handle, type of MCO you will contract with, and risk you will accept?
- Who are the key members of your practice? What roles can they assume in the negotiations and subsequent relationships with the MCOs?
- What are the minimum financial requirements of your practice? What level of revenue is needed to cover overhead expenses? What are the cash flow requirements of the practice? What are your personal financial needs and goals?

Tie the answers to these questions into a strategic plan for entering into managed care contracts—the kinds of MCOs by type and size, the kind of relationships with them, and time-based goals.

Evaluating the MCO Offering the Contract

A good contract with a poor MCO is worse than no contract at all and probably worse than a poor contract with a good MCO. Before you spend serious time going over a contract's language, do some research to see whether the MCO offering it is one you want to do business with. Here are the important questions to ask.

Who Owns and Controls the MCO?

The name of the MCO, its stationery, or its marketing literature may not give an accurate indication of its true owners—the people who ultimately will make the critical decisions. Almost anyone could be an owner, but these are the most likely candidates.

- private or publicly traded national holding company or chain
- commercial insurance company
- Blue Cross/Blue Shield plan
- physician group
- hospital or group of hospitals
- independent and self-sustaining (for-profit or not-for-profit) organization

Once you learn the owners' identities, further research can reveal a lot about

- the prior experience of the organization with managed care
- its philosophy toward dealing with physicians as providers
- the resources it has at its disposal
- its level of commitment to the business of managed care
- its reputation for business integrity and provider relationships

- other indicators of how it will implement this contract and interact with your practice

Where do you find this information? The very best source, of course, is the MCO itself. Prepare a list of your information needs and the contract-related reasons for them, and present to your MCO contact person. Be prepared to hear that the MCO does not have the time to gather some of the information for you or that it considers it proprietary and confidential. As usual, the larger your group and the more essential you are to the MCO's plans, the more cooperative it is likely to be.

The next best sources are various government agencies that have regulatory or contractual relationships with the MCO. At the state level, the departments responsible are those regulating public health, insurance, Medicaid, and licensing of medical professionals. At the federal level, the most important contact is the Health Care Financing Administration (HCFA). Additional useful sources are members of the medical community, including the state medical society. (Note: do not forget to check with other states in which the MCO may also have operated.)

Who Makes the Actual Management Decisions?

Next, try to get a feel for the people in the MCO who will make the decisions affecting your practice. Pay particular attention to the board of directors and the top management team.

- What is the composition of the board of directors? What are their names, what is their experience, and what constituencies do they represent? Are there community representatives? From what groups? Are there physicians on the board, chosen from among the physicians under contract with the MCO? What is the representation on the board committees, particularly those dealing with clinical and physician compensation matters?
- Who are the CEO and other top executives of the MCO? What is their experience and reputation in managed care?

- Who are the persons, presumably physicians, responsible for relations with participating physicians? Is there a medical director? What is her background? Is there a chance of determining how comfortable you are with this person through a meeting or an interview?
- Is the MCO entirely an independent local operation or is it part of a chain with systems and headquarters in other cities?

These are the people who will make the day-to-day decisions about the direction and operation of the MCO. They are the ones you will have to deal with as a participating provider. Your ability to influence the MCO and to make it work for you will be reflected most in the style of its managers and the access of physicians to the board of directors. It will be harder to wield such influence if the real decision makers are located in a distant city. Gather these facts from the same places you used to investigate the ownership of the MCO.

What Is the Financial History of the MCO?

The average MCO may look like a large, omnipotent organization with unquestionably solid finances. To make sure, question them.

- How long has the MCO has been in business, both in your area and nationwide?
- What has been its record of financial performance? Has there been steady growth? Has it occurred through expansion of existing operations or through acquisition of other systems? What are its projections of future growth—locally and nationally—in terms of revenues and members?
- What is its current financial condition? Is it solvent and sound? What is its credit rating? What do the traditional ratio analyses show?
- Is its stock publicly traded? How does the market rate the organization as an investment? (Note: check with a stock analyst.)
- What is its record of paying its participating providers? Is it up-to-date with the schedule

established in its provider contracts? Ask other physicians who are already working with them in the area.

The reason for gathering this type of information is that you absolutely do not want to affiliate with an organization that is financially unsound or that has trouble paying its physicians promptly. Rather large MCOs have failed and gone out of business, leaving physicians with uncollectible receivables and an obligation to continue treating current patients. In every case, there were early indicators of financial trouble. Consult the same sources for these financial data, and talk with credit agencies such as Dun & Bradstreet.

How Does the MCO Interact with the Marketplace?

Examine a good selection of the MCO's marketing materials—brochures, advertisements, signage, and the like.

- How do they describe the MCO and the services it promises to provide? Does it give any assurances about the quality of care or the physicians providing the care?
- Do the materials employ superlative language, such as "top-quality physicians" or "first-rate care," that might be interpreted as standards to which a participating physician would have to adhere?
- If the MCO has been operating in your market for some time, what are the bounds of its service area? How many members does it have in that area, and what percentage of the total managed care market do they represent? How many new members are joining each year and how many are leaving (disenrolling from) the MCO?
- How many different physicians and physician groups are under contract with the MCO? Where do they practice and what are their specialties? What are their reputations? At what rate are new physicians being added and old physicians withdrawing?

- Is the MCO using primary care physicians (PCPs) as "gatekeepers" to the other resources in its system?
- What area hospitals are part of the MCO's network of providers? What are their reputations? How recently have they joined the network? What hospitals may have withdrawn from the network within the last year or two?

Find out key utilization data about the MCO's operations in your area, such as inpatient days per 1,000 members and average length of stay. Do this for the specialties in which you will be practicing.

These kinds of information will help define the character, working environment, and performance expectations you are likely to encounter in the MCO. High turnover in participating providers may indicate problems in their relationships with the MCO, a situation you probably should avoid. Even average utilization rates will help you decide whether you can meet the MCO's performance standards. Extravagant promises made in the marketing materials may heighten the malpractice liability risks for providers.

Most of these pieces of information will be available directly from the MCO. Indeed, MCO representatives may boast directly to you about the quality of the physician panel you would be joining and the MCO's commitment to clinical standards and physician autonomy. It is important that you corroborate such assertions with physicians who have or do work for the MCO.

What Is the MCO's Standing with Accreditation, Licensing, Regulatory, and Payer Organizations?

Check to see that the MCO is licensed by the appropriate state agency and is in compliance with other applicable regulatory requirements. See whether the MCO has qualified as a federal managed care entity. Is it party to Medicare or Medicaid contracts? Determine whether the MCO is accredited by any of the leading accrediting bodies, such as the National Committee for Quality Assurance. The MCO should also make warranties in the contract about these various forms of official sanction.

Try to learn how many members have filed complaints about their treatment through the MCO—either internally within the MCO itself or externally with a government agency. Also, have an attorney research the number of lawsuits brought against the MCO by either members or providers.

Satisfaction of the standards of these independent organizations can give you some assurance that the MCO is a trustworthy, competently managed health care delivery operation. More than a few legal problems may be a signal that not everything is "on the up and up." For this information, contact the respective federal and state agencies, and the private accrediting organizations.

If your prospective MCO affiliate does reasonably well under an investigation this thorough, you can feel confident that it will be a responsible contract partner. Next, turn your attention to the language of the contract itself.

Quick Summary of All the Significant Provisions in a Managed Care Contract

The following are the typical topics covered in a managed care contract. The wording and the meaning may vary considerably, but you should be able to find most of these provisions in any contract you are offered. Some are more important than others; those will be examined next. If any of these topics are not covered by the contract, consider why the MCO might exclude them.

Basic Structural Provisions

Identification of the Contracting Parties This may seem a formality but can be the source of problems. Generally, the contract will be between an MCO and the legal entity that is your medical practice. However, there are other possibilities. The MCO may be a local subsidiary of a nationwide network. A physician may contract with a larger physician organization or PHO that then

contracts with the MCO. The physician may be practicing as a sole proprietor, a partnership, or a professional corporation. He may or may not be contracting on behalf of physician colleagues in his employ. Everyone's intentions should be clear, the proper parties identified, and the correct names used.

Date the Contract Takes Effect This is the specific date on which the physician is obligated to begin delivering services. The date is usually some time in the near future. If no date is specified, performance begins on the date the contract is signed. Be sure you understand exactly when you must begin serving the MCO and that you can be ready to deliver by that date. If you are not ready, you will be in immediate breach of the contract.

Initial Trial Period Occasionally, an MCO will offer a contract that allows the physician a trial period of practice on managed care terms with the MCO and its members. The period might last from three to six months. At its end, both the physician and the MCO review their experiences and decide whether they want to proceed with a more permanent relationship. This arrangement has advantages for a physician totally new to managed care who wants to get a feel for such a practice before making a commitment. The downside is that the MCO can refuse to continue the relationship at the end of the trial period as easily as can the physician. If you have some solid experience with managed care and follow the guidelines offered in this chapter, you should have no hesitation about entering into a contract for one year or more. The provisions for termination with and without cause and for renewal after the fixed term should provide adequate protection. In any event, most MCOs in a well-developed managed care market will not even offer this option.

Recital of Key Facts about the Parties and Their Intentions This language is a bit of fluff about the intentions of the parties and carries little legal weight on its own but may be useful in interpreting otherwise ambiguous contract terms.

Definition of Key Terms (Medical Necessity, Covered Services) This section of the contract simply defines key words and phrases that are important and are used repeatedly throughout the contract. Most do not deserve a lot of attention. However, do pay attention to the definitions of terms like *covered services, medical necessity, referral services*, and *member*.

Relationship of the Parties This simple and customary provision defines the exact nature of the relationship between the parties created by the contract. It is easy for confusion to creep in. Four prominent relationship types are employment, independent contractors, joint venturers, and shareholders. In most managed care contracts for physician services, the parties are nothing more than independent contractors.

Designation of the State Whose Law Will Govern Interpretation of the Contract This seemingly innocuous clause can have serious ramifications if legal action becomes necessary in connection with the contract. It stipulates which state's laws will be applied in interpreting the contract.[*] This sometimes make sense when the two parties are from different states and are contracting to provide services in a third state. However, in the case of almost all MCO contracts with physicians, the agreement should be governed by the laws of the state where the physicians are located and practicing medicine.

There are two good reasons to avoid the designation of a state other than your own as the source of governing law. If the MCO wants to use another state's laws for interpreting the contract, it is probably for a good reason. It has done research and has determined that the law in that

---

[*]This refers usually to state court decisions on matters of contract interpretation. It does not include state statutes on the certification or licensing of health care providers and facilities. For instance, a contract calling for the establishment of primary care clinics could not stipulate that the clinics would be licensed under the laws of another state.

state is more likely to favor the MCO in a dispute. Further, your legal expenses will be much greater if you must bring or defend a legal action in a distant state.

Other Documents Incorporated by Reference There may be a specific contract provision listing other documents that are incorporated into—that is, become a legal part of—the contract. Alternatively, there may be several references throughout the contract to external documents to which the physician must adhere. Examples of these are the benefit policies between the MCO and its enrollees, a UM manual, medical staff bylaws, and quality assurance guidelines.

Remember two things about these documents: (a) they may be just as much a part of the contract as the contract language itself and (b) if there is no provision to the contrary, the MCO can probably unilaterally change the documents. To protect your interests, seek additional language requiring advance notice to physicians of proposed changes, the opportunity to submit comments on the changes, and the option to terminate the contract if you find such changes intolerable.

Firm Rule: Do not sign any contract without first obtaining and reviewing every document referred to in the contract and without learning just how those documents may be amended.

Severability of Contract Provisions This is standard language in most every contract. If one provision or another is judged by a court to be unenforceable, this allows the remainder of the contract to remain in force.

Indemnification and Hold-Harmless Protection against the Other Party's Negligence If not properly worded, this can be one of the most dangerous provisions in a managed care contract for a physician. To indemnify or "hold harmless" another person or organization is to promise to pay for the losses or obligations it incurs as a result of your acts or failures to act. In the context of a managed care contract, this is referring primarily to malpractice or other types of negligence. If a managed care patient is injured by a physician's malpractice, that patient is likely to sue every possible defendant—the MCO as well as the physician. Under this provision, the physician would be called upon to reimburse the MCO for damages it is ordered to pay as a result of the physician's negligence.

There are three things to keep in mind about these provisions. First, avoid at all costs a requirement that you indemnify the MCO for any of its legal damages awarded in connection with the "delivery of medical services." It is fair that you should reimburse the MCO for the effects of your misdeeds. It is not fair that you reimburse it for anything that goes wrong. This issue is most likely to arise in a case where the MCO's own UM procedures produce injury to a patient. This is still an unsettled area of the law, but it is becoming clearer that the physician shall not be liable when she has complied exactly with the MCO's procedures and exhausted all alternatives.

Second, even if the contract asks you to indemnify only for your own negligence, check with your malpractice insurer before you sign. Some policies will not cover liability that you have incurred by contractual agreement. If you agree to indemnify the MCO and your insurance policy does not apply, you will have to pay out of your own pocket.

Third, make sure that there is a reciprocal provision in which the MCO agrees to indemnify and hold you harmless you for the losses and obligations you suffer as a result of its negligence. This might include negligent UM procedures and negligent selection of other providers. Further, if you will be performing administrative duties for the MCO, it should carry insurance to cover your liabilities related to those duties.

General Assurances Made by the Physicians about Their Legal Status and Authority This section of the contract includes your representations and warranties that facts you have stated during the application and negotiation process are true. This may include the information contained in the application forms you probably completed, the authority of you or your group to act on behalf of the other members of the group, the

willingness of all those members to comply with the terms of the contract, the licensing and credentialing status of your group's physicians and facilities, the absence of pending lawsuits, and similar assurances. Do not agree to representations such as these unless you are confident that they are true. If you are making representations about the members of your group, make sure that they have made similar written representations to the group. Do not ever make representations about the future (i.e., "is not the subject of malpractice lawsuits now or in the future"). It is probably a good idea to be a little nervous about provisions such as these. Try to minimize the scope of the assurances they include.

Prohibition of Assignment or Transfer of Contract Rights When you contract with an MCO after thoroughly checking out its background and credentials, you would be surprised to discover that you had actually contracted with an entirely different organization. The MCO feels the same way about its contract with you and your physician colleagues. This possibility arises if, in the middle of the contract term, the physician group or the MCO transfers its contract rights and obligations to another group or organization. It might do this for several reasons: a decision to withdraw from the practice of medicine or from the delivery of health care in a particular market, or a merger with or acquisition by another organization. Whatever the reason, you may not wish to be a partner with this new organization.

Provisions such as this one prohibit either party from assigning or transferring its contract rights to someone else. It may allow transfer in defined circumstances, such as a corporate merger, or it may require that the transferring party give notice to the other party and obtain its consent before proceeding. This kind of language is in the interests of both parties.

Written Contract Includes All Terms of the Agreement This provision states that the agreement of the parties is contained entirely within the written contract (along with its exhibits and any other documents referred to and incorporated by reference). It specifically excludes any "back room deals" and verbal promises that the parties might have made to each other but that are not reflected in the actual written contract. If a significant term is not in the contract document or other materials that it encompasses, it is not part of the agreed-upon deal with the MCO. As you are negotiating, keep track of the verbal assurances made by the MCO and make sure that they appear in the contract before you sign it.

Methods by Which the Contract May Be Amended Because the world, the marketplace, the laws, medical technology, and other forces are constantly changing, it is sometimes necessary to amend the language of a contract before it is due for renewal or renegotiation. Every good contract includes language explaining how amendment can take place. It is important that you understand this process so that you do not wind up party to a contract radically different from the one to which you originally agreed.

As a rule of thumb, it should not be possible to modify a contract without the written consent of both parties. As a practical matter, that is not always possible with the contracts between an MCO and many different physician groups. If the MCO had to obtain the consent of tens or hundreds of participating physicians, nothing would ever change. The requirements of serious integration demand a certain level of uniformity in the contracts with those physicians. So here is what to aim for in your negotiations.

First, remember that the contract includes all the manuals, policies, and other external documents referenced by the contract. You must be just as concerned with changes in them as in the contract itself.

Second, if your group is large enough or important enough to the MCO, try to negotiate a requirement that your prior approval is necessary for any significant contract changes.

Third, if you lack the bargaining power to demand a veto over changes, at least seek contract language requiring that the MCO submit proposed changes to you, in writing, no less than 30 days before they are to take effect. This should

include your right to review the changes and to make comments and suggestions, and the MCO's obligation to listen to them.

Fourth, make certain that the contract also has a provision that allows you to terminate on short notice (30–60 days) without cause or in the event of a policy change that you find totally unacceptable.

Basic MCO Commitments

MCO Obligations under the Contract One of the first things you notice about a managed care contract is that most of its provisions describe the obligations of the physician to the MCO. This is due to the fact that the MCO is the one drafting the contract and usually has the greater bargaining power. Nonetheless, that is no reason for the contract not to also describe the commitments that the MCO makes to the physician.

It would be appropriate for the MCO to promise the following:

- to market and issue contracts to enrollees, employers, or other third-party payers for the provision of services
- that a minimum number of enrollees will come under the physician's care
- to implement those administrative systems that are necessary to its contract performance
- to provide the physicians with information they need to meet their obligations under the contract
- to provide the physicians with periodic (monthly) reports and management information data related to service delivery and related issues

Get a good understanding of what information and support will be furnished to you and how often it will be provided. Clearly state those obligations in the contract.

MCO Assurances about Its Legal Status and Authority Just as the physician frequently is asked to make representations about professional legal status and authority, so should the MCO give assurances concerning its licensure, certification, accreditation, and other relevant indicators of its authority to carry on its operations. This should be expressed in the contract and should include the names of the entities granting the licenses, certificates or accreditation, such as state departments of insurance, public health, professional licensure, and Medicaid care, the federal Medicare agency, and any private accrediting bodies. Because the loss of any of these forms of authority usually prevents the MCO from continuing to operate, it should be a "good cause" for the physician to terminate the contract.

Basic Physician Practice Commitments

Although these may seem mundane, make sure in advance that you can comply with them, for they can easily become the basis for an alleged breach of contract by you.

Physician Acceptance of MCO Members as Patients Because the capacity of a medical practice to handle capitated patients is limited and because the physician must see a minimum number of patients to justify investment in managed care support systems, some contracts will stipulate the minimum and maximum number of patients that the physician will serve under the contract. It normally works this way. The contract allows the physician to turn patients away once she has reached capacity. At the lower end, if the MCO is unable to steer a minimum number of patients to the physician, it will compensate her on an FFS basis, rather than with the agreed-to capitation fee.

To properly evaluate such a provision, the physician must have a good understanding of the cost structure and patient capacity of her practice. It is essential to know the maximum number of patients you can handle, as well as the number below which you cannot make money with capitated fees. The concept of capitation works only if the patient population is large enough for actuarial probabilities to come into play—meaning that capitation fees for the patients who have no sickness are used to treat the patients who are

very sick. If a physician's patient load is too small, a few catastrophically ill patients can swallow up all the capitation revenues. These are the minimum enrollment levels recommended by David J. Kouba in an article in the *Medical Group Management Journal*[1] (Exhibit 8–1).

Terms under Which a Patient May Be Rejected When a physician is in solo practice, he can choose which patients he will and will not treat. That discretion is limited under a managed care contract. Normally, there is a provision specifying the permissible and prohibited grounds for refusing a patient. The most commonly listed grounds are

prohibited grounds

- volume or type of service the patient would utilize
- physical condition of patient
- age of patient

Exhibit 8–1 Minimum Enrollment Levels

Primary care, excluding deliveries and emergency care	500
Primary care, including deliveries and excluding emergency care	1,500
Primary and secondary care, including ancillary services and specialty consultations, and excluding surgery, hospitalization, and emergency care	3,000
Primary and secondary care, including surgery and excluding hospitalization	5,000
Primary, secondary, and tertiary care, including hospitalization and all covered medically necessary services	10,000

Source: Data from D.J. Kouba, Primary Care Providers: Managing Today's Prepaid Risk, *Medical Group Management Journal*, Vol. 38, No. 1, pp. 37, 38, and 40, © 1991.

permissible grounds

- inability to establish effective physician-patient relationship
- repeated patient failure to comply with instructions
- patient would exceed previously agreed-upon maximum capacity of the practice

Specification of Services To Be Provided by the Physician One of the most fundamental questions about a managed care contract concerns the scope of services that the physician is expected to provide as basic benefits—for each of the MCO products in which the physician is participating. This may include services in the following categories:

- inpatient
- outpatient
- elective procedures
- emergency services
- preventive services
- long-term care
- ancillary services
- home health services
- psychiatric, substance abuse services
- medical rehabilitation services

The service list should be detailed by procedure code. It should be accompanied by a similar statement of the services that are excluded from coverage. This likely will encompass services that are cosmetic, experimental, investigational, medically unnecessary, or simply not part of the benefits package purchased by the employer.

These lists are important to know because they will determine the reasonableness of the compensation offered, the services that will come under UM, and the services for which you can directly charge the patients. Pay close attention to them. Make sure that they are neither overinclusive nor underinclusive. Compare them with the service codes you presently provide. Be confident that you have the ability and resources to handle every one of the listed code items.

Watch out for contracts that use the term *covered services*, use it profusely throughout the document, yet define it in the vaguest terms. Frequently, the definition will simply refer to the underlying benefits policies between the MCO and its members. These policies can be and often are changed by the MCO and the employer, with no input from the providers. Your goal is a contract that states specifically and unequivocally the services that you must provide during its term.

Specification of the Plans or Product Lines for Which the Services Are To Be Provided To meet the diverse needs of employers, MCOs usually offer several managed care products—health maintenance organizations (HMOs), preferred provider organizations (PPOs), with or without point-of-service (POS) options, etc. Be clear about which of these products you are contracting to provide services for—they should be specified clearly in the contract. Check to see that participation in one product does not obligate you to participate in others, unless that is what you want. See whether there is language covering your participation in MCO products that may be added in the future.

Exhibit 8–2 Guidelines for Negotiating the "Scope of Service" Contract Provision

1. Prepare a list, by procedure codes, of the medical services you are capable of delivering.
2. Obtain from the MCO a list, by procedures codes, of the medical services you are being asked to deliver.
3. Obtain from the MCO utilization data on the types and volumes of services demanded by the patient population you will be serving.
4. Determine which of the proposed MCO services you are unable to deliver—due to inability or lack of resources.
5. Attempt to negotiate carve-outs in the contract for those services.
6. Obtain from the MCO a list of other medical services that are not covered and for which you may charge directly.

The number of managed care plans you agree to support will affect the volume of patients likely to choose your services or referrals you will receive from other participating physicians. Be sure that you have the capacity to handle the potential demand. The demographics and service needs of different plan patient populations can vary considerably. Stay as flexible as you can about new products or plans. In the contract, retain the right to accept or reject participation one at a time.

Hours and Locations of Member Accessibility to the Physician The MCO wants to have the right kinds of physicians in the right places at the right times to meet the medical care needs of its members. To achieve this, it may include in your contract a provision defining your availability to patients. This is even more likely if you are a primary care provider (PCP), the person patients come to first with medical problems.

The physician's "availability" can be defined in terms of several variables.

- office hour availability
- telephone availability
- emergency services availability
- appointment availability (e.g., patients seeking nonurgent appointments will be seen within a certain number of weeks; for urgent appointments, the wait will be no longer than a certain number of days)

To ensure that its members have access to a good mix of physicians at convenient locations, the MCO may require that participating physicians obtain its approval for changes in their office locations. Alternatively, the MCO may insist that the physicians give some advance written notice (e.g., 60 days) of planned relocations or may simply allow the physicians freedom to move their practices within a specified radius of their present locations.

Restrictions on Physicians' Referrals to Other Physicians and for Ancillary Services This provision restricts the selection of physicians and other providers to whom you can refer patients. The MCO's goal is to ensure that referrals for all critical components of health care delivery—physician services, hospital services, ancillary services—are made within its custom-selected referral network. The only possible exception is for patient emergencies.

This restriction should be important to you because of its impact on your existing referral and practice patterns, which, in turn, may affect your overall comfort with the contract and the relationship. Before signing the contract, learn exactly who the other participating providers are and whether you are willing to collaborate with them.

There is a small related issue here. When you are unavailable or absent, you have arrangements with other physicians to cover for you. Check to see whether this must change under the managed care contract. For instance, the MCO may accept coverage only by another participating physician or, at the least, by a physician previously approved by them. Determine also whether you or the MCO compensate the coverage doctors.

Role of PCPs as "Gatekeepers" If you are a PCP, the contract should establish clearly whether you will perform a role as "gatekeeper" to all other resources in the MCO's system. This typically includes the obligation to

- preauthorize or deny specialty care
- authorize or deny elective care
- use only participating specialists and ancillary services
- monitor, manage, and coordinate all care of assigned patients, including other physicians and ancillary care

This is not a responsibility to accept casually, especially if payment is on a capitation basis. Be confident of your ability to fully choreograph a patient's medical care.

If you are a specialist physician, you should be just as interested in the presence of a gatekeeper system. It significantly influences when patients will see you, their condition, and your relationship with the referring physician.

No Solicitation of Members by Physicians To Join Other MCOs The MCO may be unhappy if you attempt to persuade some of its members to enroll in another MCO. There may be a formal prohibition in the contract against this kind of dialogue with the members (Exhibit 8–2). When you have contracts with and a knowledge of several MCOs, there may be a strong temptation to advise your patients on plans that better fit their needs. A provision like this may inhibit your relationship with your patients Exhibit 8–2 discusses

the current status of such provisions and how you can avoid them.

Noncompetition by the Physician and the MCO Noncompete clauses are standard fare in all sorts of contracts for services. Expect to find language limiting your freedom to practice medicine after you end your relationship with the MCO.

A reasonable noncompete clause defines the time period, geographic area, and range of activities within which you may not compete with the MCO. As a general rule, the contract cannot and will not require that you effectively move out of the area to resume the private practice of medicine. Instead, you are likely to be prohibited from

---

Exhibit 8–3 Avoiding "Gag Clauses" in Managed Care Contracts

There have been rumors that some MCOs have attempted to restrict the communications of their contracted physicians with their patients. Either through contract language or unwritten threats of deselection, the MCOs try to prevent doctors from telling patients about alternative treatment options not covered by the MCO, the financial incentives that encourage them to limit services to patients, and the advantages of competing health plans or MCOs. Very few examples of such language—so-called gag clauses—have been found in managed care contracts.

Physicians wishing to avoid these limits on the doctor-patient relationship have some support. The HCFA has a policy position that prohibits health plans serving Medicare beneficiaries from including clauses in their physician contracts to prevent doctors from providing patients with information about medically necessary treatment options. The same position is taken with state Medicaid programs. The American Association of Health Plans (AAHP), representing the vast majority of MCOs, backs HCFA on this. The AAHP has gone further and urges its members to provide the following information to anyone upon request:

- Disclose physician payment policies, including financial incentives.
- Explain criteria used to determine whether experimental treatments should become covered services.
- Describe precertification and other utilization review procedures.
- Outline the basis for utilization review decisions when members disagree with them.
- Include specific prescription drugs in their formularies.
- Explain the plan's structure and provider network.
- Describe benefits covered and excluded, including out-of-area emergency coverage.

Notice any "gag" language in managed care contracts you are thinking of signing. Remind the MCO of the HCFA policy and the AAHP recommendations. Perhaps the contract was drawn up before these statements were announced. If the MCO refuses to change and you have other contract choices, take them.

taking any of the MCO's member-patients away with you.

Here is what to be worried about in a noncompete clause. When you first join the MCO, you may bring a significant number of existing patients with you. If you leave within a year or two, it should be fair for those patients to follow you.

When the contract is terminated, perhaps by the MCO, you might be concerned if the MCO immediately opens a clinic across from your office. Negotiate language in the noncompete clause that prohibits certain forms of competition by the MCO. It is only equitable.

Other than that, the clause must be narrowly drawn. It cannot cover an unreasonably large geographic area, it cannot extend for an unreasonably long period of time, and it cannot apply to an unreasonably wide range of physician activities. The law will not allow it.

Use of Physician Extenders One of the most effective tools for controlling costs without lowering quality is the use of physician extenders (physician assistants, nurse practitioners). The managed care contract may have something to say about your use of them.

The MCO may require that you employ physician extenders whenever possible and base your capitation fee on the assumption that you will. If you are not as enamored of physician extenders, try to avoid this mandate. On the other hand, you may think more highly of extenders than does the MCO, and the contract may limit your use of them. In that case, you must decide whether you are willing to change your practice style in that way and whether you can operate within the capitation fee without using extenders as much as you would like.

Physician Participation in Member Grievance Procedures The MCO almost certainly will have a mechanism for fielding the grievances of enrollees. The contract is likely to mandate your participation in that process when the grievances relate to you or your office. It would be a good idea to know in advance how involved you might become. Will you have to prepare written responses to a patient's complaint? Will you have to attend and speak at hearings on the matter? This could be expensive and time-consuming.

Financial Provisions

These contract provisions cover the primary reason that a physician enters into a relationship with an MCO—to receive payment for treating its enrollees. The payment does not make sense unless it covers your practice costs and provides an acceptable take-home income.

This must be figured out before the contract is signed. It requires analyzing the contract to learn when, how, and how much you will be paid. Some suggestions follow here. It also requires knowing the cost structure of your practice and doing some calculations to see whether you can make money on a particular contract. This is discussed toward the end of this chapter.

Although it may not be covered in the contract, you should learn the details of the billing and recordkeeping procedure you will have to follow with respect to services provided to MCO members. Find out how extensively you must document the services actually delivered. By the way, some MCOs are just as interested in these data under capitated arrangements as when payment is on an FFS basis.

Where your compensation is tied to performance factors such as cost, utilization, quality, and patient satisfaction, make sure that the MCO provides you with the data it collects to make the compensation determinations. This could be written into the contract as one of the MCO's commitments. (See section above on basic MCO commitments.)

Basic System and Formula for Compensating Physicians The obvious first step is to figure out how physicians will be compensated for the services they provide. The most common formulas used are

- FFS
- discounted FFS
- physician's usual and customary charge
- capitation fee

To a growing degree, MCOs are attempting to shift their financial risk to physicians by placing them "at risk." Common "risk-shifting" devices are withholds, risk pools, and capitated compensation schemes.

Basic Capitation Fee To Be Paid to the Physician Under a capitated arrangement, one of the most important contract provisions is the one stating the basic capitation fee to be paid to the physician. Standing alone, this figure means very little. To determine whether you can "afford" the contract, compare the capitation fee to

- your practice's existing cost structure
- the range of services you will be providing within that fee amount
- the degree of financial risk you are assuming under the contract
- the additional administrative burdens imposed on your practice by the contract
- any additional payments you may be permitted to collect from patients
- your personal financial goals and needs

Check also for a clear statement in the contract of the services that are to be included within the capitation payment and those that fall "outside the cap"—to be paid on a straight FFS or discounted FFS basis.

Accounting for Service Delivery in Special Circumstances Patients who obtain medical services from providers who are not part of the MCO's plan or are not even located in the MCO's service area present special problems. Generally, these delivery episodes are not within the control of the physician and cannot be predicted. They must be taken into account in evaluating the capitation fee or distributions from risk pools. Some MCOs are willing to reimburse the physicians for their payments to out-of-area and out-of-plan providers.

Similar provision should be made for services that members obtain on an emergency basis and that the physicians must cover from the capitation fee.

Physician Reimbursement on an FFS Basis A significant but declining number of managed care

contracts compensates physicians, particularly specialists, on variations of an FFS basis. If you are contemplating one of these contracts, obtain a copy of the fee schedule on which you will be paid if it is not included as an appendix to the contract. Compare the fees for the 10 or 20 most common services in your practice with your cost for delivering them. Factor in whatever additional costs will be incurred to comply with the MCO's billing, claims filing, and other administrative requirements.

"Most Favored Nation" Provision A "most favored nation" clause requires that the physician charge the MCO no higher a fee than he or she does to any other MCO for the same services. These clauses are common, but they should be resisted. Not all MCO relationships are the same. The demographics and risk profile of the patient population may vary. There may be different administrative requirements from each MCO. This kind of provision also limits the physician's flexibility in negotiating the best contract for his practice at any given time.

There is one setting where a "most favored nation" clause makes some sense. When your contract is with a provider-sponsored organization (such as an IPA or a physician-hospital organization [PHO]), it is in the best interests of all the participating providers to give their best prices to the organization. You might consider accepting this clause in such a case.

Changes in Compensation Levels during the Term of the Contract Check to see whether the contract allows the MCO to unilaterally change the compensation level during the term of the contract. It might try to do this to reflect changes in your utilization or quality performance. If you cannot avoid this kind of provision, insist on a clear explanation (within the contract) of exactly how your practice behavior will be tied to your compensation.

Allocations to and Distributions from the Risk Pool If the contract puts you at risk through the creation of withholds, pools, or some other device that holds back part of your compensation for later distribution on the basis of actual performance results, look for a good explanation in the contract of how it will work. In particular, be sure that you understand these points.

- exactly how much money is withheld
- the process by which the amounts in the pools will be distributed to the physicians
- the criteria to be used in deciding whether individual physicians qualify for distributions (e.g., utilization targets, quality of care, patient satisfaction)
- the formulas by which the pool funds will be distributed among all the qualifying physicians
- how frequently and by what dates the pools will be distributed
- whether the funds are distributed as a matter of contract right or at the MCO's discretion

Without these kinds of details, you will not be ensured of the terms under which you will receive an amount that can equal 10 to 20 percent of your total compensation.

Compensation for Administrative Duties of Physicians Some MCO relationships require that the physician perform certain administrative duties for the MCO, such as participation in UM and quality assurance programs or physician disciplinary hearings. It is reasonable to expect specific, additional compensation for this work, and it should be written into the contract.

Availability of Stop-Loss Insurance It has become common practice among some MCOs to provide "stop-loss" insurance or reinsurance to protect its capitated physicians against the costs of treating patients needing an unusually high volume of services. Physicians can purchase such coverage themselves, but it is much cheaper if paid by an MCO for many of its participating physicians at once. If the contract exposes you to this kind of risk, inquire into the availability of such insurance.

Stop-loss insurance can be written in several different ways. It can kick in when the expenses of treating an individual patient exceed a set amount. Alternatively, the policy may be activated in the event that treatment expenses for the entire patient pool (from that one MCO) exceed the capitation payment by a certain percentage. In some cases, the MCO will simply agree to begin paying on an FFS basis when these thresholds are passed. Often, the MCO offers this kind of stop-loss coverage as an option for which the physician must pay a premium, sometimes in the form of a lower capitation fee. Careful review of the numbers is essential.

Terms of Claim Submission by Physician and Payment by MCO Payment delayed is payment reduced. The contract should state the procedures that the physician must follow to receive compensation payments—whether capitation or FFS—as promptly as possible. This should not be complicated where capitated payments are being made. Failing some serious problem with the physician's recent care or behavior, the MCO should be able to guarantee delivery of a check at approximately the same time each month for the aggregate of the per member–per month (PMPM) fees for all the members in the physician's care.

Under an FFS compensation scheme, the physician first must file claims with the MCO for services she has provided. The MCO must verify them, then issue appropriate payment checks. The contract frequently requires that the physician submit claims within a certain time period after the service is performed. The procedure for preparing and submitting a claim likely to be paid without question should be spelled out in a document incorporated into the contract. It should include the forms, the types of information, and where the claims should be sent. The contract also should stipulate the time period (after receipt of a valid claim) within which the MCO will make payment to the physician. The provision should include a penalty, perhaps in the form of interest payments, for late payments. If these issues are not addressed by the contract, you will have no assurance of receiving payment within a reasonable time frame upon which you can base your financial planning.

Note: There is a special payments issue in the event of a contract termination—by either the physician or the MCO. The physician frequently must continue the treatment of existing patients until it has been completed or until the patients have been switched to a new provider. There needs to be a provision on how the physician will be compensated for those treatment services. Under an FFS contract, there is no reason why the same fees cannot continue to be paid. Under a capitation contract, continued capitation payments do not make sense. (At this point, the only patients in the physician's care are sick ones.) Payments under some prearranged fee schedule are usually the best answer.

No Direct Billing of Patients by the Physician Expect to find a contract provision limiting the physician's recourse to members for payments that the MCO has failed to make to the physician. Its purpose is to assure the member that the financial obligations under her managed care policy will be fixed, predictable, and established according to clear formulas. In many states, these provisions are required by law. These provisions do not apply to copayments and deductibles that the physician may be authorized to collect from a member. The physician also should be free to charge members for noncovered services.

Physician Collection of Copayments from Patients Some MCOs require their physicians to collect copayment, coinsurance, and deductible amounts directly from patients and to pass them on to the MCO. It is a small additional administrative burden. Be aware of it and be prepared to carry it out.

Coordinating Benefits with Other Third-Party Payers Because enrollees are often covered by more than one health insurance plan (through a spouse, for instance), their policies inevitably include a coordination of benefits (COB) provision, which dictates which policies will take precedence under which circumstances. In a contract

with an MCO, a physician can expect language defining his or her part in resolving these conflicts.

The language typically states that the maximum compensation the physician will receive for services is that specified in his managed care contract. In other words, do not expect higher or additional payments from another policy or plan. The contract may also require the physician to comply with and reasonably assist the MCO in administering and coordinating benefits. Be sensitive to the administrative burdens associated with this obligation.

Through either the contract or other MCO documents, get answers to a couple of COB questions. On whom does the primary responsibility fall for coordinating benefits—the MCO, the physician, both parties, or a third party? It should be the MCO. To whom can the physician turn for guidance on her role in coordinating benefits?

Program Requirements

Records and Reports Required To Be Kept by the Physician The contract will require that participating physicians maintain certain records for possible access by the MCO. It probably is a good practice to keep most of these records anyway—medical records, consent forms, referral forms, and claims forms to other payers for purposes of coordinating benefits. Just be prepared for any additional administrative burdens that these may impose.

There are other data that the MCO may want to see on a more regular basis. They usually relate to utilization review, quality assurance, and other practice monitoring programs of the MCO. Most of this information exists in patient medical records, though some effort may be required to extract it in the form that the MCO wants. This is not a provision to argue.

Just keep two things in mind. Be prepared for the administrative expense necessary to satisfy the requirement. Balance this contract provision with one stipulating the data that the MCO must provide to the physician to facilitate his performance under the contract. These would include reports on individual resource utilization, quality of care, general cost efficiency, and patient satisfaction levels.

MCOs Rights To Inspect the Physician's Facilities and Records Many managed care contracts will give the MCO a right to inspect the physician's practice facilities and records. Sometimes, the contract language may refer to "audits" by the MCO of the physician's practice. The best provisions state clearly the scope of these inspection rights (exactly what documents, records, physical spaces, or equipment may be examined), the reasons that may warrant such an inspection or audit, and the advance notice that should be required.

If your practice style has been largely autonomous, this might come as a jolt—allowing someone else to pry into the nooks and crannies of your practice. In most cases, it is unavoidable. One way to avoid nonphysician intrusions is to contract with or become part of a provider-sponsored organization first, then let that organization act as a buffer between you and the MCOs.

Patient medical records contain a lot of the information that the MCO will want to inspect. They are protected by confidentiality rights and cannot be released, even to the MCO, without proper authorization from the patient. The contract should acknowledge this fact. The actual authorization usually comes through a blanket consent in the member benefits policy to the provider's release of medical record information to the MCO for managed care program purposes. Verify that those blanket consents are being obtained. If they are not, insist on some other procedure for obtaining individual consents. Otherwise, the information cannot be given to the MCO.

The MCO also is likely to want to look periodically at financial and other information not included in the patient file.

As you view this provision, keep several things in mind. The record compilation and reporting requirements may create significant new time and expense burdens for the practice. They may require the gathering of data sensitive enough to need new security arrangements. To understand the responsibilities you will be assuming under the contract, as well as the intrusions by the MCO into your operations, it is essential to get a clear, detailed statement of the MCO's expectations and inspection rights. Too many contracts refer simply to "periodic reviews" and "reasonable access" concerning your records.

Finally, the MCO may ask for more information than it has a good reason to see. Question its motives and, where appropriate, just say no.

Physician Compliance with Other MCO Program Requirements This all-purpose provision mandates the physician's compliance with general program requirements of the MCO. There are a lot of legitimate such requirements, and they cannot all be described in the contract. Many of them will change and evolve over the term of the contract. There is no question that a physician could be caught off guard by some of these requirements or the amendments to them. So here is what to do.

1. Press to have as many of these requirements as possible explained in the contract.
2. Ask for a listing (in an appendix) of the external documents describing all other binding program requirements. All the documents should be incorporated by reference into the contract.
3. Obtain copies of all referenced documents and review them before signing the contract. As a practical matter, many physicians will not have the time, energy, or cooperation of MCOs to review all program requirements and policies prior to contract execution. At least, try to look them over after signing but before you have to comply.
4. Ask for contract language obligating the MCO to inform you 30–60 days in advance of proposed changes in the requirements and to accept your comments on them. If you have the bargaining power,

insist that your consent be obtained before the changes can take effect.

5.   Make sure that the provision on contract termination acknowledges "unacceptable program requirements changes" as "good cause" for breaking off the contract.

Procedures for Determining Member Eligibility (and What Happens When the MCO Decides after the Fact That the Member Is Ineligible) This provision describes the procedure for determining the plan eligibility of patients appearing in the physician's office and the physician's role in that procedure. This is not always as simple a process as it seems it should be. A patient may once have been an enrollee of the MCO but is no longer. The MCO itself may not provide the physician with current or accurate information on member eligibility. Look for these features in the eligibility-checking process.

- unambiguous description of the identification, document, or authorization that will constitute incontrovertible evidence of eligibility
- exact source of that evidence (in patient's possession, periodic MCO list of eligible members, eligibility contact person in the MCO)
- physician's treatment options when eligibility cannot be quickly determined
- party responsible for the cost of services provided to a patient subsequently found to be ineligible—MCO, physician, patient

Be sure you understand and feel comfortable with all aspects of this procedure. Your office will follow it thousands of times. Be aware of the financial risks of failing to properly establish eligibility.

Protection of Patient Confidentiality This very common provision requires that the physician follow certain precautions to protect patient confidentiality. This is reasonable and probably no different from what the physician already is doing.

Professional Liability Insurance To Be Maintained by the Physician This is a reasonable requirement, consistent with good business practice. It is likely to include these terms.

- physician to furnish the MCO with evidence of the maintenance of all required coverage
- types and limits of required coverage
- individuals to be covered or, alternatively, coverage of entire group
- notification of MCO within set time period of cancellation, reduction, or material change in the required coverage

This provision will be a little different in the case of MCO contracts with relatively nonintegrated conglomerations of physicians, such as IPAs or PHOs. Because these organizations are not likely to carry umbrella malpractice policies, the managed care contract may insist that the IPA or PHO make maintenance of professional liability coverage at certain minimum levels a condition for physician participation.

When negotiating this provision with the MCO, consider asking it to commit, in the contract, to maintaining appropriate insurance coverage for the losses that it may incur. In other words, all parties to the contract should be expected to keep certain minimal levels of insurance protection for the damages their acts might cause.

Quality of Care Provisions

Physician Participation in the MCO Quality Assurance Process As a concomitant to its UM program, the MCO will most certainly conduct a quality assurance process. This provision describes the physician's role in that process. It will do this in several ways.

The physician will be required to subject herself to the findings and conclusions of the process regarding the quality of care she provides. The physician will be required to cooperate with the process. In some cases, the physician also will be required to help administer the process, serving as a reviewer of the care quality of other physicians in the MCO.

Most of these requirements are little different from what physicians must satisfy in order to retain hospital medical staff privileges. The administrative responsibilities, however, can pose an additional burden. Seek additional compensation for assuming them.

Credential Standards Applied to Participating Physicians Also like most hospitals, the MCO will impose credentialing standards on the physicians with whom it contracts, and these will be codified in the contract. It will want to see evidence of the physician's current and continuing qualifications to practice medicine, including

- state licensure to practice medicine
- specialty board certification
- federal Drug Enforcement Administration registration
- staff privileges at appropriate hospitals
- malpractice insurance at specific levels

Besides a provision representing that the physician possesses all these credentials, the contract may incorporate by reference the full contents of the physician's application for participation. This is likely to include

- work history
- malpractice claims experience
- professional sanctions experience
- professional references

The contract may also refer to a credentialing manual, describing in some detail the physician application and screening process. It could include additional credentialing criteria as well. As always, try to review this manual before signing the contract.

There is a related legal matter to keep in mind. Managed care organizations increasingly are being held liable for their negligence in selecting

physicians to treat their members. As a result, their initial (and even renewal) screening of physician candidates has become much more rigorous. They will check references and may have access to the National Practitioner Data Bank (NPDB). Remember that an MCO may feel obligated to report to the NPDB the fact that it has rejected a physician's application for any reason related to quality of care. Therefore, do not apply unless you are quite confident of acceptance.

> **Note**: A growing number of MCOs are willing to delegate to a group of physicians the responsibility for selecting, evaluating, continuously monitoring, and, if necessary, terminating individual physicians. This is usually in connection with payment on a capitated basis and more likely with a large multispecialty group practice. It is extremely important to know whether this responsibility is being passed on to the physician group or organization—for both the additional administrative burden and legal liability it will impose. Besides determining whether your group is actually assuming this role, also check to see how the MCO is going to oversee your performance of the role and the terms under which they could take back the credentialing function.

Once a participating physician has established her credentials and been accepted by the MCO, she may have to meet ongoing requirements (such as continuing medical education attendance) to maintain her status. The MCO may also aggressively check to make sure that the physician's original credentials remain in effect. You should be aware of whether you will be taking on any of these obligations.

Notification to the MCO of Changes in the Physician's Credential Status This provision asks the physician to notify the MCO of changes in credential status—professional licensure, hospital staff privileges, and the like. This is a reasonable and unavoidable request. Be aware that any negative changes—that is, a lowering of a status or cancellation of a credential—are very likely to lead the MCO to terminate the contract.

Limitations on Personnel Who May Be Employed by the Physician Some MCOs may attempt to impose limitations on the ancillary and support personnel who may be used by the physician. This could include medical technicians, nonphysician clinicians, and others. The physician may be required to rely on people hired by the MCO or at least screened and approved by the MCO. The usual goal is to control the cost of employing these people, as well as the quality of work that they do.

This is a major usurpation of the physician's authority over his practice and should not be taken lightly. You may be required to let go (for lack of work) staff with whom you have grown comfortable working. You then may have to adjust to new staff you have not selected and who have no special loyalty to you.

If this provision really bothers you, it may be worth trying to negotiate its deletion. The MCO should be more amenable to this than, for example, a change in the uniform capitation rate offered to similarly situated physicians. Your chances will be improved if you can demonstrate the cost efficiency and high-quality performance of the existing staff.

Limitations on Physicians Who May Be Used by the Physician Group Through this provision in a contract with a group, many MCOs will attempt to retain the right to pick and choose which particular physicians will be allowed to provide services under the contract. Their goal is to ensure that only those physicians who practice good quality, cost-effective medicine will treat their enrollees. It can be disconcerting and disruptive to have an MCO selectively accept or exclude individual members of a physician group.

Most group practices and physician organizations believe that they conduct a reasonably vigorous credentialing procedure. Furthermore, many of these entities, such as PHOs, are built on a foundation of trust among previously independent providers. This kind of provision could undermine that trust and risk the collapse of the entire entity.

In evaluating such a provision, a group will want to review its own long-term goals, its operational style, the sophistication of its credentialing procedures, and the share of its revenues and number of its physicians likely to be affected by the contract. If the contract will be a minor source of patients and revenues, yet causes considerable upset among the physicians, pass it up. If you are a large group, probably important and desirable to the MCO, and run a tight, proven credentialing effort, push for elimination of this language. It will save the MCOs money and headaches as well.

Standard of Care To Be Provided by the Physician Many MCO contracts will stipulate the "standard of care" that the physician must meet in treating patients. They will use terms like *highest quality, reasonable and appropriate, consistent with prevailing community standards*, or *cost-effective*. The actual terminology is important for two reasons. The MCO will use it to gauge the physician's performance and, if he does not measure up, perhaps deselect him. The courts will use it as a measure of possible physician negligence when a patient suffers injury and sues.

Without other language in the contract, the standard to which a physician will be held is the quality of care provided by a comparable physician in the community under similar circumstances. Be aware of how special contract language might modify that duty. For instance, if the contract defines a higher standard, that is the one to which both the MCO and the courts are likely to hold you. This risk is compounded by public assurances (in marketing materials) the MCO gives to prospective members about the quality of care they will receive—e.g., "top physicians in the area." Agree to such higher standards only in return for much higher compensation or protections from liability and deselection. If the contract standards are different, without being clearly higher, look for two points—clear definition of the standard that you comprehend and a description of the process by which the MCO will ascertain whether the standard has been met.

Physician Adherence to Quality Review and Other Performance Standards You can expect the MCO to have a process for reviewing the quality of care provided by its physicians, as well as their conformance to other standards of performance, such as cost-effectiveness or patient satisfaction. The contract should state that participating physicians will be subject to this process. It should describe the process and identify the individuals who will implement it (medical director versus physician colleagues). The necessary detail may not be written into the contract. There probably will be a separate document describing it, incorporated by reference into the contract. Get a copy and examine it before signing the contract.

Composition and Authority of the Physician Advisory Committee Good MCOs maintain some sort of physician advisory committee to act as liaison between the MCO and the participating physicians. The body also can channel physician feedback and comments to the MCO. It is a good idea to include a description of the composition and authority of this committee in the contract. This description will give a strong indication of how effective the committee is likely to be in representing the physicians' interests to the MCO. It is also a measure of the MCO's commitment to a true partnership with its doctors.

Utilization Management Provisions

Physician Participation in the MCO's UM Process Utilization management programs are essential to MCO efforts to limit the services applied to maintain the health of their members. Managed care contracts require that providers participate in and comply with the UM program's requirements and activities. Thoroughly understand this part of the contract to be sure how the program works and affects physician practice.

The contract probably will not provide all the detail necessary to appreciate how the UM system will affect physicians. It may refer to a separate utilization manual. It is critical to see that manual and decide whether you can live with the

strictures it imposes. Whether in the contract or in a referenced manual, look for this key information.

- UM techniques employed (prior authorization, concurrent review, retrospective review, case management, gatekeeping, drug formulary)
- types of services to which the UM is applied (inpatient, outpatient, specialty, elective, ancillary)
- implementation of clinical practice guidelines, protocols, pathways, parameters, or other standards for treatment methodology
- source of such guidelines or protocols
- party responsible for the UM function (physicians, nonphysician MCO employees, independent contractor)
- information required for an informed UM decision
- party responsible for actually denying treatment
- method of communicating the denial to the physician
- availability of a process for physicians to appeal the denial
- requirement that physicians appeal disagreeable decisions
- language regarding the physician's exercise of "independent medical judgment" in all cases

The importance of understanding the MCO's UM procedures cannot be overestimated. All MCOs are practicing UM in one form or another. It goes to the heart of their claims to be able to save money for employers. The UM procedures they use can severely restrict a physician's practice autonomy and clinical decision making. They can disrupt the trust and continuity of the physician-patient relationship. They can add to the physician's administrative burden. They can place him in the untenable position of mediating between the interests of the patient and the interests of the MCO. In extreme cases, they may subject the physician to liability for injuries the patient suffers as a result of a treatment denial.

Providers have been held liable for their acts or omissions in following or attempting to follow the UM and related requirements. In negotiations, raise the question of the MCO indemnifying you for any liability imposed upon you as a result of compliance with an MCO-mandated and -operated UM program. The MCO will surely resist this proposal.

Physician Appeal of Utilization Management and Other Decisions by the MCO The physician arrangement with the MCO must include some mechanism for resolving disputes between the two parties. There should be one rapid-response procedure for appealing MCO denials of physician treatment recommendations. This should be an integral part of the UM program that produced the denial. Because so much rides on these decisions—compensation, legal liability, physician-patient relations—it is essential to understand and feel comfortable with the procedure. It may be described in the contract, but it is more likely to appear in a separate UM manual.

There also should be a grievance mechanism for dealing with less emergent conflicts between physicians and the MCO. They may not require such immediate attention but, left unattended, can be just as damaging to the relationship. They might include issues such as the imposition of more demanding reporting requirements or the MCO's contracting with a nearby physician group that competes with your own. Resorting to a grievance or conflict resolution mechanism is a good intermediary step before thinking of terminating the contract.

Term and Termination of the Contract

Term or Duration of the Contract Without this provision, there really is no contract. It should define a distinct term for the contract—in terms of a certain duration (e.g., three years) or a specific expiration date (e.g., October 21, 2003). It is possible for a contract to be terminable at will, with no clear finite term, but that is not at all a

good approach for this kind of managed care contract.

Of course, a contract term requires a beginning as well as an ending. So look for an "effective date" of the contract—the date on which your performance of the contract commitments must begin. Just be sure that you and your practice are ready by then.

The next question is, What happens when the term is up? The parties could begin negotiations for a new contract, reexamining every provision. However, this also is not a good idea for a relationship that is meant to develop into an amicable long-term partnership.

As a general rule, both physicians and MCOs should and do prefer to continue contracts with each other when they have an established relationship that seems to be working to their mutual benefits. This should lead to a desire to maintain and fine-tune that relationship, rather than to renegotiate the contract from scratch.

One way of continuing a contractual relationship is through a provision for automatic renewal unless either party gives notice that it prefers to end it. However, such language makes it less likely that the contract terms will be reexamined on a regular basis. Most physicians will at least want to reopen the question of their compensation levels. A workable compromise is an automatic renewal provision with a requirement for renegotiation of compensation (and perhaps a few other specified terms) no later than 90 days prior to the anniversary date of the contract. This approach keeps the essence of the contract in effect while adjusting some of its key conditions.

Automatic Renewal of the Contract The MCOs vary considerably in how they handle renewal of the contracts with their providers. In some cases, the renewal is allowed to happen automatically without any serious questions being asked. Other MCOs review their providers at renewal time as though they were applying for the first time. Find the contract provision that explains just how the renewal will occur, what new information will be required, and what criteria will be used.

Resolving Disputes between the Physician and the MCO Physicians are very likely to have disagreements and disputes with their MCO partners, especially during their first contact with managed care or a particular organization. They will vary from the trivial (which can be handled verbally, on the spot) to the career-threatening (which requires more serious review that is documented). It is quite important that the MCO have in place a formal mechanism for receiving and resolving physician grievances. The mechanism should include the equivalent of due process procedures and should be described in the contract.

Be wary of contract language that may limit your opportunities for redress. It is not uncommon for MCOs to require that a physician exhaust the administrative remedies afforded by the MCO before turning to the courts. In a few states, the MCO may be allowed to ask a participating provider give up its right to judicial review altogether or at least to accept serious limitations. Such contracts should be avoided unless there are rewards or protections that more than offset such a surrender of a basic right.

Rather than inhibit access to the courts, some contracts simply dictate which courts will have jurisdiction. Frequently, the MCO will choose a state either where its main offices are located or where it knows the law to be favorable to MCOs. From the physician's viewpoint, any state but the one where the physician is providing care would pose a major inconvenience if a lawsuit became necessary.

Grounds and Procedures for Imposing Corrective Action on Physicians In connection with its quality assurance, patient satisfaction, utilization efficiency, and other performance standards, a responsible MCO has a formal system for tracking physician performance and taking corrective action when indicated. That system should be mentioned in the contract and described, either there or in a referenced document. That description, wherever it is found, should include the following:

- the grounds for corrective action (quality problems, patient dissatisfaction, inappropriate utilization, costly practice style, other deviations from physician profile norms)
- the procedure for identifying problem behavior and deciding on corrective action
- the inclusion in that procedure of due process protections for the physician
- the designation of who decides when corrective action is necessary and the form it will take (medical director, committee of physicians, MCO board of directors)
- the forms of corrective action that might be taken against a physician (remedial education, restrictions on clinical privileges, limits on freedom to accept new patients, changes in compensation amounts or formulas, contract termination)

It also is good to know whether the MCO generally reports its corrective actions, at least those related to quality of care, to the NPDB. Similarly, for those physicians who might participate in the MCO's quality review process, is there sufficient compliance with the Health Care Quality Improvement Act (HCQIA) to afford them procedural protections against legal liability?

It may seem pessimistic to focus on termination issues at the beginning of what is meant to be a long, fruitful working relationship. However, MCOs are deselecting physicians in droves, and it behooves you to know how and why they might do this to you. Of course, some may dismiss you under their "without cause" provision to avoid explaining the decision at all. Others will terminate you for cause but will not allow you to defend yourself. In some MCOs, you either meet their standards or you are gone. There are no intermediate sanctions. Some may be alert enough to comply with the HCQIA, and others may not think of it.

Termination of the Contract by the Physician with Cause (Including Statement of Reasons Showing "Cause") This provision lays out the ways in which the parties can get out of the contract before its normal expiration (or automatic renewal) date. It should provide for two types of termination—with and without cause.

The language on "with cause" terminations is likely to include the following features:

- a list of the specific reasons or causes for which termination is possible (e.g., material breach of contract, bankruptcy, failure to make payments owed under the contract, failure to submit reports required by the contract)
- requirement of written notice of an alleged material breach, along with the opportunity to correct or "cure" the problems within a fixed time period (e.g., 30 days)
- provision for immediate suspension or termination in the event of quality problems with physician care, failure to maintain professional licensure or required insurance coverage, revocation of hospital staff privileges, other forms of discipline by a licensing authority, and a felony conviction

This provision should define good reasons for termination by the physician (that is, failures or breaches by the MCO) as well as the MCO.

Keep in mind that some of the above reasons for which an MCO may terminate its relationship with a physician may also require it to report the decision to the NPDB. The physician may also find himself having to explain the events to MCOs or hospitals to which he later applies. The best protection against these devastating repercussions is comprehensive due process—allowing the physician to challenge the termination before it becomes final.

Termination of the Contract by the Physician Without Cause The provision for termination "without cause" should be applied with mutual and equal time frames to both parties. For instance, either the physician or the MCO might be empowered to end the relationship without giving a reason by giving notice 90 days in advance. This advance notice period is usually longer than for terminations "with cause," which

are often 30 days. The key in setting the time periods is how long it takes to arrange for continuity of patient care.

Certainly, termination without cause language means that the MCO can leave the physician high and dry, once it has gotten what it wants out of the relationship. There is no way to avoid that. In any event, a relationship with an MCO with that attitude is not worth continuing. Just one precaution: Beware of contracts in which only the MCO has the right to terminate without cause.

Physician Responsibility for Patients after Termination of the Contract With the possibility of either party terminating the contract in midterm comes the likelihood of patients caught in the middle of treatment by the physician. The contract should deal with what happens to those patients and how the physician is compensated for services he provides them after the contract has ended.

There is not much room for debate about the physician's obligation to continue treating patients. State law, professional codes of ethical behavior, and the contract itself will usually require her to ensure continuity of care.

It is reasonable that this provision require the MCO to continue paying the physician for services rendered until the patient-enrollee is either transferred to another provider or the current treatment is completed. Payment can be on the terms defined in the contract, at the physician's usual and customary rate, according to a previously determined FFS schedule, or on some other basis. It is not reasonable, however, to continue payment at capitation rates, as the necessary actuarial principles are no longer operative.

Appendices These are the kinds of information likely to appear in the appendices of a managed care contract. They are put here because they are so voluminous. You can tell from their titles that they are just as important as any language in the body of the contract. Review them just as thoroughly.

- listing of physician's practice locations
- schedule of capitation fees by member type
- schedule of payments for certain services on an FFS basis
- detailed listing of services to be provided by the physician

Calculating Your Profits (or Losses) under a Managed Care Contract

As your physician group grows in size, through acquisition and merger, it will develop highly sophisticated management information systems to measure costs and to manage performance. However, what about now, before you can afford such systems? How can you determine whether you will make money under a particular managed care contract? Here are two simple, quick-and-dirty procedures for calculating the profits or losses under an existing or prospective contract.

Profit Calculation Procedure #1

1. Pick a recent one-year period for which you have good data on the care you have delivered, by Current Procedural Terminology (CPT) code, and the total costs for operating your practice.
2. Make a list of all the CPT codes under which you provided services during the time period and the number of times each service was provided.
3. Get the relative value units (RVUs) for each of those CPT codes. They are available from the Resource-Based Relative Value System (RBRVS) used by the federal government, as well as from McGraw-Hill and Healthcare Consultants of America.
4. Multiply the frequency of each CPT code by its RVU. Then add the resulting RVUs to get the total volume of RVUs carried out in your practice during the year in question.
5. Determine the total operating costs of the practice during the year. This includes sal-

aries, overhead, supplies, depreciation, and the income you took home.
6. Divide the total operating costs (from step 5) by the total volume of RVUs for the year (from step 4). The result is a rough approximation of the costs associated with each RVU in your practice.
7. Multiply the cost per RVU (from step 6) by the RVUs associated with each CPT code performed (from step 3). The result is an even rougher approximation of your cost of providing each CPT code procedure.

These numbers are then compared to the fees or rates you receive under a managed care contract. Here's how it works.

Under an FFS contract, the MCO will provide you with a schedule of the fees it will pay for each CPT code. It is a simple matter to compare them with the cost figures you have calculated. However, that is not the end of it. The comparison probably will show you making money on some procedures and losing it on others. So you need to multiply the profit or loss on each procedure by the number of times you perform the procedure. When the total profits and losses are combined, they will indicate whether that contract is profitable for you.

There is a small hitch if you are doing this analysis on a prospective contract—you will not know the volume of each procedure you will have to deliver. Ask the MCO for the utilization rates it should have for the population you will be serving or use your own figures for the patients you have been seeing. Then carry out the calculation.

Under a capitated contract, the MCO proposes a lump-sum fee covering all the services the physician might have to provide to each of the couple of thousand patients for whom the physician will be responsible. The MCO also will have utilization rates for that pool of patients. (The rates were necessary for the MCO to calculate its capitation rate.) Multiply the utilization rates for each procedure (from step 7 above). The result is the total cost for the physician to meet her obligations under the contract. Next, multiply the capitation rate by the number of patients in the pool. The result is the total reimbursement the physician will receive for performing her part of the contract. The amount by which the total reimbursement exceeds the total cost is the money that the physician will make on that contract.

Profit Calculation Procedure #2

This next method is more crude than the first. It uses patients as the common denominator rather than RVUs. It requires much less detailed information to support its calculations. The results will not be as accurate as those from Procedure #1. However, its sheer simplicity makes it much more likely to actually be employed. When you do not have the background data or the time required by the first method, use this one.

1. By volume or revenues, determine the top 10 or 20 procedures (by CPT code) provided by the practice over the past three years.
2. Using generally accepted practice accounting principles, calculate the cost of providing a unit of each procedure.
3. With the MCO, make an estimate of the numbers of patients likely to enroll with the practice under the contract. If there are several distinctly different groups of potential patients—by demographics, employer, etc.—make estimates for each of them.
4. From the MCO, obtain historical utilization rates for those enrollee groups. (The rates should indicate the most commonly utilized procedures and the utilization volume for each.) With luck, they may also include the statistical variability of the rates. What are the chances of them being significantly higher or lower?
5. Calculate a "most likely scenario" for utilization of physician services by the MCO enrollees. Multiply the historical utilization rates (from step 4) by the estimates of the number of MCO members enrolling

with the practice (from step 3). Do this for each different patient group.
6. Calculate the cost to the practice of treating the enrolled MCO patients. Multiply the estimate of utilization of physician services by the MCO enrollees (from step 5) by the cost of providing each unit of those services (from step 2). Add the cost of purchasing from other physicians the services that the practice is unable to provide and the cost of administering the practice's responsibilities under the contract.
7. Compare the total cost figure for serving the MCO enrollees for one month with the monthly capitation payments promised under the contract. Are the costs lower than the capitation revenues? If they are not lower, can you work to lower the utilization rates and reduce other practice costs to eventually bring the costs below the revenues? If you cannot lower the costs sufficiently in the near future, can you negotiate a higher capitation fee with the MCO? If you cannot negotiate a higher fee, is there some other benefit from this contract that offsets the losses you will incur? If not, do not enter into the contract.
8. Calculate several "what-if" scenarios, varying the number of enrollees, their utilization rates, and your costs to see what circumstances cause the practice clearly to make or lose money. At the very least, develop "worst-case" and "best-case" scenarios. This should be fairly easy to do in a capable computer spreadsheet program.

Quick Focus on the Provisions to Which a Physician Should Pay Most Attention

This is just a reminder of the contract clauses that deserve your highest priority attention.

- listing and definition of services the physicians will provide
- term of the contract and the means by which it may be renewed

- physician agreement to "hold harmless" the MCO
- methods for amending the contract, especially unilaterally by the MCO
- limits on minimum and maximum number of patients sent to your practice
- specific health plans or products the physician is committed to serve
- utilization management and quality assurance procedures
- required recordkeeping and reporting by the physician to the MCO
- required recordkeeping and reporting by the MCO to the physician
- restrictions on physician's communications with patients
- terms under which risk withholds and other risk-sharing compensation are paid to the physician
- availability of stop-loss insurance
- conditions for contract termination by the MCO or the physician
- amount of physician compensation (capitation, FFS, risk sharing)

Personal Ethical Questions To Ask Yourself before Signing Any Managed Care Contract

When entering into a contract with a particular MCO, you are agreeing to follow its rules and procedures, and you are making yourself a party to its practices and policies. Are you willing to live with the implications of that new relationship? Here are a few of the more ethical issues you might want to consider.

- Are you willing to be restricted in the medications you can prescribe by an enforced drug formulary?
- Are you willing to be restricted in the specialists to whom you can refer to those also under contract with the MCO?
- Will you be comfortable with limitations, even subtle and unwritten, on what you may discuss with your patients?
- Can you work easily under pressure to limit the time you spend with each patient?
- Will you feel contented practicing medicine under a wide array of disincentives to utilize resources in treating patients?
- How will you feel about your role as middleman between MCO and patient in denials of coverage?
- Can you live with the knowledge that at least some of the cost savings you achieve will go toward the large salaries of executives in large profit-focused corporations and toward enhancing the value of the corporation's stock?
- If your MCO affiliation is exclusive, will you miss the previous patients you can longer see?

You probably would rather not deal with any of these restrictions on your practice style. In more and more markets, there are no alternatives. These policies are becoming the norm in health care delivery.

REFERENCES

1. D. Kouba, "Primary Care Providers: Managing Today's Prepaid Risk," *Medical Group Management Journal 38*, no. 1 (1991): 37–40.

RESOURCE LIST

Contracting with Managed Care, Super Search Packet #1671. Medical Group Management Association.

Critical Steps in Managed Care Contracting: A Looseleaf Guide, vols. I, II. American Health Lawyers Association, 1996.

W. Knight, *Managed Care Contracting, a Guide for Health Care Professionals* (Gaithersburg, MD: Aspen Publishers, Inc. 1997).

Managed Care Contract Performance and Review, Book #4789. Medical Group Management Association.

Managed Care Contracting Handbook. American Health Lawyers Association, 1997.

Managed Care—Contracts, Information Exchange #4989. Medical Group Management Association.

"Ten Mistakes To Avoid When You Apply to a Managed-Care Plan," *Medical Economics*, 22 September, 1997.

"Ten Strategies for Creating Successful Managed Care Relationships," *Health Care Financial Management*, June 1997.

M. Todd, *The Managed Care Contracting Handbook—Planning and Negotiating the Managed Care Relationship.* (Burr Ridge, IL: McGraw-Hill Healthcare Education Group, 1996).

CHAPTER 9

Strategies for Negotiating with a Managed Care Organization

INTRODUCTION

Physicians do not have to accept the contract terms proposed by managed care organizations (MCOs). Depending on the bargaining power they have amassed, they may try to negotiate with the MCO for changes. Chapter 8, "Step Two: How To Analyze and Evaluate a Managed Care Contract," explains which terms to seek and avoid. There are numerous other opportunities in running a physician organization to improve your standing through negotiation. Good negotiation skills can also produce benefits in these situations.

- affiliation with practice organizations
- employment by a provider group or facility
- purchase or sale of a medical practice
- purchase or lease of medical office space
- purchase or lease of medical office equipment—both clinical and managerial

This chapter is designed to prepare a physician to conduct a successful negotiation with an MCO. It lays out important steps to take weeks or months before real negotiations begin—steps that will put you in the strongest possible bargaining position. There are suggestions on the composition of the negotiating team, planning a negotiation strategy, and special tactics for different kinds of physicians.

This is not an extended discourse on all the possible strategies and tactics available, but rather an introduction to a few common approaches that work in certain situations and some others to generally avoid. In many cases, where the negotiation is low-key or where there are few issues open to discussion, these tips will be all that the physician needs. If the transaction looks as if it will be more complex or challenging for the physician, he will be urged to let an experienced negotiator (probably an attorney) represent him.

Even where you do not get all the changes you are looking for, a good-faith attempt at negotiation will produce some benefits. It is worth the effort.

WHO SHOULD READ THIS CHAPTER

The physician most interested in this chapter is the one about to enter into her first managed care contract. If you already have executed a few contracts and want a better foundation for what you are doing, look here. Perhaps you have signed quite a number of managed care contracts but have had serious problems or were just dissatisfied with the results. There is a good chance that you never tried to negotiate at all.

If you are a seasoned contractor with MCOs, if you have a solid relationship with one or with a couple of MCOs that provide the bulk of your revenues, if you are an employee of an MCO, or if you are a member of a physician organization that handles contract negotiations on your behalf, you can safely skip this chapter.

PREPARING FOR NEGOTIATION IN THE MONTHS BEFOREHAND

In the months prior to the negotiations, take steps to increase your visibility in the community. The goal is to be known by prospective patients, other physicians (particularly those already contracting with the MCO), other providers, other professionals, local businesses (benefits managers), local business leaders, and local civic groups (including the Chamber of Commerce).

Begin gathering the data to prove that you can control costs and utilization while maintaining quality of care

- to sell the MCO on your commitment and your systems
- to sell the MCO on your competency
- for the MCO to use in selling itself to employers

Reshape your referral networks to emphasize other physicians who share your commitment to "managed care" medicine.

Do a role reversal and try to imagine what the MCO needs from its participating physicians. Draw up a list. Go through the list and determine which of those needs will be met by your group.

In addition, prepare a separate list of all the great things about your practice that should be attractive to an MCO. Describe them in some detail, backing them up with data, documents, testimonials, and research results. These are the points you will use to sell yourself to the MCO. Make sure you bring them up at appropriate points in the negotiations.

Prepare another list of your practice's weaknesses—the features that may give the MCO pause about contracting with you. Do not volunteer these facts, but expect the MCO to know or ask about them. Prepare the responses you will give (the goal is to never be caught off guard)— explain the problem away, show how it has been or will be corrected, describe the steps being taken to prevent its recurrence. (Refer to the appropriate sections in Chapter 7 on identifying

and dealing with the strengths and weaknesses of your practice.)

Assume that there is a mutually acceptable position on every contract term and that a contract will be concluded and signed. Then proceed with almost endless patience to find that position. Try not to let your negotiation decisions be influenced by time pressures—real or perceived.

PREPARING YOURSELF PERSONALLY FOR THE NEGOTIATING EXPERIENCE

Before you gear up for a particular negotiation encounter, it is a good idea to do some general preparation in negotiating skills. Start by reading a few books on negotiation. There are some good ones in the Resource List at the end of this chapter. If you have the time, it would be well spent in a negotiation training course—not the kind that advocates a "take-no-prisoners" approach. Also talk with friends and colleagues who have participated in any kind of negotiation. What did they learn, what worked for them, and what advice do they have? If you have the chance, try out your negotiating skills in a less portentous situation, for example, in buying a new car. If you feel quite unprepared for your first major negotiation, hire an experienced consultant or attorney to work with you. Watch everything this person does, take copious notes, and learn from his best practices.

> Negotiation skills are not genetic; you can learn to be an effective negotiator. You may not be able to change your basic interpersonal skills dramatically, but you can develop a negotiation style that fits your personality.

CONNECTION BETWEEN PERSONALITY TRAITS AND NEGOTIATION SUCCESS

As a general rule, special personality traits are not a prerequisite to negotiation success. All necessary negotiation skills can be acquired through training and adapted to each negotiator's personal style. The one exception may be the person who is exceptionally averse to conflict. These types of people may be more inclined to make concessions and, in the process, their apparent weakness may encourage the MCO negotiators to push for tougher terms.

Personality can become a factor in negotiations in one other way. Though the best negotiation produces a win-win agreement, there may be moments during the negotiation when one party is clearly yielding on a major issue. It is important for the long-term relationship that she be allowed to give up her position gracefully, with a minimum of embarrassment or loss of face.

WHO TAKES THE FIRST STEP: PHYSICIAN OR MCO?

If you are like the vast majority of physicians, you are flattered at the number of MCOs that have sought you out for contracting. However, there are problems with that kind of attitude.

- Your passive posture means that you will get contracts with only those MCOs that learn of your existence and decide, for whatever reasons, to approach you. These may or may not be the most desirable MCO partners for your practice. You completely miss out on all the other possible MCO contract partners, which may be even more attractive.
- Your passive posture sets the tone for the negotiations that follow: The MCO takes the lead, defines the issues, drafts the contract language, and always seems to be in charge of the process. You are constantly reacting to its initiatives. Under those circumstances, it is no surprise if the final contract favors the MCO.

Consider the possibility of taking the initiative in identifying the MCOs you would especially like to work with, approaching them to propose a long-term affiliation, suggesting the appropriate terms for a contract, demonstrating the benefits they will realize by collaborating with you, and creating exactly the kind of working relationship you want. Even if the MCO insists on starting with its draft of the contract, your assertiveness will enhance your bargaining position and probably impress the MCO. In any event, you will wind up with a better deal with a better MCO.

INITIAL CONTACTS WITH THE MCO

For most physicians, the possibility of contract negotiations arises when an MCO gets in touch with them. Remember that there is nothing preventing a physician from selecting the most desirable MCOs and taking the initiative to contact them. Seriously consider that course.

Whoever takes the first step, the physician is likely to start off talking to the MCO's contracting specialists. They will probably be your main source of contact with the MCO, even though you may need eventually to communicate with other MCO officials (e.g., medical director, financial manager, claims manager).

This is the beginning of a contracting process that can take from six months to over a year. The impressions and messages communicated during this opening stage will color the MCO's view of you and set the tone for the relationship you are trying to build. The importance is heightened even further if your goal is to persuade the MCO to switch from another physician group to yours.

From the outset, project a desire to collaborate. Talk often about "partnering" and "long-term strategic affiliation." Use words that press all the MCO's hot buttons. It is looking for partners who help give it an advantage in the competition for attracting new enrollees and keeping old ones. So tell it what it wants to hear. At this point, you are trying to get your foot in the door. Refer to the patient satisfaction surveys you conduct and the positive results they have shown. Mention your rigorous physician credentialing and utilization management (UM) programs. Share your vision for the future integration and interaction between your practice and the MCO.

Leave the MCO thinking "These people are different from the other physicians we hear from. They are the kind of group we need to do business with."

ASSEMBLING YOUR NEGOTIATING TEAM

Yes, you should be thinking in terms of going into a negotiation with some form of "team." If you are a solo or small group practice, this may consist of one physician and an attorney. If your practice is larger, there may be two or three physicians, a business or finance manager, and the lawyer.

If a lawyer is not participating on the negotiating team, at least consult one

- before entering the negotiations (what ideal terms to seek)
- after receiving the MCO's draft contract (what to change)
- during the negotiations (to evaluate proposals, counterproposals, and exact language)
- before signing the final version of the contract

In assembling your team, certainly choose people with the right combination of practical skills. Keep some other things in mind, too. You may prefer to negotiate with people who have similar backgrounds and training. At the very least, they should be people who understand the medical profession in general and your practice in particular.

Study your personal strengths and weaknesses. Choose team members who will complement or offset those characteristics.

Identify the administrative and clinical decision makers within the MCO, particularly those participating in the negotiation. Try to meet them before the negotiations begin. If you find that you have a personality or communication conflict with a key MCO negotiator, put someone on your team who can work effectively with this individual.

Ultimately, look for team members who will support you in producing the optimal outcome to the negotiation.

ALLOWING A MORE EXPERIENCED, SKILLED PERSON TO NEGOTIATE ON YOUR BEHALF

There are relatively few skilled negotiators among health care providers because they have never had reason to develop the skill. However, their numbers are growing rapidly as they are forced by market pressures to have and gain negotiating experience.

Your first significant managed care contract may not be the best place to acquire the experience. Misjudgments could lead you into an ill-advised relationship that ends up costing you money and affecting your reputation.

Whether you like it or not, some of the best negotiators around are attorneys—it is their stock and trade. If you are represented by an attorney knowledgeable in health law who also has good negotiating expertise, talk with her about assuming a role in your contract negotiations.

There are many degrees of possible involvement. You can tell the lawyer what you do and do not want out of the contract, leaving her to negotiate the best deal for you while you stay at home. At the other extreme, you can check in with the attorney after every bargaining session. The attorney can evaluate your progress and make recommendations for the next session. Perhaps the best compromise is for both you and the attorney to participate in all the negotiations, with her taking the lead. The two of you can plan strategies for each session, and she can consult with you during the negotiations about possible changes in those strategies. It is important that you be present during the negotiations so that you are able to learn from the experience. Eventually, you may feel confident enough to negotiate on your own.

SETTING THE LOGISTICAL FRAMEWORK FOR THE NEGOTIATION

There must be prior agreement of the parties on the logistical details of the negotiation. You should feel comfortable with all these practical aspects. If you are ambitious and clever, you could try to arrange some of these elements to your advantage (location of the negotiation, shape of the table, selection of the caterer), but it probably is not worth the effort.

Plan these matters with the MCO.

- identities and job functions of the negotiators for both sides
- time frame and times for the negotiation
  - number of sessions, dates, hours
  - deadlines for conclusion of the entire negotiation and, perhaps, for segments of it
- assurance that the negotiators have authority to commit their organizations
- format for the exchanges during the negotiation (formal versus spontaneous, taking turns leading on particular issues, use of a facilitator or chairperson)
- manner for setting the agenda
- frequency and length of breaks
- location of negotiation (either party's facility or a neutral site), size of room, seating arrangement, plans for refreshments

PRENEGOTIATION ANALYSIS OF THE FIRST DRAFT OF THE CONTRACT

At least two weeks, preferably a month or more, before the first negotiation session, obtain a copy of the contract proposed by the MCO. Then follow these steps. Of course, if you are bold and confident, you will send your own draft of a contract to the MCO first.

- View the contract price as just one of several issues to be negotiated.
- More than a few doctors have signed a managed care contract, or several of them, after looking at nothing more than the payment offered—whether capitation fee or fee-for-service (FFS) schedule.
- Chapter 8 should make clear that other non-financial contract terms are just as important in assessing the desirability of the contract and your chances of succeeding under it.

- Read every single provision and word of the contract until you think you understand what they mean.
- Then, review the contract in conjunction with Chapter 8 to see if you missed something.
- Then, pretend you are the top executive of the MCO and imagine how you would interpret and use each contract provision.
- Now, you should have a sense of what you like and don't like about the contract. You are ready to develop a position on each term or issue addressed in it.
- Before you enter the room to negotiate, decide how you stand on each contract issue.
  - Some terms are just fine the way they are, or are of trivial importance (and you have checked with a lawyer to make sure they are trivial).
  - For all other terms, decide two things.
    1. your ideal handling of the matter or ideal contract language concerning it
    2. your minimum acceptable position on the matter (anything less than this and you will walk away)
- Assign one of three priorities to each term.
  - A. "Critical to my success under this contract. If I do not get a change within my acceptability range, I cannot enter into this contract."
  - B. "Important to my contract success, but I am willing to bend on some of these in exchange for getting what I want on some others."
  - C. "A change would be nice, but I am willing and able to practice under the contract without a change."
- With regard to the payment terms, conduct the analysis of your practice cost structure and the likely patient volume and utilization rates under the contract (as outlined in Chapter 8) to prepare your position on the capitation fee or FFS schedule. In particular, determine
  - your minimum acceptable payment levels, below which you are not willing to participate in the contract (because

you will lose money or you will not make enough money and there are no offsetting benefits)
- a desirable, comfortable level that would permit you to meet personal financial goals

PLANNING THE ALTERNATIVE STRATEGIES IF YOU CANNOT NEGOTIATE AN ACCEPTABLE CONTRACT

- You put yourself in a weakened bargaining position if you become invested in having this contract no matter what and have not contemplated your position if the negotiations do not succeed. You are likely to make undesirable, even disastrous, concessions to secure the contract that you are not mentally prepared to live without.
- Define your "best alternative to a negotiated agreement" (BATNA), that is, the most favorable option open to you if the negotiations are not successfully concluded. For example, "If our 20-physician multispecialty group practice cannot get this contract, we will begin discussions with other similar groups to form an independent practice association (IPA) that will have greater clout in future negotiations."
- Flesh out this alternative plan of action so that you have a good understanding of its pros and cons, and what it will take to implement it. Turn it into a real possibility. If you are really ambitious, sketch out your three best alternative strategies.
- Then, as the negotiations proceed, constantly measure what you are getting under the contract against what you could get by pursuing one of the alternatives instead.
- Just knowing that you have alternatives will empower your negotiation posture and inform your negotiation decisions ("We could do better than this if we formed the IPA.").
- Your BATNA will depend on a number of factors—the size of your group (in human

and financial terms), managed care penetration in the marketplace, activities of competitors, and the dominance of the MCO with which you are negotiating. The alternatives to no contract may not be great, but there are always alternatives. Know what they are ahead of time.

FORMULATING A NEGOTIATION STRATEGY

It is essential to take the time, well before embarking on a contract negotiation, to formulate in some detail the plan or strategy you will follow. It will enhance the final outcome for you dramatically.

The strategy is composed of elements such as

- the overall packaging and presentation of the practice
- specific positions on each potential negotiation topic
- timing of concessions and the weights assigned to each
- anticipation of the tactics you will employ under various negotiation circumstances
- roles to be played by members of the negotiation team

Flexibility should be part of any negotiation plans you make. Be prepared to modify both the strategy and tactics, depending on the responses of the MCO negotiation team. Of course, the art is knowing when to stick with the original plan and when to shift to something that might work better.

> Negotiating is about knowing what your needs are from the negotiation, finding out what the needs of the other party are, and giving the other party what is necessary to meet its needs, in exchange for it giving you things to meet your needs.

In formulating the negotiation strategy, answer these questions.

- What is the overall outcome you want from the negotiation?
- What are your ideal and minimum acceptable positions on each issue in the contract?
- What is the overall image of you and your practice that you will project to the MCO?
- What features of your practice and expectations for your professional future are you willing to negotiate?
- What are your primary sources of bargaining power as you enter this negotiation?
- How will you use this power to support your negotiation strategy?
- What does the MCO have to gain by contracting with you? What does it have to lose?
- What are the primary sources of the MCO's bargaining power?
- What overall outcome do you think the MCO seeks from the negotiation?
- What overall image of itself is the MCO trying to present to you?
- What positions do you expect the MCO to take on each issue in the contract?
- Which of those positions can you accept and which must you reject?

Finally, a negotiating strategy that embodies these basic principles has a greater chance of succeeding for you.

- Identify, define, and emphasize positive features of your practice (greater patient satisfaction and member retention, superior operating efficiencies, demonstrably higher quality, reduced resource utilization, overall lower costs).
- Start with high aspirations and adopt more demanding positions on issues.
- Rigorously manage the flow of information during the negotiation (What did we learn in today's session? What information will we reveal about ourselves in tomorrow's session?).
- Gain full knowledge of the strengths, weaknesses, and power sources of both parties.
- Understand the difference between what is good for your practice and your professional

future, and what psychologic needs you might have from the negotiation process (to control, to save face, to impress colleagues), then concentrate on the former.
- Make concessions according to a plan.
- Have infinite patience.

CHOICE OF OVERALL STRATEGY FOR THE NEGOTIATION

There is a lot of lore about the best or most effective negotiation strategies. There are frequent images in American culture of clever, manipulative negotiators conniving in smoke-filled rooms to outwit their negotiation opponents. Whether or not these win-lose strategies are in regular use, they are quite inappropriate for negotiating managed care contracts.

These are some basic strategies to consider using, singly or in combination, in negotiating with an MCO.

Start High, Give Little

One of the most successful strategies for maximizing negotiation gains is to take a realistically high initial position, then to make only a few modest concessions. For this strategy to work, the initial position must be realistic—that is, it must seem plausible, if not entirely acceptable, to the MCO. This is not about making an exorbitant opening demand and allowing it to be whittled down through negotiations to something more reasonable. The strategy also assumes you have a pretty good idea of what is realistic. If you do not, for lack of knowledge about the MCO's operations and finances, forgo making an initial offer and see what the MCO proposes.

The tough opening position has a couple of advantages. First, it leaves you room to make concessions and satisfy the MCO's desire to see movement and a willingness to compromise on your part. If your first offer is much lower, perhaps closer to your minimum acceptable position, you have simply made a concession before the negotiation ever began. Second, starting high helps define the range (between your almost-final offer and the MCO's) that may become the basis for a "split-the-difference" settlement in the case of a deadlock.

Unilateral Concession in Hope of Reciprocation

Under this strategy, whatever your opening position and after a modest amount of bargaining, you make a significant unilateral concession with the expectation that it will prompt a reciprocal concession from the MCO team. It works by immediately lowering the level of distrust. However, do not surrender all your negotiating leverage in making the concession. The goal is to initiate a pattern of mutual, back-and-forth, give-and-take concessions until agreement is reached on each contract issue. If the MCO negotiators do not respond, be prepared to make effective threats.

Start High, Give First, and Give a Lot

This combines the first two strategies. It can be particularly useful if the "start-high, give-little" strategy seems to frighten the MCO and stiffen its resistance. This can prevent deadlock when you sense that the parties' real positions are not very far apart.

Equity for Both Parties

The goal of this strategy is to develop a solution based on principles of equity for both parties, rather than one winning out over the other. It requires being candid from the outset about taking this approach. Both parties must acknowledge the choice and work together to find contract language that best satisfies their needs and interests.

Often, this strategy starts with agreement on basic principles for an equitable contract. It is usually easier to build consensus around these more abstract themes. The next step is more concrete discussion about specific contract language that will flesh out the principles.

This strategy has the powerful advantage of increasing trust and reducing defensiveness for both parties by ensuring that their basic interests and goals will be recognized. It is especially useful in situations where

- the parties wish to create a long-term relationship
- a collaborative, open effort by both parties is likely to maximize the gain
- there is a desire that neither party feel it is losing out in the final settlement

It is an ideal strategy for negotiating a healthy, productive physician-MCO affiliation.

DISTINGUISHING YOUR PRACTICE FROM ALL OTHERS

In some contract situations, you may be competing with numerous other physicians for a limited number of spots on an MCO's panel. You may even be trying to displace someone currently on the panel. Here are some possible ways to define your practice and persuade the MCO that it would be a more desirable partner than the competing practices.

- Configure your services (clinical and administrative) or develop practice methods in ways that reduce the time or number of people required to deliver them.
- Show how your services mesh (geographically or by specialty) with those of existing MCO providers to offer coverage of larger geographic areas, a broader range of medical care, or a larger member population.
- Develop medical specialties or procedures that will help the MCO provide better care at lower cost while keeping members healthier and happier. This could be an advantage the MCO can promote to employers.
- Offer to assume greater risks in more aspects of the financial and legal relationship with the MCO.
- Create standardized services (clinical or administrative) or practice methods (protocols, pathways, guidelines) that reduce costs and make the MCO more efficient.

- Offer better member access (location, hours) and more satisfying attention for the MCO's members.
- Agree to assume administrative functions currently performed by the MCO (data management, claims processing, physician credentialing, utilization review), saving it money in the process.

If you can develop and present these distinctive practice features, you will stand out from the crowd.

DISTINGUISHING PERSONAL NEEDS FROM ORGANIZATIONAL NEEDS

On the surface, contract negotiations are about satisfying the objective needs of the physician organization (which may be little more than a solo practice) and the MCO. Under the surface, negotiators for those organizations often bring to the table a complex mixture of personal needs, as well. They may "need" to control the negotiation (regardless of the outcome), "win" the negotiation (regardless of the cost), impress colleagues, or avoid embarrassment.

Be conscious of the fact that both you and the MCO negotiators will have these often unconscious agendas. What to do about them?

First, try to figure out what those needs are. Think about other negotiations you have been in and how you behaved. Think about your feelings as you prepare for this negotiation and your feelings about particular contract issues. Ask a friend to join you in a probing dialogue about what you must get personally for the negotiation to seem "successful." As the negotiation proceeds, notice whether your thoughts and feelings are based on an objective assessment of your progress in representing your organization or on the moment-to-moment satisfaction of your emotional needs.

Decide for yourself whether the pursuit of personal needs is interfering with achievement of organizational goals. Often, simple acknowledgment of what is going on will lead you to the correct behavior. If not, you may have to work more deliberately to separate and suppress your personal desires in order to concentrate more fully on the organization's welfare. In rare cases, personal passions may render a person unsuited for negotiation. It may be necessary to turn the responsibility over to another member of the practice or to an advisor.

Knowing the personal needs of the MCO negotiators would be just as useful but much more difficult to do. Pay attention to what they say and how they say it (choice of words, tone of voice, facial expression). When there seem to be illogical discrepancies between a negotiator's words or behavior and the substance or weight of an issue, ask open-ended questions designed to get to the heart of his intentions. You will never be terribly successful at this, but you may get a better sense of exactly what you must do to make the opposing negotiator happy.

Do not always assume that satisfying a negotiator's personal needs is a bad thing. If the practical results of the negotiation—the contract terms agreed to—provide the foundation for a solid, long-term relationship, the binding may be even stronger if the negotiators also feel personally pleased with their role in the process. In fact, a truly successful managed care contract negotiation will also produce the following unwritten outcomes:

- The MCO develops a positive impression of you and your practice.
- You are convinced that the MCO will be an excellent strategic partner.
- A sense of mutual trust is growing between you and the MCO.
- A relationship with long-term potential has been created.

CHOICE OF TACTICS FOR THE NEGOTIATION

Tactics are the shorter-term conversational tools and methods for implementing the overall negotiation strategy. Though it occasionally makes sense to shift among strategies, good negotiators will constantly juggle tactics to optimize their outcomes—depending on the opponent's actions and the stage of the negotiation.

An understanding of tactics is essential to successful implementation of your strategy, and it is just as important for recognizing what the MCO negotiators are doing. These are the most common and traditional negotiating tactics:

- *Problem solving.* Present a position or argument as an attempt to solve a mutual problem, rather than an effort to gain a competitive edge. This tactic aims to clarify disagreements and necessary tasks to come up with a joint solution, rather than to try to change the position of the MCO negotiators. You and the MCO work together as a team to create a mutually satisfying solution.

  Problem solving is a good resort when other approaches have reached an impasse. To work properly, both parties will have to reveal some of their real preferences for an ideal agreement. This shows how far apart they are and suggests what might have to be done to bring them together.

  Note: When employing this tactic, and at any other point in the negotiation, be willing to allow the MCO to agree on a position for reasons different than yours. It does not matter whether the MCO negotiator accepts your logic and facts or not. All that matters is that you get the practical results you want.

- *Exchanging information.* A more open exchange of information is usually part of problem solving, but it also can be used as a tactic in its own right—to educate the MCO regarding certain facts or law. This should be done with the expectation that the MCO will make a favorable change in its position once it sees the information. The disclosure can be carried out unilaterally by one party or as part of an agreed-upon reciprocal exchange.

- *Trial and error.* Make an offer and see what reaction it provokes. Whether refusal or acceptance, that helps inform the next move. Gradually, through this pattern of tossing out ideas, you will begin to get a sense of what is

and is not acceptable to the MCO and what approaches do and do not work. The trial and error should not be done randomly. Try a sort of "multiple-choice" approach, offering a series of alternative solutions to the problem, each one of which requires approximately the same concession on your part. Alternatively, conduct the trials with priority C issues while remaining firm on priority A ones or expressly request or demand some feedback or response to the offer. At the very least, this will encourage a more cooperative atmosphere and gather information about the MCO's positions.

- *Traditional bargaining.* Make an offer only on the explicit condition that the MCO grants a particular concession in return. If those concessions are not forthcoming, this tactic loses its value.

- *Wielding power.* If you have some bargaining leverage (the only area physician in your specialty or a particularly large group practice), you may implicitly or explicitly threaten to walk away from the negotiation—perhaps going to a competing MCO. This is a dangerous tactic. If not used adroitly, it may lead to a breakdown in negotiations, retaliation by the MCO, or, even if it works, a poisoning of the relationship between the two of you.

HOW TO MAKE CONCESSIONS IN A NEGOTIATION

Think ahead of time about the timing of the concessions you will make, their importance (by assigned priority), and their substance. Pay particular attention to the true value of each concession—to you and to the MCO. You do not want to give away too much or too little, and you want your exchanges of concessions to be comparable.

Consider these rules of thumb in making concessions. Do not make a concession unless

- it is part of a consistent strategy,
- you are forced to by the MCO's bargaining power,

- the MCO gives a comparable concession in return,
- it is necessary to maintain the momentum of the negotiation, or
- when you are confident that you and the MCO are well on the way to forming an enduring partnership.

Make consecutive concessions on the same issue in declining amounts or degrees so that the MCO sees that there is an end to them (e.g., $1.50, $1.25, $1.15, $1.10, $1.08).

Make or request concessions on the level of services you will provide. For instance, if the MCO cannot or will not raise the capitation rate to the level you need, ask them to reduce your service obligations instead. These may be specific medical services that you effectively ask to be "carved out" of the rate or they might be administrative services, such as easing your reporting requirements.

Alternatively, give the MCO additional services in return for the higher rate. Offer to self-credential your physicians or to provide more comprehensive utilization, encounter, or outcomes data to the MCO. Have a list of these trading chips ready before the negotiations begin.

Prepare a list of all negotiating items that you could concede. Draw up a protocol for making the concession—e.g., we will concede priority C issues first, then a B issue, followed by more C issues, then an A issue, if necessary.

SOME PRACTICAL TACTICAL SUGGESTIONS FOR WINNING OVER AN MCO

The purpose of the negotiations is to create a long-term strategic partnership offering mutual benefits. Approach the negotiations with that intention.

- Talk partnership terms; use the term regularly.
- Talk about contract terms several years in the future, as though you will be together that long.

- Be willing to talk about multiyear contracts. (Exception: if you are just starting with managed care contracts or have a serious uncertainty about the MCO. After a year or two of successful affiliation, begin thinking about longer-term contracts in those cases, as well.)
- Surprise the MCO by offering utilization and financial data before they ask for them—they will be stunned and impressed, and your gesture will make it easier for you to request comparable data from the MCO.
- Express a willingness to share risk and rewards with the MCO—the true measure of partnership.
- Show respect for the MCO's unique areas of expertise and defer to its judgment in those areas. (If you think you know as much or more than the MCO about all aspects of managed care, consider starting your own MCO.)
- When you and the MCO encounter points of disagreement in the negotiations, approach them with a joint problem-solving attitude—win-win—the goal is not to win or to obtain your ideal resolution, but rather to find an answer satisfactory to both parties, even if it is not optimal for either one.

GUIDELINES FOR ONE POSSIBLE NEGOTIATION SCENARIO

- Begin the negotiations by working on several issues where you and the MCO are likely to reach quick agreement—building momentum and confidence toward continued progress. These probably are priority B non-payment issues.
- Next, tackle an A issue. If that seemed to go smoothly, if you seem to have established a collaborative rapport with the MCO negotiators, continue with the tough A issues. If you start to bog down or if the negotiations start heating up, drop back to some B or C issues. Quick agreement on C issues may get the negotiations moving again.

- Do not be afraid to put aside an issue on which no progress is being made, It is amazing how time (as little as 24 hours) can alter your perspective, and the MCO's, on an issue.
- Tackle the payment issue last.
  - Focusing on nonprice issues first projects your balanced interest in all aspects of the new relationship—rather than a myopic fascination with nothing but the money. This will impress the MCO with your concern for issues important to it.
  - The payment issue can be daunting. It will be a lot easier to resolve after you have built a foundation of trust and cooperation through negotiation of everything else. It also will be more difficult to let the payment issue stand in the way of concluding a contract that is 95 percent settled.
- Do not change your previously agreed-upon positions on issues in the middle of negotiations. Do not trust your judgment in the heat of the moment. Express your strong interest in the new position; promise to seriously consider it with your negotiation team members before the next negotiation session. Discuss it privately among yourselves—unpressured and candidly. If it still seems like a good strategy change, adopt the new position and announce it at the next session.

WHEN THE NEGOTIATIONS ARE AT AN IMPASSE OR DEADLOCK

The majority of negotiations proceed with few hitches. However, sometimes, in unpredictable ways, the talks will just bog down. Occasionally, this is an indication that you and the MCO will not be able to reach agreement. More often, a little remedial action will loosen things up.

The first step is to take a break. This could be for minutes, hours, or days. The passage of time frequently changes the parties' perspectives on knotty issues. Both sides should begin looking for really creative solutions to the impasse.

Engage in some free-form brainstorming. Consider bringing in an experienced facilitator to lead you in that process. Both parties should be encouraged to consult with other people—to check their facts, bolster their positions, reexamine their viewpoints, and seek new approaches. In a totally intractable situation where the parties, nonetheless, need or want to reach an agreement, it may be advisable to employ the services of a mediator or arbitrator.

There is always a path to agreement between two parties that truly want to affiliate with each other.

TIPS FOR SOLO OR SMALL GROUP PRACTICE PHYSICIANS

1. Track closely the trends in managed care penetration into your area. Seek out the first reputable MCOs to enter the marketplace for a contract relationship.
2. Develop aggressively the clinical and administrative techniques and methodologies required to prosper under managed care.
3. Identify and promote to the MCO the characteristics of your clinical competence, general practice style, and practice management that distinguish you from other similarly situated physicians and that offer clear benefits to the MCO.
4. Take steps to enlarge the size of your practice before you enter negotiations—by adding new partners, employing additional physicians, acquiring another practice, merging with another practice, or allowing your practice to be acquired by another practice.
5. Consider participating in an IPA, physician-hospital organization (PHO), or management services organization (MSO) (reviewed in other chapters of this book.) that emerges in your area after determining that it has a competitive managed care strategy and before beginning your contract negotiations.

6. Consider forgetting about a direct contract with an MCO and work instead to become a subcontractor or member of a larger physician organization that does the contracting with the MCO.

It is a real challenge for solo practice physicians to even attract the attention of established MCOs, not to mention negotiating a decent contract. The best strategies are to get in early, demonstrate your uniqueness, and grow larger as fast as you can.

TIPS FOR PRIMARY CARE PHYSICIANS

1. Determine how many other physicians in your primary care specialty there are in the area served by the MCO. In other words, define the competition.
2. Determine the primary care services covered by the MCO.
3. Determine the fees or rates paid by the MCO to other primary care physicians for those services.
4. Determine key practice and outcomes data for your practice and the competing practices (resource utilization, admissions, lengths of stay, and costs). Demonstrate the superiority of your practice. Describe the mechanisms you have in place or are implementing to improve those data even further.
5. Prepare your practice in other ways for handling the compensation system offered by the MCO, especially if it is capitation.
6. Identify the high-quality, cost-efficient specialist physicians who are part of your referral network.
7. Lay out the service, cost, and quality advantages and disadvantages of your practice in contrast with competing primary care practices.
8. Talk to the medical director and UM personnel within the MCO to learn what they expect from their primary care physicians.

9. Find out whether the MCO will be willing to guarantee certain enrollment levels for your practice.
10. Seek higher fees or capitation rates when you offer demonstrable advantages, particularly cost savings, over competing primary care physicians.

In most areas of the country, the demand for primary care doctors exceeds the supply. Exploit this fact in contract negotiations. If you also present a strong gatekeeper capability and a cost-efficient practice style, you will have little trouble securing attractive contracts.

TIPS FOR SPECIALIST PHYSICIANS

1. Determine how many other physicians in your specialty there are in the area served by the MCO. In other words, define the competition.
2. Determine the specialty services covered by the MCO.
3. Determine the fees paid by the MCO to other physicians in your specialty for those services. Determine also whether the MCO wants to capitate physicians in your specialty. If it is doing so now, find out what the rates are.
4. Determine key practice and outcomes data for your practice and for the competing physicians. Demonstrate the superiority of your practice. Describe the mechanisms you have in place or are implementing to improve those data even further.
5. Prepare your practice in other ways for handling the compensation system offered by the MCO, especially if it is capitation.
6. Identify the high-quality, cost-efficient primary care and other specialty physicians who are your leading referral sources.
7. Lay out the service, cost, and quality advantages and disadvantages of your practice in contrast with competing specialty practices.

8. Talk to the medical director and UM personnel within the MCO to learn what they expect from their physicians in your specialty.
9. Find out whether the MCO will be willing to guarantee certain enrollment levels for your practice.
10. Seek higher fees or capitation rates when you offer demonstrable advantages, particularly cost savings, over competing physicians in your specialty.

In many areas of the country, the supply of specialty doctors exceeds the demand. The actual discrepancy varies greatly, especially among the specialties. The result is greater competition among specialists for the best managed care contracts. This, in turn, can lead to a decline in their practice revenues. To secure the contracts, specialists must try even harder than their primary care colleagues to distinguish themselves from competing specialists. To maintain their existing income levels, specialists may have to develop a new, unique subspecialty, procedure, or treatment. At the least, they are likely to have to serve a higher volume of patients at a lower unit price or per capita rate.

The specialists who prepare thoroughly for negotiations stand a much better chance of overcoming those adversities and making a good long-term connection with an MCO.

TIPS FOR LARGER GROUP PRACTICES

The more physicians in the group practice, the stronger its bargaining position in a contract negotiation with an MCO. It has the capability to treat larger numbers of enrollees over a wider geographic area, is likely to be better managed, and is better able to afford more professional management and more efficient, up-to-date control/reporting systems. Most of the recommendations in this chapter and throughout the book are aimed at getting such groups into the most favorable relationships with MCOs. To make a good organization even better, consider the following:

1. If yours is a largely primary care group, add specialists (through merger, acquisition, employment, or subcontract) to build into a larger multispecialty group practice.
2. If yours is a largely specialty group, add physicians in primary care and other specialties to build into a larger multispecialty group practice.
3. If yours is a multispecialty group, expand the total number of physicians in all specialties to enable you to cover even broader geographic areas and member populations served by the MCO.

Your group already is a prime candidate for strategic contract partner with an MCO.

FUNDAMENTAL REASONS THAT MANAGED CARE NEGOTIATIONS FAIL

The Physician Does Not Understand the Needs of the MCO

With all the media attention on MCOs' cost cutting, it is easy to believe that their only interest in contract negotiations with physicians is getting the lowest possible fee or rate. This is simply not true of any responsible, forward-looking MCO. Such a belief can create problems for a physician during the negotiations. She is likely to neglect addressing the MCO's genuine interest in other areas, such as quality assurance, patient satisfaction, and staff credentialing. Further, the MCO may conclude that the physician is interested only in the highest possible fee or rate if that is the first and primary issue she raises.

> **Lesson:** Through general research about MCOs (such as reading this book) and specific research on this one MCO, discover the full range of expectations it has for its physicians. Determine how your practice can meet them, and put this forward during the negotiations.

The MCO Does Not Understand Why Your Practice Is Any Different or Better Than Another Practice

The MCO is choosing which of many physician practices to accept as contract partners. It wants only those that offer the MCO and its members something unique, something not available from other practices—a geographic location, a medical specialty or procedure, an elevated reputation, or an ability to minimize utilization. To win a contract with that MCO requires understanding how your practice will benefit that particular MCO and presenting that information during the negotiations. It also requires that you spend time listening carefully to what the MCO team is saying (they are probably trying to tell you what they want from the relationship) and asking thoughtful questions (to make sure you know what they want).

> **Lesson:** Increasingly, in markets heavily penetrated by managed care, the negotiation is really a sales pitch on your part to the MCO. View it that way.

The Physician Has Not Figured Out Who the Real MCO Decision Makers Are and What Their Needs Are

This is less a problem with MCOs experienced in contracting honestly with physicians. Time can be wasted and your negotiation position compromised if the MCO representatives must regularly seek the approval of another officer in their organization for their bargaining concessions.

> **Lesson:** Establish at the outset that both parties' negotiators have the authority to commit their respective organizations. Find out who the members of the MCO negotiating team will be and try to learn what they hope to gain from the negotiations—both for themselves and for their organization.

The Physician's Practice Format and Service Offerings Are Not Suited to Managed Care

A physician will make this mistake only once—the first time he tries to contract with a health maintenance organization. He will then take steps to reform his practice style and operations to bring them up-to-date with the demands of managed care. Alternatively, the physician will watch his practice wither away. Persuading an MCO to contract with you because of the unique features of your practice assumes that such features exist.

> **Lesson:** If you are approaching your first managed care contract, be sure that you have shifted to a "managed care" frame of mind and style of practice. Determine that you offer to the MCO products and services that help it meet its objectives. If you do not, don't waste your time in the negotiation.

The Physician Is Not Prepared To Offer the Kind of Pricing Structure the MCO Wants

You may feel that you have made great progress by moving to discounted FFS schedules. You may have begun to think about how you would operate under capitation. However, you may be stuck if the MCO states a preference for a complex structure of withholds and risk pools.

The basic pricing structures used by MCOs are

- fee for service (FFS)
- discounted FFS
- case rates
- episode rates
- capitation
- risk-sharing pools and withholds
- per diem (hospitals only)
- outcome based (coming)

> **Lesson:** Know and understand the pricing structure demanded by the MCO. Be prepared to practice effectively under it.

The Physician's Practice Does Not Cover the Right Geographic Area or a Broad Enough Geographic Area To Satisfy the MCO

The MCO is looking for physicians located where their members live or will travel. The MCO also will prefer to contract with groups of physicians who are able to service a wide area—reducing the total number of contracts it must execute. If your practice is in the wrong area (where there are no MCO members or there are other MCO physicians) or simply covers too narrow an area (requiring contracts with a lot of small practices such as yours), you may have trouble securing a good contract.

Lesson: Find out where the MCO's members live and go for their health care. If you don't really cover that area, forget about that contract and search for another MCO with members closer to you. Even better, start combining with other practices to form a larger integrated network with a wider service area.

THE GOLDEN RULES OF NEGOTIATING

- Know exactly what you want.
- Know exactly what you are getting into.
- Don't promise anything you can't deliver.
- You do not get what you deserve, you get what you negotiate.

RESOURCE LIST

Books

R. Fisher et al., *Getting to Yes*, 2nd ed. (New York: Penguin Books, 1991) (best introductory book on general purpose negotiation skills).

"Make Your Practice Irresistible to Health Plans," *Medical Economics*, 7 March, 1994.

L.J. Marcus et al., *Renegotiating Health Care: Resolving Conflict To Build Collaboration* (San Francisco: Jossey-Bass, Publisher, 1995) (best book on negotiations in a health care setting).

H. Raiffa, *The Art & Science of Negotiation* (Cambridge, MA: Harvard University Press, 1982) (best advanced book on general purpose negotiation skills).

D. Robbins, *Integrating Managed Care and Ethics.* (Westchester, IL: Healthcare Financial Management Association, 1997).

P. Sperber, *Fail-Safe Business Negotiating, Strategies and Tactics for Success* (Englewood Cliffs, NJ: Prentice-Hall, 1983).

Courses

L.J. Marcus, *Program for Health Care Negotiation and Conflict Resolution.* Harvard School of Public Health.

Gerard Nierenberg's Art of Negotiating Seminar Workshop. Negotiation Institute, (800) 747-8802.

Videotape

The Art of Negotiating. Negotiation Institute, (800) 747-8802.

Computer Software

The Art of Negotiating. Negotiation Institute, (800) 747-8802.

CHAPTER 10

Step Three: Forming or Joining a Small, Single Specialty Group Practice

INTRODUCTION

If you are a solo practitioner or sharing a medical suite with a couple doctors you barely know, this will be your first step toward integration, toward allying with like-minded colleagues, in order to present a slightly larger group of providers speaking with one voice to any hospital, managed care organization (MCO), employer, or insurance company you may need to deal with.

This will be your first step toward sharing information about your style of practice, how you utilize resources, the quality of the work you do, and its cost to you and the ultimate payer. This probably will be the first time your practice methods have been exposed to the close scrutiny of peers, with cost-effectiveness as a major motivating factor.

For the first time, you probably will have to compromise some of your desires in order to accommodate those of your partners. To that degree, this will be the beginning of an inevitable, but not necessarily terminal, erosion of your autonomy. The key is that, by taking this step, you are controlling exactly how and when you will yield the autonomy, rather than being forced into it through a managed care contract you cannot afford to turn down.

WHO SHOULD READ THIS CHAPTER

If you are a physician still surviving in a solo practice, or are sharing the costs of a medical suite with a couple other doctors, or are the member of a two- or three-person single specialty group practice, you definitely should read this chapter. It outlines the simplest, most basic, least intrusive form of consolidation you must consider if you are to survive the health care industry upheaval with any degree of professional autonomy.

BASIC UNDERSTANDING

What we are talking about here is the prospect of two or more physicians, currently practicing actively and independently of each other (though they may be occupying the same office facilities), merging their practices—legally, administratively, and clinically. It could involve two physicians coming together or the combination of six or seven practices, some composed of two or three physicians.

WHY WOULD DOCTORS WANT TO MERGE THEIR PRACTICES?

This question is important for two reasons. It is the first question that should be asked of all physicians considering merging their practices. Their answers will determine whether individual physicians should be included or whether the group should proceed further with its discussions. To be blunt, there are right and wrong answers to the question. The right answers may also give you encouragement to begin thinking about this first move toward integration.

Here are examples of some answers to avoid:

- *"Because everyone else is doing it."* That may be an indication that something is going on in your market that you ought to pay attention to, but it does not mean that you should slavishly imitate the actions of other physicians. They may all be making the same mistake. Your decision to merge, or not, should be based on an independent analysis of market trends in your area and your personal goals for the future.
- *"The state medical society says we should do it."* A responsible medical society will not make specific recommendations of this sort to its members. It certainly could not give one piece of advice that was appropriate for all its physicians in their diverse practice settings. Again, your decision needs to be based on the merits of your situation.
- *"To fight back against managed care."* There may be comfort in numbers, but there is no long-term advantage in trying to resist the national movement toward managed care. Certainly, support medical society lobbying efforts to restrain, legislatively, the worst abuses of managed care—like "gag rules." Reactionary motives will poison the work atmosphere in a merged entity, dooming it to eventual failure. The point of combining practices is to be able to increase the chances of success under managed care.

Even responses like these might be misguided, even though they look good initially:

- *"The economies of scale will reduce our overhead."* In some cases, this may be true—particularly where the merging practices have not been well managed in the past. Some practices, however, are already tight, efficient operations and leave little savings to be gained through consolidation. In fact, larger group practices often see an advantage in adding certain patient-friendly services, so their overhead may actually go up.
- *"Expanded demand for group-owned ancillary services will increase income."* It may indeed accomplish that. However, trying to raise income by providing more services is a direct contradiction of the purposes behind managed care. Furthermore, if the increased service use is due to self-referrals and cross-referrals by group members, it may violate the Stark laws.

And here are the kinds of answers that bode well for the future of a new group practice:

- *"To gain a competitive advantage in a rapidly changing marketplace."* The new health care marketplace is based on a competition model. You don't have to like it; it is simply a fact of life. Those players win who do a better job of competing. By merging with other like-minded physicians, you increase the number of strategic alternatives available to you and the resources you can use to implement them.
- *"To learn how to practice high-quality, low-cost medicine."*
- *"To learn the new skills I need to survive under managed care."* The practice techniques expected of physicians under managed care are significantly different from much of what is still taught in medical school. It is easier to acquire these new skills in collaboration with other physicians. You can share experiences and new knowledge. The group can better afford the systems required to support the new techniques.
- *"To position myself and my practice optimally for the future."* Looking forward to the future is always a positive rationale for change. Even if you are not sure exactly which direction you ultimately want to go (e.g., become part of a large multispecialty group practice, evolve into an integrated delivery system (IDS), develop a for-profit model in which your investment grows), you are ahead of the game by taking this modest

first step.

Each physician's answer to this question should be personal and from the heart. A desire to follow the crowd or turn back the clock or seek revenge will not sustain a group striving to compete in a superheated marketplace. Use this question as a litmus test for evaluating candidates for participation in the merged group.

The process of putting together even a modest-sized group practice from among physicians who have little experience in collaboration is complicated, time-consuming, frustrating, and expensive. Be ready for this. Here's how to start.

OPENING PHASE: EDUCATING, ANSWERING QUESTIONS, AND CHECKING COMPATIBILITY

Exploring the Possible Interest of Physician Colleagues

The conversation about possible merger can begin in any number of ways. If the initiative comes from you, do a little advance research and reading. (Consult some of the resources listed at the end of this chapter.) Approach the physician you share an office suite with or a colleague with a separate practice in the same specialty. Seek doctors you believe are primed to consider some kind of serious integration and with whom you think you could work. Begin a discussion group that holds a few informal meetings.

The first step, probably the hardest of all, is reaching a rough consensus among this group on the objectives for whatever initiative you might put together. If your minds cannot meet on the reasons for doing this, do not proceed! Fundamental differences now will not fade away and could sabotage all your subsequent efforts.

You need to hear from each prospective merger participant on these issues:

- What do you need from your professional life?

- What do you want from your professional life?
- What do you find disagreeable about the merger idea?
- What could we do to overcome those disagreements?

A full expression of feelings is essential at this point. Do not assume that silent members are silently acquiescing. Force everyone to speak up.

Once everyone seems to be pointed within 90 compass degrees of the same direction, begin the serious examination and planning.

Your first expenditure of money should probably go toward hiring an experienced outside consultant or facilitator to guide this education and planning process. He or she can help tremendously to streamline and moderate a difficult task. He or she can ask and say things without sacrificing personal esteem with the group.

Hiring a consultant means having the money to pay her. Ask group members to make modest contributions, perhaps $250 each, to support the study process. Their willingness to do this will be a measure of their commitment to the venture.

During the early discussions, get to the bottom of these questions:

1. *Why do we want to form a group and merge our practices?*

This is the same question you raised when you first approached your collaborators, but this time the answers need to be more specific and committed. They will become the basis for a medium-term strategic plan that will guide the new group through its first two or three years.

2. *What do we expect the proposed group practice to look like in three years?*

This question further illuminates the founding physicians' aspirations for the group. If their intentions are not this focused, it forces them to begin thinking in such terms. The answers will help flesh out the strategic plan. Here are some possibilities:

- "The group will be concentrated on the clinical practice of medicine."
- "Some group members will be pursuing interests in teaching or research."
- "A few participating physicians will demonstrate managerial skills and begin to emerge as leaders."
- "The size of the group will be much larger and still growing."
- "The group will have added new members in other subspecialties."
- "The group will be in the process of evolving even further along the path toward greater integration and risk sharing."
- "The group will no longer exist, having been acquired by or merged with another provider entity, such as a multispecialty group or an integrated delivery system."
- "The group physicians will be much more skilled at delivering minimum cost, maximum quality medicine."

3. *What is our view of the local managed care trends and the relationship the group practice should have with them?*

Expect lots of unproductive opinions on this issue. Consider these two extremes:

- "I hate it. It is a plague on the practice of medicine. The group practice should be a vehicle for helping to protect physician-guided medical practice as long as possible."
- "It is here to stay and we might as well get good at it. Let us set out to create the dominant IDS in this area."

There is a healthy, reasonable middle ground between these two polar positions, but individual attitudes may vary so much that it would be a mistake to practice together under the same roof.

4. *Do we recognize the importance of collecting data and understanding every aspect of the practice—in order to teach ourselves how to manage care and prove to MCOs, payers, and patients that we know how to do it?*

5. *Are the practice styles and cultures of the merging physicians compatible?*

The key characteristics to examine and compare are

- the focus of the physicians' practices (academic versus clinical)
- the hours worked per week and the number of patients seen
- the time devoted to research or teaching
- the desire of each physician to be involved in management details
- the rigor of administrative and clinical control
- the effectiveness in managing other people
- the experience and effectiveness in working on teams
- the experience in practicing under managed care
- the willingness to learn and change
- the use of resources (drugs, tests, specialists, and physician extenders) for comparable diagnoses
- the personalities of the physicians
- the procedures and other services capable of being provided within the specialty

These are some of the hardest characteristics to decipher. Many people have trouble talking about them, not to mention asking others about them. Nonetheless, they are critical matters that can make or break a new group. It is worth spending the time necessary to discover these traits about your prospective partners.

6. *How much will each physician have to invest to get the group started and to keep it going in the future?*

The amount can range from as little as $2,000 per physician to set up a lightly affiliated independent practice association (IPA) to as much as $20,000 to $25,000 per physician for a highly integrated physician-run MSO. See Chapter 27, "Financing Strategies To Support Your Integration Plans," for more information on financing strategic plans.

Look at the investment question this way. Depending on the number of physicians initially interested, count on spending at least $1,000 each to get educated about the possibilities and to figure out how much you will really have to spend before it is all over. Furthermore, view any money spent on these issues as an investment in the re-creation of your medical practice.

ACTIVE PLANNING PHASE

Once it is reasonably well established that the physicians in the group have common, responsible goals for merging and seem sufficiently compatible with each other, the next step is to begin more practical, detailed planning of the new venture.

Fitting the Merger into the Local Market Scene

Conduct a market feasibility study to determine how well the merger idea fits with what is going on in the local health care market. If you have some time, you can do a rough job of investigation yourself, using information generally available and your own professional contacts. You might also consider hiring a knowledgeable consultant for a more thorough study. The study should look at issues such as

- the geographic distribution of providers and specialties (especially yours) in the area
- the market penetration of managed care and capitation arrangements
- what is known about the strategic plans of MCOs and insurance companies
- what is known about the strategic responses of hospitals, clinics, group practices, and other provider entities

Now, in the face of all these gathered facts, what are the compelling reasons for affiliating your practice with the other physicians' practices?

There are, in fact, circumstances where it will not make sense to take even this preliminary step toward integration.

- If the market is being rapidly taken over by managed care, there may not be enough time to form a group practice, gain experience in managing care, and grow steadily larger until you are a major player in the marketplace. Instead, look around for an existing or forming multispecialty group practice, probably of significant size and preferably experienced in doing well under capitation. Gain membership with it on the best terms possible.
- If the vast majority of the best providers in the market have already gathered themselves into a few, quite large IDSs, there may be no point in going through the motions of forming a group practice. Each physician might be better off approaching one of the existing groups or systems, and negotiating the best possible deal for joining them.
- The provider-sponsored groups in the area may have all the physicians in your specialty that they need. You have waited too long to ally yourself with a physician-run organization. Your only option may be to seek membership in a delivery system dominated by a hospital or an MCO. It may even be necessary to sell your practice to a physician practice management company (PPMC) and accept employment with them.

In most markets in the United States, it is still competitively feasible to create a larger single specialty group practice. Among the market advantages you may find that you gain by this move are

- broader geographic coverage to qualify for managed care contracts
- ability to handle the larger patient populations necessary to succeed under capitation
- resources and mutual support for learning the techniques of practicing "value" medicine
- strategic positioning for negotiating better deals in affiliations with still larger delivery systems
- ability to provide a wider range of services in your specialty
- critical mass of physicians may enable the group to secure an exclusive contract to provide specialty services to a hospital, IDS, or MCO

Do not forget that your strategic move in the marketplace, in forming even a modest-size group practice, will be noticed by other physicians and providers. Be prepared for reactions at all levels—emotional, political, and competitive. Colleagues, particularly those in your specialty left out of your group, may be resentful. That will pass. Many may envy you and your groupmates. Some may seek your advice on forming their own groups.

However, you should pay closest attention to the competitive responses you provoke. Other providers who feel threatened by your move may seek new strategic affiliations of their own. Some examples are:

- A local hospital concerned that your larger group might be able to dictate contract terms to it could attempt to acquire the practices of the other physicians who did not join your group.
- Worried about being left out, those other specialists could decide to sell out to a PMC or merge with a large multispecialty group practice—and now your group is the one feeling left out.

- Feeling that your group represents too powerful a force in your specialty, the local hospital and a good part of its medical staff may decide to form a physician-hospital organization (PHO)—without your participation.
- A new MCO entering the market prefers to contract only with solo and small groups, at least in specialties like yours, so excludes your group from its physician panel.

On the other hand, some of these same players may be so cowed or impressed by your strategic initiative that they seek out beneficial relationships with you. Finally, if the market is large enough, your merger may not create a ripple. Generally, however, do not expect to make your competitive moves unnoticed. See Exhibit 10–1 for more information on how to analyze your group and its market area.

Is a Merger the Best Structural Alternative?

With a better understanding of the local marketplace dynamics, it is time to ask whether, of all possible strategic choices you could make, merger into a group practice is the best one.

The simplest way of making this decision is first to break it down into three broad choices.

1. Move as slowly toward integration as the market will allow, preserving traditional physician autonomy as long as possible.
2. Proceed as aggressively as possible toward integration using provider-sponsored organizations.
3. Sell assets to or merge with an existing organization, becoming one of its physician employees.

The first choice seeks a looser affiliation with other providers. This might involve participating in an IPA composed of a variety of physicians in the area. Initially, it serves as a managed care contracting vehicle and allows its participating doctors to continue in their separate practices. Eventually, it may introduce some utilization

Exhibit 10–1 SWOT Analysis

Special Tip: A popular mechanism to prepare for strategic planning is a SWOT analysis. "SWOT" stands for Strengths-Weaknesses-Opportunities-Threats and those are the elements you review for your group and its market area.

Strengths may include specialty training, locations, affiliations, managed care experience, or unique staff or equipment. Strengths are exploited and enhanced.

Weaknesses may include little investable capital, poor specialty mix, disadvantageous office locations, or minimal managed care experience. Weaknesses are corrected and improved.

Opportunities may include an invitation to form a physician-hospital organization with a leading local hospital, an invitation to contract exclusively with a leading MCO in the area, or a chance to form a perfectly positioned physician group that will dominate the local provider market and any negotiations with MCOs. Opportunities are to be seized.

Threats may include a leading MCO contracting with another physician group, the local health care delivery market increasingly dominated by profit-motivated MCOs, growing restrictions on physician clinical decision making, or declining practice incomes combined with increasing practice expenses. Threats are defended against, attacked, or avoided.

management measures and begin offering centralized practice management services. Read more about IPAs in Chapter 11, "Step Four: Joining an Independent Practice Association."

You might also consider becoming part of a PHO being formed by the medical staff and the hospital where you have privileges. A PHO also will start out seeking managed care contracts. The hospital's capital resources then can be applied to integrating and growing the PHO into something resembling an IDS. Read more about PHOs in Chapter 15, "Step Six: Forming a Physician-Hospital Organization—An Affiliation between Your Group Practice and a Hospital."

The third choice is the easier way out of the turmoil that is going to exist in the health care industry for several more years. It avoids the time, money, and anxiety expended in creating new organizations and affiliations, negotiating new contractual relationships, worrying about reliable sources of investment capital for the organization and income for you, going to numerous planning meetings, and making endless policy and management decisions. Instead, the practice assets are transferred to an existing organization (by sale or merger), and the physician becomes an employee, member, or partner of the

organization. The organization has a solid financial future and handles all the management decisions, leaving the physician to the pure practice of medicine.

This choice is implemented by joining a PPMC or selling your practice to some other larger provider organization. For more information on these options, read Chapter 16, "Step Seven: Partnering with a Management Services Organization or Physician Practice Management Company," and Chapter 18, "Step Nine: Selling Your Practice to a Hospital, Physican Group, Managed Care Organization, or Physician Practice Management Company."

The second choice leads to the formation of a single specialty group practice, as described in this chapter. There are other possibilities in this category—such as organizing a large multispecialty group practice or foundation or equity-model physician organizations—but these presume access to considerable investment capital and management expertise. They probably would be beyond the means of physicians just trying to move out of a solo or small group practice.

The premise of this book is that physicians will do best by pursuing integration as vigorously as possible, through physician-dominated organizations. Only unique market conditions in your area should persuade you to make choices in the first and third categories.

> **Reminder:** Go for all the integration you can handle at the moment.
> Always keep your eye on the future—at least three years out.

Getting the "Deal-Breakers" out in the Open

As the group becomes more serious about merging practices, take the time to find out each physician's "nonnegotiable" issues—the points on which she says, "If this doesn't change, count me out." What can you not live with? What must you absolutely have?

Common areas of irreconcilable disagreement are

- valuing and combining the assets of each practice
- formulas for physician compensation
- physician retirement plans
- governance of the new group
- routine management of the new group
- physical location of the new group
- required levels of malpractice insurance coverage
- official name of the new group

Exposing these issues may result in some physicians having to leave the group, if sufficient compromises cannot be made. Still, it is better to do it at this early stage rather than later when merger commitments have been made.

Agreeing on Common Strategic Objectives (Three Years Out)

Before the group starts planning the details of operating the new practice entity, it is logical that it should first lay out the strategic objectives it aims to achieve in the first few years. Such objectives are mandatory to give long-term direction to the day-to-day operations.

Eventually, the group will develop more ambitious, long-term goals. Initially, while they are gaining experience doing this kind of future thinking, the physicians should look no further than three years out with more modest goals like

- integrating specified aspects of clinical and administrative operations
- increasing revenues from managed care contracts to a specified level each year
- increasing revenues earned on a capitated basis to a specified level each year
- acquiring and becoming familiar with information technologies and systems for specified business functions
- adding specific numbers of certain categories of physician extenders

After learning to collaborate in pursuit of such predetermined goals (for perhaps two years), prepare longer-term, more enterprising strategic objectives like

- adding specific numbers of physicians in designated specialties
- increasing the size of the group practice to specified levels—in terms of number of physicians, total revenues, number of capitated patients, or other similar indicators
- forming strategic affiliations or partnerships with other specified providers or organizations
- developing new practice sites at designated geographic locations
- improving specific resource utilization rates or quality indicators to designated levels each year

You will be amazed at how much more progress you make when your energies are focused on specific, measurable targets on the visible horizon.

Escape Hatches for Doctors Wanting To Leave

From the time you first start talking about creating a merged practice and for as long as it stays in existence, there is the potential for participating physicians to become uncomfortable with the decisions and actions being taken. If their discomfort becomes intolerable, they will want to leave the group. It is a good idea to plan for these departures in advance.

The implications of a sudden departure by one or more physicians can be serious, depending on how far along the group practice is in its development. If several go at once, they may reduce the group size below a useful level. Some of the departing physicians may have been carrying out important planning tasks for the group, perhaps because they had unique expertise. Once the new group is operational, it has patient care responsibilities that are impacted when one or more doctors leave. The most difficult issue is how to compensate a physician who has merged her practice assets inextricably with the group's and may have made additional capital contributions, loans, or investments. Full payback at the time of leaving could bankrupt the fledgling group.

Early in the planning process, probably with the help of a lawyer, set up "escape hatches" for physicians wishing to leave at key stages in the group's history. This needs to be put in writing and agreed to by all physicians who join the group. Different escape terms should be defined for these circumstances:

- When conversations have just begun, a few meetings have been held, some decisions reached, but no commitments made.
- The physicians have made some modest monetary contributions (a couple hundred dollars each), a consultant has been hired, and each physician has signed a letter of intent.
- The group practice has been in operation for no more than two years, a new legal entity has been created, individual practice assets have been transferred to the entity, the physicians have made substantial monetary investments in the new organization, and it is rapidly developing its own identity, but is still a little shaky financially.

- The group practice has been operating for over three years and is now on a solid fiscal foundation. Based on a reliable core of physicians, it is growing and expanding.

If you are lucky, no physicians at all will leave for the first 10 years. But, the odds are that some will want to back out, for any number of reasons. Knowing the terms of their departure ahead of time will minimize the cost, confusion, and disruption.

Signing Agreements of Commitment

At periodic intervals during the discussion and planning process, document the progress made and decisions reached, and ask physicians to commit by signature to the actions and to the organization. Moving from the complete autonomy of a solo practice to the intimate collaboration of a modern group practice is a scary prospect for many doctors. Some may get cold feet as they get closer to the final commitment. Documents of commitment give the group confidence that it has a large enough mass of engaged physicians to keep moving forward. They also impress upon the physicians the seriousness of their undertaking.

Throughout the education and planning process, give participating physicians hard copy on the issues being discussed. Take minutes of the conclusions reached, type them up, and get copies to everyone involved. Although nobody has signed off on these records, they are powerful evidence if disagreements later arise.

Once the group reaches the point where it has a good, rough outline of the kind of organization it wants to create and is about to make legally binding commitments and serious expenditures of money (in the thousands of dollars), request that the physicians sign letters of intent. These are quite detailed documents that lay out most of the terms under which the parties propose to merge. They look a lot like legal agreements, but have nothing like the same effect. They often will include a clause stating that the letter "does not constitute a binding contract of the parties" but is "only to confirm the Practices' mutual understandings and is subject to negotiation of a definitive agreement among the parties with respect to the creation of the Group Practice."* Signing the letter solemnizes the verbal conclusions the group members have reached.

Eventually, the final decision to bring the new group practice into existence (while dissolving the individual component practices) will be made. At this point, a number of formal, legally binding agreements will be executed. What they are will depend on the type of legal organization being formed. Expect documents like these:

- documents forming the new legal entity under which the group practice will operate (typically articles of incorporation)
- agreements transferring title to practice assets from individual physicians to the new legal entity
- shareholder or lender agreements documenting monetary investments made by the physicians in the new legal entity
- employment agreement between each physician and the new legal entity

Once these are signed, there is no turning back.

Concentrating on a Single Specialty?

There may be a temptation, even an opportunity, to include physicians in other subspecialties among the group planning the merger. There are good strategic reasons for considering this some day. Ultimately, your single specialty group will have to graduate to a multispecialty group practice to remain competitive. So, why not make that move now rather than later?

As a general rule, if your practice history has been in solo or small group practice, it is advis-

_____

*This is language from an actual letter of intent for the merger of practices to form a single, multispecialty clinic.

able in forming this first substantial group to concentrate on physicians within a single specialty—your specialty. You probably are already familiar with most of the potential candidates. It will be challenge enough learning to work with them, without having also to adjust to entirely new specialties and practice technologies. Multiple specialties add a whole range of complications in the areas of governance, financial contribution, compensation, and utilization management. It is not worth trying to tackle those until you have gained more experience working with physicians in your own specialty under the rigors of managed care.

Only in a few exceptional cases should you consider leaping directly to the formation of a larger multispecialty group practice.

- You and several members of your merging group have solid prior experience working with other specialists, working in a group setting, and working with managed care.
- The availability of several top physicians in different specialties offers a unique opportunity to assemble a premier multispecialty group, and if you do not take them now, they will go elsewhere or form a group without you.
- The consolidation and integration of providers in your market area is moving so rapidly that there is no time for the luxury of learning to collaborate with other doctors and manage care in a single specialty group practice.

If you feel that your situation falls within one of these exceptions, the next chapter you read should be Chapter 13, "Step Five: Growing into a Larger, Multispecialty Group Practice."

> **Remember**: A free-standing single specialty group (of any size) is a transitional stage—you must eventually affiliate with your referral sources (i.e., primary care doctors in a multispecialty group practice).

ORGANIZATION IMPLEMENTATION PHASE

Legal Organizational Form To Take

Your attorney will advise you on the options available in your state. The most common forms are standard for-profit corporation, professional corporation, limited liability corporation (LLC), limited liability partnership (LLP), and traditional partnership. The straight partnership device should be ignored for its problems with personal liability. Other forms, like the LLP, offer the same advantages without those problems. The several corporate alternatives, many of them designed with professionals in mind, are all improvements over the general-purpose for-profit corporate form. In some states, you may be required to organize as a professional corporation to avoid violating the doctrine against the corporate practice of medicine.

The key criteria and concerns in choosing among the available organizational forms are these:

- minimizing taxes to the physicians in their transfer of assets to the practice and subsequent compensation by it
- insulating the physicians from liabilities incurred by the practice
- facilitating the attraction or accumulation of investable capital
- allowing for an effective governance structure
- accommodating future expansion through acquisitions, mergers, or affiliations
- minimizing recordkeeping and reporting requirements
- encouraging effective integration by the physicians

Valuing and Merging the Assets

Merging several physician practices into one group practice means that the physicians must give up individual ownership and control of their practice assets and turn them over to the new group entity in which they share ownership and control. This transaction raises several key issues.

- *Exactly which assets will pass from the physician to the group?* While it is possible to acquire a practice as a complete business entity, this is rarely done. Normally, only specific assets are transferred—things like equipment and supplies. The physician may own an office or have a leasehold on one, but, if the new group will operate out of a new central location, it may have no use for that property. If the physician enjoys a positive reputation in the community and will bring a good number of patients to the group, there may be a desire to acquire the soft asset of "goodwill" from the practice, or at least to acknowledge it.
- *What values will be placed on those assets?* For tax purposes (of both the physician and the group) and for determining how the physician will be compensated for the assets, dollar values must be placed on them. Because of the risk of fraud and abuse legal charges, the valuations must be fair and reasonable. They should be carried out by professionals with experience in assessing those kinds of assets. The gold standard for asset valuation is usually "fair market value." The difficulty in accurate valuation, as well as the legal implications. is aggravated in the case of goodwill.
- *How will each physician be compensated for the assets he or she transfers to the group practice?* The group clearly will not be paying cash for the assets. It likely has very little. What the physician receives in return for the assets is an ownership interest in the new legal entity—probably measured in shares. The challenge is deciding how much each will receive. Some physicians may bring more valuable assets to the group. If the shares they receive are proportional, they will have greater control over the group's affairs. If all the physicians are given an

equal number of shares—so no one physician dominates—some of them may feel inadequately compensated for their asset contributions. Some hard choices have to be made.

Through loans from the group to high-asset physicians, special classes of shares, and special majority voting arrangements on the board of directors, it should be possible to work around these problems. If mishandled, however, they could seriously alienate important group members.

For more detailed information on this topic, read Chapter 18, "Step Nine: Selling Your Practice to a Hospital, Physician Group, Managed Care Organization, or Physician Practice Management Company."

Allocating Revenues or Compensating the Physicians

Another make-or-break issue for most of the physicians will be the method and amount of their compensation in the new group. Initially, the physicians may be inclined to think about the revenues each of them has brought to the group and wonder how the group's total revenues will be allocated back to them. Try to steer them away from this kind of thinking as quickly as possible.

Concentrating on the revenues a physician might have earned if she were still in solo practice is contrary to the group welfare ethic that must prevail if the group is to succeed. Very soon, that physician will not be able to bring in such revenues on her own. That is the primary reason she is moving to a larger group setting. In addition, managed care effectiveness requires maximizing net profits through minimizing utilization of resources, even if this must be done at lower revenue levels.

Initially, each physician should receive compensation very close to what she earned in independent practice. Then, gradually, introduce compensation formulas that reward desired behaviors—reduced utilization, improved clinical outcomes, and satisfactory patient ratings, among

others. For more information on this sensitive issue, read Chapter 25, "The Kinds of Physician Reimbursement Systems You Can Expect under Managed Care," as well as the sections on "Formal, Regular Evaluations of Physician Performance," "Align Incentives among Physicians, Ancillary Staff, and Other Employees," and "Shape Physician Compensation To Produce Desired Behavior" in Chapter 19, "Step Ten: Increasing the Level of Integration in Your Provider Organization."

Resolving Retirement Plan Differences

The physicians joining together in the group are likely to have a variety of arrangements for their pension or retirement plans. Some will have made no provisions at all. Others will have plans with different retirement payment amounts, under different terms, purchased from different vendors. It will be in the group's interest to have all its members eligible for approximately the same pension benefits. There also are savings available if everyone's plan is contracted with the same insurance source. Since no one will accept decreasing his pension payment amounts, it probably will be necessary to duplicate the most attractive plan for everyone in the group.

Creating a Governance Structure

This is another hot button issue. It relates to the amounts, in money and assets, which each physician has contributed to the group enterprise and the resulting influence he will have over the group's decisions. A well-designed governance system also goes a long way toward assuaging the nervousness the physicians will have in giving up their independent practice autonomy.

There are a number of variables in governance that can be used to accommodate the concerns of participating physicians. The primary governance vehicle is the board of directors. Here is how it can be custom-tailored.

- It can vary in size. In a small group, all of the physicians can be directors. Eventually, only a subgroup of doctors will represent the others by serving on the board. Generally, the larger the board, the more diverse interests that can be represented and the slower the decision-making process.

- There are different mechanisms that can be used to choose the physicians who will be directors.
- The terms of office and opportunities for re-election can be defined.
- The size of the majority necessary for approval can be varied for different types of issues.
- Certain seats on the board can be reserved for certain constituencies (i.e., particular subspecialties, geographic areas, nonphysician managers, or component practices).

In addition, considerable decision-making authority can be delegated to the various committees that can be set up subordinate to the board.

It also is possible to start the new group off with certain protections in place to reassure the merging physicians that no significant decisions will be made without their input. Then, over time, as leaders emerge who have the confidence of the whole group, the protective mechanisms can be removed.

The shape of the governance system can make the difference between a group of physicians functioning confidently as a team and a disjointed, suspicious group constantly in disagreement.

For more information on governance structures, read Chapter 22, "Creating an Effective Governance Structure for an Affiliated or Integrated Physician Group."

Setting a Management Structure and Framework

The new group organization you have created needs structure, personnel, and procedures for managing its larger, more complex operations. This is done to maximize its efficiency and to give people who work in the organization or have to deal with it (as patients, payers, providers, and vendors) a sense of predictability in its actions. There are several standard pieces to this management infrastructure.

Hiring a General Business Manager

The first of these measures should be the hiring of a full-time business manager. Ideally, this person will have some business training and managerial experience, preferably in a physician practice. It is possible that one of the administrative staff people from one of the merging practices may qualify for this position.

The business manager's first responsibility is to take over the design and implementation of the new infrastructure. As he or she demonstrates the ability to handle these tasks and, eventually, manage the group's continuing operations, the physicians must be prepared to delegate many of the practice management duties they previously handled themselves.

Common Administrative Policies and Procedures

Like any business venture, a medical practice is governed by policies and procedures. These cover topics like medical recordkeeping, claims filing, purchasing, scheduling, human resource management, and general accounting. Policies and procedures need to be written down and publicized to those who must implement them and those who are affected by them. It is likely that each of the participating practices followed rather different procedures. Except where there is a very good reason for maintaining the difference, standard policies and procedures should be established for administrative matters throughout the organization, across all practices.

Common Clinical Policies and Procedures

This is a more sensitive area than the administrative tasks. It could include issues like the creation of a drug formulary, collection and dissemination of data on quality and utilization, preliminary efforts to apply treatment guidelines, and implementation of physician productivity standards (measured by number of patients seen). Move more tentatively toward establishing common policies of this sort. Within the first year, once the group seems to gel as a unit, as its members gain confidence in each other's clinical skills, and as the demands of MCO contract partners become apparent, begin to propose some unification of clinical policies. Start with those to which there seems to be the least resistance. But, move with all deliberate speed, for it is these kinds of initiatives that will determine the group's ability to practice the kind of medicine demanded by managed care.

Types of Data Gathering and Reporting

Control and management of inputs, processes, and outputs in the practice of medicine is essential to meeting the requirements of managed care programs. Promptly, upon creation of the new group, begin to define the kinds of data that will be gathered and from whom, how, and to whom they will be reported; and what actions they are intended to influence.

This will probably start with the basic financial accounting that all the practices have been carrying out. Establish a standard list of accounts and bookkeeping procedures to be used by all the practice sites. This will enable comparisons of cost data.

Other areas for early data systemization include

- claims filed with particular payers
- patients seen by practice site, by payer, and, as soon as possible, by physician
- resources (drugs, tests, referrals) utilized by physician
- complaints of any sort from patients or payers

This is just the beginning of what will become a sophisticated system for gathering data from all practice sites and analyzing and structuring them for redistribution to key decision makers throughout the organization, including the physicians. You can expect to be expanding and refining this

system for the indefinite future. Very quickly, it will become apparent that a modern computer technology will be needed to support the growing information system. That technology will consume a major portion of the group's capital spending for several years.

Which Existing Staff To Keep and Which New Staff To Hire

The merger of several practices, the centralization of some services, and the addition of others will result inevitably in a reshaping of the work force employed by the new entity.

Certain tasks, such as claims filing, will be performed by fewer people. As the group steadily improves its operational and clinical efficiency, it will be possible for more work to be done by a smaller staff. Hard decisions will have to be made about which people to let go.

Each physician is likely to argue for retaining the staff she brought with her to the new group. This will be done out of loyalty and preference for working with that person. In fact, some physicians may insist that certain of their employees be continued as a condition of joining the group. If you accept such a condition, agree to retain the person only for a fixed period of time (perhaps a year at most) until his or her effectiveness can be established.

Uniform performance appraisal standards and procedures should be introduced across the organization as soon as possible. Their findings will support the decisions on which staff people to dismiss.

As some old members are being let go, new ones will be hired. These generally will be people with the skills required by the new operational and clinical procedures the group has adopted. Operators for the new computer system, analysts to interpret the data that accumulate, and new physician extenders are some possible examples.

Discretion Left to Individual Physicians

The crux of integrating physicians is deciding how much discretion and authority to leave with the individual physicians and what responsibilities to put in the hands of professional managers and trained technicians working at a central location. Ideally, the decisions should be made for objective business reasons—usually having to do with improved business efficiency. Like the choice of which staff to keep and which to let go, the physicians will have powerful feelings about yielding even small pieces of their autonomy. However, the need for these changes should have been discussed and accepted early in the education and planning stage.

The first tasks taken away from individual physicians should be those that they will miss the least and which offer the greatest potential for improved efficiency and effectiveness. Be sure to explain thoroughly the nature of the change and the benefits it will produce—particularly for the physicians. Further shifts in responsibility should take place according to a steady, progressive schedule.

In deciding whether to centralize a task or not, keep an open mind to the possibility that there are unquantifiable advantages to handling it at a local level. It may permit a quicker response to a patient's request or give a physician more immediate feedback on an action she has taken.

Name of the New Group

The new group practice organization will need a name, at least for legal purposes. A well-thought-out name serves a couple of other purposes. It can further the unifying effect among the physicians. It is helpful if they feel proud saying that they belong to the "Happy Valley Medical Group." The name can also have a valuable marketing effect.

It is not worth getting too wrapped up in finding the perfect group name. Within two or three years, the physicians and the market will have accepted it and will no longer be concerned with it.

Central Location of the Group

Issues of geographic location will come up in two ways. The new group entity will need a primary office, if only for legal purposes. This also

is likely to be the site where the growing number of centralized group functions is performed. In addition, the question may come up about the desirability of moving some or all of the participating physicians into a single practice location.

Initially, the main office can be based at the facilities of one of the larger merging practices. Eventually, as management services are centralized and new ones added, it probably will be necessary to move these operations to separate quarters.

Whether to consolidate the individual physicians into one or more practice sites is a complex question. The answer will turn on several factors.

- possible synergies, administrative and clinical, from physicians practicing in close proximity to each other
- advantages in securing and serving a particular patient population (e.g., under a managed care contract) through geographically dispersed sites
- the appropriateness of the physicians' current locations—in terms of geographic location; modern, efficient office configuration; and room for expansion

As the group evolves over the year toward a multispecialty group practice, and its revenues from managed care and capitation grow, one of its goals should be the development of a more rational pattern of office locations. This may mean bringing everyone together into one large clinic facility that also includes the management offices. Or it may make more sense to place the practice sites strategically throughout the service area.

Do not overlook the simple overhead savings that may be available by combining separate practices into one physical space. At the same time, do not feel an automatic urge to centralize all group activities. Do so only as far as it makes business sense.

Levels of Professional Liability Insurance

The group needs to be sure that it has sufficient professional liability insurance coverage, acquired as inexpensively as possible.

Most MCOs require that their contract providers carry specified minimum amounts of coverage. The levels are usually reasonable and the chances are that one or more of the merging physicians already has coverage at those levels. Some of the physicians, however, may carry less coverage or even none at all. Common sense and liability protection for the group says that all physicians should have the same, responsible coverage amounts. The simplest approach usually is to accept the highest coverage level of all the physicians as the standard for everyone. There should not be much protest since the group together will be paying the premiums.

The joint purchase of the liability insurance also offers the opportunity to obtain a group discount by using one vendor, rather than the several probably used by the independent physicians.

Capital Assessments or Contributions from Participating Doctors

To plan and carry out the merger of several physician practices into a single specialty group practice, with the intention of moving rapidly along the path of integration and modern care management, will cost a minimum of $200,000 for a group of 10 doctors. This is before the doors of the new enterprise open. This covers attorneys' fees, consultants' fees, filing fees, clerical expenses, and the hiring of a business manager. It does not include the value of the physicians' time spent in planning meetings. It does not include the cost of a new central office for the management staff—if one is desired. It does not include the ongoing costs of integrating the practices after they have merged.

During the first several years of the group's operation, capital spending needs are likely to exceed the amount of investable capital generated by the business. The participating physicians will be the primary, perhaps the only, source of start-up and ongoing capital for the group.

Serious thought must be given to the amount and method of those capital contributions. When the education and planning discussions are just starting, each physician should be asked to contribute a couple hundred dollars toward incidental costs. If the discussions go nowhere, the money will not be recouped. Otherwise, from that point on, all physician contributions to the venture must be recorded and, eventually, recognized formally.

The financial projections will give some idea of how much money must be injected by the physicians and when. Their contributions can take three forms.

1. *An investment.* The exact nature of the investment will depend on the kind of legal organizational form adopted. It may be an interest in a partnership or shares in a stock corporation. If the organization does well, the worth of the investments may increase, and the physicians may be able to realize a gain at some time in the future.

2. *A loan.* This characterization of the contribution may be necessary to accommodate larger contributions from some physicians than others without giving them a greater share of ownership and control in the business. The loan would be made on fair market terms, including interest and requiring repayment according to a schedule.

3. *Payment of dues.* In some cases, groups have asked their physician members to simply pay a form of dues to cover the cost of certain benefits they receive from participation in the group. As these amounts are not recovered, they usually are not very large, no more than one might pay in annual dues to a country club.

Clearly, the plans for physician capital contributions must be well understood by everyone going into the merger. There can be no surprises. If the plan for the new group is well conceived, there should be no possibility of these contributions being lost and, in most cases, their value will only grow.

Financial Planning

A major purpose of the group practice being created is to make money and certainly not to lose any. To ensure that your strategic and operational plans have a reasonable chance of achieving that purpose, it is important to do some financial planning before you get too far along toward implementation. With the help of an accountant or business planner, draw up these projections:

- income statements (revenues and costs) by month for the first three years
- balance sheets by quarter for the first three years
- capital spending budget for the first three years
- cash flow statements by month for the first two years

Although the group's finances are unlikely to develop exactly according to these projections, they provide both targets and benchmarks against which to measure the group's actual performance. Variances should be studied to learn what did and did not work. If nothing else, the process of preparing the projections will force the physicians to examine the financial implications of their contemplated merger. It may cause them to revise or even abandon the plans. It will give them experience in budgeting. These statements are a key ingredient of a good business plan that precedes the formation of a new venture.

Tie All This up in a Formal Business Plan

As the group moves through the design of the new entity and prepares for its implementation, all key decisions, expectations, and intentions should be documented. This all then should be tied together in a formal business plan, of the sort that entrepreneurs must show to prospective capital investors.

The act of preparing the plan will virtually guarantee that the group looks at all the important issues. The preparation of an internally logical and consistent business plan dramatically improves the chances of success for the new organization. And, at some point, the plan or a variation of it may come in handy if the group does approach outsiders for funding.

When it comes time to formalize the business plan, the services of an appropriate business consultant could prove helpful.

Legal Review of the Group Plans

There are several types of legal checks that should be performed before the group practice enters the final implementation stage. These should be handled by a skilled health lawyer.

1. *Due diligence.* A standard review of all possible legal implications, impediments, or liabilities in connection with a transaction resulting in the creation of a new organization. For instance, are there outstanding malpractice claims against any of the physicians that might be carried over to the new group? Or, are any of the assets being acquired pledged as security for a physician's debt?
2. *Tax advantages and disadvantages.* The transfer of valuable practice assets from the physicians to the group needs to be structured in a way that minimizes the tax liabilities—particularly capital gains.
3. *Antitrust.* It is possible that a merger among physicians in a narrow specialty in a smaller market could concentrate enough market power to create an antitrust law violation. Normally, the only answer will be to involve fewer physicians than originally planned. This should not be an issue for modest-size groups in larger markets.
4. *Fraud and abuse. Stark laws.* These laws are implicated when referrals are either bought or sold, or made to an entity in which the group has a financial interest. As long as the merger of the practices is genuine and not a sham, there are not likely to be legal problems in this area. Some scrutiny should be given to independent ancillary services facilities the group may own.

Legal Steps in Formation

At a certain point, when you and the other physicians have fully negotiated the terms of your union and they have been committed to writing, and all legal implications have been reviewed, your lawyers will lead you through the formal final steps in creating the new organization. This primarily entails the physicians signing documents and the lawyers filing at least some of them with appropriate state agencies.

When this stage is completed, the individual practices will no longer exist, and the new group practice will spring into existence.

Key Elements To Worry about in Forming a New Group Practice

- agreeing on a common vision for the group
- allowing enough time to hear everyone out and to identify barriers to achieving the goals of the group
- forming the group for the right reason
- determining whether the new group has a viable, competitive role in the marketplace
- having common views on the utility of the group in addressing managed care challenges
- determining if the formation of the legal entity of a group practice is the best way to meet the physicians' goals in the context of the existing market environment
- determining the initial level of integration within the group
- assessing the compatibility of the personalities and cultures of the practices being joined
- addressing the "core" anxieties that the physicians will have about this first attempt at combination
- determining the cost to each physician of starting and then sustaining the group

---

RESOURCE LIST

"The Best Ways To Group Up—Group Medical Practice," *Medical Economics*, 23 September, 1996.

"Choosing a Group Where You'll Be Happy," *Medical Economics*, 13 February, 1995.

The Development and Management of Medical Groups (Englewood, CO: Medical Group Management Association, 1996).

Implementing a Physician Organization (Chicago: American Medical Association, 1996).

"Is There a Future for Single-Specialty Groups?" *Medical Economics*, 28 October, 1996.

K. Korenchuk, *Merging Medical Practices*, part of a series on Integration Document Design and Analysis (Englewood, CO: Medical Group Management Association, 1994).

Medical Group Management Association, *Medical Group Practice, Legal and Administrative Guide* (Gaithersburg, MD: Aspen Publishers, Inc., 1998).

## CHAPTER 11

Step Four: Joining an Independent Practice Association

INTRODUCTION

For many physicians, the first move away from the absolute individualism of a solo or small group practice is participation in an independent practice association (IPA). After joining a very basic IPA, there are no noticeable changes to the physician's practice or life. She operates out of the same office, follows the same practice style, and still controls every clinical and business aspect of her practice. What is different is the flow of new patients from the managed care organization (MCO) with which the IPA has negotiated a contract on the physician's behalf. It is a deceptively alluring picture, with all the pleasure and none of the pain of managed care.

This chapter examines the IPA model, noting what is good and bad about it. It explains how to use the IPA model as a positive transitional form leading toward the more integrated structures demanded by managed care. There are practical guidelines on setting up an IPA that serves physicians' short- and long-term interests. After reading the chapter, a physician will have a better idea of whether an IPA is a useful step on his strategic path or a wasteful detour.

WHO SHOULD READ THIS CHAPTER

A physician who has little experience with any kind of managed care or in collaborating with other physicians, or who is simply nervous about

making a big jump into a new, more integrated practice entity might consider joining an IPA. It is a first tentative step away from the total autonomy and isolation of solo or small group practice and toward some kind of affiliation with other providers.

If you are reluctant to try any of the other new practice forms described in this book, you must at least allow yourself to participate in an IPA. It does not require that you change the ownership or location of your present practice, it gives you a minimal feeling of collegiality with other physicians, and it will steer you toward working with MCOs.

On the other hand, if you are eager to expose yourself as quickly as possible to the new integrated, value-based ways of practicing medicine, you are likely to be impatient with even a few months in an IPA. You are better off moving ahead to a merger with other physicians or participation in a management services organization (MSO).

BASIC DEFINITION OF AN IPA

An IPA is the loosest possible network of physicians, formed for the purpose of negotiating and securing risk-sharing contracts with payers—either MCOs, insurance companies, or employers. The contracts generally use capitation or withhold arrangements. The participating physicians maintain their independent medical practices. Each physician stays at her original practice location and retains control over her practice operations. Aside from their IPA involvement, the physicians continue to compete with each other.

Only physicians are accepted as IPA members. The IPA negotiates contracts for the provision of only physician services. As a rule, IPAs offer little opportunity for operational integration of the practices of its members. However, exceptions to that rule are possible. Sometimes, the term independent practice organization (IPO) is used to describe exactly the same practice form.

IPAs provide very limited integration of medical practices. Each practice participating in the IPA remains a separate business enterprise, often in competition with the other medical practices participating in the IPA. Commonly, the revenues received by a practice through the IPA represent only a small share of total practice revenues and the attention of IPA physicians is usually more focused on their still existing fee-for-service business.

The only element of structural integration created through an IPA takes the form of the capitated revenues distributed by the IPA to each member practice. Without actual combination of the practices, very little operational integration occurs either. At best, there is limited centralization of billing and collection functions and quality assurance procedures. Since the basic operations of each practice remain unchanged, an IPA will not provide the significant benefits to physicians that might result from full or partial operational integration.

An IPA is typically formed by physicians who are unwilling, at least initially, to surrender individual practice autonomy to a group practice. As a result, the IPA has little chance of modifying the practice patterns of a physician through quality control or utilization management. The IPA does not own or control the member practices, so it has minimal ability to impose organizational discipline on its members.

In the worst case, physicians join an IPA grudgingly, hoping to gain access to capitated business without otherwise changing the nature of their practices. The IPA is formed as a defen-sive reaction to managed care rather than as an assertive competitive strategy, more for political than sound business reasons.

In the best case, the IPA is viewed as the first step in physicians becoming comfortable working together and then, eventually, combining their practices into one. If the IPA is successful, the next step is for the physicians to merge their practices into a partially or fully integrated group practice.

The IPA lies at the low end of the continuum of physician practice integration. It involves structural integration only to the extent that it negotiates joint payer contracts that funnel patients and revenues to the economically separate private practices of the physicians. The IPA usually has no serious operational integration.

A certain minimal level of integration is necessary to protect against antitrust allegations. This requirement normally is satisfied if the IPA and its owner-members share risk, which means that the IPA is paid on a capitated basis. Any IPA that accepts fee-for-service payments, even discounted ones, has significant antitrust exposure.

WHAT AN IPA CAN DO FOR A PHYSICIAN

Participating in an IPA gives a physician the opportunity to take a tentative. nonthreatening step in the direction of managed care. It instills a sense of forward movement. Through its activities, the physician may gain knowledge and confidence to inspire her to accept even more integration with the other physicians. And that would be a good thing.

Even without the integration, the IPA consolidates many separate physicians into a much larger critical mass with a common purpose. Participation provides experience in working with other like-minded colleagues toward that goal. The physician must also become accustomed to delegating authority to, and taking direction from, other trusted individuals—both physicians and nonphysicians.

A physician member of an IPA gains access to managed care contracts and patients he would never otherwise see. In addition, the IPA provides the physician with a range of administrative services that can alleviate his administrative burdens, freeing him to concentrate on practicing medicine.

For all of this, the physician still owns all of her practice assets and is legally independent. She can withdraw from the IPA and resume unaffiliated solo practice at any time.

WHO CREATES AN IPA AND WHY

An IPA typically is founded by doctors of foresight in the community responding to the entrance of MCOs into their marketplace. One or more MCOs may already be active in the area, signing contracts with large multispecialty group practices or a physician-hospital organization (PHO) created by a local hospital. The MCO may also be negotiating agreements with individual physicians—on less than optimal terms. Or, there may be no substantial MCO presence at all, but physician leaders see the IPA as a low-risk, low-threat, low-commitment, and low-cost way to ease area physicians into a "managed care" practice style.

In some cases, hospitals have chosen to sponsor or encourage formation of an IPA as a prospective partner in managed care contracting. The IPA form does not entail the degree of hospital domination that can scare physicians away from a PHO. Nonetheless, one of the most useful contributions a hospital can make to IPA formation is providing start-up capital, and it will certainly want something in return. In those situations, the financing is better configured as a loan rather than a purchase of ownership shares—to avoid yielding any control to the hospital.

VARIATIONS IN THE IPA MODEL

The primary distinction among different kinds of IPAs lies in the degree of their operational integration. In the simplest, most recognizable archetype, the IPA does nothing more than contract with payers, contract with physicians, and transfer payer payments to the physicians.

There is potential complexity in even so simple a model. For the IPA to pass legal muster, there must be some degree of risk sharing among the physicians. If this takes the form of a capitation rate, the payment of that rate can be passed through more or less intact to the physicians. (Although, see the section on "How an IPA Distributes Net Earnings to Physician-Owners" later in this chapter.) But, what if the risk sharing involves withholds and risk pools, perhaps coupled with a discounted fee-for-service (FFS) payment schedule? Suddenly, the IPA is concerned with filing and collecting claims, as well as managing the risk-sharing mechanism.

As the local managed care market heats up and competition develops among too many physicians for a limited amount of managed care business, the IPA may come under pressure to accept lower capitation rates. To do this profitably, it probably will be necessary to embark upon some manner of utilization management and quality assurance programs with the IPA physicians. In addition, the IPA will have to start dropping from its ranks those physicians who cannot practice at the levels of cost efficiency and outcome quality demanded by the MCOs. These activities obviously require that the IPA employ more people, expend more money, carry out more tasks, and generally expand the scope of its operations. These activities also intervene more directly in the clinical and administrative decision making of the participating physicians.

This is a summary of the services that an IPA might offer to its physicians.

- negotiation of nonprice contract terms
- negotiation of contract price terms (requires significant risk sharing to avoid antitrust problems; the level of risk sharing required is a strong motivator for real structural integration as well)
- billing and collection
- utilization management and quality assurance (difficult to enforce utilization restrictions and quality standards against free and autonomous physicians)
- bookkeeping and accounting

- tax accounting
- employee hiring and supervision
- supplies purchasing and other vendor relations
- various other business services

Imagine the IPA moving inexorably into these new areas—because it is the only way to survive as the local market for physician services becomes more competitive. Eventually, the IPA will reach the point where its operations are so intertwined with those of the physicians that the only remaining step toward full integration is for the physicians to sell their practice assets to the IPA, which then transmutes into an MSO or a large, fully integrated, multispecialty group practice. The evolution is then complete.

CASE STUDY: LANE INDEPENDENT PRACTICE ASSOCIATION (EUGENE, OREGON)*

A good example of an IPA is the Lane Independent Practice Association in Eugene, Oregon. It was founded in the late 1970s in order to staff the provider panel of a new health maintenance organization (HMO) that was being developed. Nearly all the 450 physicians in Lane County surrounding Eugene joined the IPA. The IPA was paid on a capitation basis. The physicians, in turn, were reimbursed on the basis of a discounted fee-for-service schedule accompanied by a 15 percent risk withhold. The system worked fine through the early 1980s. The physicians were serving between 20,000 and 25,000 covered lives. They always received the risk withhold, sometimes even more.

Like most IPAs, however, they were not aggressively managing the utilization of resources and the associated costs. The amount of withhold returned steadily declined before disappearing

---

*This case study is based on information in the book, "Integrated Health Care: Case Studies," by Dean Coddington and Barbara Bendrick, Center for Research in Ambulatory Health Care Administration, pp. 150–151, 1994.

altogether. In 1986, in order to get a grip on the costs, some of the physicians proposed capitating the primary care doctors in the group. The proposal stirred strong feelings. When it was rejected, many of the primary care and specialist physicians left to form the Oregon Medical Group, a multispecialty group practice dedicated to care management.

By the mid-1990s, the Lane IPA was still in operation, serving about 60,000 lives. The risk withhold was still not being paid in most years.

DISTINGUISHING AN IPA FROM A PPO

At first glance, an IPA looks a lot like a PPO (preferred provider organization). In fact, the differences between them are so significant that a PPO does not deserve consideration in a physician's long-term practice strategy.

A PPO contracts with MCOs or employers to deliver physician care to their members or employees and contracts with many solo and small group practice physicians to provide that care. Unlike the IPA, the PPO contracts involve no risk sharing; their payments all are on a FFS or discounted FFS basis. Due to the antitrust implications when risk sharing is not present among the physicians, the PPO does not negotiate prices for them—either as a group or individually. It simply acts as a "messenger" between the payers and individual physicians, relaying price offers that the physicians accept or reject without consulting with each other.

The PPO generally does not offer a significant number of additional business services to the participating physicians. As long as it is dealing in FFS contracts, there is little incentive to develop utilization management programs. There is not much potential for building a PPO into a more operationally integrated entity, as required by managed care market forces.

The most common PPO model involves independent physicians accepting a somewhat lower fee schedule than they normally charge (the "discount") in return for being designated as a "preferred provider" in the enrollees' health insurance policies, which presumably leads to a greater increase in patients than they otherwise would realize. These PPOs are most often started by MCOs, insurance companies, employers, and even profit-seeking entrepreneurs. It is an important distinction that their primary mission is to serve the interests of payers, while an IPA, by design, acts for the primary benefit of its physicians.

FINANCING THE START-UP AND OPERATION OF AN IPA

The IPA is one of the least expensive forms of new physician organizations, but it still requires a hefty up-front investment and some way to finance ongoing operations. A good estimate of IPA start-up costs is $200,000.[1] The level of operating expenses that must be covered varies widely, depending on the range and depth of services provided to the physicians. An IPA that negotiates and administers contracts, conducts utilization management and quality assurance programs, oversees billings and collections, and engages in some practice management, all for a collection of 100 or more physicians could easily spend $1 million a month. A brand new IPA that is keeping its activities to a bare minimum, doing little more than the basic contracting function, and serving a more modest number of physicians (say 50), may be able to get by on a monthly budget of $50,000.

The start-up capital usually comes from the sale of ownership interests in the IPA to the participating physicians. (If the amount needed to start an IPA composed of 50 doctors is $200,000, each of them will have to pay in $4,000.) Additional capital might be sought from other parties interested in the development of an IPA. These may include a hospital that sees the IPA as a managed care contracting partner, an MCO that prefers to execute one contract with a collective of physicians rather than many contracts with many individual physicians, or a self-insured employer that wants to assemble a diverse mix of physicians willing to share some risk in exchange for serving its employees.

The important question is with the form of the financing transaction. Even though it immediately burdens the IPA with regular interest payments, a loan arrangement is the best way of securing the required capital without yielding control of the IPA to nonphysicians.

The alternative is selling shares in the IPA. The problem with this approach is that, at start-up, it would be necessary to hand over an unacceptably large control interest in the IPA to parties (hospital, MCO, etc.) whose goals may not coincide with those of the physicians. Once the IPA is well established and significantly larger, a much smaller ownership share can be traded for the funds necessary to finance an expansion of the IPA.

Operating revenues for the IPA come from the physicians, in a couple ways.

- Member physicians make monthly payments to the IPA. The payments may be the same for each physician, may be lump sums varying by specialty, or may be calculated as a percentage of each physician's earnings for that month.
- The IPA deducts a fixed or variable (depending on its range of activities) percentage from the MCO payments before they are passed on to the physicians.

As the IPA grows and develops needs for additional capital, it may request that the physicians make further investments or contributions. This may even be seen as an opportunity. If the IPA is thriving financially, its shares of stock may actually increase in value, making them a desirable investment for physicians.

RECOMMENDED LEGAL ORGANIZATIONAL FORMS FOR AN IPA

An IPA can take almost any legal organizational form, such as a business corporation, professional corporation, limited liability company, nonprofit corporation, or partnership. The key factors in choosing among them are

- the presence of a "corporate practice of medicine" doctrine in the state
- whether the IPA will contract to actually provide physician services or will simply serve as a conduit or messenger to the physicians actually delivering the services (in the manner of a PPO)
- the need to allow the purchase of ownership shares in the organization (either by physicians for control reasons or nonphysicians for capital financing reasons)
- whether participation in the IPA will jeopardize the favorable tax status of individual physicians' pension plans
- the number of potential owners (shareholders) and the securities law requirements that must be satisfied
- the desire to limit exposing the personal wealth of the physician-owners to the IPA's liabilities
- the desire to avoid double taxation of net earnings that may be passed through to the physicians as dividends
- the level of regulation and oversight of nonprofit organizations in the state

Barring unusual legal circumstances, the best choices of legal form are the business corporation or the professional corporation.

An IPA organized as a traditional *for-profit business corporation* limits the financial liability of participating physicians to the amount of their original investments. This form allows the sale of ownership interests to raise capital and to give physicians legal control of the entity. If the IPA contracts to actually provide medical services, as most do, in contrast with the PPO messenger model, and if there is a legal ban on the corporate practice of medicine, a straight business corporation will not work. A professional corporation or a partnership entirely owned by physicians will have to be used.

A *professional corporation* functions very much like a business corporation except that it

can be owned and, therefore, controlled entirely by physicians. This may be the ideal solution as long as the IPA never needs, at some point in the future, to sell shares in the corporation to nonphysicians for new infusions of capital.

The *partnership* alternative fails for its inability to shield the participating physicians from unlimited liability for organizational activities. It avoids double taxation of organization income reaching the owners, but it does this by funneling all income through to them. Of course, they will have to pay taxes on all the income received. The partnership form also makes it hard to sell or transfer ownership interests to nonparticipating individuals.

In the many states that offer the option, organization as a *limited liability company* can be quite attractive to an IPA. It combines the liability limitations of a business corporation with the income pass-through of a partnership.

Organizing as a *nonprofit corporation* is the least desirable alternative. While it does minimize certain securities law restrictions, the form presents several disadvantages for IPAs. It is unlikely to qualify for federal tax-exempt status, so normal income taxes will still have to be paid. It will be prohibited by state law from distributing earnings to owners and, as a result, will not be able to function as the entrepreneurial, equity-building entity an IPA needs to be. State regulatory agencies also tend to watch nonprofits more closely than for-profits.

HOW AN IPA DISTRIBUTES NET EARNINGS TO PHYSICIAN-OWNERS

After negotiating one or more managed care contracts, the most basic function of the IPA is to distribute the revenues produced by those contracts. The formula for the distributions should be set out in the professional services agreement with each IPA physician.

Earnings distribution is not a simple matter. It can be complicated if the IPA receives different types of revenue from its contract payers—capitation, FFS, discounted FFS. It may take a sophisticated accounting system to keep track of how much is owed to physicians who see patients from those different plans. Under capitation, which should predominate, decisions must be made about the following issues:

- allocating revenues to primary care physicians who are more productive than others; that is, they see more patients in the same period of time
- allocating revenues to physicians in certain specialties that traditionally have been higher paying than other specialties
- allocating revenues to specialist physicians who have stronger referral relationships with primary care physicians in the IPA
- allocating revenues to physicians who are more efficient in utilizing resources in treating comparable numbers of patients
- using withhold accounts or risk pools to spur desired physician behavior (i.e., using specialty, hospital, and ancillary services in a manner consistent with IPA goals)
- compensating specialist physicians on the basis of subcapitation rates versus straight FFS reimbursement
- employing cost control mechanisms for the ancillary services included in the IPA's capitation rate

It is certainly possible to devise a quantitative distribution formula that takes into account all of these factors, as well as any others that may come up. For instance, the IPA could allocate capitation revenues to physicians according to

- the percentage of total enrollees assigned to each physician
- the percentage of total patient encounters attributable to each physician
- the percentage of total referrals received by each physician

However, no matter how precise and logical the methodology may be, there are bound to be some unhappy physicians. Indeed, the biggest problems with the distribution system probably will be political and emotional. After all, these are practitioners who have spent most of their careers receiving every cent of the fruits of their labors. They have not had to share earnings with other physicians or rely on formulas devised and administered by someone else.

Some IPAs also do a certain amount of FFS business with payers.* It might seem natural to send the money directly to the individual physicians performing the services that generated the fees. However, it is a better idea to apply some risk-sharing overlay even to these payments. This further reduces any possible antitrust risk and helps encourage practice efficiency.

See Chapter 25, "The Kinds of Physician Reimbursement Systems You Can Expect under Managed Care," for a more thorough discussion of physician compensation options.

SUCCESS FACTORS IN THE FORMATION OF AN IPA

When the track record of IPAs up until now is examined, several factors emerge as clear indicators of potential success. In planning or evaluating an IPA, it is worth keeping them in mind.

1. Organized as a separate business or professional corporation for the primary purpose of contracting with MCOs.
2. Physician practices remain legally and physically independent.
3. Participating physicians are composed of the appropriate numbers, specialties, and practice locations required to serve the enrollees of the MCOs contracted with.
4. Participating physicians view the IPA as an evolutionary step in their progress toward greater integration.
5. While governance of the IPA remains always in the hands of physicians, the bal-

---

*This must be a rather modest part of total revenues if the IPA is to minimize the risk of antitrust complaints. Fortunately, FFS payments are a rapidly declining revenue source throughout the health care system.

ance of power is tilted in favor of primary care doctors.

6. Initially, the IPA implements the minimum operational infrastructure (employees, facilities, and expenses) required to perform its contracting function.

7. As market conditions dictate and physician wishes permit, the IPA steadily expands the range of services provided to its physicians.

8. Governed by a board of physician directors with vision, leadership skills, and the respect of the participating physicians.

9. Participating physician group is steadily winnowed down to only the most cost-efficient, high-quality, team-oriented practitioners.

DEFINING PHYSICIAN CONTROL OVER THE IPA

Governance is an important issue for IPAs, but in slightly different ways than for other new provider organizations. In PHOs, MSOs, and integrated delivery systems (IDSs), physicians often are concerned with making sure that they get enough seats at the board table. In IPAs, it is a given that physicians will dominate; the question is how much authority, if any, will be granted to nonphysicians in return, say, for their capital investments. There is the further matter of allowing all the participating physicians a direct say in some more crucial decisions.

Some of the key issues that may come before an IPA board are these:

- bylaws enactment and amendment
- election and removal of directors
- admission and termination of physician shareholders
- sale of shares to nonphysicians
- approval of new MCO partners and contracts
- expansion of range of services offered by the IPA
- approval of financial matters (budgets and fund-raising)

The board will pass on all these issues, but some may be subjected to a supermajority (e.g., two-thirds) instead of a simple majority (51 percent) vote. A few of them may be put to a vote of all the physician shareholders. This kind of veto power should be reserved for only the most vital strategic issues—such as movement of the IPA toward further integration. Resist the pleas of any physicians seeking the right to approve or reject new managed care contracts.

See Chapter 22, "Creating an Effective Governance Structure for Affiliated or Integrated Physician Group," for additional ideas on the board of directors of the IPA.

INCLUDING AND EXCLUDING PHYSICIANS AS IPA PARTICIPANTS

One of the most controversial decisions in forming an IPA concerns which area physicians will be permitted to participate. There will be a temptation and pressure to accept anyone who wants in or, at least, all interested members of the physician community creating the IPA (for example, a local hospital's medical staff). Accepted physicians may request special treatment for their friends and colleagues.

Giving in to these desires compromises the IPA's mission and chances of success from the very beginning. The IPA should be rigorously selective in screening and credentialing physicians—within the limits of antitrust constraints. It should rely on objective clinical, economic, and practice style standards drawn up in advance and applied without exception. (Physicians in competition with each candidate should be excluded from the accept/reject decision.) In addition to ensuring each physician's clinical competence, it is important to assess whether she is adaptable to new economic realities, capable of practicing cost-effective medicine, and open to learning new skills and collaborating with others.

A new IPA also needs to be sensitive to the specialty requirements of its MCO partners. Most will prefer a predisposition toward primary care, and such doctors should predominate in the IPA group and on its governing body.

If the IPA is as selective as it should be, there will be problems with the physicians who are excluded. They may be integral parts of accepted physicians' referral networks and collegial relationships. These may be threatened. The best response, the only response, is to use objective criteria in excluding them—criteria that clearly serve the long-term interests of the total organization. Communicate openly to them about the purpose of the IPA and why every physician in the community simply cannot be a part of it.

Exhibit 11–1 shows the standard steps in putting together an IPA. Whether you are a leader in the process or just expect to be one of the participating physicians, use this list to follow and evaluate the progress in creating the IPA.

Give These Issues Special Attention in Evaluating or Planning an IPA

In forming or evaluating an IPA, there are a few key issues that should be the focus of your attention:

- the existence in your market area of an IPA you would be willing to join
- if no appropriate IPA exists, your willingness and ability to work to establish one
- if an IPA does exist, the fit of the IPA's mix of specialties to the market's needs
- the adequacy of the IPA's capitalization to meet current and projected operating requirements
- the presence of strong, informed, and respected physician leadership of the IPA
- day-to-day management of the IPA in the hands of experienced administrators or executives
- IPA enforcement of utilization review and other cost control mechanisms with its physicians
- form of physician compensation for services performed through IPA contracts
- freedom of IPA physicians to operate under other risk sharing contracts apart from the IPA

- whether you view the IPA participation as the end point or the beginning of your involvement in managed care and provider integration
- whether the IPA physician-owners view the IPA as the beginning or the ending of a strategy toward increased integration, utilization control, cost-effectiveness, and quality emphasis

HAZARDS TO WATCH OUT FOR

IPAs have not been an overwhelming success in the marketplace. The primary reason is the fallacy in their very conception. They are an inadequate half step toward physician collaboration and provider integration. As a final form of organization, they have no future.

The physicians remain in separate competitive practices. They lack the unity of economic interests that truly minimizes costs and propels the organization toward real operational integration. Each IPA physician works in the best interests of her practice, not the IPA as a whole. Because of lack of physician commitment and the geographic dispersion of the practices, the IPA cannot exercise the clinical discipline necessary to modify physician practice styles in the way MCOs are demanding.

In addition, IPAs have been plagued by some more commonplace failings. Try to anticipate and avoid these pitfalls:

- undercapitalization
- lack of physician leadership
- absence of management expertise
- absence of effective cost control mechanisms (no utilization management or effective economic incentives to reduce costs)
- overemphasis on specialty physicians in markets that need more primary care physicians
- inability of physicians to agree on a compensation system that is consistent with the goals of the IPA (e.g., specialists simply bill fee-for-service against the IPA's revenues, or physician impulse/desire to withdraw any net earnings remaining at the end of the year)

Exhibit 11–1 Step-by-Step Process for Creating an IPA

1. Form a cadre of physicians with the need or desire to begin a physician-originated response to managed care.
2. Once you have settled on the IPA form, define its mission, strategic goals, and the range of activities it will offer initially.
3. Assess the state of the local market and the mood of the competition.
4. Define the market (in terms of MCOs, employers, or services) and the geographic area the IPA will target.
5. Determine the IPA's start-up capital requirements, ongoing operating expenses, and the sources of capital and revenue to meet them.
6. Capture those financial data in formal budgets and projections.
7. Draft a formal strategic plan for the development of the IPA over the coming five years.
8. Combine the plan, budgets, and projections in a formal business plan for the IPA—a document that can be shown to prospective physician-owners and financing sources.
9. Decide on the legal organizational form of the IPA.
10. Determine the makeup of the IPA's physician leadership, along with a candid evaluation of its strengths and weaknesses.
11. Plan the initial composition of the IPA's administrative staff.
12. Define how the IPA will package itself and the image it will present to potential contract partners.
13. Make a preliminary identification of the MCOs or employers that will be approached for contracts, and the types of contracts that will be preferred.
14. Figure out the systems and procedures the IPA will need to operate under the reimbursement schemes likely to be used by the MCOs.
15. Check for securities law compliance required by the ownership structure the IPA decides to employ.
16. Prepare the necessary organizational documents, including
    • articles of incorporation or partnership agreement
    • corporate bylaws
    • shareholder agreements and securities law filings
17. Sign professional services agreements with the physicians.
18. Choose the initial members of the board of directors.
19. Appoint members to the board committees (finance, planning, credentialing, contracts, nominations, etc.).
20. Secure appropriate insurance coverage (professional liability, personal liability, directors, and officers).
21. Hire the personnel necessary to conduct the IPA's planned activities, including a qualified business manager.
22. Set up the credentialing system with criteria, procedures (including due process protections), and staffing.
23. Lay out the formal lines of communication between the IPA and the participating physicians.
24. Formulate the methodology for distributing IPA income to the physicians.
25. Design and acquire the financial and other management information systems needed to properly administer the IPA relationships with payers and physicians.
26. Identify the number of desired physicians—by specialty and practice location—to be recruited into the IPA.
27. Hold a series of meetings for physician candidates to explain the IPA concept, purpose, and goals and to answer questions.
28. Obtain preliminary commitments from targeted and interested physicians.
29. Describe a schedule, with deadlines, for the targeted physicians to become part of the IPA network.
30. After securing all necessary background information, apply the credentialing procedure to the targeted physicians.
31. Sign professional services agreements with the targeted, credentialed physicians, issue stock or other ownership interests to them, and receive payment of their stock purchase prices or membership fees.
32. Begin operations by negotiating and concluding the first managed care contract.

REFERENCE

1. "Can Integrating Organizations Support Their Future Capital Needs?" *Medical Group Management Update 35*, no. 12 (1996): 1.

RESOURCE LIST

D. Bachrach and S.B. Berkow, "Building a Sustainable, Risk-Bearing IPA," *Healthcare Financial Management 51*, no. 12 (1997): S5.

IPAs & Physician Networks, Super Search Packet #4920, (Englewood, CO: Medical Group Management Association, updated annually).

"The Second-Generation IPA: Will It Save Independent Practice?" *Medical Economics*, 11 August, 1997.

Todd, Maria K. *IPA, PHO and MSO Development Strategies: Building Successful Provider Alliances* (New York: McGraw-Hill Healthcare Education Group, 1997).

McGraw-Hill Healthcare Education Group: (800) 262-4729. Copublished with The Healthcare Financial Management Association.

"Will the Big, Bad Antitrust Wolf Blow Your IPA Down?" *Medical Economics*, 7 April, 1997.

Organization:
The IPA Association of America
333 Hegenberger Road, Suite 305
Oakland, CA 94621
   (510) 569-6561

CHAPTER 12

Participating in a Group Practice without Walls

INTRODUCTION

Many physicians are searching for an organizational structure that provides just enough integration to make them competitive in the managed care marketplace yet retains as much of the traditional style of medical practice as possible. The group practice without walls (GPWW) is one of the more attractive possibilities—at least in the short run.

The GPWW concept allows individual physicians to integrate their solo and small group practices into a single practice entity while maintaining their original separate medical office locations. A new legal organization is created, usually a professional corporation, although partnerships are possible. The participating physicians are the owners of the organization and merge their practices into it. This arrangement allows the doctors to continue practicing in their own offices, preserving a lot, though not all, of the autonomy solo practitioners value so highly.

WHO SHOULD READ THIS CHAPTER

Solo practitioners and members of small group practices (2 to 3 doctors) who are planning their first serious move toward integration and learning a managed care style of practice should read this chapter, along with Chapter 10, "Step Three: Forming or Joining a Small, Single Specialty

Group Practice." These are the first, least revolutionary strategic changes they should be considering.

If some colleagues have been talking about forming a GPWW, reading this chapter will help you evaluate their proposal and make an informed decision about whether to go along with them. If you already have your mind set on creating a GPWW, this chapter will provide some tips on how to make it work best for you. You can learn the steps in a good process for getting one started.

There is no point in reading this chapter if you are committed to collaborating and integrating with other doctors in the boldest, most aggressive fashion. If you want to be a part of a large, high-performing physician group with a dominant position in an integrated delivery system (IDS), a GPWW will not get you there. If anything, it will distract and delay you from the assertive strategic moves necessary for managed care success.

WHAT IS A GPWW AND HOW IS IT DIFFERENT FROM OTHER PHYSICIAN ORGANIZATIONS?

A GPWW is simply a framework that allows physicians in established practices to create a corporate relationship without moving in together. They form an organization, usually a professional corporation, which becomes their employer. They practice as much of their medicine as possible through managed care contracts negotiated by the group. Their services are billed under a uniform fee schedule set by the group. The physicians use a common provider number assigned to the organization.

Initially, each participating physician's practice may be operated as a profit center. After covering the practice's direct costs and paying a share of the central management and services overhead, any remaining revenues go to the individual physician. Later, more innovative revenue allocation formulas are implemented.

Technically, the physicians are employees of the new group practice, into which they have merged their separate practices. Their support staffs become employees of the group practice as well. In some cases, their employment may be transferred to a separate management company (also owned by the physicians) that contracts with the GPWW to provide management services.

The physicians continue to work in their own offices. They retain operational control over their support staffs, equipment, medical records, and clinical relationships with patients. Management staff and other personnel performing centralized functions usually work at a separate location.

The group practice may be owned entirely by physicians in a single specialty, by only primary care physicians, by only specialty physicians, or by a market-appropriate mix of physicians. The individual practice sites are run as subdivisions of the overall organization.

The GPWW format offers a mechanism for linking physicians at multiple sites. They reap the economies of scale that come from centralizing and sharing services. Through the GPWW, the doctors contract as a single unit with managed care organizations (MCOs) and other payers. And still, they have the satisfaction of staying and practicing in their own offices.

Since a GPWW is set up as an independent legal entity, ultimate control over its operations lies with a single unified governing board—typically a board of directors in a professional corporation. The board makes all the strategic "big picture" decisions for the group, including development of fee schedules, approval of payer contracts, negotiation of affiliations with other organizations, and selection of employee benefit and pension plans.

Because of the added complexity of uniformly directing operations at several scattered practice locations, the group employs a professional management staff. These people take over many of the day-to-day administrative tasks previously handled by the physicians in their individual practices.

LEGAL BENEFIT FOR ANCILLARY SERVICES

If the GPWW physicians are truly integrated—particularly through risk sharing—they are likely to avoid liability under the Stark laws against self-referral. Although the laws restrict a doctor's ownership of ancillary medical services to which he refers patients, they make an exception when the services are owned by the physician's truly integrated group practice. Revenues from ancillary services are often a significant source of income for groups in highly competitive markets.

The organization is not a GPWW when the physicians retain ownership of their practices, maintain separate cash flows, and merely allow some of their revenues to be channeled through the group entity. The arrangement will further fail the group practice test by allowing physicians to opt out of contracts, choose which central services they will use, hire and fire their own staff, and buy equipment without central office approval. This kind of physician structure more closely resembles an independent practice association (IPA).

The GPWW looks a lot like the traditional group practice described in Chapter 10, "Step Three: Forming or Joining a Small, Single Specialty Group Practice." The main differences are that the single specialty group practice tends to be composed of fewer physicians gathered together in a single facility. The GPWW usually starts off with a larger number of doctors who have a strong desire to remain physically autonomous, even if not legally or financially.

The primary problem with a GPWW is that it does not require physicians to change their behavior. The primary value of a GPWW is as a transitional model, allowing physicians to ease into collaboration and integration.

ADVANTAGES AND DISADVANTAGES OF THE GPWW FORM

These are the good and bad features of GPWWs.

Advantages

- Some economies of scale are gained through centralized services, for example, instead of one accountant servicing each of 10 practices, it may be possible for two accountants to handle all 10 at a central location.
- Requires less up-front capital investment than more ambitious organizational forms, like management services organizations (MSOs), which entail the purchase of practice assets.
- Offers multiple, geographically dispersed practice sites that may be more attractive to an MCO and its patients.
- Facilitates the negotiation of equity or debt capital by pooling working capital and other assets and by creating a unified entity whose shares can be sold to outside investors.
- Provides physicians with a foundation for engaging in relatively large-scale managed care risk contracting.
- Allows the participating physicians greater leverage in their negotiations with hospitals and MCOs for inpatient risk pools.
- Creates a basis and procedure for physicians selling their practices upon retirement.
- In its more advanced forms, can develop control systems that reduce resource utilization with accompanying cost savings.
- Provides a vehicle for participating specialty physicians to restrict their earnings in order to maintain the income and survival of the primary care physicians who are their source of referrals.
- By taking advantage of the group practice "safe harbor" under Stark, permits referrals to and collection of profits from ancillary services and other medically related ventures.
- Efficiencies and professionalism of centralized billing, accounting, claims filing, and financial management reduce costs and increase revenues.
- Makes it easier for the group to recruit new physicians to provide new services or replace a retiring physician.
- Centralized human resource management (compensation, recruitment, training, performance appraisal, and personnel policies) reduces costs and increases productivity of nonphysician staff.
- Joint marketing programs enhance the physicians' presence in the marketplace.
- Delegation of administrative tasks to central management frees physicians to concentrate on practicing medicine.
- Physicians can continue to treat their patients in a familiar setting with minimal interference in their practice methods.
- Physician compensation still depends largely on each doctor's personal productivity.
- Physicians can select their own support staff and reward them within broad groupwide guidelines.
- Physicians set their own office hours and hospital schedules.

Disadvantages

- Multiple locations limit the economies of scale available through integration.
- While dispersed, the physician practice sites may not be optimally located for the patient population served by the group.
- Only partial integration of the practices prevents development of the discipline and culture necessary for managed care success.

- For political reasons, the group founders often leave the governance and decision making too diffuse.
- For all the above reasons, the GPWW will be less competitive with more fully integrated group practices.
- The appeal of continued physician autonomy may attract physicians who will resist further efforts to integrate the practices and tighten control over utilization and quality.
- When the group begins to manage utilization and quality more closely, it may be necessary to negotiate the departure or even the dismissal of poorly performing physicians.
- Even if they spend less time on administrative matters, the physicians will spend more time on governance and setting policy.
- Although the physicians retain considerable independence, there is still some loss of autonomy.

COMPROMISES TO BE MADE WHEN JOINING A GPWW

Most members of a newly formed GPWW will be leaving solo or small group practices. The move will require some major shifts in attitude, even if the new group is only loosely bound together.

Compromise. Solo practitioners are accountable to no one but themselves. In a group, physicians must reach consensus on a variety of operational issues, from pension plans to medical supplies vendors. Individual doctors will not always get the outcomes they would prefer. They must learn to compromise.

Community. The participating physicians must begin thinking as a group or community of individuals with common interests. Toward that end, they must develop a shared vision for the future and accompanying strategic objectives. Each physician must be willing to sacrifice some of her personal interests for the welfare of the larger group.

Uniformity. In the pursuit of integration and in order to present a common face to the world, the group will need to create uniformity in many of

its policies and procedures. One way this shows up is in a standard fee schedule that the group offers to medical care payers—like insurers, MCOs, and employers. Physicians in the same specialties must agree to accept the same fees. Frequently, this results in some doctors receiving more than they did in solo practice while others are paid less.

Limits. In solo practice, the physicians had control over almost every aspect of the business. In a group, they must subject themselves to limits, in the interests of efficiency and uniformity. Most contracts and leases will be in the group's name and signed by a group representative. The group's business manager will control many routine operational matters, and the group board of directors will make all the strategic and policy-level decisions.

> **Caution**: If you are especially anxious about turning over control of certain practice decisions to directors or managers you do not know, investigate the GPWW before you join. Check two things. Look into the business backgrounds of the people in those positions, to find out their experience and attitudes regarding physicians and managed care. Talk with others who have worked with them before. Treat them as though you are interviewing them for their jobs. Next, study the new organization's bylaws to see what powers have been granted to the directors and what chance you have of influencing their decisions. In your investigations, bear in mind that these people will be deciding crucial questions such as: How will the group manage risk sharing in capitated contracts? With which managed care payers will the group contract? When will the group shift from basing physician compensation on revenue generation to practice efficiency?

Liability. In solo practice, a physician bears substantial legal liability, but primarily for her own actions. In a group, the corporate structure protects the physician from unlimited liability, but she simultaneously becomes responsible for the acts of all her colleagues. If a few physicians have poor malpractice histories, the insurance premiums of all will rise. If the organization must pay damage awards resulting from the negligence of its employees (causing employment discrimination or personal injury, for instance), it ultimately comes out of the salaries of the member physicians.

Expenses. One of the arguments in favor of GPWWs is that centralizing many administrative functions lowers the cumulative costs of the group. Be wary, however, of a structure that actually creates an even greater overhead load in the central office. Examine the group's proposed expense makeup. Look out for excessive, overpaid executives and unnecessary added services.

PRACTICAL STEPS IN FORMING A GPWW

The process of setting up a GPWW is similar to that for creating a single specialty group practice, with a few differences. The GPWW is likely to involve more physicians from the outset. This will make it harder and take more time to reach agreement on the founding principles and continuing operations of the new organization. Because the participating physicians will remain scattered at their individual practice sites, the cost of moving them all to a central facility will be avoided. However, it will be necessary to install systems and implement procedures for linking them to some degree.

The following reviews the key steps in the formation process.

Education and Commitment

- Hold initial meetings among interested physicians to learn how a GPWW works, along with its advantages and disadvantages. Assign tasks and responsibilities. Lay out plans for next steps in study and development.

- Request monetary contributions from each physician toward development costs. During the planning period leading to actual start-up, either one large contribution or several smaller ones can be sought. The initial amount should be at least $500.
- Ask each physician to sign a letter of intent, indicating her willingness to participate further in the process, abide by the decisions made, and disclose necessary information about her practice to facilitate the planning.

Analysis and Planning

- Hire a consultant experienced in working with physicians to plan provider group ventures like a GPWW.
- Gather detailed information about each physician's practice operations, particularly cost data, revenue sources, patient volumes, and utilization rates. Use questionnaires, interviews, and site visits.
- Aggregate and analyze the data from all the practices. Determine the potential for cost savings and revenue improvements. Estimate the additional overhead expenses for the new combined organization.
- Prepare *pro forma* financial statements, including balance sheets, income statements, cash flow projections, and capital budgets.

Formation and Implementation

- Retain an attorney experienced in working with physicians forming group practices.
- With the attorney's assistance, reach agreement among all participating physicians on the legal form of the organization (i.e., professional corporation), governance/committee structure, compensation plan, cost-sharing formula, and initial operating procedures.
- Design and begin acquiring the control and reporting systems needed to operate the group. These will impact cost accounting and assessment, revenue accounting, physician and staff compensation, centralized bill-

ing and collection, and general reporting to the physician shareholders and the board of directors.

- With the assistance of experienced accountants or valuation specialists, place values on the practice assets that will be transferred to the GPWW.
- Calculate the stock shares that each physician will receive for her assets, plus the loans that will be made to or from the physicians to account for different amounts of assets transferred to the GPWW.
- Bring the GPWW into existence by signing and filing the documents that incorporate the organization, merge the practice assets, issue shares to the physicians, and acknowledge any other initial capital financing.
- Hire a general manager and other staff necessary to provide the centralized services.

The money and time consumed in creating a GPWW will depend on how many physicians are participating and whether they have worked together previously. Count on the process taking nine months to a year. The costs expended to get the new group off the ground will be at least $50,000 and could exceed $250,000 if many unrelated physicians are coming together. This money goes primarily toward consultants, filing fees, and clerical assistance.

KEYS TO MAKING A GPWW WORK WELL

There has been enough experience with GPWWs to know what factors are most important in determining their success and failure. Pay attention to these.

Patience and Haste

Allow the physicians enough time to learn about GPWWs and each other and to become comfortable with the idea of giving up their prac-

tice assets to work more closely with each other. Also, move with all deliberate speed to begin this collaboration so that all physicians can acquire managed care skills—especially in markets that are evolving rapidly.

Common Vision and Values

Do not proceed very far with the planning of a GPWW (or any other physician organization) without reaching consensus among all participating physicians on exactly what kind of organization they are creating, how it will operate, and what it will evolve into in the future. It is particularly important to decide whether the GPWW is viewed as the final step toward managed care or a transitional stage in the building of a larger, more comprehensive, integrated delivery system.

Governance

Devise a governance structure (board of directors and committees) that gives all the participating physicians confidence in the decisions being made in managing the organization, but also does not impede speedy decision making. Key questions that will have to be addressed are

- whether to allow all participating physicians on the board or only a representative group of them
- what procedure and criteria to use in selecting board members
- whether to reserve board seats for specific constituencies (certain subspecialties, geographic areas, or community representatives)
- whether to require special majorities to approve decisions on certain sensitive issues

Participation

A decision that must be made very early in the discussion process is what kinds of physicians are to be included in the group and who will be left out. If the founding physicians are all based at the same hospital, there may be a temptation to open the GPWW to the entire medical staff. Alternatively, the GPWW membership could be restricted to primary care physicians, doctors in a particular subspecialty, or a market-appropriate mix of specialties. Within these categories, the group might impose criteria for reputation, compatibility, or managed care experience. In making these choices, bear in mind the repercussions among those doctors excluded.

Withdrawals

The novelty of a GPWW may attract some physicians who then find they do not like it and want to leave to return to their original practice arrangement. It would be wise to plan in advance to make such departures as painless and undisruptive as possible. Even if they never use it, such a withdrawal provision may help all the physicians feel more comfortable joining in the first place. Do not forget to include a noncompete clause in the original shareholder agreement to prevent departing physicians from taking group patients or setting up a competing organization.

It might also be a good idea to define a procedure for requiring a participating physician to leave, for a variety of reasons (incompatibility, poor-quality medicine, inability to reduce utilization, etc.). Do it before the situation arises. This procedure will be needed especially if the GPWW started with an open, nonselective panel of physicians who will be culled as the group gains experience.

Compensation and Cost-Sharing

Physicians joining a GPWW do so with the expectation of maintaining and, eventually, increasing their incomes. So, the ways in which revenues are allocated and costs shared will make a big difference to them. The profit-center approach described earlier may be adequate to

get started. But, very soon, the group should be thinking about bringing all revenues in through the GPWW and compensating the physicians on the basis of relevant performance criteria. Other factors to take into account might be administrative duties, community services, and seniority. Finally, there is the matter of allocating any ancillary income that may be received. This probably should be pooled with the other revenues.

Physician Pensions

The primary decision here is whether to keep all existing pension plans that physicians bring with them separate from the group or to combine them into a single group-sponsored plan.

Centralized Management Services

Begin operation of the GPWW with as few practice management services centralized in the main office as are required by the Federal Trade Commission (FTC) to demonstrate integration and avoid antitrust problems. This will minimize the change and disruption to the individual practices and the overhead cost assumed by the central office. At the same time, have in place a firm schedule for expanding the range of services that will be integrated over the entire group.

Workforce Changes

As more and more practice management services become centralized, there are bound to be shifts in the composition and location of the support staff. Long-standing employees of some physicians may lose their jobs while others can be reassigned to the central office. New employees with new skills will be hired. This can create turmoil and upset. Make all employment decisions on sound business grounds. Keep open communications with all staff about the changes taking place.

CASE STUDIES: THREE GPWWS AND THE PROBLEMS THEY ENCOUNTERED[*]

Premier Medical Group (Denver, Colorado)

This primary care group has faced and surmounted several classic problems that can occur to a GPWW.

The participating physicians could not agree on the use of specialists. Some wanted to refer only to a limited number of selected specialists under contract to the group. They felt this arrangement gave them greater control in meeting the capitation rates under their managed care contracts. Other doctors preferred to continue using the specialists they had referred to for years.

There was disagreement over whether every doctor had to use the administrative services provided by the central office or could continue to handle administrative tasks within each practice. The effect was to reduce the savings possible by centralizing the services.

Some physicians in the group did not want to share inpatient coverage, preferring to work a fixed number of hours each day without any additional group responsibilities.

The continuous dissension and inefficiency made it hard for the group to win many managed care contracts. Ultimately, 30 physicians withdrew to form their own group.

In the words of the group's executive director, all these problems could be traced to the failure to find "a common vision among its doctors as to what it means to be a group." Every one of the disagreements (referrals, coverage, and centralized services) should have been resolved before the group began operating.

Premier faced one other daunting problem of a very different sort. The state attorney general saw the group's scattered practices sharing in managed care contracts and suspected that their network was nothing but a price-fixing scheme. After an investigation, he exonerated the group for the reasons that the doctors shared in any losses incurred by the group, gained efficiencies through shared administrative services, and marketed themselves as a unified group. Their one weak spot was in basing each physician's compensation solely on her personal productivity. Their risk sharing could be improved by distributing at least part of the group's revenues according to factors like patient satisfaction or utilization rates.

Cascade Physicians (Portland, Oregon)

This is another primary care group composed of over 30 physicians. It has experienced start-up pains similar to those faced by many GPWWs, though not as traumatic as those of the Premier group.

The 13 founding members took 10 months to organize themselves, but still had a hard time changing old practice habits. The early installation of a new computer system quickly led to centralized billing and collection. Both the physicians and their staff had trouble adjusting to the computer system and were reluctant to give up control of these important revenue-related functions.

As members of a more interdependent group, the Cascade doctors had to communicate with each other regularly. Not only was this a departure from their previous practices in isolation, but the phone system they were using was not up to the task.

The group discovered that the initial $10,000 capital contribution from each founding physician was not enough to cover the start-up and early operating costs. A $100,000 loan later had to be taken out to pay for the computer system.

Other problems emerged when new physicians were added to the group. Cascade learned the hard way the importance of orienting prospective new members to the philosophy and goals of the group. When this wasn't done, later conflicts

---

[*]*Source:* Adapted with permission from D. Mangan, The Rapidly Changing World of Clinics Without Walls, *Medical Economics 72*, no. 9, pp. 130–132, 134, 137–138, and 140, © 1995, Medical Economics Publishing Company.

arose—particularly over submission to utilization review and referrals restricted to panel specialists.

In one case, a two-physician practice left after 11 months over disagreement with changes that were expected of them. They preferred their previous geriatric, Medicare patient population to the more age-diverse patients they would have to see through the group. To accommodate the group's patients, the two doctors would also have had to relocate their practice. Finally, they were not comfortable shifting from their traditional fee-for-service reimbursement to the group's expanding capitation arrangements.

Was the move to a GPWW format worth all these headaches? The Cascade doctors report that their larger combined mass has "opened the door to business opportunities that would have passed us by had we all stayed in our individual small practices." They are seeing more patients and enjoying annual revenue growth of 5 to 10 percent. Their greater bargaining clout has enabled them to negotiate higher reimbursements from existing managed care contracts.

The long-range goal of Cascade Physicians is to become a major component of an IDS. It aims to do this by building arm's length strategic affiliations with a hospital or insurance company, rather than surrendering its independence to a physician-hospital organization (PHO).

New Mexico Medical Group (Albuquerque, New Mexico)

This GPWW enjoyed the good times early in its history. It used a $300,000 loan in 1986 to set up a variety of ancillary services. The revenues from these services (which reached $2.8 million a year), along with $250 a month contributions from each doctor, paid for the central administration, payroll for the 175-person workforce, and retirement of the debt.

Things began to change with the appearance of the Stark II regulations. The group had to sell its medical equipment business. It expects to lose even more of these revenues as it accepts more and more capitation and implements tighter utilization review.

To adapt to these changing conditions, the group is scrapping the old profit center revenue allocation system. Instead, all revenues are being pooled before administrative expenses are deducted. The amount remaining is distributed to the physicians on the basis of utilization, productivity, and equal shares.

The group also is centralizing more business functions and standardizing its personnel procedures. Its future plans include installing a more sophisticated information system and growing in size from 30 to 50 physicians. To fund this expansion program, the physicians are willing to sell as much as 49 percent of the shares in the organization to an investor.

In the words of the executive director, "We're making a transition from a loose group practice without walls to a tighter one."

EXPECTED COSTS TO PLAN AND ESTABLISH A GPWW

The costs to expect when forming a GPWW can vary widely. They depend primarily on the number of physicians participating, their familiarity and comfort with each other, the number of separate practices they represent, the number of different specialties they practice, their experience with and sympathy to managed care, and how long it takes them to reach consensus on the founding principles of the new organization.

For example, a group of 10 primary care doctors who have covered for each other and shared knowledge and experiences may be able to get a GPWW up and running in just six months with a total start-up expenditure of $20,000 to $30,000. In contrast, 50 or more physicians from several different practices and specialties with little previous joint working experience may need well over a year and nearly $150,000 to form a GPWW.[*]

---

*The members of Cascade Physicians in Portland, Oregon, contributed $10,000 each in return for equal ownership shares in the GPWW. The larger than usual amount funded a reserve used in connection with the group's capitation contracts.

Monthly contributions toward the GPWW's administrative overhead rarely exceed $1,000 per physician. In the Premier Medical Group, a GPWW in Denver, Colorado, each doctor makes a monthly payment of $300 or 3 percent of monthly gross revenues, whichever is greater.*

SOURCES OF FINANCING FOR A NEW GPWW

If the participating physicians are all closely affiliated with a particular hospital, there is a good chance that it will be willing to grubstake the new organization. Resist the temptation. A GPWW is normally the physicians' first move toward consolidation and integration. The hospital's interests are unlikely to be aligned with those of the physicians. Do your best to grow as large as possible while still a physician-dominated organization and before accepting significant nonphysician partners.**

The best financing alternative is contributions from the personal or practice funds of the participating physicians. This may be coupled with a line of credit from a local bank, which is likely to ask for personal guarantees from the physicians. The next best funding source would be a practice management services firm willing to provide up-front capital, generally in return for a ownership interest in the practice assets. If, however, the physicians were willing to part with those assets,

it would make more sense to think specifically about becoming part of a full-blown MSO.

Insurance companies and MCOs may also be willing to invest in the physician group. Like the hospital, they will want a share of control in return.

ANTITRUST ISSUES WITH LOOSER GROUP PRACTICE MODELS

As physicians move from independent practices competing with each other toward large groups or networks in which they are partners or employees, there is a murky, twilight zone in which they are both competitors and collaborators. GPWWs and IPAs are examples of this transitional state. There are significant legal risks for physicians while interacting in this way.

- By jointly negotiating on discounted fee-for-service contracts while continuing to function as independent, perhaps competing, practices, the physicians might be accused of conspiring to fix prices in violation of antitrust laws.***
- By making referrals to ancillary services jointly owned by the "group," the otherwise independent and nonintegrated physicians would appear to be violation of the Stark II prohibitions against self-referrals.****

A top FTC official states that a GPWW or any other physician combination will run into trouble if it "involves fixing fees without legitimate economic integration." What forms should that inte-

---

*This is not a place to save a few dollars. The New Mexico Medical group in Albuquerque, New Mexico, began with low initial physician contributions ($1,600 each) and minimal monthly payments ($200). They now need to add physicians to compete, but lack the capital to recruit them from out of state. A group member said recently, "If I were to do this again, I'd have the doctors put in more money up front and pay more each month."

**If a hospital helps to fund a GPWW, it could look as though the hospital is paying the doctors to refer patients to it. A not-for-profit might place its tax-exempt status in jeopardy. The federal government may look at the hospital's seed money as an indirect payment for referrals, in violation of the Fraud and Abuse Act.

***A physician group was held to be restraining trade in 1991. The FTC ordered the dissolution of the Southbank IPA, a group of 23 obstetricians and gynecologists in Jacksonville, Florida. The FTC said the group was actually an "anti-competitive conspiracy" to fix fees charged third party payers and to boycott insurers who did not accept its fee schedule.

****This problem is highlighted by the exception in Stark II for referrals to ancillary services owned by truly integrated group practices, whose terms are not satisfied by the typical GPWW.

gration take? The following group characteristics will not guarantee freedom from antitrust liability, but their absence will attract the FTC's attention:

- *Economic integration.* The doctors are employees of the group and earn salaries. The costs of running their practices are incurred by the organization, not the individual physicians. Most administrative functions are performed centrally by the organization—including payroll, billing, collecting, claims, accounting, personnel, and purchasing.
- *Shared economic risk.* The risks inherent in capitated contracts are spread among all the doctors in the group. This means that the cost of providing catastrophic care to one or more patients is borne by the entire group. The physicians also have joint exposure to any other unexpected liabilities, such as legal damage awards against the group.
- *Equity capital at risk.* Every member physician has invested personal funds in getting the group started and will lose those funds if the group fails.
- *Added efficiency.* As a result of consolidating their practices, the physicians are able to produce efficiencies beyond what they could accomplish separately. They are able to offer more services, higher quality care, greater accessibility, or lower costs to their patients.

TIPS FOR MAKING THE GPWW A SUCCESS

1. Be selective in allowing physicians to participate in the GPWW. Look for the right primary care-to-specialist mix and a positive attitude toward working constructively under managed care.
2. View the GPWW as no more than a transitional stage toward developing a much more tightly integrated physician system. Use it as a tool for organizing area physicians who have never collaborated in this way before.
3. From the outset, plan the incremental steps the physicians will take to integrate their

practices with each other. This means integration along several scales—clinical practice, quality assurance, utilization management, administrative services, cost allocation, and compensation.

4. Become adept at managing care and take in as many qualified physician members as market conditions will allow before exploring affiliations with other providers, particularly hospitals. The bigger and more experienced you are, the more leverage you will have entering into any strategic partnership.
5. Do not even consider creating a GPWW in anything but an immature managed care market. The lack of MCO presence will give your group some breathing room, in which you can get used to working with each other and changing some of your practice behaviors. You also can make some mistakes (e.g., miscalculation of acceptable capitation rates or purchase of an inadequate information system) without suffering fatal consequences. If managed care is already well established in your area, move immediately to a more advanced form of physician integration such as an MSO, a foundation, or a fully integrated multispecialty group practice.
6. Require substantial up-front capital contributions from participating physicians. Explain that they should expect to make even further investments in this, their organization. Impress upon them the need to tighten their belts, accept lower compensation growth, and avoid any unnecessary expense. During the first few years, until the group is on a sound financial footing, reinvest all net earnings in the business. When businesses fail, the most common reason is inadequate financing.
7. Be clear and specific about the group's strategic goals and values. Give prospective physician members a thorough indoctrination. Obtain their full agreement with everything that the group plans to do.
8. Move immediately to begin developing a group culture. Hold frequent meetings

among the physicians and the full support staff. Plan regular social gatherings of the entire group. Periodically publish a friendly and informative newsletter reporting on group events and progress. Conduct educational programs to help all group members perform their jobs better. Get used to using the pronoun "we."

## CHAPTER 13

Step Five: Growing into a Larger, Multispecialty Group Practice

INTRODUCTION

The large, multispecialty group practice represents the culmination in the evolution of integrated physician-owned organizations delivering a full spectrum of physician services. Once this point has been reached, if the physicians wish to develop further into an integrated delivery service (IDS), the next steps are to build connections with other kinds of providers, particularly hospitals. This can be accomplished by acquiring, being acquired by, or merging with other provider entities such as a hospital or hospital system. Of course, physicians who have come this far without giving up their independence are likely to prefer contract-based strategic affiliations that do not require yielding control. For more information about how to build an IDS, read Chapter 21, "Step Eleven: The Final Step–Evolving into a Regionwide Vertically Integrated Delivery System."

WHO SHOULD READ THIS CHAPTER

This is the chapter for physicians who are very serious about succeeding in a managed care system, who are willing to take risks in shaping their professional futures. It will be useful to physicians in several categories.

Physicians who have moved within the last couple years into their first group practice, probably single specialty, should be wondering what their next steps will be. This chapter explains where they should be headed ultimately.

Physicians who now practice in a physician-hospital organization (PHO), independent practice association (IPA), or group practice without walls (GPWW), who see those systems evolving further, who appreciate the need for tighter integration, will want to look closely at the group practice model described in this chapter.

This chapter is must reading for a physician at any stage of her strategic evolution who wants to stay in charge, and perhaps is seeking a leadership role for herself, but does not want to sell out to any nonphysician-controlled entity (physician-run management services organization [MSO], investor-owned physician practice management company [PPMC]).

Some physicians are only now contemplating their first proactive efforts to engage with managed care and want to lay out a complete step-by-step strategic path. In this chapter, they will learn about what may be the final stop on that path.

Those doctors who know already that they want to sell their practices to an amicable MSO or PHO and concentrate on practicing medicine need not spend much time here. Considering participation in a large, multispecialty group practice presumes a sense of ambition and entrepreneurship on the physician's part.

CHARACTERISTICS OF A LARGE, MULTISPECIALTY GROUP PRACTICE

Start with an image of the small, single specialty group practice described in Chapter 10, "Step Three: Forming or Joining a Small, Single Specialty Group Practice." Then, imagine adding, over time, the following features:

1. A large, multispecialty group practice includes physicians practicing in several different specialties. The physicians and their specialties are chosen to match the medical needs of the patient population the group is serving through the several managed care contracts it has negotiated. Whether functioning as gatekeepers under capitation or as referral sources under some fee-for-service (FFS) variant, primary care doctors usually predominate. They compose 40 percent to 60 percent of the total.

    This market-appropriate mix of physicians is not assembled overnight. It is built up over a period of time—years if the market allows it, months if there is competitive pressure and sufficient capital. The physicians may be added by direct hiring, by acquiring selected individual practices, and by merging with or absorbing larger specialty groups.

2. This group model employs considerably more physicians than the single specialty version. The actual number will depend on the volume of patients they have contracted to be responsible for and the group's willingness to subcontract with outside physicians for care in the narrower specialties. To cover the most common specialties and back them up with a commensurate panel of primary care doctors, it would be hard for a well-developed group serving even a modest population to number less than 50 physicians. Numerous multispecialty groups employ 100 to 200

physicians, and some of the very largest have panels of several hundred doctors. These are among the largest and best known multispecialty groups:

*   The Nalle Clinic, Charlotte, North Carolina
*   Lovelace Clinic, Albuquerque, New Mexico
*   Scott & White Clinic, Temple, Texas
*   Marshfield Clinic, Marshfield, Wisconsin
*   Park Nicollet Clinic, Minneapolis, Minnesota
*   Summit Medical Group, Summit, New Jersey
*   Mayo Clinic, Rochester, Minnesota
*   Fargo Clinic, Fargo, North Dakota
*   Carle Clinic, Urbana, Illinois
*   Lahey Hitchcock Clinic, Worcester, Massachusetts
*   Geisinger Clinic, Danville, Pennsylvania
*   Great Falls Clinic, Great Falls, Montana
*   West Florida Medical Center Clinic, Pensacola, Florida
*   Cleveland Clinic, Cleveland, Ohio

3. Decision-making authority is concentrated in the board of directors and a staff of professional managers and technicians. No administrative tasks are left in the hands of physicians and, to the extent required to manage care effectively, there is some intervention in clinical decision making. The board of directors is small and maneuverable.

4. There are opportunities for qualified physicians to assume leadership and even managerial roles. They must demonstrate competence for the positions and a willingness to devote the time necessary to do the work well. All physicians are compensated for the administrative tasks they perform, whether large or small.

5. Individual physician compensation is set by the group's management, usually according to a predetermined formula applied uniformly to all group physicians. The formula is designed to reward behaviors that benefit the group as a whole—low utilization, high quality, high patient satis-

faction, productivity, perhaps seniority. As much as possible, the compensation criteria are measurable, objective, and preferably quantitative. Physicians no longer think in terms of the revenues that they, personally, are bringing into the group or the income they might be able to earn if they still were in private practice.

6. Financial management and controls, particularly budgets, are developed centrally for the entire group, including separate practice sites and physicians. Individual doctors may have input to the financial planning process but, once budgets are set, they are fully subject to them.

7. All operating systems are, to the fullest extent possible, consolidated and run centrally. These include billing, collections, general accounting and reporting, payroll, benefits, maintenance, facility management, data processing, medical records management, utilization management, quality assurance, and general information gathering. The systems use common stand-ards, formats, and procedures that are applied uniformly to all physicians and staff.

8. All human resource management decisions (hiring, compensation, performance management, firing) are made centrally according to uniform standards and procedures.

9. Each physician is an employee of the group. Individual physicians are not personally responsible for the expenses of the group or their practice within the group. Each physician has an opportunity, at some point, to acquire ownership shares in the group. Every physician with ownership shares may seek a position on the board of directors.

10. All revenues from ancillary services (laboratory tests, imaging centers, emergency clinics, etc.) are pooled with other group revenues and applied to the expenses of the entire group.

11. All contracts with third party payers (managed care organizations [MCOs], insurance companies, employers) are negotiated by the group, in the name of the group. Individual physicians do not enter into payer contracts on their own. Physicians see only patients who come to them through the group and its contracts. They do not have any significant number of private patients.

12. The board and management of the group prepare all strategic plans and objectives. They approve the capital budgets, including any significant expenditures on equipment and facilities.

13. The group's services are marketed entirely under the group's name. Considerable marketing effort and expense goes toward creating a unified and appealing group identity in the eyes of its stakeholders.

14. The group is organized legally as a professional corporation. At some time, if it sees an advantage in selling ownership shares to nonphysicians in order to raise capital, the group will convert to traditional for-profit corporate status.

15. The group has developed and implemented an aggressive utilization management program in which all physicians participate. It already has accumulated several years of experience in reducing the costs of health care delivery. It has documented its capability and record in this area and is prepared to demonstrate them to payers.

16. The group has developed and implemented an aggressive quality assurance program that covers all its physicians. Documented results for the last several years show that quality of care has been improved in several important areas and has been at least maintained in all others. The group is able to demonstrate to others the quality assurance machinery it has in place and the positive results it has produced.

17. The group is in the process of implementing clinical protocols or guidelines to encourage its physicians to practice uniformly high quality, cost-effective medicine. For the diagnoses it encounters most often, the group may use its clinical outcomes research results to develop its own

protocols. Otherwise, it carefully selects from among the protocols designed by third parties like specialty boards and the National Institutes of Health.

18. The group has begun gathering the clinical data that will permit it to accurately assess the outcomes of various treatment decisions made by its physicians. It will compare these data with the resources utilized in the treatments that provide the greatest value—quality balanced against cost. The outcomes data alone may also be useful in evaluating the competence of individual physicians and the risk profile of certain patient populations.

19. The group systematically measures the levels of patient satisfaction with all aspects of their encounters with the group (scheduling, phone contacts, interpersonal dealings, quality of care, physical layout, etc.). It responds promptly to legitimate patient grievances and strives constantly to raise patient satisfaction.

20. Great progress has been made in installing sophisticated management information systems for gathering data and reporting on the group's financial and clinical operations. The system's outputs are used to great advantages to measure, understand, and demonstrate the value of everything the group does. Clinical outcomes are compared with utilization data and patient satisfaction levels. Profitability of specific managed care contracts or patient populations is calculated. The risk factors inherent in particular patient populations are determined. The clinical capability of member physicians is appraised and used as the basis for credentialing decisions. The suitability and value of outside referral targets (hospitals and subspecialists) is regularly examined. The information systems permit the group to monitor and fine- tune every nuance of the organization and demonstrate to contract and strategic partners how well managed it is.

CASE STUDY: MARSHFIELD CLINIC (MARSHFIELD, WISCONSIN)[*]

The most successful multispecialty group practices quickly become enmeshed in integrated provider systems—often of their own making. The best examples of still independent multispecialty groups are Scott & White (Temple, Texas), Lovelace Clinic (Albuquerque, New Mexico), Mayo Clinic (Rochester, Minnesota), Carle Clinic (Urbana, Illinois), and the Marshfield Clinic (Marshfield, Wisconsin).

The Marshfield Clinic ("Clinic") could be a model of the kind of group to which physicians might aspire. It is one of the largest medical groups in the country. Over 530 physicians practice in a central diagnostic treatment center and 39 regional centers and satellite clinics. Over one-quarter are primary care doctors. They are supported by nearly 3,700 ancillary personnel. Together, they serve some 3,000 patients a day and over one million each year. This produces annual operating revenues of nearly $300 million.

About one-third of the Clinic's patients comes from a clinic-owned health maintenance organization (HMO), the Security Health Plan, with approximately 80,000 subscribers. Another one-fourth has commercial insurance and about 20 percent are Medicare recipients. The remaining patients are covered by Medicaid or fee-for-service.

The Clinic maintains and funds its own research division, the Marshfield Medical Research Foundation. It also sponsors a variety of outreach programs that collaborate with over 1,200 hospitals, clinics, and other institutions throughout the upper Midwest. Among the services they provide are off-site physician consultation, 24-hour electrocardiogram (EKG) interpretation via computer, mobile echocardiography, reference laboratory, regional blood banking, radiology, electroencepha-

---

*Source: Adapted with permission from the Center for Research in Ambulatory Health Care Administration, 104 Inverness Terrace East, Englewood, Colorado 80112-5306; 303-799-1111. Copyright 1994.

lograms (EEGs), orthotics/prosthetics, radiation physics, pulmonary function, and biomedical electronics.

Once a new physician has completed two successive one-year contracts, he is invited to become a shareholder in the Clinic. As such, he will have one vote like every other physician and will himself be eligible to run for the board of directors. The board, in turn, annually elects all the Clinic's executive officers, including the nine members of the executive committee. The board meets monthly to review the actions of the executive committee, make major decisions, and set policy.

Until 1980, all Marshfield Clinic physicians were paid identical salaries, regardless of their specialties. Even now, their salaries fall within a narrower range than prevails in the open market. Most fall between $150,000 and $250,000. Primary care physicians receive more than they would in private practice, while specialists receive somewhat less. One of the products of this frugality is that the Clinic has been able to accumulate significant financial reserves. It does not follow the tradition of paying out all revenues left over after expenses are paid in physician compensation.

This compensation policy has not discouraged a steady stream of physicians and small group practices from seeking Clinic affiliation. The Clinic has proved adept at integrating primary care physicians from solo practice backgrounds, employing them after purchasing their practice assets.

STEP-BY-STEP PLAN FOR EVOLVING FROM A SMALLER SINGLE SPECIALTY GROUP PRACTICE TO A LARGER, INCREASINGLY INTEGRATED MULTISPECIALTY GROUP PRACTICE

It is conceivable that a large multispecialty group practice could be built at once, by consolidating physicians from many small practices. That strategy would take a great deal of capital financing and present serious challenges in melding the disparate career goals and practice styles of so many physicians. It is more likely that one or two single specialty groups with physicians with ambition and foresight will take deliberate steps to build themselves into the larger, more integrated model. These are some of those important steps.

1. *Form a physician task force to plan and lead the group building process.* This task force is the catalyst for the several-year process that will transform your small single specialty group practice into a larger, more integrated multispecialty group practice. It will be composed of a few or all of the members of the current group practice, perhaps joined by ambitious doctors from one or two other group practices. If more than one group is involved, it would be nice if one of them was composed of subspecialists and the other was all primary care physicians.

   At this stage, the task force members need two qualities before all others: vision and curiosity. This means that they understand the need for their practice settings to become something different and have open minds to new organizational forms, practice methods, and operating procedures. Some of them are likely to be the physician leaders of the group that emerges.

   It is helpful, but not essential, that they represent a mix of specialties. They need to be able to work effectively with a wide variety of people—physicians of all specialties, hospital administrators, MBAs from MCOs, insurance company executives, attorneys, and bank loan officers. They must have persistence and endurance.

2. *Do a rudimentary market assessment.* At this point, it probably is adequate and more resource efficient to do this yourselves. Later, certainly within a couple years, you should hire a professional market analyst to conduct a thorough review

and description of the market area in which you expect to compete.

For now, do the best you can on the following points:

- Define a geographic market area that makes common sense to you. This should be the region from which the larger group you are assembling will attract most of its patients. If you are in a large city, the area may be a few defined neighborhoods, an area bounded by certain streets, or just "the east side of town." If you practice in a smaller city, your market could be the entire municipality. If you are located in a more rural area, the market area may encompass one or more counties. Don't worry about absolute accuracy; you can adjust the boundaries later.

  Inventory the health care providers in that area. This includes all the traditional players in the health care delivery system—physicians (noted by specialty), hospitals (noted by classification), long-term care facilities, home health care organizations, other ancillary care entities, laboratories, clinics, pharmacies, and the like. If you are truly visionary, you might want to include alternative medicine sources.[*]

- Evaluate these providers for their strengths and weaknesses, financial assets, apparent strategic intentions, affiliations with other providers, forms of reimbursement, and geographic location. This information is more subjective and proprietary. Check the same sources as above. Start to clip media articles on any of these organizations. Gather anecdotal information from col-

leagues, vendors, and any other relevant sources.

- Identify and describe the payers in the area. These will primarily be MCOs, insurance companies, employers, Medicare, and Medicaid. To the best of your ability, determine their overall market shares, as well as their percentage of your current revenues.

- Make a rough approximation of the extent to which different reimbursement schemes are used in the market (FFS, discounted FFS, capitation, subcapitation, global capitation, specialty capitation, case rates).

- Evaluate the patient population in the market area. These are the people who will be treated by the organization you are forming. Look for their demographics, place of residence, place of employment, incidence of illness, and sources or means of payment for health care.

Read Chapter 14, "Assessing the Market for Managed Care and Integration Opportunities" for a more detailed discussion.

3. *Sketch out a tentative strategic growth plan.* The task force members should go over the market data they have collected, especially noting trends and strategic plans. Conduct a healthy discussion and debate on what these mean for the future of health care delivery in the area and what sort of new systems seem to be evolving. Look for opportunities that an ambitious physician group could seize and exploit. The task force's goal is to begin imagining how they fit into the local delivery system of the future and the ideal organizational vehicle to take them there.

The plan starts with a vision of the kind of organization the task force physicians want to be part of five years from now, presumably something like a large, integrated multispecialty group practice. If their deliberations lead to a different kind of organization, such as an MSO or IPA,

---

[*]Get this information from the government agencies that regulate them, trade and professional associations, (state and county medical societies, hospital associations, chambers of commerce), and provider directories that may be published.

they should turn to those chapters of this book.

In the plan, describe as fully as possible the sort of organization you will create, who will own and control it, where it will be located, and what services it will offer. Then, specify the following characteristics of the organization:

- The geographic and patient catchment area. The geographic area from which the group will draw its patients and, within that area, the types of people the group aims to serve (e.g., Medicare, employees of certain companies, etc.).
- The numbers of patients the group will serve. This is a figure projected for each of the next five years, reflecting the growth of the group and its service capabilities. It also can be broken down by type of patient or payment source. These numbers will be quite speculative, but nonetheless are valuable as growth goals and motivators for the group.
- The annual growth in group revenues, from what sources and on what reimbursement terms. The sources are the typical payers—MCOs, insurance companies, direct contract employers, and government financing agencies. The group might also think about subcontracting with still larger IDSs. The reimbursement terms are the usual FFS and capitation variations, along with any innovative approaches like "percentage of premium." The proportion of revenues derived from risk-sharing arrangements should increase every year.
- The number and size of managed care contracts and direct contracts with employers. Also, try to indicate with whom the contracts will be negotiated. In the case of areas with little or no managed care, make your best guess of when a MCO might decide to move in.
- Numbers, geographic location, and specialty mix of physicians needed to serv-

ice the numbers and kinds of patients you have projected in the areas you propose to cover. This is probably the most crucial strategic objective, as it defines the overall size of your organization and is a variable over which the group has the most control.

Keep in mind that the group's initial managed care contracts do not have to cover the full range of physician services. Contract for only what the group can currently provide. Gradually move toward broader, more encompassing contracts under which the group subcontracts with outside specialists. Depending on the optimal economic model, the group may eventually provide through it own physicians all specialty services under a global contract.

The next step in putting together this strategic growth plan is to look over the inventory of area physicians and determine which ones would fit into the group's plans to serve the proposed patient population. The preliminary selection criteria are medical specialty, geographic location, and expressed interest in managed care.

The preferred method of incorporating the selected physicians into the organization is merger with no exchange of cash. This assumption is critical to the next planning step—roughly calculating the capital that will be needed to cover the planning and start-up costs, plus overhead personnel and services for the first year or so. A merger does not require the expenditure of cash and normally brings in the entire practice, including its existing accounts receivable.

When you have done all this, you will have a detailed enough plan to carry you through the initial process of planning the new organization and recruiting its members.

4. *Approach and negotiate with physicians and physician groups as prospective merger candidates.* Put together a written

description of your vision for the group practice you are trying to build. This includes most of the elements of the strategic growth plan just outlined. Frame it in terms that will be most appealing to the physicians who will see it and entice them to want to learn more about your ambitions.

Hold informal meetings first, with the doctors to whom you feel closest and believe to be most sympathetic to your ideas. Gauge the response you receive from them and make some minor adjustments to your plans. Enlist as many as possible in continuing discussions. Next, hold more formal meetings with other physicians you know less well. Attendance at all these meetings is by invitation only. Remember, these are doctors selected within your target area as most suitable for the specialty mix you are trying to assemble.

The group founders, probably the task force, plus any consultants or attorneys you may already have drawn into the process, will attend these meetings to explain your intentions and answer the many questions that will come up. Be prepared to conduct multiple meetings with the same participants if necessary to win their confidence.

When physicians or groups become comfortable with the precepts of the proposed new organization and show interest in being included, have them fill out application forms seeking information on basic credentialing criteria and practice backgrounds.

5. *Obtain a letter of intent and an initial membership fee from most interested and qualified physicians.* Review the application forms submitted by interested physicians. Sort them into three categories.
   (a) those you would like to enroll in the group immediately
   (b) those who look like good merger candidates when the group is further along in its development

   (c) those who do not meet the group's requirements under any circumstances

   From the physicians in the first group, request a letter of intent, which is an informal, nonbinding, yet detailed, statement of each physician's commitment to affiliation with the group you are proposing. The letter will explain the type of organization being planned, the merger of the physician's practice into it, and her subsequent role in its ongoing operations. It will include the physician's agreement to provide more comprehensive information about herself and her practice, to permit the group to assess thoroughly her suitability and to begin incorporating her practice into the group.

   This is about the time that the group will need an infusion of money to keep the planning process going and cover the expenses of consultants and clerical help. All involved physicians—whether founders or recent enrollees—should be expected to pay an initial membership fee (or initiation fee, enrollment fee, capital contribution, or whatever term makes sense). Normally, the amount will be between $500 and $2,000, with an average of $1,000.

   If the organization finally takes shape and these physicians still are members, this money will be considered part of their investment in the organization. If they drop out for any reason before the new organization is created, the money should be returned if at all possible. If the proposed entity never sees the light of day, these will be spent funds for everyone concerned.

6. *At some point, make a decision about physical facilities and geographic locations.* There are definite clinical and economic advantages to primary care physicians (PCPs) and specialists practicing together in one cliniclike building. If this is the group's preferred practice arrangement, as it expands rapidly by adding physicians, it almost certainly will become necessary to

move into new, larger quarters. Such a move may be made more than once while the group is growing. Anticipate the capital costs of the moves.

At the same time, there is a marketing/accessibility advantage in having some of the physicians, particularly the PCPs, at smaller satellite facilities situated more strategically throughout the community being served. It would be nice if physicians newly added to the group were already located in good proximity to the group's patients. But, not all of them will be and their practice sites may have to be moved.

Eventually every participating doctor may have to relocate—either to a central clinic or to a carefully planned primary care access site. During its early history, the group's doctors may practice out of a single facility, for the sake of convenience and efficiency. Then, as the group becomes truly multispecialty and accumulates greater capital resources, and as competition in the local market increases, new satellite practices can be established out in the community.

7. *As the number of physicians in the group grows, refine the governance structure.* It may be possible to steer a small, single specialty group practice through occasional, informal meetings of all its physicians. This clearly will not work for a group of over 30 physicians, from several different specialties. As new physicians come into the group, unfamiliar with its founders, one of their leading concerns will be protection against arbitrary decisions that damage their interests. Install a more formal and sophisticated governance structure—consisting primarily of your board of directors and associated committees.

Pay attention to the representation of various specialties on the board. The current rule of thumb is to maintain a PCP/specialist ratio among the group's physicians in the range of 50/50. It should be possible to carry that same proportion over to the board of directors. However, while the group is in its early growth stages, it is unlikely to have this ideal mix of specialties. For instance, picture a group of six cardiologists who decide to grow into a large, multispecialty group practice. Their first mergers are with a three-physician neurology practice and a group of seven ophthalmologists. At this point, the board of directors is bound to be all specialists. The next merger candidate may be a loose collection of 22 doctors in primary care fields. Suddenly, they constitute a majority that could dominate the board.

The best approach is to move toward assembling a physician group that is approximately 50 percent primary care (the actual percentage depending on the demographics of the patient population being served). Once there is a significant number of PCPs on board, even though they may not be close to a majority, many groups grant them an influential, if not dominant, position on the board.

Other important features of a responsible group practice governing structure are

- a formal procedure for electing board members
- regular meetings with predetermined agendas
- recorded votes on all decisions
- minutes taken, transcribed, and approved

As governance responsibilities grow, spin off some standard physician board committees, such as executive, contracting, membership/credentialing, compensation, operations, and finance.

For more information on governance issues, read Chapter 22, "Creating an Effective Governance Structure for an Affiliated or Integrated Physician Group."

8. *As the number of physicians in the group grows, restate the requirements and rights regarding ownership and capital contribu-*

tions. Before the group gets very large, some basic questions about ownership must be answered, questions that intersect with the governance issues just discussed. Will every member physician be an owner or entitled to ownership? On what terms? With what voting rights?

At the beginning, it may be essential that every physician joining the group become an owner—both for the commitment this elicits and for the capital contributions that are part of ownership. Once the group is better established, it probably will want to redefine its ownership policy.

A mature group practice might provide that physicians newly admitted to the group may not become member-owners at all for the first two years. At that time, they may automatically have the option to purchase an ownership interest or the group may make a judgment on whether they are qualified to become owners. In the latter case, the criteria used could include the physician's time spent on group work, particularly the interest she has shown in leadership, management responsibilities, and committee work. Some physicians might also be employed with the understanding that they are not interested in ownership and will never be more than perfectly contented employees.

This raises some additional questions. May some physicians purchase larger ownership shares than others? What is the connection between a physician's ownership interests and the voting power he has on group issues such as electing board members? Does a physician with a larger ownership interest have more votes? At what price do physicians purchase their ownership shares? If the group requires further capital investment from its owner-members, how will they be assessed?

The best policy is usually to restrict all physicians to equal size ownership interests. This minimizes possible feelings of inferiority and superiority, coupled with an insistence by larger owners that they have a larger say in group decisions. If a physician has actually made a larger capital contribution to the group that might seem to warrant more ownership shares, there are three things that could be done. The physician could effectively donate the excess to the group (without being table to take a tax deduction) and accept a one member–one vote policy in the interests of group homogeneity and harmony. Excess capital contributions could be exchanged for a separate class of nonvoting ownership shares in the organization. The organization could issue long-term modest-interest notes to the donors of large capital sums.

Likewise, the best policy on voting rights is one person–one vote, regardless of the amount of capital contribution. Specialists have traditionally done better, financially, in their practices. As a result, they are able to invest more money in the new organization than PCPs. If voting rights are proportional to capital invested, specialists will always control the organization. In any event, those physicians less able to contribute can come to resent their wealthier colleagues who bought more influence in the group. This is not the way to start off a challenging new venture like this one.

The price of ownership shares in the business will depend on factors like the number of physicians participating and the total amount of capital required to get it operational. (This capital investment is something well beyond the $1,000 the first doctors might have chipped in to get the planning process started. For more information on amounts and sources of start-up capital for physician organizations, read Chapter 27, "Financing Strategies To Support Your Integration Plans.") A formula must also be devised for determining the appreciation in value of ownership shares as the group grows and prospers. This is to permit new physicians to buy into the group and retiring physicians to sell out. An attorney knowledgeable in corporate law will be helpful in sorting out questions of numbers, classes, and prices of ownership in the group organization.

One of the most challenging issues facing a group of physicians trying to go it alone in a rapidly changing, competitive market is finding the capital necessary to get a substantial new business organization started and then to keep it growing. If these funds, often in the hundreds of thousands and even millions of dollars, do not come from the physicians, they must be sought from third parties like banks, well-heeled hospitals, MCOs, venture capitalists, or entrepreneurs. They will want something in return—normally a share of the ownership, and the control, of the organization. Then, the physicians will have lost the thing they were trying hardest to protect—their autonomy.

It must be made clear to all physicians joining the group that significant capital contributions will be expected of them. An initial investment will be required when they first join and additional investments may be called for in the future. Eventually, the organization will grow to such a size that all its capital needs can be met through retained earnings, loans in the organization's name, and stock sales in subsidiary entities or in such small amounts that physician control of the business is not threatened.

Another sensitive issue is the method of electing members of the board of directors. Start with the premise that each physician will have just one vote. In order to ensure adequate board representation, it may be desirable to reserve certain board seats for certain specialties, such as PCPs. Even if an important subgroup, like PCPs, is in a minority on the board, it can be assured a minimal level of influence through voting devices like supermajorities and co-majorities. Remember to maintain the appropri-

ate specialty ratios on board committees as well.

Until the group becomes quite enormous (hundreds of physician members), it should be possible to maintain a high degree of collegiality and consultation, if not actual participation, of all members in all key decisions.

9. *As the number of physicians in the group grows, develop a modern, coherent, and generally accepted physician compensation system.* Among many fractious issues, the one of physician compensation may be the most divisive. It is important to move newly joined physicians away from a focus on what they were earning (or could be earning) in private practice or what revenues they are generating (or think they are generating) for the group. This is to avoid debates over whether the specialists are subsidizing the PCPs. The primary reason for physicians to leave small, private practices for larger, better managed group practices should be the belief that, in the medium to long run, they will be better off financially.

Very quickly, if not immediately after forming the new group organization, all revenues received through the group should be pooled for application to group operating expenses. Physicians should be paid salaries tied to group-oriented performance factors.

As a practical matter, PCP income will probably rise more rapidly than that of the specialists. Do everything possible to make sure that no one suffers an income decline.

To read more about alternatives in physician compensation, see Chapter 25, "The Kinds of Physician Reimbursement You Can Expect under Managed Care."

10. *As the group grows, seek greater risk-sharing in relationships with all payers.* In your strategic growth plan, set annual targets for increasing the group's number of managed care contracts or, to use a better

measure, the share of the group's revenues coming from managed care contracts. Even if the contracts call for discounted FFS reimbursement and leave most of the utilization management authority in the MCO's hands, you will gain experience operating under a managed care regimen. You will learn how discomforting it is to have a third party intervene in your clinical decision making. A good MCO partner will also work with your group to help it develop or acquire its own care management capabilities.

Set strategic goals, probably a little bit further in the future, for entering into more managed care contracts that reimburse on a capitation basis or for increasing the percentage of group revenues from capitated sources. To prepare for the rigors of capitation, begin installing the care management systems you will need (e.g., utilization management, quality assurance, patient satisfaction, clinical outcomes measurement, treatment guidelines, strict physician credentialing, etc.) before capitation fees have become a major source of group revenues. In other words, practice the art of managing care when the group's fate is not riding on it.

As the group's ability or willingness to provide a wider ranger of medical services expands (by adding physicians in new specialties to the group or subcontracting with outside specialists), negotiate with your MCO contract partners to have them included under the capitation rate. Do not hesitate to do this even in the middle of a contract term. Many MCOs will welcome the inclusion of additional services in the contract and be more than willing to renegotiate it. Of course, the capitation rate will be adjusted upward to take into account the group's expanded service responsibilities.

A golden rule of delivering health care under risk-sharing arrangements is to seek and assume as much risk as you can han-

dle. "Risk" in this context is measured by the variety of medical services the group is committed to provide, in uncertain amounts, to a designated patient population. The larger the share of those patients' total health care needs the group can take responsibility for

- the greater the control it has over the health care delivery process and over its own destiny
- the greater the opportunity for maximizing profits by managing the risk well

Whether or not the group is being reimbursed on a capitated basis, negotiate with managed care contract partners to take over whatever utilization management and quality assurance tasks they may previously have carried out themselves. In fact, aim to take over as many of the traditional MCO functions as they are willing to let you have and you are capable of handling. Every increase in the group's responsibilities and risks assumed should be matched by an increase in its reimbursement rates.

The goal is to take over as much of the MCO's work as possible, leaving it doing little more than marketing, enrollment, and collecting premiums. The group then will be perfectly positioned to assume those remaining functions, dispense with the MCO, become an MCO itself, and deal directly with the employers.

11. *Begin collecting more and more comprehensive data on*
    - quality of care delivered by the group
    - utilization of all kinds of group resources
    - cost of care delivered by the group
    - satisfaction of patients seen by the group
    - clinical outcomes of the treatments provided by the group

    These data will be used by the group for at least two purposes—to manage the value of the medical care it is providing in order to maximize the profits it earns under capitation and to demonstrate the results of its management efforts to MCOs, employers, and other payers.

Initially, use whatever data gathering systems and methods are currently available within the group. They may be rudimentary and so may be the data they report. They are better than no data at all.

Steadily, upgrade the sophistication of the group's equipment and systems for collecting these kinds of information. This will mean purchasing new computer hardware and software, as well as proprietary data gathering, recording, and reporting systems. It also will be necessary to hire specially trained people to operate the equipment and systems.

You can expect that acquiring this capability will consume a major portion, probably over half, of the group's capital expenditures during the first two to three years.

12. *Develop and implement a formal mechanism for managing the utilization of all resources within and by the group.* Utilization management is the key to success in managed care. Even if you resent it, you will need it to operate within increasingly tighter capitation rates and your MCO partners will be looking for it. Make no mistake, "utilization management" means finding safe ways to reduce the utilization and the cost of all the resources that go into your delivery of health care.

Cost reduction is carried out through the kinds of budget controls employed throughout American industry.

- Budget planning and enforcement requires all employees to be always conscious of the costs they are incurring by their actions and decisions.
- Centralized, negotiated purchasing policies ensure that the group pays the minimum for the goods and services it acquires.
- Centralized, professional human resource management maximizes em-

ployee productivity and minimizes wage, salary, and benefits costs.

Resource utilization by physicians in the course of providing care is the primary focus of this effort. This is with good reason, as it frequently is claimed that decisions by physicians influence the spending of as much as 80 percent of the health care dollar.

There is a great deal of literature on the design and operation of effective utilization management. In addition, it would be a good idea to seek the advice of your largest or most cooperative MCO partner. It will appreciate your interest and ambition. It should have some specific suggestions and be able to provide valuable technical assistance.

The strategies you adopt for controlling utilization are various and must be tailored to the sensitivities of the group's physicians and the demands of payers. Here are some examples.

- *Mere publication of key utilization rates can have a moderating influence on outlier physicians.* This can be as simple as posting a list of key utilization rates (e.g., lab tests for a common diagnosis) for all physicians, so that each one can compare himself to his colleagues without knowing specific names.
- *More rigorous physician profiles.* These are more comprehensive data pictures of each physician's practice style.
- *Traditional utilization review, as practiced by MCOs but now carried out by the group.* The review may be before (prior), during (concurrent), or after (retrospective) the treatment decision in question, such as a hospital admission or a surgical procedure.
- *Financial incentives designed to encourage desired behavior*—not just lower utilization, but the same or improved quality and patient satisfaction. These need to be fine-tuned; they

are not blunt instruments and can produce unexpected, undesirable results.
An incentive plan might also raise
some issues under the "fraud and
abuse" and Stark laws.

• *Direct, mandatory consultation with
outlier physicians.* This will include an
expression of the group's concern discussion of correction strategies and
negotiation of improvement goals. The
consultation typically is carried out by
members of a utilization committee.

• *Continuing medical education (CME)
opportunities (voluntary and mandatory) in new practice techniques and
styles that are more cost-effective.* The
group gathers and disseminates information about appropriate CME workshops and pays the tuition for
physicians who voluntarily attend. The
utilization committee may also require
a physician to attend a designated
workshop as part of her remedial work.

• *Disciplinary action against physicians
who do not or cannot correct utilization
problems.* There are not many options
at this stage. The physician may be
given verbal or written warnings.
Sometimes, simply telling someone
that he is being "disciplined" for poor
performance is enough to get his attention. The group might also assess a
monetary penalty against incorrigible
doctors. Discipline is applied only as a
last resort, after the above less severe
corrective measures have been tried.

• *Deselection of the physician.* This ster-
ile euphemism for "firing" has upset
many physicians when used by their
MCOs against them. Normally, in those
cases, the MCO has failed to give a reason for the dismissal. When carried out
responsibly, it is a discrete means for
removing from the group a member
who is behaving in a way contrary to
the common interests of all the other
members. The deselected physician is

given ample opportunity to adjust and
is told the reason for his departure. You
may be surprised how your feelings on
deselection change when your income
is directly impacted by the costs of
excessive utilization by another physician.

If the marketplace allows you the time,
do not frustrate and antagonize the physicians in your group by introducing the full
range of utilization management mechanisms at once. Start loose and informal,
then get tighter and more systematic.

13. *Develop and implement a formal process
for monitoring, ensuring, and improving
the quality of care provided by individual
physicians.* This is the necessary counter-
balance to the aggressive utilization management described above. Working together, these processes help the group to
deliver the highest "value" care.

The quality assurance (QA) process
depends on some traditional quality control measures like tissue, medical records,
and peer review committees. While these
try to catch distinct problems after they
have occurred, QA goes several steps further. Through the measurement of clinical
outcomes, QA aims to rate care quality on
a full spectrum from good to bad. By
developing and applying clinical pathways
or protocols, QA attempts to define, prospectively, a model of high quality care.

This is not an optional function of the
group. Nearly all payers—MCOs and
employers—will insist that providers
have a proven QA program or will themselves conduct quality review of their providers. Here, too, it makes sense to consult
with an MCO partner to learn what systems work best for them.

14. *Develop and implement a capability to
measure the clinical outcomes of individual physician treatment decisions.* The
group's ability to measure clinical outcomes serves several purposes.

- The results can be shown to prospective contract partners (MCOs and employers) as powerful evidence of the quality of care delivered by the group. Eventually, most payers will want their larger providers to have this capability. Outcomes results also may be used one day to prepare "report cards" on your group, which are useful in attracting patients.
- Clinical outcomes can be used for assessing the quality of care of individual physicians. In this way, they act as part of the group's QA program. They become a sound basis for corrective action with mispracticing physicians.
- When outcomes results are combined with detailed utilization and cost data, it becomes possible to show which treatment decisions produce the greatest patient value. These can be codified as clinical protocols or guidelines.

This is a science that has just begun to develop in the last decade. It is not yet a simple matter to evaluate clinical outcomes with accuracy. For one thing, the results must be adjusted for the risk posed by the patient. This is an initiative being pursued primarily by the largest well-financed teaching hospitals, provider groups, and research organizations.

Measuring clinical outcomes should be a low-priority task for a developing, modest-size multispecialty group practice. Just keep it in mind as a goal for some time in the future.

15. *Begin to develop or acquire and implement clinical treatment protocols, guidelines, or pathways.* There are two steps to the effective use of clinical protocols: first, finding relevant and reliable guidelines and second, encouraging or enforcing their use by physicians.

Within your group, try to develop some guidelines for the conditions seen most often. It may take some time and perseverance to come up with treatment models you are willing to commend to other physicians. In the process, however, you will learn what the characteristics of accurate, trustworthy guidelines are. This knowledge will help in your acquisition of guidelines from outside sources. Furthermore, physicians exposed to the process of developing clinical protocols will have more confidence in them and will be more inclined to use them.

Clinical protocols or pathways are being developed in a variety of places for general application by physicians and other providers. Some of the more common sources are the National Institutes of Health, medical specialty boards, and insurance companies. The American Medical Association (AMA) also has launched a Clinical Practice Guideline Recognition Program, which will identify and approve those clinical practice guidelines that are developed and evaluated in accordance with scientifically based criteria.

The group that employs protocols or guidelines receives several benefits. The care that it provides is more uniform, generally higher quality, and generally lower cost.

Somewhat related to a program of clinical guidelines is the development and implementation of a drug formulary. It offers similar benefits.

It is not always easy to get physicians to accept either clinical guidelines or drug formularies. They are likely to feel that their clinical authority is being usurped and replaced with standardized medicine. Certain measures will smoothe the introduction of these new initiatives.

- To the extent that the physicians can be involved in the design of the guidelines or formulary, they will better understand their usefulness.
- If the guidelines are properly risk adjusted, physicians will be less likely to resist them on the grounds that their

patients presented unique conditions that required unique treatment.

- Enforcement of the guidelines or formulary should allow the physician the opportunity to explain the circumstances that warranted a deviation from the recommended norm.

Even with these preparations, it probably will be necessary to put in place a procedure for enforcing use of the guidelines and formulary. It might look something like this:

- Begin with a thorough explanation and indoctrination. Describe the origins of the guidelines, how they were prepared, how they should be applied, the expected benefits to be gained from using them, and the experience with guidelines of other similar group practices.
- Start off slowly. Make the guidelines or formulary available and ask the physicians to try steadily to increase their use of them. Continue this for six months to a year.
- Then, begin tracking the compliance of individual physicians with the guidelines or formulary. Provide physicians with comparative data on their performance. Take no action at this time. Give the physicians another six months or so to begin making practice adjustments on the basis of the data.
- Finally, begin following up on those physicians who seem to stray unnecessarily from the guidelines too often. Seek explanations and negotiate corrective measures. Initiate disciplinary action against those doctors who persist in unwarranted deviations from the guidelines.

16. *Develop and implement a system for measuring patient satisfaction, responding to patient grievances, and correcting physician or staff behaviors that may be causing dissatisfaction.* Patient satisfaction is different from clinical outcomes and must be assessed separately. A patient receiving excellent clinical outcomes may be unhappy with her overall treatment experience, and vice versa.

There are a variety of good instruments available for checking directly with patients on their satisfaction levels—phone or mail surveys and focus groups are among the most popular and effective. But, do not rely solely on these measurements. Pay attention as well to other useful indicators like

- formal patient complaints
- change of physician
- withdrawal from MCO membership
- malpractice suits

Just as important as gathering this information on patient satisfaction is how you respond to the problems it uncovers. There should be a formal system in place for correcting the problems and improving satisfaction levels. Include components like these:

- Address patient grievances immediately, perhaps by making a monetary payment in return for a signed release form. Go a little bit overboard to prevent the situation from worsening into a lawsuit and to build a reputation for dedication to patients.
- Make changes in systems and personnel to effect long-term solutions to underlying problems.
- Where appropriate, educate, discipline, and deselect physicians who prove unable to deliver acceptable levels of patient satisfaction.
- Look for other ways to make patients' interaction with the group more comfortable, even without hearing a specific complaint. Notice what other physician groups are doing to cater to their patients. Copy the successful ideas.

17. *Develop and implement a formal mechanism for evaluating the performance of physicians.* Physicians are the key players

and decision makers in the group's complex of systems that produce health care. It is essential that they all perform in ways and at levels that serve the group's overall interests.

This requires defining group expectations for each physician, evaluating how well she meets them and holding her accountable when she does not. This is best done through a formal performance evaluation process that combines reviews of several key indicators that can be traced to specific physicians, like utilization rates, clinical outcomes, patient satisfaction, compliance with group policies, interactions with staff, productivity, and other relevant variables.

18. *Hire a medical director.* When the group becomes large enough, perhaps 40 to 50 physicians, it will make sense to employ a medical director. This person is a physician, often a member of the group interested in assuming some leadership responsibilities. Her primary role is as steward of the community of physicians who make up the group and of the medical care they deliver to patients. She also acts as liaison to the lay management of the group.

This person sits at a pivotal point in the group's evolving management infrastructure. She must

• have the personal and clinical respect of the other physicians in the group
• have a good grasp of the fundamentals of professional business management and medical practice in a competitive managed care setting
• be able to strike a balance between the demands of business survival and ethical medical practice
• be able to communicate back and forth between the doctors and the managers

This is a role that a group member could begin filling on a part-time basis (while the group has 25 to 30 physicians) with a growing time commitment until he is

working at it nearly full time or someone else is hired for the position

It is clear that any physician must be compensated for the time he spends as medical director.

19. *Upgrade the sophistication of the group's management of its human resources.* As the size of the group grows, so will the number of nonphysician ancillary, support, and clerical personnel it employs. Idiosyncratic and ad hoc personnel management decisions that worked fine with a small staff are no longer acceptable when the workforce approaches 100.

This is largely a matter of establishing policies and procedures, and installing systems to apply them—in areas such as

• job description and classification
• wage and salary administration
• employee benefits
• performance management
• employee discipline
• hiring and firing

The goal is to ensure that the treatment of all employees is fair, uniform, and predictable.

The upgrade process will be facilitated greatly as soon as the group is able to hire a full-time human resource manager.

20. *Reexamine, tighten, and systematize the group standards for selecting and retaining physician members.* Once the group begins to face serious competitive pressures, it will realize that it cannot afford to accept as members any interested physician, nor can it simply take those it "likes." Rather, it must apply rigorous, objective standards that result in acquiring the right physicians at the right time. This requires a multistep program composed of

• a strategic manpower plan, based on the group's long-term strategic growth plan and objectives, that specifies how many of what kinds of physicians (specialty, experience, skill level, location)

will be required by which month and year for the next five years

- job descriptions and specifications for the physician positions to be filled
- formal procedures for identifying candidates, recruiting them, and screening them for clinical and nonclinical criteria, and hiring them, or where necessary, merging their practices with the group
- a system for monitoring each physician's continuing satisfaction of and compliance with the criteria or standards, initiating corrective measures when necessary, and deselecting the physician when she proves unable to meet the group's expectations

21. *Upgrade the sophistication and professionalism of the operations management structure.* As the group grows and takes on new functions, managing its operations becomes increasingly complex and challenging. To deal with this, the group needs to

- Devise a formal management/organizational structure that assigns clear-cut work responsibilities to individual managers and establishes appropriate reporting relationships among them.
- Recruit and hire managers into that structure with the right kinds of training and experience. They may be a sort of people you have never dealt with before—professional managers, more likely to have MBAs than MDs, and more inclined to think in terms of interest rates than pulse rates.
- Look for managers experienced in working in the health care field and with physicians who are willing to try to balance clinical efficacy with cost-effectiveness and are willing to learn from health care professionals.
- Be willing to learn something about business principles from management professionals.
- Delegate virtually all administrative responsibilities to the managers you hire.

22. *Develop a focused and increasingly aggressive marketing campaign.* Without being unethical or tasteless, gradually build up a program that defines the group's "identity" and promotes it to its various stakeholders (patients, payers, employers, affiliated providers, and government agencies).

This is not a priority in the early years, while the group is still growing and deciding on its final shape. Once it becomes clear what kind of physician-run entity is emerging (including its mission and objectives), it will be just about the time to devote money and personnel to publicizing its existence, its values, and its salient characteristics.

The first promotional effort will be a basically objective communication to important audiences that the group exists and possesses certain health care delivery capabilities that may interest them. Someday, when you feel the pressure of close competition, you may choose to engage in more subjective advertising, that is, subtle efforts to shape people's thinking about your organization.

The marketing will encompass creating a unique name for the group, perhaps a logo or other special graphic symbols, facility signage, stationery, brochures, discreet ads in print media, perhaps broadcast media and billboards, direct mail promotional materials, and educational workshops.

The initial marketing budget will be well below 1 percent of gross revenues. In a more competitive marketplace, it could reach 2 or 3 percent.

23. *Upgrade numerous other operating systems.* Whenever the group improves the functioning of some parts of its operational infrastructure, this often will reveal the shortcomings in other areas. For instance, greater effectiveness at managing care and the addition of new specialists in geographically desirable locations may win the group new contracts for larger patient pop-

ulations, which the existing phone communications, scheduling, and medical records systems are not capable of handling.

Every operating system of the organization cannot be expanded and improved at once—the group probably does not have the resources. Remember, we have already discussed improvements in the management information systems (MIS) and the human resource management (HRM) system, plus the addition of systems for utilization management, quality assurance, physician performance management, patient satisfaction, and clinical treatment guidelines. However, a vision for how the organization will look when fully developed (or, alternatively, by a certain time in the future, perhaps in five years) can be planned now.

A good executive manager will work with the physician board of directors to define and prioritize the tasks necessary to take a smaller, somewhat disjunctive group practice and build it into a larger, more integrated group practice, and then manage the phased completion of those tasks over several years. There is almost no facet of the group's operations that may not benefit from some kind of upgrade or improvement.

WHY THIS STEP IS IMPORTANT

For several reasons, it is the purpose of this book to encourage most physicians to move to this stage of strategic development.

- A large, multispecialty group practice is the only way to grow beyond a certain size. There are a finite number of physicians in your specialty in your marketplace. This expanded size will be necessary to wield bargaining power in negotiations with large MCOs, insurance companies, and employers.
- It is the most efficient way to offer the full spectrum of medical services demanded by most MCOs, employers, and other payers.
- The greater size results in a larger mass of human and financial resources to be applied to the more professional management of the practice, particularly for the purpose of information gathering, which is critical to success under managed care and capitation.
- The integration and shared risk taking of virtually all the physicians required to service a managed care contract provides much greater control over the utilization, costs, and quality of the services delivered.

RESOURCE LIST

A Guide to Forming Physician Networks, Atlantic Information Services, (800) 521-4323.

A Guide to Forming Physician-Directed Managed Care Networks (Chicago: American Medical Association).

Creating a Financially Sound Primary Care Network (Westchester, IL: Healthcare Financial Management Association, 1997).

Implementing a Physician Organization (Chicago: American Medical Association).

Mergers, Super Search Packet #0995 (Englewood, CO: Medical Group Management Association).

Merging Medical Practices, Book #4619 (Englewood, CO: Medical Group Management Association, 1994).

Physician Equity Model, Book #4908 (Englewood CO: Medical Group Management Association, 1996).

Satellite Clinic, Information Exchange #4903 (Englewood, CO: Medical Group Management Association, 1996).

CHAPTER 14

Assessing the Market for Managed Care and Integration Opportunities

INTRODUCTION

Just because you have a great idea for creating a new multispecialty physician group that will move quickly to integrate with other providers does not mean you should go ahead with implementation. No matter how well the idea is conceived, other factors may prevent its success.

Aggregate national statistics clearly show a rapid trend in the direction of integration and managed care. However, local and regional conditions vary considerably around the country. The entrepreneurial physician's own practice or organization may not be as ready for as bold a move as she has planned.

Sometimes, the success of the new venture may depend on something as simple as timing. The window of opportunity for a particular idea may have passed. For instance, if most of the physicians in an area, or at least those in key specialties, are already part of existing integrated delivery systems (IDSs), it may be too late to think about forming another integrated system. Or, the window of opportunity may not have opened yet. In certain parts of the country, there may not be a sufficient number of physicians psychologically prepared to join an integrating system.

Of course, even though the market or an organization may not be ready for one kind of strategic initiative, there still may be room for another proposal better suited to local conditions.

This chapter outlines the steps in assessing both the external and internal environments for a new physician-sponsored strategic venture. It defines the kinds of information that need to be gathered, as well as possible sources. There are recommendations for criteria to use in deciding whether to proceed with the original proposal. The chapter also looks at ways to adjust an inappropriate proposal to better fit the current circumstances and enhance its chances for success.

WHO SHOULD READ THIS CHAPTER

This chapter describes an assessment process that is preliminary to the execution of most of the strategies laid out in the other chapters. The most likely approach is for a physician to read several of those chapters and begin to focus on one integration strategy or one type of organization. Then, that physician might come here to learn about techniques for determining the plausibility of the strategy or organization in his market area.

Alternatively, this could be one of the first, best chapters to read. When a physician has a vague notion that a new physician entity is desirable and that she might be a catalyst in getting it started, it may seem premature to concentrate on a particular organizational form. It could be more sensible to first conduct a thorough workup of the critical factors within the local geographic area and within one's own organization. A good strategy often emerges naturally from such an exercise.

The only person who can safely ignore this chapter is the member of an organization large enough that it will simply hire consultants to carry out the various environmental assessments and analyses.

BENEFITS OF CONDUCTING AN ENVIRONMENTAL ASSESSMENT

An environmental assessment will consume both time and a certain amount of money. It may seem like a step than can easily be omitted. That would be a serious mistake. Here is why.

1. The only worthwhile reasons to implement the strategies in this book are to create a new, more rewarding relationship between physicians and the world around them—particularly patients and payers. An environmental assessment describes the world that the physicians intend to influence and evaluates the resources they hope to use to exert that influence. As a result, they are more likely to be successful.

2. The environmental assessment will identify the local stakeholders of the physicians—those people and organizations that have a stake in how well the physicians operate their practices. They begin with the patients and payers, and will also include employers, hospitals, referral physicians (both incoming and outgoing), competitors, ancillary providers, community groups, and governmental agencies.

3. The environmental assessment will give the physicians some feedback on how they and their practices are viewed by their various stakeholders.

4. The environmental assessment will tell the physicians exactly where they fit into the local competitive market scene.

5. The environmental assessment will reveal something about the current and potential strategies of the physicians' competitors.

6. The environmental assessment will describe the demographics of the popula-

tions that the physicians are serving or might aim to serve.

7. The environmental assessment will project trends in the demands for the kinds of services that the physicians provide or might provide.

8. The environmental assessment will identify opportunities for the physicians to satisfy unmet market needs.

9. The environmental assessment will determine the reimbursement rates being paid for different kinds of medical services.

10. The environmental assessment will determine how far managed care and capitation have invaded the local market place.

11. The environmental assessment will get a sense of patient and payer awareness of managed care and their acceptance of it.

12. The environmental assessment will identify potential coventurers with the physicians in a new managed care initiative.

13. The environmental assessment will lay out the cost structure of the physicians' practices, as well as their revenue sources. By combining these data, the environmental assessment also will calculate the profitability of different aspects of the practice—product lines, contracts, and demographic groups.

14. The environmental assessment will evaluate the practice's systems and procedures, the elements of the physicians' practice styles, and which are particularly suitable and effective for managed care. By the same token, it also will reveal those practice features that do not work well with managed care.

15. The environmental assessment will provide a statement on the practice's overall readiness for managed care, capitation, integration, or any new strategic practice initiative being considered.

16. The environmental assessment will likely reveal, without a lot of effort, some of the most obvious and appropriate strategic moves the physicians might make in their marketplace.

17. The environmental assessment will identify the best potential partners and financing sources for those strategic moves.

Without these benefits, which an environmental assessment provides, physicians may very easily wind up with a strategic plan that is ill suited to the local market conditions and that their organization is incapable of implementing effectively. After much time and money is expended, the result can wind up in failure.

STEP-BY-STEP PROCESS FOR CONDUCTING AN ENVIRONMENTAL ASSESSMENT

The scope of the environmental assessment, and the process by which it is conducted, will depend on the size and complexity of the physician group. A larger group can afford to devote the resources to a more thorough assessment, including the possible hiring of a consultant. A smaller group, even a solo practitioner, might be able to do nearly as well, at least with the assessment of the external environment, by combining resources with a few other similar practices.

The larger group also requires that a more sensitive and open process be followed. The environmental assessment needs to be viewed as the first step in a formal strategic planning effort that culminates in new directions and initiatives for the physicians. This can include the formation of new integrated entities described in this book. Because the implications of the process are so far-reaching, all the physicians must feel involved and invested. They must be kept up to speed on the findings of the assessment, they must participate to some degree in the discussions of the strategic alternatives raised as a result of the assessment, and they must have a meaningful role in decisions about actions to be taken.

Of course, if only a handful of physicians are participating, they all probably will be involved in every step of the process. Where more physicians are concerned, say 10 or more, a more elaborate set of inclusive procedures should be employed.

But, first, some basic principles about the environmental assessment itself:

- There are primarily two components—an assessment of the external environment outside the practice and one of the internal operations of the practice.
- The two assessments can and should be conducted simultaneously.
- It is possible to hire qualified professional health care consultants to do all or part of each of the two assessment components.
- It is possible to accomplish a major part of the assessments, probably enough to serve the purposes of this chapter, through the efforts of a business-savvy researcher—a member of the practice's administrative staff, a local business school student, a lower-cost generalist business consultant, or the physician herself.

These are the steps to follow:

1. *Form a task force.* The first step is to assemble a task force to oversee the assessment and, eventually, the planning and implementation process. Staff it with both senior and junior physician members of the group. If nonphysician or nonprofessional personnel will have key roles in implementing any strategic proposals, give them representation on the task force.

2. *Decide whether to hire a consultant.* Next, decide whether or not to hire a consultant to carry out all or part of either assessment. It probably will be necessary to use different people to examine the marketplace and the physician's practice operations. The available resources will determine whether or not, and for which of the assessment tasks, a consultant might be appropriate. Expect to pay between $50 and $150 an hour for the consultant's time, depending on her qualifications and experience, or a lump sum for an entire course of work.

   To find a good consultant, check with institutions (e.g., hospitals) or colleagues who may have used one recently; ask among the faculty at a local university's business school; see if the state or local medical society has any recommendations; or consult the Yellow Pages under "health care consultants," "marketing consultants," "management consultants," and "market research and analysis." Look for a person who has conducted this kind of work before, preferably for physician clients.

One way to approach this decision is to start off doing some of the research yourself or through a staff member. See how much can be accomplished that way; the results may be surprising. When you get to issues you feel unqualified to handle, or when you run out of time, energy, or patience, turn to a consultant.

3. *Lay out a schedule of tasks and deadlines.* Prepare a list of the kinds of information that will be gathered and the sources of that information, name an individual to be responsible for gathering the information, and set a deadline for completion of each information gathering task. The task force should meet regularly, weekly or biweekly, to review progress, hold people accountable, and make new assignments. The list of information topics and sources can be developed from the outline in the sections that follow.

4. *Analyze and reach conclusions.* As the information begins to come in, you will learn new things about the market in which you practice and the workings of your practice. Immediately, start to decipher and categorize the information. Write brief analyses of the findings, noting especially the meaning and importance for your practice; the relationships, affiliations, and other links among organizations; the likely impact on those organizations of the data observed; and further research suggested by the findings. It should be possible to draw up useful profiles of some of the key players in the

local marketplace, such as hospitals, physician groups, employers, and managed care organizations (MCOs). Try to speculate on how these entities might affiliate with each other if they decided to form one or more integrated systems.

Begin to tie disparate pieces of information together, as in, "With what we know about utilization rates at hospital A, what we have heard about employer B's concerns with its employee health costs, and the likelihood of new state legislation next year authorizing provider-sponsored MCOs, it seems reasonable to conclude that. . ." Wherever possible, note the trends that may be taking place. The better you can predict the future, the more you can benefit from it.

The overriding purpose of this data gathering exercise is to enable your practice to interact more profitably with the world around it. One way to frame the new knowledge about the practice is in terms of the traditional SWOT (strengths-weaknesses-opportunities-threats) analysis. As you learn more about your internal operations and how they compare with the competition and changes occurring in the market place, describe in some detail

- the **strengths** of the practice that give it an advantage over the competition, that would appeal to prospective strategic partners, and that can be leveraged to exploit developments in the marketplace.
- the **weaknesses** of the practice that must be improved or circumvented or, at the very least, explained. These characteristics should be taken into account when planning any strategic move, to ensure that not too much reliance is placed on them.
- the **opportunities** available for exploitation by the practice now or in the near future. Timing is often critical in taking advantage of opportunities.

- the **threats** posed to the practice by its competitors, by new entrants to the marketplace, by trends in the demand for its services, and by changes in government regulation or financing programs. In some cases, they can be turned into opportunities. Otherwise, some form of counteraction must be taken.

5. *Decide whether or not to document formally the assessment results.* The final stage in the assessment process should be to write up completely the findings, analyses, and conclusions. This could be a very time-consuming task, on top of the work that already has been done. And, like all time-sensitive data, it will become increasingly out-of-date the moment it is completed.

   The physicians may feel that enough documentation has been prepared in the course of accumulating and studying the information. They may be confident that they have a good grasp of the realities they face within and without their practices. A written final report may seem superfluous. If that is the case, skip it.

   On the other hand, these data and the conclusions drawn from them will be the basis for the strategic visioning and planning to follow. The physicians are likely to make repeated references to this material. In dealing with potential partners or investors, they may want to show them the factual grounds for their strategic thinking. A lot of time and money will have been expended in gathering it. It is an information resource of some worth. It would be a shame if its usefulness was reduced because it was scattered among a collection of many different small reports prepared by different people. These could be good arguments for making the effort to synthesize and combine them into a single, accessible summary document.

6. *Sketch out the strategic possibilities that emerge from the assessments.* Even as the assessment information is coming in, strategic possibilities and directions will begin to suggest themselves to the physicians. A more rigorous analysis of the data will reveal even more opportunities. They could take the shape of the following kinds of fact situations:

- A local hospital is planning to form a physician-hospital organization (PHO), primarily in conjunction with its own medical staff. However, that staff is not well represented with physicians from the practice's particular specialty. The hospital and staff may be receptive to participation by the practice's doctors.
- Two significant local employers intend to offer managed care options to their employees for the first time during the next open enrollment period. As a result, the demand for provider services through the local MCOs is likely to increase dramatically. The providers will have the upper hand in contracting with the MCOs.
- A significant local employer has indicated dissatisfaction with the cost of health care services from local MCOs, as well as the difficulty in getting reports on outcome quality and patient satisfaction. The employer might be open to the possibility of contracting directly with a well-organized provider group more sensitive to the employer's concerns.
- Well over half the providers in the market area (physicians and hospitals) are part of some form of integrated network or system or are actively planning to join or develop one. Within three years, the local provider market could be dominated by two or three integrated systems with a full complement of physicians. Now (and within the next six months or so) may be the time for the physicians to join (or lead) one of the integrating groups, or get left out.

- Managed care has made very little penetration in the local market area. Employers have indicated a general desire to enroll more of their employees in health plans based on managed care principles. It is reported that a couple commercial indemnity insurers, as well as Blue Cross/Blue Shield, are contemplating the formation of rudimentary provider networks. A few physicians have heard that an MCO active in an adjoining state is thinking about moving into the local market. There are the usual rumors about new strategic initiatives being discussed by various groups of providers. The time seems optimal for a group of dedicated, entrepreneurial physicians to take the lead in assembling a physician-controlled provider system that can negotiate from strength with either MCOs or employers.

FORM A STRATEGIC VISION FOR THE PRACTICE

The environmental assessment will probably suggest more strategic alternatives than the physicians could possibly implement. In fact, some may conflict with each other. Simply choosing from strategic options (e.g., join an independent practice association [IPA], merge into a multispecialty group practice, collaborate in a PHO, form a group practice without walls [GPWW]) is not the most rational way to plan a practice's long-term future. A better, more systematic approach is a strategic planning process with three more steps to it: Form a strategic vision, create a strategic plan that fulfills the vision, and take actions to realize the plan.

A strategic vision is a picture of what the practice will look like approximately five years from now. How large it will be? Who will be part of it? Where will it be located? How will it be structured? With whom will it be affiliated? What kinds of services (or products) will it offer? Who will it serve? How will it be paid? What will be its reputation in the community and the profes-

sion? What kinds of systems will it use to support its activities? The vision is often stated in rather abstract terms; it does not have to be as precise as the above list may suggest. More than anything else, it needs to be clear enough to serve as a guiding light to the physicians for some years to come. When the physicians start arguing about different strategic plans and objectives, the vision is there to ground their discussions.

The vision is not cast in stone. It can be adjusted as changing conditions, external and internal, warrant. Just remember that a vision that is constantly, radically changing is no vision at all.

A practice of a very few physicians may be able to agree fairly quickly on a vision for the group. If more than, say, 10 physicians are involved, it might be wiser to carry out a facilitated retreat to reach consensus.

CREATE A STRATEGIC PLAN THAT FULFILLS THE VISION

The strategic plan is a series of five to seven initiatives, or individual strategies, designed to bring the reality of the practice closer to its vision. The term "strategic" usually applies to activities that are expected to take longer than a year to complete. Each strategy consists of

- a clear description of what is to be accomplished
- a measurable, preferably quantitative, objective that will indicate when the strategy has been carried out
- a specific date by which the strategy will be completed
- the connection between completion of the strategic initiative and realization of the strategic vision

There often is a temptation to create an omnibus strategic plan with a "wish list" of 15 or 20 objectives that the organization would like to achieve in the next five years. Resist this. Keeping the number to seven or so will better focus the energies of the organization and improve the chances of successful implementation.

A strategic plan for a four-physician single specialty group might look like this:

1. Expand the number of same specialty physicians in the practice to
   - 8 (in two years)
   - 12 (in four years)
   - 16 (in five years)
2. Identify and merge with a 10 to 15 primary care physician group (within three years), with a view toward assembling a multi-specialty group practice (within six years).
3. Begin investment in and implementation of a state-of-the-art financial and clinical information system that will be fully operational within four years.
4. Identify three key measures of resource utilization unique to the group's specialty and meaningful to MCOs (e.g., specialty referrals, hospital admissions, drug prescriptions) and track them for six months and take steps to reduce them (by 5 percent within one year, by 10 percent within two years, and by 12 percent within three years).
5. As the geographic distribution of the group's patients warrants it, set up additional primary care practice offices throughout the primary service area (one within four years, three within five years).
6. Increase the take-home income of each group physician by an average of 5 percent each year for the next five years.

There are a couple things to keep in mind about strategic plans. There is not one "right" or even "ideal" plan for a particular group. There is a multitude of plans that will bring a group to more or less where it wants to be in five years. They may just take different routes. Strategic success has more to do with thoroughly researching the plan in advance (through the environmental assessment), creating it with thoughtfulness and the participation of all responsible for its execution, and then executing it well, than with choosing the right one.

All strategic plans embody a substantial element of risk. The group will commit money and other resources in an effort to influence events in the future. Without a crystal ball, they cannot be certain that circumstances and assumptions will not change and confound their best intentions. It is necessary to assume risk (and not just the risk inherent in capitation) in order to achieve success in a business venture. Do not make the mistake of wanting and waiting for a virtual guarantee of success before committing to a plan. If you take a strategic initiative, there is a small but significant chance that you will fail. If you take no strategic initiative, you are almost bound to fail.

TAKE ACTIONS TO REALIZE THE PLAN

The strategic plan, though practical and specific, is usually not nearly detailed enough by itself to be implemented. What is required is the definition of a set of even more concrete, short-term actions which, when carried out, will achieve each of the strategic objectives. It is a little impractical to try to specify all the necessary actions for a strategy that is planned to be completed three or four years in the future. So, here is how most business organizations manage the strategic planning function.

The necessary meetings and discussions are held to prepare the initial strategic vision and strategic plan, with objectives. A commitment is made to an annual planning process, scheduled for the same time each year, usually two to four months before the beginning of the next fiscal year. During that process:

1. The vision is reviewed and, if current conditions have changed sufficiently, amended. Amendments happen rarely.
2. The strategic plan is also reviewed. Those objectives that have been achieved are removed. Other objectives that have become irrelevant or no longer desirable are also removed. Some of the remaining objectives may be adjusted in their content or time schedule. New objectives are added. The entire plan is extended another year into the future.

3. On the basis of the revised strategic plan, an annual operating plan is prepared for the coming fiscal year. This usually is done by the organization's chief executive officer (CEO) or general manager. In a small practice, the physicians themselves would draw it up. The operating plan sets out the actions and goals that will be worked on over the course of the year, with the intention of progressively implementing the multiyear strategies in the strategic plan. The operating plan is accompanied by an annual budget, whose expenditures fund the plan.

At various points in the strategic planning process, the group will be forced to take into account its limited resources. In the very long term (10 to 15 years), almost anything is possible. In the near future (0 to 3 years), the group's ambitions will be constrained primarily by the availability of two factors—financial capital and the time physicians have to spend on planning for the future versus practicing medicine today. Money to invest in strategic ventures is probably the biggest complication in physician efforts to remain autonomous and in control of clinical decision making. At some stage in its development, almost every business is faced with the choice of trading control for capital. This issue is discussed in greater detail in Chapter 27, "Financing Strategies To Support Your Integration Plans."

For the moment, in their planning, physicians should make at least rough estimates of the resources required to implement the several strategies in their strategic plan. The annual budget serves as the cost estimate for carrying out the operating plan.

TYPES OF INFORMATION GATHERED DURING AN ENVIRONMENTAL ASSESSMENT AND WHERE TO FIND THEM

These are the types of information that should be gathered in the optimal, most comprehensive environmental assessment. There are several reasons why a group might not meet this ideal. They may not have the time or money to do as thorough a job as they would like. Instead, they set priorities among the information categories and concentrate on those most relevant to them and their situation. In some cases, the information simply may not exist. For instance, there will be no information on managed care if no MCOs are active in the area. Or, the information may never have been assembled in a usable form. Even where the information clearly exists, the group may be denied access to it. Certainly, competitors will not freely reveal their strategic intentions.

Whenever the group especially wants to incorporate certain information into its strategic thinking, but cannot find it in an accurate form, it need not give up. It should gather whatever data can be located, even if they seem rather subjective or biased. Then, make the best, well-reasoned assumptions it can about the subject of the data. It could also postulate several alternative scenarios (best case, worst case, most likely case) and make calculations for each of them. As the future unfolds and real-time information starts to come in, appropriate adjustments in the strategic plan can be made.

Assessment of the Internal Operations of the Physician Practice

1. *Prepare a narrative description of the practice's history since its founding.* This should be a little bit of fun for the physicians. The description traces how the practice got started and developed over the years to where it is now. Remembering this history can remind the physicians of their greatest strengths and the aspirations they had when they began practicing. This description becomes the backdrop against which future plans are made.

2. *List procedures performed by Current Procedures Terminology (CPT) code.* This information will indicate the specific kinds of medical services provided by the practice and their volume. If possible, record each procedure and its frequency or volume for each physician in the practice.

You may be surprised at the mix of services (physician specialty is not always determinative), their frequency, and variations among physicians. This information can be useful in evaluating the group's ability to perform under a managed care contract. It will offer clues on the types of new physicians to recruit into the practice or merge with in other practices in order to fill service gaps. The information should be readily available through the practice's claims system.

3. *Calculate some key clinical performance ratios* (e.g., patient visits per physician per week, annual physician encounters per patient, hospital days per 1,000 patients, referrals per 1,000 patients, key diagnostic tests per 1,000 tests, number of midlevel providers (MLPs) and nonprovider support staff per full-time equivalent (FTE) physician, and other relevant utilization data for each physician). Pick at least three of these indicators for which the data are most readily available. Gather information on as many other indicators as time permits. If there are still others more relevant to your kind of practice, concentrate on them. What you are looking for is a few good measures of your performance of clinical tasks. Try to find indicators in at least these areas: the physicians' direct contacts with patients, the physicians' referral of patients to other forms of treatment (e.g., specialist physicians, medications), and the physicians' use of nonphysician personnel in treating patients. You may want to check the published American Medical Association (AMA) or Medical Group Management Association (MGMA) survey data and make comparisons in order to ensure comparability. These data may be available in summaries of the claims filed by the practice. If not, it may be necessary to search individual claim forms or even patient medical records and then make some simple calculations to come up with the desired ratios.

4. *Compare clinical performance data with survey data averages compiled by groups like the AMA and MGMA.* The main reason for gathering these clinical data is to compare the clinical performance of the practice and its physicians with the averages for others like them, as published in the annual surveys conducted by the AMA and the MGMA. The comparisons may reveal differences that can be explained by regional variations or different levels of risk presented by patients. Quite often, however, the differences will mean that the practice is not as clinically efficient as it could be. The data comparisons will direct the physicians' attentions to those areas of clinical behavior that need improvement. If the physicians are entering into managed care contracts, the need for improvement may be even more immediate—under pressure from the MCO.

5. *Compare clinical performance data with averages or norms from the existing providers of MCOs in the area.* Once the internal clinical data have been gathered under the previous section, there are several bases for further comparison and analysis.

   • MGMA, *Cost Survey 1997 Report Based on 1996 Data* (A superb compilation of cost and utilization data for different size group practices. Cost is $200 for members, $250 for affiliates, and $300 for nonmembers.)

   • AMA, *Physician Marketplace Statistics 1997–1998* (Cost is $299 for members and $399 for nonmembers.)

   • AMA, *Socioeconomic Characteristics of Medical Practice 1997* (Cost is $99.95 for members and $159.95 for nonmembers.)

   • AMA, *Medical Groups in the US, 1996 Edition* (Cost is $59.95 for members and $79.95 for nonmembers.)

   • AMA, *Practice Characteristics of Physicians in Medical Groups* (Free with other purchases.)

• Local MCOs, particularly those with which you might contract or affiliate, will have a variety of performance data on their current providers. Try hard to obtain these data from them, as they are the standards against which they will measure your performance.
• If the group's data can be collected over a period of time, even two or three years, they can be compared with themselves to show trends. Even without an external incentive, the physicians in the group would be well advised to take steps to begin reducing some of these performance indicators.

The collection and practical application of these kinds of data is essential to the group's success under managed care. They provide the basis for determining how the practice stacks up against the competition and against the MCO-imposed standards. They show exactly where the physicians must make some improvements.

6. *Gather financial and claims data for the last two to three years.* The financial data on a practice's operations are the other half of the story, with the clinical data. They are important both standing alone and in combination with the clinical information. The financial data should include, at a minimum

• basic financial statements for the last three years—balance sheet, income statement, cash flow statement
• expenses related directly to patient care and administrative overhead expense
• personnel expenses, separated into direct salary and employee benefits
• physician salary expenses, whether recorded as such or simply taken home after all other expenses are covered
• costs attributable to midlevel (non-physician) providers
• cost of providing each procedure or service for which a coded claim is filed (to the extent it is possible to determine)

• aggregate cost of providing services to all the lives covered under each managed care contract
• expense of performing the non–patient-specific tasks required by a managed care contract (quality assurance, peer review, supervision)
• revenues received for each procedure or service on which a coded claim is filed
• total revenues received through each managed care contract and through each member program, if each contract covers more than one program

Properly compiled, these data will give the physicians a good picture of where their practice money is coming from and how they are spending it. More specifically, it will begin to tell which procedures are moneymakers and, overall, which managed care contracts are most profitable. Prospectively, the data can be used to analyze and project which new contracts might be financially worthwhile for the practice.

Most of these data can be pulled out of the standard bookkeeping records of a good practice. Some, like the financial statements, will already have been prepared for other purposes (e.g., tax reporting). Others will require manipulation and recalculation of the existing data. Information from claims forms may have to be retabulated manually. In many cases, the greatest revelation will be that the practice's accounting system is not sophisticated enough to generate the data required. Upgrading that system may become the first order of business.

7. *Indicate all major revenue sources and their trends (up or down)*
• by payer
• by major employer
• by demographic group (age and sex), if easily isolated

It is important to know the absolute amount of revenues earned from particular payers (specific MCOs, specific commercial insurers, Blue Cross/Blue Shield, Medicare, Medicaid, direct contract employer, patient out-of-pocket) in order to figure out which are profitable. Such knowledge informs decisions on whether to participate with a certain payer. The relative amounts (percentages) coming from each payer also indicate how dependent the practice is on particular revenue sources.

If similar calculations can be made for demographic groups, or even patients located in certain geographic areas, the group can make adjustments in the services it offers and the accessibility to its practice.

8. *Calculate some key financial performance ratios.* These are simple, standard indicators of financial performance, like revenues per FTE physician, net income per FTE physician, personnel costs as a percentage of revenues, current ratio, debt-to-equity ratio. These are easily calculated from numbers in the simplest practice bookkeeping system.

9. *Compare financial performance data with survey data averages compiled by groups like the AMA and MGMA.* The financial performance data are the basis for comparison with the practice itself, as it develops over time, and with other similar practices. The sources of comparative financial data are the same as those mentioned earlier for comparative clinical data.

  • the practice's own historical bookkeeping records, going back two to three years
  • data available from MCOs for their current provider organizations (these may be less readily available than the clinical data)
  • AMA practice financial survey results
  • MGMA group practice financial survey results

In the most sophisticated analysis, the financial data will be integrated with the clinical data, eventually demonstrating the cost-effectiveness of particular treatment alternatives or pathways. Work to develop that capability. For the present, use the data to evaluate the operating efficiency of the practice—in terms of economic productivity per physician and costs of delivering certain standard medical services.

10. *Document all hospital affiliations and most frequent referral patterns.* This information indicates who the physicians' current operational partners are—the other area providers they trust enough to care for their patients. As such, they are also prospective strategic partners of the practice, in joint ventures, mergers, or the creation of entirely new entities.

Each physician should note the hospitals at which she has admitting privileges. Since there are not likely to be too many, list all of them. Indicate any differences in the class of privileges or limitations on clinical privileges. Each physician should also review his records for the last couple years to determine which other physicians have been referral targets for his patients. Unless the number is extremely large, try to list all of them. Make subjective judgments about each referral doctor concerning two things: the clinical quality of his medical care and the resource utilization intensity of his practice style. Give each one a grade ("A" to "E") on both counts. If you feel able, also rate how receptive each physician might be to overtures about new strategic organizational initiatives or affiliations with your practice.

11. *Describe the demographic and socioeconomic characteristics of the patient population primarily served by the practice.* These data will be available only if they have been regularly collected for some legitimate reason. (If the data are not available, the best alternative is to skip two sections down to the data item on "drawing patient profiles.") There are several reasons for breaking out the demographic and socioeconomic information on current

patients: (1) It tells you something about the kind and volume of medical services patients require; (2) it may be an indicator of additional services that you might offer patients or ways to improve the services currently offered; (3) it will be a measure of how easily the practice will adapt to serving the patients under a new managed care contract (whose demographic characteristics may or may not be the same); and (4) in combination with financial data, it will show which demographic subgroups are being served profitably by the practice.

12. *Attempt to calculate the net income (revenues over expenses) for each service or service group provider, each major payer, and each substantial demographic group.* These are probably the most essential of the internal data that will be gathered. They demonstrate clearly where the practice is and is not making money, by its most obvious and most manageable components. If it is shown that a particular payer relationship is not profitable, the practice has several choices—drop the relationship, renegotiate its monetary terms, or stay with it as it is for nonmonetary reasons.

If certain procedures or procedure groups appear to be money losers, the physicians can take several different approaches. They could choose to no longer perform that procedure, they could consciously refer the patient out for that procedure, they could continue to offer the procedure as a sort of loss leader essential to getting and keeping certain patients, or they could investigate further to find out why the procedure is not economical and take corrective steps.

Discovering patient groups that are unprofitable to serve is another matter. Generally, they cannot simply be dropped for that reason. At the very least, it would be unethical to do so and perhaps even a form of illegal discrimination. Further, it would be prohibited by the contract under

which the physicians are serving them. The options are to stick with them, with the knowledge that the profits made on other groups in the contract are more than offsetting them, look for ways to treat the group more profitably, or if the losses on these groups make the entire contract untenable, drop it.

Many practices will have trouble calculating this kind of information. Remember that profits are basically the result of subtracting expenses from revenues. There should be no problem determining the revenues from various payers. Figuring the costs expended under the contract with each payer requires totaling the services or procedures provided to that payer's members and then totaling the costs of those services and procedures. If the practice cannot figure out the costs of performing specific individual procedures, it will never be able to know whether a particular payer contract is profitable or not. This ability to quickly ascertain the costs associated with practice activities is crucial to success under managed care.

A practice that lacks the systems or data to compute its profitability by payer will have just as hard a time in figuring out whether it is making money on a particular medical procedure or group of patients.

13. *Draw a profile of three or four categories of typical patients seen in the practice, in terms of demographics, conditions presented, and services required.* What you are trying to do here is to define a few types of typical patients seen by your practice. The purpose is not particularly to understand the diversity of your patients in any detail, but rather to create a picture of the practice in terms of its most common patients. For instance, there may be a predominance of geriatric (Medicare) patients or patients from new families (mother, father, and young children). If the physicians have not thought about this before or have never discussed it, they

may be surprised at what they learn.

The results of this typology may suggest that the group should expand the number of patients that it serves in these existing categories, perhaps by contracting with MCOs that enroll similar populations. If the physicians are already adept at treating this group, there is logic in doing more of the same. On the other hand, the group may feel that it is overly dependent on certain patient groups or their information may indicate that some significant demographic shifts are occurring in their marketplace. Perhaps, new MCO or government entitlement programs have created new opportunities among different patient groups. The physicians might reasonably decide to develop the clinical skills and practice presence necessary to attract and serve some of these newer groups.

The patient profiles should be prepared for the three of four types most often seen by the practice. They can be selected by intuition or by systematically reviewing patient medical records. A good profile will include the following characteristics:
- gender
- age
- geographic location of residence
- medical conditions most frequently presented
- income level
- employer
- source of health care coverage or payment

Add in any other factors that might affect the kind of clinical services the patients usually require.

14. *Define each physician's history of resource utilization.* If the practice has not done so already, it should begin gathering data on the rates at which individual physicians utilize critical and costly resources. For some practices, it may be necessary to install a system that does this for the first time.

Look at the following kinds of resource utilization, as well as any others unique to your specialty or practice:
- **Hospital utilization.** How often do you admit patients and how long do they stay there (ALOS)?
- **Specialist physician utilization.** How often do you refer patients to other physicians? How long do they stay engaged with that physician or what expenses do they incur for the physician's services? What would it take for your practice to provide those services itself?
- **Diagnostic test utilization.** How many and what kinds of diagnostic tests are prescribed for the average patient of each physician? What expenses are incurred as a result of these tests?
- **Medication utilization.** How many, what kinds, and what dosages of medications do you prescribe for the average patient? What are the costs of those medications?
- **Supplies utilization.** What volume and kinds of other supplies does each physician consume in treating her average patients? What is the cost of those supplies?
- **Personnel utilization.** How much time of nonphysician providers and non-provider staff are consumed, at the physician's direction, in treating the average patient? What is the cost of that personnel time?
- **Physician time utilization.** How much personal time does each physician spend with her average patient? To put it another way. how many patients does each physician see per hour, day, or week? Based on the physician's take-home income for the previous year, what is the worth of the time spent on each patient?

Many practices today will be challenged to collect and report these kinds of data on physician utilization rates. There are numerous incentives for doing so.

- Increasingly, MCOs want to see this data-gathering ability in their contract partners.
- The MCOs may specifically ask to see, on a regular basis, the practice's data on utilization rates, and base its reimbursement policies on them.
- The MCO may collect its own utilization information on the physicians' utilization rates. It behooves the practice to do the same thing, as a check on the accuracy of the MCO's figures.
- Even if the MCO were totally disinterested in the utilization rates, it would make sense for the practice to gather this information. With this knowledge, it can manage the utilization of resources and intelligently reduce them. When fewer resources are used to deliver the same units of care, expenses go down and profits go up. More specifically, it can focus on individual physicians who are unnecessarily high utilizers. Through education, feedback, and counseling, it can attempt to modify their practice behaviors.

15. *Describe the quality of each physician's and the practice's relationships with hospitals, physicians, and payers in the area.* These are largely subjective descriptions of the relationships between the practice and its physicians, on one hand, and other providers and payers in the market area, on the other. They may include some numbers—age in years of the relationship and revenues that pass between the parties. The most important information, however, is the kinds of information shared, the projects worked on together, the degree of dependency of one party on the other and for what, the impressions of the physicians of the quality of services provided by the other parties, the competence and integrity of their personnel, the modernity of their equipment and physical plant, the basic

trust and reliance between the parties, and the prospects for the two of them collaborating in the future.

The descriptions are most easily produced by listing the key providers and payers and then interviewing the practice's physicians about them. A good way to start might be to ask separate physicians to prepare drafts of the descriptions. After the whole group has read and discussed them, they can be amended.

The value of these descriptions is that they give the practice a better grasp of the other players in the marketplace with whom it will have to contend. Some will have to be fought as competitors; others are potential strategic partners.

16. *Note the practice's experience or familiarity with the most common care management devices*—utilization review, capitation, drug formularies, clinical protocols or guidelines, clinical outcomes data, quality assurance, patient satisfaction surveys, and the like. These are the mechanisms that a modern physician group must employ to thrive in a managed care environment. Prepare summary descriptions of the practice's current experience with or implementation of these and any other relevant care management devices. Does the practice have the requisite systems in place? Are they modern, state of the art? How effectively have they been working until now? What plans does the practice have for acquiring new care management systems and competencies in the next two to three years? Has the practice set any goals that it aims to achieve through application of these mechanisms, such as reduced utilization, reduced costs, improved quality of care, greater uniformity in treatment patterns, and improved patient satisfaction.

When contracting with MCOs or negotiating affiliations with other providers, the practice will use these summaries to demonstrate its ability to manage care. They will strengthen its position in such negotiations.

17. *List the practice's current MCO contracts, including*
    - mix of services provided under each contract
    - number of patients served under each contract
    - previous years under each contract
    - reimbursement methodology and rate under each contract
    - resource utilization rates (outpatient visits, hospital admissions, ALOS) under each contract and their trends for the last three years
    - utilization and quality management programs implemented under each contract
    - percentage of practice revenues from each contract
    - profitability for the practice of each contract

These data offer some of the best insights into the practice's ability as a manager of care. For most practices, their work under contracts with MCOs sums up their total experience with managed care. Their success here augurs well for the future. If there have been problems with their performance (financial or clinical) under these contracts, they can be recognized now. The physicians can take corrective measures before managed care has completely taken over their professional lives—through more contracts, through affiliations, and through integration.

Most of these data should be available directly from the contracts themselves. However, some interesting problems may emerge. The contract may not specify as clearly as it should the services to be provided by the physicians, and they may never have asked. No one may be keeping track of how many patients are being seen under each contract. If the number is small, it may not be worth the administrative cost to continue the contract. There is

a good chance that the practice will not have good information on the utilization rates for individual physicians under each contract. However, one of the benefits of working with a responsible and supportive MCO is receiving the reports that it often compiles and supplies to its physicians on their performance under the contract. Ask your MCO partners for any data they may have on you that would help you improve your performance for them.

Knowing the proportion of total revenues generated by each contract indicates how dependent the practice is on a particular MCO. This information can lead to several actions. Where substantial revenues come from one MCO, the physicians may try to reduce that dependence (by building up other revenue sources) or instead develop it into a closer, even more rewarding long-term relationship. Smaller volume contracts may be dropped altogether or given greater attention because of their strategic value to the practice.

18. *List the nonclinical professional activities of the physicians, particularly those that have placed them in managerial or leadership roles.* Interview each physician for this information. A large range of nonclinical professional activities (research, teaching) may suggest that a physician will not have the time to contribute to preparing the practice for the future. Effective service as a manager or leader could qualify the physician as a catalyst and guide for new strategic initiatives the practice must take.

The goal of this part of the assessment is to determine how prepared the practice is to
- practice medicine under a risk arrangement
- operate efficiently under a capitated contract
- deliver medical care at a cost within a specified capitation rate or fee schedule

- design, acquire, and implement effective, coordinated care management systems and procedures
- gather, interpret, integrate, and apply a broad set of clinical and financial data
- provide medical services to a larger, more diverse, geographically dispersed population of patient-enrollees
- work collaboratively with physicians in other specialties, ancillary personnel, and managerial personnel for the common good of the entire organization
- take a leadership role in forming a comprehensive physician-controlled provider network
- enter into affiliations, joint ventures, and even mergers with other organizations for the strategic advantage of everyone involved
- provide or find elsewhere the substantial financing for new strategic initiatives both within the practice and in partnership with other entities

Assessment of the External Environment of the Physician Practice

1. *Define the service area of the practice, in terms of geographics and populations served (including primary and secondary areas) and classify existing patients by ZIP code, age, sex, and payer.* The first step in assessing the external environment is defining it. The environment that concerns the practice does not include the whole country. Initially, the practice should be most interested in the area from which most of its patients come.

   The definition will be a geographic one—lines on a map. Review the current patient lists for residence addresses. If possible, note the exact street address. At least, take down each patient's ZIP code. Plot this information on a map—by hand drawing or computer. Putting pins in a large map can give an interesting graphic

perspective.

It should quickly become plain that the bulk of patients live in certain sections of the city and not in others. They may be so conveniently clumped that no further classification will be necessary. If they are more scattered, focus on those in the most common ZIP codes. They often will account for 80 percent of all patients. The goal is to draw a line around the densest concentration of patients. This can be referred to as the practice's "primary service area." Neighborhoods that are homes for significant numbers of other patients are the "secondary service area." The delineation of the areas does not have to be superscientific, as long as the physicians are satisfied that most of their patients reside in the primary area and quite a few others are living, less densely, in the secondary area.

2. *Describe the demographic and socioeconomic characteristics of the service area (primary and secondary), as well as any plausible larger market area into which the practice might expand.* The next step is to prepare a simple, practical description of the people (not just the practice's patients) located in the defined service areas. Look mainly at the demographic and socioeconomic information about them.
   - age, gender, and ethnicity
   - stage of life and family unit size
   - annual income levels
   - predominant housing type

   As these data come in, notice differences among neighborhoods within the service areas, as well as between the service areas themselves. Pay particular attention to the contrasts in characteristics between the practice's patients and other residents of the service area.

   The differences may reveal untapped markets for the practice within each area. They may indicate that the practice has been focusing on the needs of a patient population that is only a minority in the area, with no prospect of growing larger. Through the data, the practice may learn better ways of appealing to and serving even its current patients.

This is a good time possibly to sketch out a third area that extends beyond the primary and secondary service areas—a larger area into which the practice might expand in the future as it grows and merges. Call it a potential market area. Take the same approach with it. Define the area precisely in geographic terms. Conduct a similar demographic and socioeconomic analysis. Look for similarities to the current service areas, which would make expansion easier by serving an already well-understood patient population. Even if the residents seem quite different, the new knowledge will facilitate the practice's move into that area, whenever it comes.

3. *Count the numbers of physicians in the practice's service areas and the larger market area—by specialty and practice setting.* The practice rarely will be lucky enough to be the only provider of its kind or specialty in a particular area. There are three good reasons for knowing what other providers are operating in the area.

- Some may be competing for the same patients and managed care contracts as the practice.
- Some may be excellent prospective strategic partners.
- Even those who are neither competitors nor potential partners are capable of making strategic moves that affect the practice and must be anticipated.

Concentrate on tabulating the physicians in the primary and secondary service areas and in the prospective market area. Get their numbers by practice setting (solo, group, hospital-employed) and specialty. Note the size of the groups, if possible.

4. *Draw a profile of three or four categories of area physicians, practices, or groups that could be considered competitors of your practice.* These are meant to be more detailed pictures of the most common types of competing physician groups faced by the practice. Occasionally, in the case of very narrow specialties, they may be single physicians in solo practice. More often, they will be groups of physicians gathered into various types of integrating organizations. They can be descriptions of actual real-life physician groups or a collage of features from several similar or related groups.

The purpose of this exercise is to focus the physicians' attention on the primary competition or types of physician competition they will encounter as they integrate in a quest for patients and contracts. It might be summed up in the homily "know thy competition."

Note: Some physicians may feel uncomfortable talking about "competition," particularly among physicians. It just does not seem right that providers should be fighting with each other, figuratively, for the opportunity to deliver health care services to needful patients. Nonetheless, competition is what is occurring in the health care marketplace (another discomforting term) today. Physicians have the choice of ignoring the presence of market forces; in which case, they will shortly lack sufficient patients to keep their practices going. If it makes it easier, look at it this way. Your physicians develop a superior ability to meet the cost, quality, and accessibility needs of patients and payers. They become better at it than any other physicians. Competition is simply a planned series of proactive steps to communicate that ability to the patients and the payers. It certainly is in the patient's best interests to be treated by the best available physician—and that happens to be you.

The competitor profiles should include as much of the following information as can be obtained:

- number of physicians in the group and their subspecialties
- ages of the physicians and their plans for retirement
- total revenues of the group
- primary types of patients seen by the group
- primary sources of revenue
- primary payers dealt with
- primary forms of reimbursement
- any direct contract relationships with employers
- primary hospital affiliations of physicians in the group
- subjective description of the "kind" of practice the group operates (exclusive/inclusive, high/low cost, friendly/austere, ambitious/relaxed, sloppy/efficient)
- subjective assessment of the cost and quality of care provided by the group, unless more objective data are available (i.e., malpractice suits)
- subjective assessment of the group's reputation with patients, payers, employers, hospitals, and other physicians
- geographic area from which the group's patients primarily come
- subjective assessment of the group's ability to manage care, with specific reference to procedures and systems that may have been installed
- any information on the group's strategic plans, intentions, or discussions
- particular ways in which the group may pose a threat to your group

It probably is impossible to obtain all this information, in accurate form, about any physician group. If they are truly competitors, they will not want you to have it. The goal is to do the best you can. Keep eyes and ears open for any pieces of information about these groups—from colleagues and vendors, in newspapers and medical society publications. If precise objective data are not available, settle for subjective, impressionistic knowledge.

5. *Identify major employers in the area, the approximate number of covered lives (employees) they represent, the geographic distribution of those lives, their current source of health care coverage and the types of products offered.* Information on area employers should be a little easier to come by. These data will help the practice think about several issues.

- By knowing which MCOs are most popular with employers, the practice can concentrate on wooing and contracting with them.
- By knowing where a business's employees reside, the practice might plan the strategic location of new primary care offices or clinics.
- By knowing about an employer's plans for growth or expansion (or retrenchment), the practice can prepare in a variety of ways to meet its increased (or decreased) demands for health care.
- By becoming familiar with an employer's experiences with its health care coverage, the practice can consider more realistically the possibility of direct contracting with it.

Frequently, it will be possible to obtain much of this information about an employer by simply calling its human resource or employee benefits manager. They have no reason to hide it. If you explain that the data will help you better meet the needs of the employees, the employer should be happy to share it with you.

6. *Plot historical trends among these data and project them into the future—particularly for population, demographic, provider, and managed care figures.* Health care data that are simply slices in time are not terribly helpful to a physician group planning for the future. They are better than nothing at all. However, everything in health care is changing so rapidly that

today's data will be obsolete tomorrow. It is important to track trends in all these data that are part of the environmental assessment. That number on managed care penetration becomes much more meaningful when you know that it is going up or down.

There are two basic methods for plotting data trends. If you are lucky, you can obtain the relevant information from a source that has already been collecting it for several years. It will be instantly obvious which way the data are headed. This is the most likely method for identifying trends in the external environment.

The alternative is for you to begin gathering the data you want at regular intervals. After as short a period as two years, some rudimentary trends may become evident. This is usually the only way to assemble trend data about the internal operations of the practice. In fact, most practices presently have a wealth of historical data (in medical records, in general bookkeeping records, and on claims forms filed) that can be manipulated to reveal important trends.

7. *Count other key nonphysician providers, particularly acute care hospitals and any integrated systems that may be taking shape (PHOs, IPAs, GPWWs).* This is a continuation of the census of key players in the local health care marketplace. Previously, the physician population has been surveyed and described. In this part of the assessment, the other pieces of the health delivery (as opposed to financing) system are identified. Because of their importance and size, the acute care hospitals are the primary targets. In addition, do a rough job of enumerating the other providers in the area—long-term care, rehab, and specialty hospitals; free-standing outpatient facilities and emergency centers, and high-level ancillary providers. It is useful to know about these people and institutions for several reasons.

- Foremost, some of them may be potential strategic partners or participants

with the practice in a joint venture or integrating system.
- If they are not affiliating with you, they may be affiliating with other physicians (your competitors) to form a system that poses a threat to anything you might have in mind.
- Whatever they do, they will be a factor in the cost structure and development of the local delivery system—even if they achieve their major impact by simply going out of business.

This is probably a good point to also start keeping tabs on physicians and other providers who have aggregated themselves into significant (more than 20 physicians) group practices, particularly multispecialty groups, PHOs, IPAs, GPWWs, and IDSs. Look for any conglomeration of providers that appears to be integrating its operations for competitive purposes.

Try to learn the following information about these entities:

- exactly what people and institutions are involved
- how far along the path to integration they have progressed
- how tightly bound or committed they are to each other
- what their current size is—in terms of revenues, number of beds, provider staff, and covered lives
- what is known about their future plans for strategic change and growth

This knowledge is a direct look at what the provider community is doing to adapt to managed care. The number of providers involved and the pace of their integration efforts is a good indicator of how rapidly the marketplace is evolving. It is a key to how quickly you and your colleagues must begin to move. You can see what integration models are being used and how well they are working.

8. *Identify the primary health care coverage sources (insurance companies and MCOs) operating in the market area.* These are the

practice's primary customers. It is the patients who ultimately must be served and satisfied, but the insurance companies and MCOs are the ones who pay the providers.

In most markets, the number of payers is not likely to be overwhelming. They must file a considerable amount of publicly available information with the insurance commissioner or another state regulatory agency. If they are publicly traded for-profit companies, they must also have made substantial annual filings with the federal Securities and Exchange Commission (SEC). Here is what to look for:

- the official name of the organization, which may be different from the name it is using locally for marketing purposes
- other states in which the organization is providing health care coverage
- the size of the organization, both locally and nationally, in terms of revenues, employer contracts, covered lives, and provider contracts
- geographic distribution of enrollees
- rough estimate of its local market share
- number of primary care physicians, specialty physicians, and hospitals in the network
- list of primary employer contracts, as well as other managed care contracts (Medicare or Medicaid)
- list of primary provider contracts
- sample copy of typical managed care contract with physicians
- nature of relationships between the MCO and providers (exclusivity, other contract terms, amicability, "long-term partners," negotiating style)
- open or closed provider network
- typical payment methodology for each provider category (e.g., discounted/capped fee-for-service [FFS], salary, capitation, bonus, risk pools, withholds)

- care management methods imposed on providers
- reputation with employers and patients for quality of clinical care and patient satisfaction
- reputation with physicians for integrity and tenor of its dealings with them
- usual negotiating style (firm but fair, hardball, long-term partners, short-term exploitation)
- financial performance (balance sheet, income statement, reserves, medical loss ratio)
- willingness to provide financing for strategic initiatives (such as acquisition of a state-of-the-art information system or the construction of primary care satellites) by its participating providers

These kinds of data will enable the physicians to target certain MCOs for closer examination and possible affiliation. The knowledge will give them a stronger position in their negotiations with particular MCOs. Prior familiarity with the MCOs allows the physicians to build the right kind of care management system, demonstrate a sufficient ability to manage care, perhaps locate some of its practice offices more conveniently to an MCO's members, determine whether it can make money at the fee or rates paid by an MCO, prepare an appropriate negotiation strategy, and decide whether they want to deal with a particular MCO at all.

9. *Determine the rough percentages of health care revenues accounted for by managed care and capitation, the number of patients covered by managed care and capitation, and the number of physicians under managed care and capitation contracts—within the market area. Track the historical trends for these data (last three years, if possible) and project them into the future.* After accumulating the above data, it should be possible to prepare these aggregate figures on the penetration of managed care and capitation into the local

market. They may not be absolutely accurate, but they will be close enough to provide a basis for strategic planning. In some cases, an existing organization (like a state health maintenance organization (HMO) trade association or a faculty group at a local university) may already have compiled the necessary historical data and projected them into the future. These data, plus the information on the formation and growth of integrating organizations, and on the strategic intentions of key providers in the area, will tell your group how quickly it must move to grow larger and acquire care management skills. Check the section below on model market development stages, which might help you understand what is going on in your market.

COMPETITION IN THE MARKET AREA

If it is not already a product of the environmental assessment, now is the time to define more clearly the competitive interrelationships in the local market. Using the data gathered, specifically the lists of providers, determine who competes with whom—perhaps grouping those providers who are clearly in competition with each other (e.g., most of the primary care physicians on the north side of town, all seven of the cardiologists located throughout the city). Especially identify those who might be considered competitors of your group.

The next step is rather speculative. At several points, the assessment has gathered precise and not so precise information about the long-term strategies considered by players in the local health care market. Here is where those fragments get tied together.

Define and, where necessary, make guesses about the proposed or likely near-term strategic moves of key competitors in the market area, particularly those faced by your practice. Focus on those physicians and physician groups, along with their possible strategic partners, whose actions could cause you the most harm. Could they secure managed care contracts that you were

seeking? Could they take away contracts you currently hold? Do they dominate a specialty or geographic area that you will need to survive? Do they have a primary relationship with a hospital or physician group that is essential to your strategic plans? Does their access to capital permit them to acquire systems and practices and form strategic joint ventures that give them a significant strategic edge over you? Have they already entered into strategic affiliations or partnerships that may preempt the integrated system you had in mind?

Postulate two or three alternative strategies for each of your primary competitors. "If I were in their shoes, I would first try to build a multispecialty group and, if that was not immediately feasible, I would form or join an IPA. My next best strategy would be to affiliate with the local hospital in a PHO."

Try to anticipate what other players might do in response to each of your competitor's strategic moves. For instance, if a leading primary care group formed a PHO with a key hospital, what would the other primary care physicians do?

Engage in a little bit of "what if?" scenario analysis. Describe a possible or likely set of strategic moves by several competitors and make an informed guess about the responses of the rest of the market.

HOW ENVIRONMENTAL ASSESSMENT RESULTS MIGHT AFFECT STRATEGIC DECISION MAKING

The purpose of conducting all or part of that comprehensive environmental assessment is to inform the strategic decisions that the physicians must make. These are some of the ways to translate that information to the practice's benefit.

- Conclude how quickly it appears that managed care is penetrating the market. Estimate what percentage of market area residents with health insurance will be covered by managed care in three years.
- Conclude how dominant a factor managed care is becoming in the practices of area phy-

sicians—in terms of revenues and patients attributable to managed care. Estimate where it will be in three years.

- Do the same thing for capitation.
- Conclude how quickly the physicians in the market area are developing the ability to manage care, through the implementation of systems that measure cost, quality, and patient satisfaction; to offer incentives to physicians who minimize cost and maximize quality; to screen and credential physicians for their attention to quality, cost, and patient satisfaction; and to follow practice guidelines. Estimate what percentage of the physicians will be practicing under capitation contracts within three years.
- Conclude how quickly the physicians in the market area are moving to integrate their practices with each other and with other providers. Estimate what percentage of physicians in the market area will be locked into one kind of integrated system or another within three years.

USING ENVIRONMENTAL ASSESSMENT RESULTS TO FINE-TUNE AN EXISTING PROPOSAL OR ENGINEER A COMPLETELY NEW ONE

Finally, use this market knowledge to shape your own strategic plans.

- Look for market niches that are not being filled—in terms of geographic area or medical procedure or customer service—and take steps to occupy them.
- Anticipate when a new opportunity is looming on the horizon, one that other market players do not seem aware of, and beat them to exploit the opportunity. When it arrives, you are ready to take advantage of it while the competition is still figuring out what is happening and making plans.
- Anticipate a competitor's move and prepare your organization to counter it immediately, perhaps before it is even announced or

implemented. Do not wait to read about these events in the media and then react. See them coming and be proactive.

- Notice when the supply of a critical resource is running short and grab up what is left. This could be physician practices, space in a favorably located medical office building, or positions on an MCO's provider panel.
- When a new law is enacted affecting health care delivery, quickly interpret it, looking for new opportunities it may create, and move to take advantage before the competition does.
- Recognize weaknesses or vulnerabilities in competing organizations and exploit them. Your action might be a marketing campaign that emphasizes a service or a geographic location that they do not offer. You might raise those weaknesses, with your offsetting strengths, in negotiations with an MCO for an exclusive provider contract.
- After identifying local demographic trends, begin assembling the resources to better serve the coming new population subgroups. This may involve hiring physicians in new specialties (pediatrics or geriatrics) or staff with new language skills, or planning satellite clinics in areas of anticipated population growth.

MODEL MARKET DEVELOPMENT STAGE CLASSIFICATION FOR COMPARISON WITH YOUR MARKET

In order to appreciate how rapidly or slowly your market area is developing, it sometimes is helpful to place it along a model continuum of development stages. Although this model is divided into neatly defined stages, keep a couple things in mind. Few markets will fit completely into any one of these stages—characteristics of a market are often at different stages of evolution. Actual market development is truly continuous. It flows more or less smoothly over time, with occasional abrupt bellwether changes or events. See where your area fits into this framework.

Stage 1. *Living in the past and denial of the present.*

- Physicians practice in traditional settings (solo or small groups).
- Free choice of specialists for referrals.
- Specialists dominate the medical community.
- Hospitals are independent, free-standing entities, which still emphasize inpatient care.
- Employers purchase care from major indemnity insurers.
- Minimal exposure to managed care in contracts, reimbursement, practice style, or organizations.
- Managed care plans are beginning to show up (0 to 10 percent market penetration).
- Reimbursement is on an FFS basis.
- When managed care is discussed, physicians argue with hospitals, and primary care doctors argue with specialists—over control—and nothing changes.
- When MCOs arrive, they will exploit these divisions, playing one party off against another.

Stage 2. *Fish or cut bait: the MCOs arrive.*

- Physicians form and join IPAs that lack serious utilization management.
- Managed care plans begin to proliferate (10 to 30 percent market penetration) and a few leading plans emerge.
- Larger physician groups take shape to cater to the MCOs.
- Demand for hospital beds is declining.
- Employers are forming coalitions to evaluate providers.
- Hospitals are forming alliances with other providers.
- MCOs and provider networks begin contracting with employers, promising more for less and taking patients out of the FFS system—and away from the physicians who have relied on FFS reimbursement.
- It is definitely time to begin affiliating with other practices. If the managed care pressure

is not yet too intense, a loose arrangement with other physicians may be enough for a while. Consider an IPA—you will hang on to your assets and your practice. If large, heavy-hitting MCOs are moving in, no delay is possible. A legal consolidation of assets and integration of clinical practices must be implemented promptly.

- "You'll be able to negotiate more favorable rates and terms with payers if you grow from 6 doctors to 40 or 50, rather than from 6 to 10."[1]
- Whatever the form, your plan needs to emphasize the development of primary care expertise and exercise discrimination in invitations to specialists. Establish and maintain the right ratio of primary care to specialists doctors (1–1 or 2–1 in a fully capitated market).
- Furthermore, you must be able to demonstrate that your group is cost-effective and quality conscious. "Demonstrate" means two things. The physicians must in fact practice cost-effective quality medicine, and the group must regularly collect the data to prove it.

Stage 3. *Here come the hospitals—they want a role in the game.*

- The IPAs implement utilization management procedures.
- Physicians groups are forming rapidly and growing dramatically.
- Physician groups are building linkages with hospitals.
- Formalized provider systems are taking shape.
- Employers establish strong incentives for managed care coverage, and are exercising a strong influence over the health care market.
- Marginal MCOs drop out and a few dominant MCOs emerge (30 to 50 percent market penetration).
- Alliances between provider systems and payers are developing.

- When MCOs become a dominant force in the market (representing 40 to 50 percent of covered lives), their utilization management measures begin to take effect. In particular, hospital admissions and stays decline. The result is predictable and pervasive. Hospitals start to shrink and disappear.
- The hospitals cannot afford to watch idly as managed care takes over and physician groups grow larger. They must and do demand a role in shaping the new health care system. Their inclination is to propose affiliations with doctors—through devices like a PHO—as the sole means of survival for both them and the doctors.
- In the right market situations, physician-hospital affiliations may be the right strategic move. But, caution is necessary.
  - You are likely to affiliate with just one hospital.
  - If the arrangement does not work out, you and the other physician participants will be left in the lurch.
  - Think seriously about the hospital's life expectancy.
  - Hospitals are closing, merging, going bankrupt, and being bought out—all events that could mean the end of the PHO.
  - Many PHOs have not been successful ventures in their own right and have closed down.
  - The key seems to be this: If physicians and hospitals affiliate without doing more, they will fail; if the PHO is viewed as a transitory form as the providers steadily integrate and become adept at managing care, they are likely to succeed.

    There is an assumption that any payer—MCO or insurance company—will prefer to deal with a single integrated group of hospital(s) and physicians or will feel compelled to do so. This is not necessarily true!
  - Some payers want the greater bargaining leverage they have with smaller groups and, if they do have such

groups to negotiate with, may avoid your PHO.
  - More significantly, some payers may simply prefer your group of physicians but a different hospital than the one you are affiliated with.

This is where prior environmental assessment becomes vital and why the shaping of new integrating organizations (PHO or otherwise) must be based on valid strategic considerations.

Look at it this way: It probably is easier for a payer to replicate a hospital, personnel and all, than a group of physicians of varying specialties. Put bluntly, in most situations, the hospital probably needs you more than you need it—but you may still need it.

Stage 4. *Providers start to share risk.*

- More sophisticated and integrated physician-hospital unions have developed.
- Physician groups are larger, more integrated and involve a multitude of specialties.
- Generalist physicians dominate the numbers, the governance, and the management of the provider entities.
- Several regional provider systems compete with each other as an oligopoly.
- Relationships between providers and payers are firm and nearly permanent.
- Regional market is dominated by a few strong, surviving MCOs that operate more and more like structured HMOs (50 to 70 percent market penetration).
- Direct contracting between employers and providers takes place.
- By now, the doctors have come to see managed care as inevitable. They are now integrating wholesale with each other and with other providers, like hospitals.
- At this stage, the way physicians are paid and, therefore, the way they practice starts to change dramatically. Providers (physicians and hospitals) are reimbursed on bases that reward cost-effectiveness and penalize excessive service delivery.

- For many physicians, the new reimbursement form is capitation.
  - Initially, capitation affects mainly primary care physicians.
  - Increasingly, there are capitated payments to practitioners in specialties where utilization is reasonably predictable.
  - Larger groups are more likely to have the resources and expertise to manage risk, and the size necessary to cover enough lives to spread the risk widely.
  - "Many managed care plans are reluctant to offer capitation to individual doctors and smaller groups."[2]

  Note on capitation: Under capitation, a group of physicians assumes responsibility for a given number of "covered lives," not for providing certain kinds of medical services or maintaining certain accessibility (practice hours). Carried a conceptual step further, physician groups see themselves as obligated to meet a full range of health care needs for a "community" of covered lives for a single aggregate lump sum fee (e.g., 1,000 covered lives × $1,250 per year = $1.25 million to meet most all their health care needs).

  > **Hint:** Do not think in terms of, "If I deliver more than $1,250 worth of care to a single patient, I am in a losing position." Do think in terms of, "Even though I may deliver more than $1,250 worth of care to one patient, that patient almost certainly is balanced by another patient who needs no more than $400 worth of care during the same time period. As long as our group is meeting the legitimate health care needs of our 1,000 covered lives through the delivery of no more than $1.25 million in medical services, we are in a winning position."

- Many MCOs prefer to manage and coordinate care themselves (through various forms of utilization and quality management) rather than allow physicians to handle this under capitation or some other form of risk sharing.
- Few providers are yet fully proficient at accepting the risk of potential loss (along with the gain) under a capitated arrangement.
- Few providers and few geographic areas have reached this stage of market evolution. Markets at this stage include California (especially Southern), Minnesota, and Massachusetts. In these areas, some physicians are treating three-quarters of their patients under managed care.

Note for success: At this stage, the groups that are succeeding are

- rather large—100 or more physicians
- focused on primary care—one-third to one-half of all their doctors
- accessible over a wide geographic area
- experienced in managing risk with operating programs, policies, and procedures that control both cost and quality
- able to demonstrate the cost-effectiveness of their practice methods
- able to document the quality of their care (generate outcomes data) and patient satisfaction (collect survey data)

> **Caution:** As the pace of consolidation and integration quickens and spreads to all areas of the country, some markets will move more quickly through these stages—perhaps taking just a year or two to develop from Stage 1 to Stage 4.

Stage 5. *Physician-run IDSs—doctors start to control all the providers.*

- Managed care, usually based on capitation, fully dominates the market place (70 to 85 percent market penetration).
- Physicians are creating large, integrated, multiprovider systems that they own and control.
- Physicians are moving into preponderant positions of governance.

- Physicians are moving into leading positions of management.
- Hospitals are accepted primarily as "brick and mortar" buildings and secondarily as possible sources of capital. Their traditional role of industry leadership disappears almost completely.
- Employers are more sophisticated and insistent in what they expect from the providers and payers of their employees' health care—in terms of performance, systems, and reporting.
- Employers buy health coverage from any entity that can meet their requirements, including physician-run organizations.
- There is resentment from other providers toward the physician-run systems and apprehension from the payers.
- Several physician-run IDSs exist now, but they are not yet a major force in any part of the country.

Stage 6. *Physician-run MCOs—doctors control all delivery and financing.*

- Managed care has advanced about as far as it can in most parts of the country (90 percent market penetration).
- Physician-run IDSs have dominant, and even controlling, market shares in many areas.
- Many of these physician-run systems choose to eliminate the middleman, take on the financing function, contract directly with end payers (employers, as well as Medicare and Medicaid), and essentially become physician-run MCOs.
- Physician entities of all types have acquired the entrepreneurial and business skills, and the access to capital, to compete directly with investor-owned IDSs and MCOs.
- Steadily, health care delivery and financing organizations that are owned, or governed, or managed by physicians are emerging as the standard in the U.S. health care system.
- Today, there are a few physician systems that offer HMO products or have direct contracts with employers, but they are a minority. Lack of capital, business expertise, and ambition currently prevent others from joining them.

REFERENCES

1. D. Murray, "The Four Market Stages and Where You Fit In," *Medical Economics 72*, no. 5 (1995): 44.
2. Murray, *Medical Economics 72*, 44.

RESOURCE LIST

The Center for Healthcare Information publishes a variety of materials and information useful in determining the providers and payers in key marketplaces. They are expensive but probably worth the price if you need such thorough and detailed information. Their offerings include these:

  "1998 Directory of Physician Groups & Networks—IPAs, PHOs, MSOs, PPMCs, Group Practices"

  "Managed Care Local Market Overviews" (available for 71 U.S. markets)

  "Healthcare Provider Mailing Lists"

  "HMO & PPO Database & Lists"

They can be ordered from the following address: Center for Healthcare Information, 4000 Birch Street, 112, Newport Beach, CA 92660, (800) 627-2244.

Feasibility Studies for Practice Expansion, Super Search Packet #4277 (Englewood, CO: Medical Group Management Association, updated annually).

D. Patterson, *Indexing Managed Care, Benchmarking Strategies for Assessing Managed Care Penetration in Your Market* (Westchester, IL: Healthcare Financial Management Association, 1997).

## CHAPTER 15

Step Six: Forming a Physician-Hospital Organization—An Affiliation between Your Group Practice and a Hospital

INTRODUCTION

A very popular way to move toward integration and make oneself a more attractive contracting partner for managed care plans is to deliberately form or join a physician-hospital organization (PHO). This chapter describes the different forms a PHO may take, lists the advantages and disadvantages for participating physicians, reviews the critical issues in the creation of a successful PHO, and lays out a step-by-step formula for putting one together.

WHO SHOULD READ THIS CHAPTER

A solo practitioner or member of a small group practice considering some tentative moves in the direction of collaboration with other providers and more aggressive managed care contracting would be wise to become familiar with PHOs. This is a viable alternative for market areas not yet heavily penetrated by managed care. The PHO is a reasonable first step for a physician who feels uncomfortable selling her practice assets to a management services organization (MSO), integrating her practice with other physicians, or practicing as an employee of a hospital.

When the hospital where you have staff privileges begins talking about a PHO, or physician colleagues suggest working together to obtain managed care contracts, read this chapter for an introduction to the possibilities. If you are looked to as a leader in the local medical community, you may want to propose the formation of a physician-initiated PHO. Learn what that takes in this chapter.

If managed care organizations (MCOs) already are very active in your market, if you accept the need to immediately pursue close integration and risk sharing with other providers, or if you are part of a primary care group that wants to play a leading role in a new integrated delivery system (IDS), a PHO probably is too primitive and tentative a form for you. Read the material on multi-specialty group practices and medical foundations.

WHAT IS A PHYSICIAN-HOSPITAL ORGANIZATION?

A PHO is just what the name says—an organization of physicians and, usually, one hospital who have come together to pursue common purposes. The name has been attached to almost every conceivable combination of physicians and hospitals, including MSOs and medical foundations. For this chapter, PHO refers to the first, often tentative, affiliation of physicians and hospital in response to the threats and opportunities of managed care.

The typical PHO is a joint venture between physicians and one or more hospitals for the purpose of securing managed care contracts. It is a separate organizational entity from its physician and hospital participants. It may take the form of a for-profit business corporation, taxable nonprofit corporation, tax-exempt nonprofit corporation, limited liability company, or general partnership. The participating hospital may be for-profit or not-for-profit. The physicians frequently are organized into their own entity, such as an independent practice association (IPA).

Ten or fifteen years ago, the first PHOs were created by hospitals to organize their medical staff physicians and bond them more tightly to the hospital. Together, they often hoped that this new unity would help them maintain their patient volumes and, if they were lucky, slow the spread of managed care into their markets. Sometimes, they functioned as genuine joint ventures in the acquisition or establishment of ancillary service facilities—such as imaging centers, home care programs, clinical and diagnostic laboratories, or ambulatory surgery clinics.

The hospital often handled most of the start-up tasks and supplied the majority of start-up capital. The most responsible PHOs split their ownership 50-50 between the hospital and the doctors. They were governed by typical boards of directors with equal representation from the two participant groups. Committees of physicians and administrators also were established to deal with credentialing and membership, utilization review and quality assurance, and contract review.

Credentialing standards were no more than the bare minimum necessary to avoid major malpractice problems (acceptable professional liability legal history, current staff privileges at the hospital, and peer reputation for quality practice). Membership in the PHO was open to any physician who met these standards and paid the initiation fee.

The contract review committee made sure that contracts were negotiated to fit the fee schedule guidelines it defined. This particular practice is now legally unacceptable for antitrust reasons. (See "Legal Problems with PHOs" below.)

The utilization review committee usually was not given the authority necessary to have any serious impact on physician practice patterns.

The typical PHO is staffed by hospital employees assigned on a part-time basis, some independent contractors, or a small cadre of full-time staff. Their primary responsibility is the negotiation and maintenance of managed care contracts, some superficial quality assurance work, and general support of physician-hospital relations. Processing of claims is generally handled by a third-party administrator.

Most PHO operating expenses are covered by a 10 to 15 percent withhold on the revenues from the contracts it negotiates. Additional funding may come from ancillary services set up by the PHO or a direct contribution from its managed care partners.

PHO physicians usually are compensated on the basis of a discounted fee-for-service schedule. Risk sharing has not been a part of the PHO tradition.

POSITIVE AND NEGATIVE FEATURES OF PHOS

There are good and bad things to be said about PHOs. Some features may be more pronounced in certain locations and under certain proposed arrangements. This may make the PHO option much more or much less attractive to you. Evaluate and weigh your unique circumstances.

Advantages

- The PHO is relatively easy and inexpensive to form.
- Where there are purchasers currently interested in contracting with such a network, the PHO can have almost immediate success.
- The PHO's contracts and credentialing criteria can be structured in a flexible way to allow for relatively more or less physician risk sharing and a relatively more or less selective (open or closed) physician panel.
- The PHO gives the parties the opportunity to establish an effective working relationship on a contractual basis that may lead to more integrated approaches as necessary.
- The PHO form gives the physicians access to the hospital's capital and management expertise, if it has any of either.

Disadvantages

- There may be antitrust issues if the PHO physician network is too large, is structured to be exclusive, or does not take risk.
- There will be state insurance licensure issues if the PHO seeks to take global capitation.
- Concerns of the Internal Revenue Service (IRS) and the Office the Inspector General in the Department of Health and Human Services will need to be addressed in financing the PHO, particularly the IRS insistence on equal funding between the hospital and physicians in the aggregate.
- A contracting network alone may not be a sufficient competitive strategy in the market. Messenger-model provisions, either to address physician unwillingness to grant the PHO full agency authority or to address antitrust concerns, may render the structure ineffective.
- Because of its overall sponsorship and funding of the PHO, the hospital may end up dominating the relationship.
- There can be substantial political problems if the PHO restricts its physician participation to something less than the entire hospital medical staff.
- The parties to the PHO may feel that formation of this new entity is the only adjustment they need to make to managed care and forget about further integration and changes in their delivery methods.

WHY PHYSICIANS AND HOSPITALS ARE FORMING PHOs

Hospitals have traditionally pursued PHOs in a reaction to declining occupancy rates. They believed that a closer relationship with physicians who do a lot of admitting—that is, specialists—would ensure a steadier flow of patients. The PHO also seemed like a noninvasive, tolerable way of acquiring an increased share of the revenues available through managed care contracts. The fact that the hospital and physicians together could negotiate in a single, louder voice with the managed care organizations also had appeal.

The physicians often joined the PHO for lack of a better idea for responding to managed care pressures. PHO membership offered the promise of maintaining the status quo of independent physician practices, while organizing them into a loose network that, with the participation of a hospital, could bargain more forcefully with MCOs.

These motives would have been viable five years ago. They are completely outdated now.

WHAT PHOs ARE DOING RIGHT NOW[*]

There are PHOs operating in over 40 states. Predictably, they tend to be concentrated in states with greater managed care penetration. Half of the PHOs were less than a year old in 1994. Half had no full-time employees. Two-thirds had medical directors who spent less than a quarter of their time at the PHO. Most of the PHOs are beginning to implement utilization management and case management systems. However, few of them are currently tracking utilization data by physician or payer.

The primary reason (80 percent) providers form PHOs is to **improve their clout in managed care contracting.** Only 72 percent are content that they are achieving that goal. The larger the PHO's number of covered lives, the happier it is likely to be.

About half of the PHOs have a secondary purpose of finding **direct contracting arrangements with employers.** This has been a troublesome road for them.

- State insurance-type laws prevent many PHOs from entering into risk-sharing arrangements with employers. Some have simply insisted that the PHOs obtain licenses as health maintenance organizations (HMOs), with the attendant financial reporting and monetary reserve requirements.

---

[*]The data under this heading are based on an Ernst & Young survey conducted in 1994 and reported in the August 1995 issue of *Healthcare Financial Management.*

- A few PHOs encountered resistance from their current managed care partners, who see the direct contracts as direct competition.
- Some simply overestimated the interest of local employers in direct contracting.
- Other PHOs found that they did not have in place the information and enrollment systems necessary to compete with full-blown managed care plans.
- Most PHOs also do not have the experience or flexibility to offer the full continuum of care sought by many employers, to offer care in the multiple markets where some employers operate, or do not have the variety of managed care products (point of service and indemnity) still popular.

Most of the covered lives served by PHOs come through **low-risk contracts with preferred provider organizations (PPOs).** Over 86 percent of PHOs with PPO contracts did not involve capitation. Still, 52 percent of the PHOs also had contracts with one or more HMOs. Evidence shows that, as PHOs mature, a greater concentration of their covered lives come through HMO contracts. (19 percent of PHOs had HMO contracts covering more than 12,000 lives.)

In measuring the success of their joint ventures, more than 90 percent of PHOs cited performance indicators such as number of covered lives, number of payer contracts, and the profits earned under the contracts by the participating providers. In other words, their primary concerns are **maximizing revenues.**

So far, most of the PHOs are less interested in the more difficult task of reducing costs through economies of scale and tighter operational integration. In over 70 percent of the PHOs, the participating hospitals were not using the entity as a vehicle for **acquiring physician practices.** Although hospitals independently are buying up practices in many parts of the country, this is not an important goal for 70 percent of PHOs.

Today's PHOs are more concerned with the objectives of improving collaboration between medical staff and hospital (60 percent) and assuring the quality of care (63 percent). The happiest

PHOs seem to be those that have created the best working relationships between their doctors and hospitals.

About two-thirds of PHOs have the intent of **sharing financial risk.** Approximately the same percentage has accepted capitation payments under their HMO contracts. The compensation of the participating providers is rather traditional: The primary care physicians and the hospitals stand at risk through capitated fees, fee-for-service withholds, and per diems. Specialist physicians are primarily paid through fee schedules.

The physician component of PHOs is predominantly specialist.[*] Almost 75 percent of PHOs had more than 50 percent specialists. In over 50 percent of the PHOs, specialists composed more than 65 percent of the physician membership. Nearly 60 percent of the PHOs have fewer than 35 percent primary care doctors. Only 21 percent have more than 50 percent.

The PHOs are generally split between open and closed physician panels. The prerequisites to membership on the closed panels include accreditation, board certification, staff membership at the participating hospital, and malpractice protection. Less than half of the PHOs use economic credentialing in screening its physician members.

The future plans of PHOs may be overly ambitious. Almost two-fifths of them intend to merge with other organizations within the next three years, and 40 percent of those expect to evolve into full health plans.

WHY PHOs DO NOT WORK

Historically, PHOs have not been very successful. They have not secured the number of additional managed care contracts originally anticipated. They have not generated the additional revenues expected by their physician and hospital providers. Their operations often are

---

*The common wisdom is that a managed care–driven delivery organization will do best with a 50–50 or even 60–40 primary care to specialist physician ratio.

subsidized by the participants. And, in their original, nonintegrative forms, they are unlikely ever to satisfy the growing demands of MCO partners for tight management of care.

The reasons for PHO failure are these:

- They offer a specialty-dominated, relatively undifferentiated physician panel that lacks the primary care emphasis demanded by managed care.
- They usually are started and largely controlled by the hospital, whose motives are not necessarily attuned with those of the physicians.
- Their original goals are often defensive and designed to somehow get the "goodies" from managed care while maintaining the status quo in hospitals and physician practices.
- There is no commitment to learn and satisfy the desires of the managed care payers.
- There is no commitment to modify physician practice patterns in order to reduce utilization.
- There is no intention to gather the cost, utilization, and quality data needed to understand and manage the care being provided.
- The participants in the PHO are unwilling or unable to invest the capital required for modern information systems, utilization and quality control functions, and future expansion.
- They have few or no full-time operating staff.
- They are managed by chief executives with limited experience managing integrated health care delivery organizations.
- They try to perform with too small operating budgets.
- They have limited capacity to accept and successfully manage capitation and other risk-sharing arrangement with payers.
- Because of the distorted original mission, capital restrictions, and a history of failures, they are limited platforms for growth and evolution.

The critical question for PHOs is whether these faults simply reflect immaturity in the PHO development process or a fundamental belief by PHO participants that they can get by without ever becoming more integrated and ambitious.

FORMING A PHO THAT DOES WORK

The PHO model still has a role to play in strategic plans for some physician practices. Local market dynamics and a physician's current reservations may make a more ambitious venture unworkable for the moment. In such a case, a PHO could be an excellent first step down the path toward physician-controlled integrated provider entity. These are the key steps in putting together a PHO.

Finding a Common Strategic Vision among Prospective PHO Participants

The first step in forming a PHO is defining a common strategic vision that works for both the physicians and the hospital, which is suited to the current competitive climate. It also is the most critical step. Without common ground at the outset, all further efforts will be compromised.

Physicians must overcome their distrust of hospital administrators. Specialist physicians must overcome their disdain for primary care physicians. If the parties start with suspicions, they will only get worse, not better, under the PHO relationship.

A "common strategic vision" means a long-term purpose for the organization that transcends the individual, short-term needs or desires of the participants and that reflects the market realities of the new American health care system. It especially takes into account the competitive dynamics of the PHO's service area. The vision must eventually lead all the participants toward greater integration of their delivery efforts. Simple managed care contracting can only be an evolutionary step toward that final objective.

Deciding Who Takes the Lead in Forming the PHO, Who Will Invest in It, and Ultimately Who Will Own It

The traditional pattern of hospitals conceiving, planning, and implementing the PHO is unacceptable to physicians. This early initiative shapes the entire future of the entity and inevitably produces a bias toward the hospital.

As a physician, if the idea of a PHO seems attractive, do not wait for an area hospital to raise the issue. Begin discussing it with a small group of forward-looking colleagues. Begin the work of gradually mobilizing the best physicians on the hospital medical staff or in your market area into a loose network of practitioners. During this process, identify physician leaders who can speak on behalf of the medical community. Do your best to include a healthy contingent of primary care doctors. Seriously consider pulling the network into a formal organization like an IPA.

Take these initiatives before you have any conversations with the hospital about forming a PHO. If the hospital raises the issue before you start organizing, hold them off until you can gather even a cadre of committed physicians and have a few strategy sessions. Even better is to get organized, get focused, form an IPA, and approach the hospital first about some kind of strategic partnership.

Securing sufficient capital (see Exhibit 15–1) to get the PHO started raises a major problem. Almost invariably, the prospective hospital partner will have more investable capital than an informal group of physicians. Ownership and control of organizations frequently parallels the original investment sources. Physicians must not allow the hospital to buy a dominant position in the PHO, even by default.

As soon as a coherent physician group begins to take shape, commit the physicians to begin accumulating capital individually. Set time-based goals. Establish that the accumulated amounts will be used as initiation fees or to purchase interests in the IPA that is developed. Those IPA funds will constitute the physician contribution to the PHO's capital needs.

The PHO may still have to rely disproportionately on the hospital for start-up capital. In that case, the best solution is to restrict the hospital equity investment to no more than the physician group is able to invest so that ownership of the PHO is divided 50-50 between the doctors and the hospital. The additional money that may be required should be obtained through loans at market terms from a bank or the hospital.

Choosing an Organizational Model: Hospital Ownership, Physician-Hospital Ownership, Physician Participation

The choice of PHO organizational model is a major factor in determining the kind of partnership that will develop between the physicians and the hospital.

Some PHOs are created, owned, and controlled by a hospital, with physicians connected through "participation agreements." The decisions about which physicians may participate and on what terms always lies with the hospital. This model makes no sense for physicians. Reject it.

A large number of PHOs are jointly owned and controlled (often on a 50–50 basis) by a hospital and the several small group practices and solo practitioners that compose its medical staff. This arrangement is tolerable, but suffers from the fragmentation of the physician component. On key issues, the hospital, speaking with one voice, is likely to overwhelm the numerous physicians and physician groups, speaking with many voices.

The ideal model is a PHO owned and controlled equally by the hospital and a single unified physician organization (such as an IPA). The IPA can establish internal procedures for selecting physician members and allowing them to choose their representatives to serve on the board of the PHO. The important difference is that the physicians decide which of their colleagues will participate in the PHO and are able to speak more consistently and forcefully in dealings with the hospital.

Be aware that a hospital that is not accustomed to working with physicians who are organized and assertive may feel threatened by the new solidarity of your IPA. Its response will be the first test of its commitment to a true partnership with physicians.

Exhibit 15–1 Finances of Starting and Running a PHO

The amount of money it takes to form and maintain a PHO depends very much on the number of contracts it negotiates and how aggressively it pursues integration. These are some rough estimates of the costs involved:

Research and preparation	$50,000 to $200,000
Start-up	$1,000,000 to $2,000,000
Ongoing operation	$500,000 to $5,000,000

Source: Data from D. E. Goldstein, Organizational Options for Intergration, *Alliances: Strategies for Building Integrated Delivery Systems*, p. 112, © 1995, Aspen Publishers, Inc.

Designing a Governance Structure That Satisfies Both the Physician and the Hospital

The 50–50 ownership ratio does not guarantee a workable governance structure. The primary governing body is the board of directors. Any arrangement that gives the hospital control of the board or the final vote in case of a tie is unacceptable. Even a formula that gives the hospital and the physicians each half of the board members should be avoided. The hospital representatives will always vote as a bloc. They only need one physician board member on their side in order to prevail.

There is an alternative governance structure used by many PHOs that better protects the interests of the physicians and the hospital. The board is composed of two separate and equal groups—the hospital representatives and the physician representatives. Board votes require the majority approval of both of these groups.

Almost as important as making sure that physicians have a clear, influential role in the PHO is ensuring that primary care physicians are properly represented among the physician group. Keep in mind the current rule of thumb that any provider organization catering to MCOs should maintain a roughly 50–50 ratio between primary care and specialist physicians. Some PHOs have addressed this concern by reserving seats for primary care doctors on both the IPA board and the PHO physician bloc—regardless of the proportion of primary care physicians in the IPA as a whole.

Choosing between For-Profit and Nonprofit Status

Although the PHO is most likely to wind up as a standard for-profit corporation, there may be some arguments for seeking tax-exempt nonprofit status. The trade-offs can be critical.

It is relatively easy and inexpensive to incorporate under state for-profit corporate law. This affords the key benefit of the ability to issue shares of stock in return for investment capital. Sale of stock can be an effective device for raising capital unavailable by other means. Formal ownership interests in the PHO may be an important incentive for participating physicians. The downside of selling stock is the time and expense of complying with federal and state securities laws. Depending on the number and location of prospective shareholders, it often is possible to gain an exemption from these laws. Of course, for-profit corporations also must pay taxes on their earnings.

The appeal of nonprofit corporations is that they do not pay taxes on their income and can accept donations that are tax-deductible to their donors. As a general rule, this organizational option will not be available because the purposes of most PHOs will not qualify for charitable status. Only if the PHO can demonstrate that it is serving a substantial community interest and is willing to restrict physician membership to 20 percent of its governing board might it even consider seeking such status.

Deciding What Physicians and What Kinds of Physicians Will Be Invited To Participate

For many PHOs, deciding which physicians will be invited to participate is a moot question. If the hospital has a dominant role, it is likely to prefer an open panel PHO including any interested physician on its medical staff. This also may seem preferable to avoid the resentment and antagonism that often result when only selected physicians are permitted to join. The hospital also is likely to be quite happy with a large proportion of subspecialists in the PHO, since they will admit more than primary care doctors will.

For serious competition in a managed care world, an open panel PHO does not work. Do not bother joining one. MCOs are attracted to provider organizations that take aggressive steps to manage the cost and quality of the care they deliver. One of the mechanisms MCOs look for is a policy of using only physicians who have a demonstrated ability to practice cost-effective, high-quality medicine. Not all physicians meet these requirements. The MCOs also want to see a primary care/specialist physician ratio in the neighborhood of 50/50. No hospital medical staffs currently have such ratios.

The PHO you join should maintain a **selective panel** of physicians with a primary care focus. The selection criteria should screen in those practitioners who have or show promise of developing the ability to deliver high-quality, low-cost medical care.

It will take more money and time to create and operate a selective PHO. The enrollment and credentialing procedures will be more complex and drawn out. Legal issues must be carefully weighed to avoid violating the rights of the excluded doctors. Even if the selection process is carried out with great care and sensitivity, there are likely to be emotional and political repercussions. Do not underestimate them. Document the need for the screening through market research on the needs of payers. Put the definition of the selection criteria in the hands of respected, knowledgeable leaders in the physician community.

A selective panel PHO must be the ultimate goal. If that is not an immediately workable possibility, consider these approaches. In a market that has not been deeply penetrated by managed care, where there may be two or three more years before competition really heats up, form an open panel PHO right now. But, do it with the understanding and expectation that all physicians will train in delivering managed care, friendly medicine, and that those who do not measure up will have decreasing roles in the organization.

Alternatively, do not even talk about a PHO for the moment. Instead, concentrate on forming an organization of physicians committed to gradually bringing their practices into unison. (This may be an IPA.) They, too, will develop skills that prepare them for managed care. This organization may not necessarily include all members of the medical staff. It may initially execute some physician-only contracts with MCOs. Then, when the group is strong, more experienced, with greater bargaining power, propose to the hospital the formation of a PHO.

Developing PHO Systems for Utilization Review, Quality Assurance, and Physician Credentialing

As an end in itself, the PHO will not succeed. It is a sensible strategic choice only if it moves the provider-members along the path toward managing the care they deliver. From the very beginning, the PHO founders must plan for the restriction of PHO membership to cost-effective physicians, coupled with formal mechanisms for controlling costs and maintaining quality. Managed care plans in an immature market may be more tolerant initially, but they will eventually demand that their contracted providers implement such features. It is preferable to create your own effective credentialing, utilization management, and quality assurance programs and persuade MCO partners to accept them. If you do not take the initiative, the MCOs will tell you how to do it or simply take over the responsibility themselves.

Format through Which the PHO Contracts with Managed Care Plans

Technically, the PHO does not contract with managed care plans. It negotiates the contracts that are entered into between the managed care plans and the hospital and the physicians, individually. The providers are the only entities with the legal authority to deliver medical care. The PHO acts as a sort of broker. Frequently, there is an agreement between the physicians and hospital and the PHO that they, the providers, will accept automatically managed care contracts negotiated by the PHO. Some PHOs give their members a limited opportunity to opt out of certain contracts. That is not a good idea, as it vitiates the PHO's ability to negotiate with MCOs on behalf of a unified, broad-service provider network. It will dilute the market success of the PHO.

Contractual Agreements That Will Be Needed To Connect and Bind the Parties to a PHO

Your lawyer will explain the legal steps required to set up a PHO in the configuration you have chosen. These are the contractual agreements and other legal documents that you are likely to encounter.[*]

Your **first step** is the formation of a physician organization. (If you know that this organization will be an IPA, read Chapter 11, "Step Four: Joining an Independent Practice Association," for more detailed information.) The documents involved in this step are

- Articles of Incorporation—the formal document filed with the state Secretary of State to create the for-profit corporation that is the physician organization.
- Corporate Bylaws—this is the set of rules that you create to govern the working rela-

tionships among the owners, directors, and officers of the physician organization.
- Shareholders' Agreement—this is a contract between the physician organization and its owners (physicians, obviously) controlling how their ownership shares may be transferred, resold, or repurchased. Its purpose is to ensure that the shares remain in the hands of physicians, normally those of the organization's choosing.
- Subscription Agreement—this is the document required by state securities laws setting forth the terms under which the physician members of the physician organization commit themselves to purchasing its shares. It defines the method for determining the purchase price and the necessary qualifications of anyone who purchases shares.

The **second step** is the formation of the PHO itself. This involves a similar set of documents, as follows:

- Articles of Incorporation—the formal document filed with the state Secretary of State to create the for-profit corporation that is the PHO.
- Corporate Bylaws—this is the set of rules that are created to govern the working relationships among the owners, directors, and officers of the PHO.
- Shareholders' Agreement—this is a contract between the PHO and its owners controlling how their ownership shares may be transferred, resold, or repurchased. The owners are the hospital and the physician organization, or if a physician organization has not been formed, independent solo practitioners and medical groups. Its purpose is to ensure that the shares remain in the hands of physicians, normally those of the organization's choosing. It may also restrict the ability of the shareholders to participate in and own any other PHO.
- Subscription Agreement—this is the document required by state securities laws setting forth the terms under which the physician

---

*For model language for these documents, see *Physician-Hospital Organizations*, by Keith M. Korenchuk (Medical Group Management Association, 1994).

organization and the hospital commit themselves to purchasing its shares. It defines the method for determining the purchase price and the necessary qualifications of anyone who purchases shares.

The **third step** is the binding of the hospital, the physician organization, and any independent physicians to provide care to the members of MCOs with which the PHO may negotiate contracts. This is accomplished through documents under which the provider members commit to participating in the contracting network led by the PHO.

- Physician Participation Agreement—through this document, individual physicians or group practices agree to provide medical services to MCOs through participation in the PHO or, if an intermediary physician organization has been established, through participation in that organization. Often, these documents will include basic managed care contracting provisions (e.g., credentialing, quality assurance, capitation reimbursement) in order to preempt the issues in later negotiations with the MCOs.
- Physician Organization Participation Agreement—through this document, the physician organization (if one exists) agrees with the PHO to assemble and contract with individual physicians and group practices to provide medical services to the members of the MCOs with which the PHO contracts. The individual physicians and group practices connect with the PHO through this document. If there is no physician organization, this document is not necessary and the PHO will rely entirely on the Physician Participation Agreements.
- Hospital Participation Agreement—through this document, the hospital agrees to provide hospital services to members of MCOs with which the PHO contracts. It is the counterpart of the Physician Participation Agreement.

The **fourth and last step** is execution of a services contract between the PHO and its member providers, and an MCO. Many states have enacted laws governing the terms of these contracts. Furthermore, the MCO frequently will want to use its own standard contract language, so there may not be much room for negotiation.

- PHO Services Agreement—this document defines the relationship through which the PHO providers deliver health care services to the MCO's plan members. It is a contract between the PHO and the MCO under which the PHO agrees to arrange for the necessary provider services. The PHO does not commit itself to deliver the services; it normally is not authorized or licensed to deliver health care services. Some MCOs may be satisfied with this agreement and the participation agreements that the PHO has with its hospital and physician members.
- Physician Services Agreement—this document is a contract directly between the physician organization and the MCO under which the organization agrees to arrange for its physician members to provide medical services to the MCO's enrollees. This direct link may be required by the fact that only the physicians organization (and not the PHO) is authorized under state law to deliver such services.
- Hospital Services Agreement—this document is a contract directly between the hospital and the MCO under which the hospital agrees to provide hospital services to the MCO's enrollees. This direct link may be required by the fact that only a hospital (and not the PHO) is authorized under state law to deliver such services.

Depending on the nature of the structural relationships making up the PHO and on the range of functions it intends to perform, there may be numerous other documents required. These are the most fundamental and the ones most likely to be encountered.

Case Studies of PHOs*

These are a few examples of more ambitious, successful PHOs.

Akron City Health System (started in 1987)

140 primary care physicians

310 specialist physicians

Started by the medical staff at Summa Health System, a major area hospital. The physicians and the hospital were encouraged by the largest employer in the area, Goodyear Tire & Rubber, which wanted to contract directly with a full-service physician/hospital system.

In addition to dealing directly with self-funded employers, Akron City contracts with a number of HMOs, PPOs, and insurance companies. It also runs its own HMO. The PHO has defined criteria for the kinds of contracting relationships it will accept.

Ownership of the PHO is divided into two classes of stock—one for the physicians and one for the hospitals. It costs a physician $250 to join when she first becomes eligible. If she waits until later, the entry fee is $1,500.

The PHO is governed by a 16-member board, composed of

- 4 primary care physicians
- 4 specialist physicians
- 4 community representatives (chosen by the hospital)
- 4 hospital representatives

Prior to the formation of the PHO, relations between the medical staff and the hospital administration were so good that the physicians did not feel the need to create their own organization before entering discussions with the hospital.

Initially, the PHO allowed all members of its medical staff to join without restriction. However, the organization now is top-heavy with specialists and is considering methods for limiting their

Source: Adapted with permission from "What Makes a PHO Go?," *American Medical News*, © 1994, American Medical Association.

numbers. Economic credentialing is a very serious possibility.

The PHO has both fee-for-service and capitation contracts with its payers. The member physicians are compensated according to a fee schedule. Primary care physicians receive a small increment per member per month for their gatekeeping responsibilities. Physician reimbursement within the PHO will eventually be capitated.

The PHO maintains a 12-physician utilization review committee to assure quality of care. Certain specific procedures require precertification by this committee before they may be performed. Physician "report cards" are in the works.

The PHO has invested nearly a million dollars in a modern information and claims processing system.

California Pacific Medical Services Organization (started in 1992)

150 primary care physicians

250 specialty physicians

The formation of California Pacific followed the merger of two San Francisco hospitals and the integration of four previously independent physician groups that had been affiliated with them.

Its stated mission is to provide cost-effective management services for the participating providers while building a partnership between the physicians and hospital system. It also intends to create an opportunity for physicians to practice high-quality medicine together in a managed care environment.

California Pacific is composed of the hospital system and an organization of the physicians called the California Pacific Medical Group. It is governed by an eight-member board with four representatives each from the hospitals and the physicians. The chairperson of this board is a physician. Certain critical voting issues before the board require a majority of each of the two components (i.e., three physicians and three hospital representatives).

The 400 or so members of the California Pacific Medical Group refer to it as an "IPA plus." It is governed by a board of 14 physicians—8 primary care and 6 specialists. The group maintains no staff of its own, contracting instead with the PHO for any needed services.

The Medical Group includes about 90 percent of the 1,500 physicians on the medical staff of the hospital system. It is facing challenges in trying to integrate department heads from that medical staff into its governance structure without compromising their leadership roles on the staff.

The group recognizes that it has a disproportionate number of specialist members. A moratorium on enrollment of new specialists is in place while it considers options for actually reducing their numbers. One possibility is requiring board certification of all new physicians.

California Pacific is a party to 12 managed care contracts under which it treats over 100,000 enrollees. These contracts account for about 20 percent of the case load for a typical member of the medical group.

Primary care physicians are compensated under their choice of three arrangements—fee-for-service, individual capitation, or group capitation. Specialist physicians are compensated according to a Resource Based Relative Value Scale (RBRVS)-based fee schedule with a risk withhold. There is not complete satisfaction with these arrangements, and they are under regular review.

California Pacific provides a package of utilization management mechanisms to its physicians, including prior authorization, inpatient concurrent review, case management, and performance evaluation. Primary care physicians act as gatekeepers for the specialists, who cannot be seen independently.

The hospital system provides a computerized information system that not only handles appointment scheduling and claims submissions, but also tracks charges and payments by payer and physician reimbursement.

Spectra Health System (started in 1992)

34 primary care physicians

no specialists

After the Chandler (Arizona) Regional Hospital and some of its primary care physicians almost simultaneously tried to enter the market for Medicaid managed care, they saw some value in joining forces in seeking such contracts. The physicians created an IPA, which then joined with the hospital to form the for-profit Spectra Health System corporation. The hospital agreed to channel all its managed care contracts through the PHO and to allow 50 percent of the contract proceeds to go to the physicians. In addition, the hospital contributed most of the start-up capital for the PHO, with the understanding that the physicians would repay 50 percent of that amount from their PHO contract earnings.

The PHO is viewed as only an evolutionary step on the way toward an integrated delivery network. Eventually, Spectra intends to accept financial risk in a managed care setting and maintain a strong market position, while continuing the tradition of local health care provided by local providers.

The PHO is governed by a board made up of three physicians from the IPA and three representatives from the hospital.

All 34 of the IPA's shareholders are primary care doctors. Other physician members practice through contracts with the PHO. The initiation fee for joining the PHO is $1,250. Membership in the IPA is currently closed unless a physician fills a needed specialty, practices in a vital geographic area, or can bring a significant number of managed care patients with him or her.

Physicians belonging to the PHO generate 80 percent of the hospital's revenues. The PHO's contracts account for 52 percent of the hospital's revenues.

Spectra has three capitation contracts that include over 20,000 covered lives. The typical contract is based on a percent of the premium paid to the managed care organization. Spectra also participates in PPO arrangements with three different insurance companies. The PHO receives nearly $80 million in capitated premiums each year.

The primary care physicians bill the PHO at the RBRVS rate with a 15 percent withhold. The specialists used by the PHO are paid a capitated rate.

Spectra operates a utilization management program that includes prospective review, admission and concurrent review, retrospective review, and case management components. Keeping utilization management in-house was a decision calculated to foster physician support.

The PHO has plans to spend nearly a million dollars on a computerized central information system to link its providers and manage utilization data.

Hartford Physician Hospital Organization (started in 1987)

190 primary care physicians
390 specialist physicians

This PHO is a joint venture between the Hartford Hospital and over half of its medical staff. The PHO's stated mission is to "develop an integrated business strategy for selective contracting and medical management." In pursuit of the mission, it is implementing advanced medical management procedures and developing market-focused service products—specifically, arrangements that result in economic risks and rewards shared with the participating hospital and physicians. It also has been establishing strategic alliances with managed care plans that have compatible clinical and business goals.

The Hartford PHO runs on an annual operating budget of about $300,000 that supports $44 million in annual revenues from at-risk contracts.

The PHO is governed by a 12-member board of directors—6 are physicians and 6 represent the hospital. A majority vote (four votes) of each component is required to approve any proposal.

The physicians participating in the PHO are organized into the Hartford Physicians Association. It includes 580 of the 700 doctors on the active staff of the Hartford Hospital. About 60 percent of those 580 physicians are in solo practice. Initiation fees for membership are $1,000 followed by annual dues of $200 to $300. The Association's six-member board is made up of a minimum of two primary care practitioners and at least two specialists.

In order to join the Physicians Association, a physician must be an active member of the medical staff, have a primary affiliation with the hospital (75 percent of each specialist's admissions must be to the Hartford Hospital), be board certified in her specialty, and present testimony from three current Association members that her practice style is compatible with the PHO's mission and medical management goals.

The PHO's current capitated contracts cover 75,000 lives, and the PHO continues to sign more. It also is beginning to engage in direct contracting with area employers. Under most of its managed care contracts, the physicians are reimbursed on a fee-for-service basis with a 15 to 20 percent withhold.

The Physicians Association maintains a Medical Management Committee that monitors quality assurance and utilization review. The committee's 14 members include practicing physicians, clinical chiefs, the hospital vice-president of quality management, the associate director of quality management, the PHO's executive director, and associate executive director. The utilization review procedures employ data provided by insurance companies that identify specific physicians. Counseling is provided to outlier physicians to help them alter inappropriate practice patterns.

Although the hospital is developing a new computerized management information system, the PHO intends to install its own system to ensure that the data it collects are used only for PHO purposes, and not those of the hospital or insurance companies.

LEGAL PROBLEMS WITH PHOs

Because of their combining independent providers into a joint contracting entity, and the lack of integration that follows, PHOs present some real legal risks.

Tax problems: If the participating hospital is tax-exempt and if its capital contributions to the new organization are disproportionately greater than its ownership interest, it may be held to have provided a "private benefit," thereby threatening its charitable status.

Fraud and abuse problems: Hospital contributions or payments to the PHO that exceed its ownership interest may also suggest that it is paying for the referrals that it hopes the PHO physicians will make to the hospital.

Antitrust problems: In conducting compensation/reimbursement negotiations on behalf of many otherwise competing physicians, the PHO may be committing the antitrust violation of price-fixing. Adopting the "messenger model" of negotiation will cure this. In addition, if the PHO is started by the only hospital in town signing up its entire medical staff, it may be engaging in a prohibited form of monopolization.

WHO SHOULD AND SHOULD NOT JOIN A PHO

The chances are that you will not be involved intimately with the formation of a PHO. The hospital where you have privileges and a subgroup of its medical staff will probably offer you the opportunity to join. Whether you accept or not depends to a large degree on your personal circumstances.

Join a PHO if…

- You are a specialist who needs increased access to managed care patients.
- You are under the age of 50.
- You are any age and want to get on the path to managed care.
- You want an increased flow of managed care patients, but want to remain in a solo or small group practice as long as possible.
- You practice in a market that is moving rapidly toward managed care.

Avoid a PHO if…

- You are a specialist serving a unique clientele of private-pay patients.
- You are a hospital-based or employed physician with a guaranteed income.
- You are over the age of 50 and expect to retire before managed care becomes dominant.
- You feel uncomfortable working or collaborating with administrators or other physicians.
- You immediately see the inevitability of managed care and want to move immediately to a more advanced form of provider integration.
- You practice in a market with no managed care on the horizon, or with only one hospital and minimal competition among physicians.

ACTION STEPS FOR PHYSICIANS THINKING ABOUT A PHO

You have come to the conclusion that you are among that group of physicians who might benefit from participation in a PHO. You are open to the possibility of joining a PHO when invited. Here are a few strategic tips to maximize the benefit you gain from such an affiliation.

- Do not join a PHO as a solo practitioner or a member of a small group practice.
- If possible, join a PHO as a member of a large, preexisting physician organization like an IPA.
- Seek a PHO that allots at least 50 percent of the ownership and governance to physicians.
- Seek a PHO that currently restricts provider membership to those who can demonstrate an ability to deliver low-cost, high-quality care or plans to do so in the near future.
- Seek a PHO or a physician organization component of the PHO that allots at least 50 percent of its physician membership and governance to primary care physicians.
- Join a PHO only as an intermediate step toward creation of or participation in a fully integrated, physician-led delivery system.

PATHWAYS TO SUCCESS FOR PHOs

So many PHOs have been in operation for so many years that it is possible to generalize about what the prerequisites are to their success. You are better off avoiding any PHO not committed to these principles:

- The hospital and the physician group share a common vision, agreed to beforehand.
- Neither party (hospital or physician group) pursues MCO contracts, integration initia-

tives, or strategic affiliations outside the context of the PHO.
- The joint entity includes a substantial portion of primary care physicians.
- The participating physicians maintain offices well distributed among the region's population centers.
- The PHO moves quickly to install systems to measure and adjust utilization rates of all participants—individual and institutional.

- The PHO starts with sufficient capital to support ongoing operations and planned further growth.
- The PHO moves quickly to enter into capitation contracts binding both the physicians and the hospital.
- The PHO participants have demonstrated skill in delivering high-quality, cost-effective medical care. If they do not currently possess the skill, they move quickly to acquire it and gather data to show that fact.

RESOURCE LIST

Hospital Affiliated IDS: Formation, Operation and Contracts Handbook (Washington, DC: American Health Lawyers Association, 1995).

Hospital Group Affiliations—Contracts, Information Exchange #4800 (Englewood, CO: Medical Group Management Association, 1995).

"In Managed Care Markets, Deals between Hospitals and Doctors Take Some Unexpected Forms," *Hospitals & Health Networks*, 5 January, 1998.

Integrating Healthcare Information Systems: A Strategic Development Approach for PHOs and Other Physician-Hospital Alliances (Alexandria, VA: Capitol Publications, 1995).

T. Murphy and T. Hardy, *Hospital-Physician Integration, Strategies for Success* (San Francisco: Jossey-Bass, Publishers, 1994).

Physician Hospital Organizations, Book #4541 (Englewood, CO: Medical Group Management Association, 1994).

"Physician-Hospital Organizations: The 'Training Wheels' of Tomorrow's Provider-Sponsored Networks?" *Journal of Health Care Finance*, 22 June, 1996.

CHAPTER 16

Step Seven: Partnering with a Management Services Organization or Physician Practice Management Company

INTRODUCTION

A lot of media attention recently has been given to physician practice management companies (PPMCs)—because they are a visible, new form of for-profit health care delivery venture that seem to have some respect for physician control over clinical decision making. But, is this enough to offset the PPMCs need to produce bottom-line results that satisfy investors?

Under the independent practice association (IPA) and physician-hospital organization (PHO) option, participating physicians and group practices retain management responsibility for virtually all aspects of their medical practices. By entering into a management relationship with a management services organization (MSO) or PPMC, physician groups take an active, yet partial, step toward integration by turning over the business management, but not the patient management, of their groups to professional managers. Sale of the physicians' assets to the MSO/PPMC is usually part of the deal. A whole variety of benefits flow from this commitment, not the least of which is the opportunity presented to reorganize and reenergize the group, make adjustments to its structure and governance, fund essential new capital projects, and introduce a new sense of business discipline.

This chapter describes the basic MSO/PPMC concept, how it often is initiated, and the relationship physician groups have with it. The types of services provided by the MSO and how they can be expanded to foster closer integration are examined. Some of the pitfalls in MSO/PPMC negotiations and dealings are identified.

The purpose of this chapter is to help physician groups see the incremental benefits of an MSO/PPMC connection and how it may move them further along the path toward participation in a true integrated delivery system (IDS).

WHO SHOULD READ THIS CHAPTER

An MSO or PPMC will have appeal mainly for physicians who are willing, immediately, to surrender legal and practical control over many aspects of their practices to an organization with nonphysician management. In return, they are relieved of virtually all practice management headaches, and they receive a substantial cash payment for their assets. If such an arrangement with an MSO seems like a good, quick answer to the increasing pressures of billing procedures, claims filing procedures, and general practice management, read this chapter.

Involvement with an MSO/PPMC also has strategic value as a positive step along the path toward consolidation and integration of physician practices. Whether the step makes sense for you depends upon the ownership and governance structure of the MSO/PPMC, your preferences for physician control of health care delivery, and your group's ability to generate investment capital. This chapter explains these variables.

Even if you have reservations about the basic MSO/PPMC format, read the chapter to learn about the several MSO/PPMC variations that may accommodate your concerns.

If you and some physician colleagues are looking for an organizational form that streamlines the management of your practices while providing an integration vehicle for developing managed care skills and contracting with managed care organizations (MCOs), consider starting your own MSO. If you are committed to competing actively in the managed care marketplace, but lack the capital for growth and systems development, the MSO/PPMC may be the answer. For that reason, definitely read this chapter.

Perhaps you have seen the media reports and journal articles about PPMCs like PhyCor and MedPartners. You really are not interested in selling your practice just now, but are intrigued by all the fuss about this new integration model. This chapter will tell you what you need to know.

If you already are a member of a highly integrated group practice or a medical foundation, or otherwise no longer have independent responsibility/ownership of your medical practice, this topic is moot. You have moved beyond this stage. Skip it.

WHAT IS AN MSO?

The term "MSO" is often used generically to describe both MSOs owned by physicians, hospitals, or MCOs and PPMCs owned by private investors. The vast majority of the largest of these entities have been formed by either hospitals or private investors.

In its most basic form, an MSO is an independent organization that purchases the physical assets of a physician's practice, leases them back to her, and provides her with comprehensive practice management services for a fee.[*] The MSO may be owned entirely by a hospital, jointly by physicians and a hospital, or entirely by a group of physicians, or it may be operated as a

for-profit corporation owned by shareholders and dedicated to profit maximization.

The physician continues to own the "practice"; that is, the provider number, the medical records, the patient list, and the overall goodwill. The relationship with the MSO is a contract for management services. The physician still practices as an independent provider; she is not employed by the MSO. All of the physicians participating with the MSO in a particular area usually organize themselves into a separate incorporated group.

An MSO offers three primary attractions to a solo physician or a small group physician. First, it provides a full range of practice management services. By using these services, the physician relieves herself of the responsibility of functioning as a business manager for her practice. She often is not well trained for this duty, does not especially enjoy it, and would prefer to be directly delivering medical care. The MSO employs experienced practice managers with skills in all phases of operating a medical practice. Solo or small group practitioners could not independently afford such expertise.

A second major feature of an MSO is the access to capital it offers. As a for-profit investor-owned organization large enough to manage many physician practices, it is able to raise substantial funds through the sale of shares or the negotiation of loans. The proceeds may then be invested in the expansion of those practices or the acquisition of the new systems required by managed care—information, quality assurance, or utilization management.

When she initially sells her practice assets to the MSO, the physician often receives a substan-

---

*There are two more basic forms of MSO that do not at all involve the purchase of practice assets. The first type offers nothing but management services, on an a la carte basis. You may purchase and separately pay for accounting services, billing services, claims filing services, coding services, and the like. The second kind of MSO offers complete packages of services for managing an entire practice. They are purchased for a single all-inclusive price.

tial lump sum of money in payment. Some MSOs, particularly those owned by hospitals, have been willing to pay handsome amounts to bind physicians to their facility. This can be an unique opportunity for a physician to cash in the equity in her practice. With the movement toward managed care, it is not easy to sell a physician practice to another physician.

Finally, an MSO can connect the physician practice to a network of hospitals and other practices for the purpose of managed care contracting, as well as conducting the contract negotiations in expert fashion. This third feature is generally the only one a physician enjoys when participating in a PHO.

Generally, an MSO concentrates on providing practice management and managed care contracting services. Participating practices may also enjoy some economies of scale as a result of consolidation of their operations and purchasing through the MSO. Physicians under contract with an MSO usually view the management fee they pay as an overhead expense.

There is one added benefit of dealing with an MSO. It frees you and your practice group colleagues to rethink your strategic plans for the future. Some of the opportunities that may become available are

- reorganizing the way the physicians in the group interact with each other
- redefining your long-term goals for the group
- calculating a new compensation formula for the group
- identifying new affiliation paths and partners beyond the MSO connection
- placing renewed emphasis on quality measurement and assurance
- deciding to build the kind of information-gathering system that enhances your managed care marketability
- committing to significant changes in practice style

The breathing room to do this fresh thinking may be the greatest appeal of the MSO.

Recommendation: The most constructive attitude toward joining with an MSO is that it is the beginning of your collaboration with other like-minded physicians and professional practice managers to position yourselves optimally for a managed care future. It is not an end in itself. You will have a lot more work to do in adjusting your practice style and integrating more closely with other providers.

WHAT IS A PPMC?

Look at a PPMC as an MSO on steroids. Many of them resemble MSOs in that part of their business is based on management services contracts with IPAs. They do not purchase the assets of the physicians belonging to the IPA. The contracts typically run for 5 to 15 years. Under them, the PPMC provides management services and negotiates managed care contracts in return for a regular fee. In addition to a possible reduction in operating expenses and increase in practice revenues, the physicians are able to deal with one entity, the PPMC, rather than multiple MCOs when dealing with preauthorizations, referrals, and formularies.

On the side of the PPMC business that has attracted so much attention, the PPMC acquires the tangible and intangible assets (excluding real estate) of solo and group practices for a one-time payment of cash, stock in the PPMC, or a combination of the two. The PPMC simultaneously forms a professional corporation that signs employment agreements with the physicians. The nonphysician staffs of the practices become employees of the PPMC.

The physicians elect the board of directors that run the professional corporation. They also are left in charge of all clinical decision making. Business decisions, on the other hand, are handled by a separate board composed equally of physicians and PPMC officials.

There is a service contract between the PPMC and the professional corporation through which the PPMC provides practice management expertise, strategic planning, infrastructure and systems development, access to managed care contracts, and capital. The PPMC will also try to bring some economies of scale by centralizing employee benefits, purchasing, malpractice insurance, and the recruitment of staff and physicians. In return for this, the physicians pay the PPMC a management fee equal to 15 to 20 percent of their practice profits. That is profits, not revenues. The contract may run for 20, 30, or even 40 years. At the end of that term, the contract may be renewed or, if not, the practices and their nonphysician employees revert to the physicians. The assets may be bought or leased back.

MANAGEMENT SERVICES TYPICALLY PROVIDED BY AN MSO/PPMC

The actual services available from a particular MSO/PPMC depend on the scope of its own expertise. They can include some or all of the following:

- billing and collection
- utilization management
- quality assurance
- physician recruitment and credentialing
- shared laundry services
- organizing CME programs
- general accounting (A/R and A/P)
- supplies purchasing (clinical, office)
- vendor contract negotiations
- management of payroll, benefits, and workers' comp
- employment and supervision of nonprofessional staff
- information system installation and management
- payer contract negotiations (including managed care)
- medical records management
- marketing and public relations
- financial management (budgets, MIS, reporting, debt management)
- equipment purchase and maintenance
- facilities planning and management

In many cases, these services are available in various combinations, up to and including complete turnkey practice management packages.

METHODS OF PAYING THE MSO/PPMC FOR ITS MANAGEMENT SERVICES

Physicians and groups obtaining services from an MSO/PPMC will pay for these services according to several different formulas.

- A fixed monthly fee is charged for each service or bundle of services.
- The physician group is charged a percentage of either its gross billings, its collected revenues, or its capitation revenues.
- The MSO/PPMC charges a fixed amount per capitated member served by the physician group.
- The physician group covers all the operating costs of the MSO/PPMC plus an additional percentage as "profit."
- The MSO/PPMC receives a fixed amount according to one of the above formulas, plus an "incentive bonus" if its meets certain performance objectives, such as reducing costs by a certain amount or adding a number of new physician practices.
- The MSO/PPMC receives all revenues, minus a predetermined amount for physician compensation paid to the physician group.
- Out of total revenues, the physicians receive a predetermined compensation figure and the MSO/PPMC has all of its actual or budgeted costs covered. Any remaining revenues are divided between the physician group and the MSO/PPMC according to a predetermined formula. Any shortfall revenues causing the physicians to earn less compensation or the MSO/PPMC to operate at a loss is taken into account in the next year's budget negotiations between them.

One important factor to keep in mind about any compensation arrangement is that any payments made by the physicians to the MSO must be at or near fair market value. To do otherwise risks violation of the fraud and abuse and Stark laws. This danger is heightened if a hospital is a sponsor of the MSO.

Caution: Think about where the money comes from to pay the management fee of the MSO/PPMC. If the PPMC's management of practice operations is unable to reduce expenses and its negotiation of managed care contracts does not produce additional revenues, every dollar of management fee must be taken out of physician compensation. It is possible for a physician's income to decline after selling out to a PPMC. This makes it very important to check the PPMC's financial track record in managing the other practices it has acquired.

ALTERNATIVE ORGANIZATIONAL MODELS FOR AN MSO

Joint Physician-Hospital–Owned Model

A new for-profit MSO corporation is formed and jointly owned by a hospital and physicians. The MSO provides practice management services to solo physicians and physician groups. The physicians contribute their tangible practice assets to the MSO in return for up to a maximum of a 50 percent interest in the MSO. The hospital makes a capital contribution equal to the total value of the assets contributed by the doctors.

If additional funding is needed, the hospital may make further capital contributions and receive more than a 50 percent share in the MSO. It might also loan money to the MSO, at fair market rates and terms. The physicians usually are formed into a single, large professional corporation, or several medical groups, owned entirely by the physicians. The MSO manages the practice of the professional corporation, bills for the medical services it delivers, leases the equipment and space it uses, employs the nonclinical personnel needed, and provides a variety of administrative services. The professional corporation employs the physicians and other clinical personnel. The physicians and the hospital share in the profits and losses of the MSO in proportion to their ownership interests.

Hospital-Owned MSO Model

A hospital forms or uses an existing subsidiary as an MSO to provide practice management services to individual physicians, group practices, or a single, large professional corporation. The hospital provides all the capital funding for the MSO. The MSO purchases the tangible practice assets of the physicians for cash and may assume their space leases. The MSO also manages the physicians' practices and bills for their medical services under a management contract. While the MSO is owned and controlled by the hospital, the physicians may be permitted a minority role in the governance of the MSO.

Investor-Owned PPMC*

A group of entrepreneurs sets up a for-profit PPMC. They hang on to most of the corporate stock themselves, but reserve plenty of shares to trade with physicians for their practice assets. The PPMC aggressively acquires new practices, which produces a steady growth in revenues. At the same time, it uses a combination of professional management expertise and judicious capital investment to reduce the expenses and increase the revenues of already-acquired practices. The expectation is that when the PPMC becomes large and successful enough, it will have a public offering of its shares, and the founders and affiliated physicians will realize substantial appreciation in the value of their shares.

---

*There is an interesting, brief discussion of physicians forming their own PPMC in the article, "Practice Management Companies Improve Practices' Financial Position," in *Healthcare Financial Management,* November 1997, p. 56.

MOTIVES FOR THE FORMATION OF AN MSO

The circumstances facing some physicians may encourage them to play a active role in forming as MSO. Even if your desire is simply to use the services of an MSO, it is a good idea to understand the motives of those who started and manage the MSO to which you will assign your practice.

- *Facilitating physician organization and consolidation*

Hospitals have an interest in helping their physicians, those on their medical staffs, to begin consolidating their practices in preparation for joint managed care contracting. Of course, the hospital hopes and expects that the physicians will want the hospital as a strategic partner in most of their contracting. A popular tool of support is an MSO sponsored by the hospital. The hospital typically creates the MSO as either a separate corporation or as a division of the hospital corporation. The hospital invests in the MSO the capital that is used to purchase the physicians' practice assets.[*] The management services that are provided by the MSO to the physicians improve operating efficiency and make the physicians more effective managed care partners. The physicians do not have to spend the often-considerable sums of money required to reengineer their practices. A number of hospitals have established MSOs in conjunction with a PHO.

---

*The hospital may subsidize many aspects of the MSO's operation and, through it, the development of the physician group's infrastructure. However, it is essential that the amounts paid by the MSO for the physicians' practice assets and the amounts paid by the physicians for the MSO's management services be fair market values. Any significant deviation threatens violation of the fraud and abuse laws and the tax-exempt status of the hospital, if it has so qualified.

- *Enabling physician recruitment by a group practice*

Large or growing physician group practices can have difficulty recruiting new members when the value of the assets are so large that often young recruits cannot afford the capital investments required to join the group as a partner or shareholder. This problem can be reduced if the hard assets of the group are moved into a separate organization—the MSO—that simply leases them to the group. The physicians in the group form a separate corporation for this purpose and will own interest shares in it. Without the large and expensive fixed asset overhead, the group needs much smaller capital contributions from the new physicians it recruits.

There is the potential of an added benefit. If the MSO is run efficiently and grows, it may turn into a money-making venture for the physician owners. Shares in the MSO may be offered as inducements for new physicians who have the money to invest.

- *Cashing in physician investment in their practices*

The notion that a physician-owned MSO can be a profitable investment is carried a step further in what is known as the "physician equity" model of an MSO. The goal here is to create an organization that acquires enough physician practices, manages them so efficiently, and perhaps steers them into so many remunerative managed care contracts that ownership shares can be sold to outside, nonphysician investors at a capital gain to the physician investors. The challenge is to earn enough profits to attract the outside investors without depriving the MSO of operating capital it needs to do its basic job—managing physician practices.

- *Earning a profit for nonphysician investors*

In this case, the MSO also is founded and operated for the primary purpose of earning profits and creating capital gains. The difference is that the investors reaping the gain are nonphysicians. Indeed, to facilitate the liquidity of their MSO investments, its shares of stock may be publicly traded. These entities are more commonly referred to as PPMCs. Physicians affiliating with this kind of MSO should bear the same caution: Will profits be emphasized at the expense of proper support for their practices?

- *Channeling of physician referrals to the hospital*

Candidly, the bottom-line reason most hospitals develop MSOs for their medical staff physicians is to lock in the referrals they make to the hospital. They are simply trying to survive and referrals are their lifeblood. Keep this in mind as you discuss PHO possibilities with them. Look for the fewer, more enlightened hospitals that seek true partnership with their physicians in forming modern, integrated delivery organizations—even if it means reduced admissions in the short-term.

- *Maximization of profits for the shareholders*

All the largest, most successful PPMCs have been formed by private investors with one intention—to maximize the return on their investments. This is not necessarily a bad motive if they are looking at returns in the long run. In that case, they usually will see the need to build respectful working relationships with their doctors. The wisest PPMCs welcome physicians into positions of authority, particularly over clinical matters.

Be aware of those PPMCs put together by entrepreneurs in for the quick kill. They begin buying physician practices for company stock rather than cash. They tell the doctors that their reward will come when the company goes public and the stock price appreciates. The founders are not especially adept at managing the practices to improve their efficiency. Instead they generate increasing revenues by acquiring more and more practices. When the market looks ripe, there is an initial public offering (IPO) of stock. The entrepreneurs sell all their stock and bail out. The market quickly realizes that the PPMC is just a collection of poorly managed practices with no long-range plans. The stock price plummets. The physicians are left with near-worthless stock and uncompetitive practices.

REASONS FOR SELLING YOUR PRACTICE ASSETS TO AN MSO/PPMC

The prospect of selling all the tangible assets of your medical practice (even for a healthy sum of money) should give you pause. You are giving up possession and control of the most visible manifestation of the practice—the real estate, equipment, and materials essential to delivering medical care. If the MSO fails or you become unhappy with its services, you generally will be unable to recover title to your assets. It makes sense to understand the good reasons for selling in the first place.

- *You are tired of spending more time managing your practice than delivering medical care.* You would be quite happy placing that responsibility in the hands of a professional practice manager, particularly if you are able to cash in your assets at a good price at the same time. You are not especially concerned with assuming a leadership role in all these changes. You may see retirement on the horizon and want to concentrate on being a doctor until then.
- *You want to cash in the value of your tangible practice assets.* Either because you are looking forward to retirement or just realize that the days of free-standing solo or small group practices are numbered, you may decide that now is the best time to turn the hard assets of your practice into cash. Depending on your specialty, you are likely to have difficulty simply selling out to another physician. The MSO offers the opportunity to realize that cash without really giving up your clinical practice at its present location.
- *You would like to invest in a rapidly growing business in a booming industry about which you have special knowledge.* If you have the

chance to become a shareholder in the MSO to which you sell your assets, you might view the entire transaction as primarily an investment decision. You should expect to receive those shares instead of money in payment for the assets. This option requires a strong belief that the MSO is more than just a competent practice manager, but that it also has the vision and resources to grow and prosper financially. If this is your motive for selling, you should give the MSO the same scrutiny you would any other venture to which you entrust your life savings.

- *You wish to affiliate with people and organizations that have strategic plans to embrace and exploit the managed care revolution. Rather than simply practice medicine in a low-profile, low-risk setting for as long as you can, you intend to aggressively shape your future role as a health care provider. Knowing your own limitations, you wish to become part of a larger, more influential provider group and gain access to greater managerial expertise and financial resources. You find all of this in an MSO and its associated physician group.*

ADVANTAGES AND DISADVANTAGES OF THE MSO/PPMC OPTION

As you are considering the possibility of selling your practice to an MSO or PPMC, that is, to a hospital or a group of private investors, weigh these pros and cons.

Advantages

- It is the simplest form of some kind of meaningful integration.
- It also can be a significant first step toward much more comprehensive integration.
- It allows physicians to affiliate and begin integration with a hospital without becoming major investors.
- It addresses corporate practice of medicine prohibitions in states where this is an issue.

- The physicians retain ownership of their practices, medical records, patient lists, and provider numbers.
- Where the purchase price is paid in cash, the physician realizes a significant capital gain on the investment in her practice.
- The physicians have a vested interest in the MSO/PPMC's success because management of their medical practices is involved.
- The physicians have a further vested interest in the MSO/PPMC's success when they also have an equity interest in the organization.

Disadvantages

- Depending on the level of MSO services provided, it often requires large capital investment.
- The MSO relationship cannot compel physicians to refer to the sponsoring hospital.
- It offers less integration than more advanced options like a Medical Foundation or an IDS.
- Once the tangible practice assets are sold, the physician loses a lot of leverage with the MSO/PPMC and the option of easily reestablishing her original practice.
- An unreliable or insensitive MSO/PPMC management can steer the practice development strategy for its affiliated physicians in unplanned directions unacceptable to them.
- The strategic advantages that PPMCs offer to their participating physician groups do not always materialize because of cultural incapability and lack of shared vision and values among the groups.
- The specialist oversupply may lead to declines in specialist referrals and revenues that create financial difficulties for single specialty or disease-focused PPMCs.
- It does not provide a vehicle for physicians and hospital to align their incentives and share in cost savings from managed delivery of inpatient and outpatient care.
- There is little evidence that PPMCs have been able to improve the operating efficiencies or create significant new revenues for the practices they acquire.

- The management fees of those PPMCs that cannot reduce operating expenses and increase revenues for their physicians will simply come out of the physicians' compensation.
- It normally will not qualify for tax-exempt status and, therefore, enjoy tax-exempt financing.
- There are potential inurement and private benefit issues in connection with tax-exempt hospital funding or subsidization of ongoing operations.

GUIDELINES FOR NEGOTIATING WITH A PPMC

The sale of your practice assets to a PPMC should entail detailed negotiations. After all, it means giving up control of the tools of your profession, the means by which you earn your livelihood. Here are some tips for planning and conducting those negotiations.

- Do not sign a Letter of Intent with language that restricts you from talking with other PPMCs.
- Do not give the PPMC detailed financial data about your practice until you are very near to closing a deal.
- Hire professional advisors (at least an attorney and an accountant) with knowledge of physician practices and PPMCs and experience in helping physicians negotiate with PPMCs. Count on them for:
  - general business advice
  - conduct of the negotiations with the PPMC
  - review of the contract language
  - conduct of the due diligence process
  - evaluation of references from the PPMC
  - assessment of the PPMC's senior management
  - analysis of the PPMC's past performance and financial stability

- Conduct a thorough version of the traditional "due diligence" process, gathering as much information as possible about the PPMC and its prior history.
- Ask the PPMC to lay out in detail its corporatewide long-term strategic plan. Is it simply trying to buy up as many practices as it can or does it also intend to improve the operating performance of those it has acquired?
- Ask the PPMC to explain its strategic plan for your particular market.
- Ask the PPMC to propose the business plan it will implement for your practice, if you agree to sell.
- Ask the PPMC to point to the competitive features that distinguish it from other health systems and PPMCs in the market.
- Review in detail the financial history of the PPMC, both in your market and nationwide.
- Review the career histories of the top executives of the PPMC, as well as those persons who will directly manage your practice.
- Get the names of physicians already affiliated with the PPMC and interview at length as many of them as possible.
- Make site visits to the PPMC and spend time (even social time) with key PPMC officials to see if the organization's culture and personalities match yours.
- Look very closely at how the PPMC handles utilization management, risk management, quality assurance, and the role of primary care physicians.
- Research the current value of the PPMC's stock, its historical trends, and experts' opinions on where it is headed in the future.
- Check the Form 8-K that all publicly traded PPMCs must file with the Securities and Exchange Commission (SEC) to learn the prices they have paid for other practices.
- Ask these hard questions of the PPMC officials:
  - When will their efforts at reducing practice expenses and increasing revenues at least offset the management fees you will pay them?

- What recourse do you have if, in fact, the practice expenses increase and revenues decline under the PPMC's management?
- If a major share of the purchase price for your practice assets will be paid in PPMC stock shares and the value of that stock will depend largely on a public offering so it can be publicly traded, what assurance can the PPMC give that the offering will take place?
- What assurance can the PPMC give that its current policy of physician control over clinical decision making will be maintained?
- What assurance can the PPMC give that any of its policies or promises will not change if it merges with or is acquired by another PPMC?
- Since so much of the success of the deal depends on competent performance by the PPMC of its managerial duties, can you pull out if its performance does not measure up?
- In general, under what circumstances and terms can you withdraw from the agreement with the PPMC (including recovering your practice assets)?
- How does the PPMC aim to balance the clinical needs of doctors and patients with the profit needs of investors and the stock market?

• You will never again have as much negotiating leverage as you do just before you sign with the PPMC. Use it to full advantage.

Key Advice: There are two pieces to a deal with a PPMC. One is the large sum of money you will receive immediately for selling your practice assets. The other is the potential for future growth in the performance and value of the practice. Unless you expect to retire within five years, it would be a serious mistake to focus on the sell-out price and ignore the PPMC's ability (or inability) to grow your practice over the long run.

BASIC QUESTIONS TO ANSWER BEFORE SELLING OUT TO AN MSO/PPMC

As you examine the usefulness of the MSO/PPMC model for your purposes, gain an understanding of these critical issues:

• Who or what owns and controls the MSO/PPMC?
• What is the purpose for which the MSO/PPMC was formed?
• What are the functions and services the MSO/PPMC offers to perform?
• Can you live and work with them for the remainder of your career?
• How do you feel about being wedded to a particular hospital or group of managers for the indefinite future?
• How do you feel about practicing medicine under the aegis of a purely profit-driven business corporation?
• What are their future plans for the management of the practices like yours, especially in the way that they will interface with the managed care industry?
• Will the MSO/PPMC and its owners still be able to meet your needs five years from now?
• Will further integration and even risk sharing be possible under your MSO/PPMC model?
• How do physicians fit into the governance structure of the MSO/PPMC?
• What procedures are in place to protect physician authority over clinical decision making?
• Are you willing to give up the security of owning all the assets of your practice?
• How onerous have your business duties become and how much do they take away from your enjoyment of clinical practice?
• How much capital does your group need to carry out the growth strategy you have in mind, and what capital sources do you have access to?

CHOOSING THE RIGHT MSO/PPMC PARTNER

There are two decisions to make regarding the owner or sponsor of the MSO/PPMC to which you sell your practice. The first concerns the type of partner. Do you feel more comfortable selling out to and having your practice managed by a hospital, a separate group of doctors, a doctor group to which you belong, or a profit-motivated group of nonphysician investors? Then, within your preferred category, which hospital, physician group, or investor group would you like to affiliate with?

In choosing the type of partner, there are some biases to look out for. If the MSO/PPMC is owned by a hospital, do they have physician interests at heart or are they simply trying to fill beds? If the MSO/PPMC is jointly owned by physicians and a hospital, do the physicians have a prominent role in the governance? If physicians are the exclusive owners of the MSO/PPMC, do you know them, are they competent managers of a large organization, and are their strategic goals for the MSO/PPMC network of practices consistent with yours? If the MSO/PPMC is owned by nonphysician investors, pay close attention to their long-term plans for competing in the managed care marketplace. Are they out to maximize short-term profits at all costs or do they see the value of building an enduring relationship with their physician partners?

Once you have settled on a type of MSO/PPMC, check the following characteristics of each potential partner:

- its cultural and philosophical fit with you and your group
- its financial history and current condition
- the personnel and other resources it will apply to the management of your practice

- its operational history in managing physician practices
- its understanding of general physician concerns and values
- its familiarity with the market in which you compete
- its management style—how it reaches decisions and solicits the views of its physician clients
- the incentives built into the MSO/PPMC relationship and the goals they encourage
- if the MSO is hospital-owned, a willingness to give appropriate emphasis to ambulatory over inpatient care
- if the MSO is hospital-owned, operational and strategic management of the MSO is handled apart from the management of the hospital

Of course, in smaller markets, you may have a more limited choice of MSO/PPMC options. When it comes to negotiating the acquisition price, bear in mind the rules of thumb in Exhibit 16–1.

RELATIONSHIP OF THE PHYSICIAN GROUP TO ITS INDIVIDUAL MEMBERS

Affiliation of a physician group with an MSO or PPMC requires rethinking the ways that the group relates to its member physicians. This is because the management of physical assets is no longer a concern of the group, while planning for ongoing integration is now a primary focus.

The organization and direction of the group must move from protection of the interests of individual physicians to enhancement of the good

---

Exhibit 16–1 Typical Terms of Practice Acquisitions by PPMCs

- Typical purchase price for physician practices is five to seven times its estimated profits.
- Payment is typically one-half in cash and one-half in stock, though the formula can vary dramatically depending on the PPMC, the group being acquired, and the market location.
- The practice price will include the tangible and intangible non–real estate assets of the practice. Goodwill is the primary intangible asset.
- There is a potential tax benefit in that the sale proceeds will be taxed at a lower capital gains rate.

of the entire group. The documents binding each physician to the group (the partnership or employment agreement) must prevent activities that might threaten the group's long-term success.

Specifically, the physician group should make the following requirements:

- Physician group has the sole authority to establish policies and procedures regarding the acceptance and treatment of patients.
- All work performed by the physician will be subject to review by the physician group.
- Physician group will establish each physician's work schedule.
- Each physician will devote his full time and attention to practicing medicine within the group; moonlighting in any way that might compete with the group will not be allowed.
- Physician group will set and adjust, as it finds appropriate, the professional fees charged for the physician's services.
- All revenues produced by the physician's work will accrue to the group rather than the individual physician.
- Physician group will have the sole authority and responsibility for managing the business side of the physician's practice.
- Physician group is the owner of the medical records and client lists generated by the physician's practice.

Special attention should be given to the duration and renewal of these agreements. In the case of new physicians unknown to the group, terms should be kept short (one or two years) and renewal should require deliberate action by the group following assessment of her performance. Once a physician has established her competence and reliability, it is possible to consider longer terms with automatic renewal.

The biggest problem for an MSO/PPMC-based physician group is departing physicians. The long-term prosperity, stability, and reputation of both the group and the MSO/PPMC depend on building a cadre of committed doctors. Each time a physician leaves, the group must bear the costs of lost revenue, lost market share in her specialty, replacement recruitment costs, and start-up costs for the replacement physician. It creates an image, with patients and payers, of instability and unreliability. The problem is compounded if the departing physician stays in the area and competes directly with the group.

The group addresses this problem by making a noncompete clause part of the employment or partnership agreement. In most states, the law will permit the group to require that the physician, as a condition of joining, promises to avoid competing with the group if and when she leaves. "Competing with" is defined in terms of providing certain medical services within a relevant geographic market area for a reasonable period of time. Noncompete clauses must be drawn up carefully to stay within the law.

In the few states, which prohibit noncompete clauses in physician service agreements, the employment or partnership agreement may specify a predetermined amount of damages that a physician must pay the group if she leaves and enters into direct competition.

The group will also want to review the stock ownership arrangements with its members. With the sale of all tangible assets, ownership is much more related to choosing the board of directors and various committee members whose role in shaping the group's future is now much more important. Procedures for electing directors must ensure the selection of respected, forward-looking people, not simply the most popular.

PREPARING FOR THE TURNOVER OF GROUP ADMINISTRATIVE RESPONSIBILITIES TO THE MSO/PPMC

Once you have made the decision to enter into a relationship with an MSO or PPMC, there are several preparatory steps necessary.

Compile a list of creditors, suppliers, landlords, and other parties to whom you have financial obligations. As part of its purchase of your practice assets, the MSO/PPMC will assume responsibility for most of these debts. This fact will be reflected in the asset sale agreement. However, it is necessary to obtain from each of these parties assent to the transfer of the obligations to the MSO/PPMC. The MSO/PPMC's larger size and resources should make it an even more attractive debtor than you were.

The MSO/PPMC also will take over most of the contracts you have with third parties such as equipment leases, equipment service contracts, janitorial and waste collection agreements, and a variety of insurance policies. All of these people must be contacted to make appropriate changes in the contracts.

It also is possible that other third parties have security interests in some of the assets that you will be selling to the MSO/PPMC. For instance, if you buy a piece of medical equipment on an installment basis, the vendor is likely to retain a right to the equipment until it is completely paid for. These parties must be identified so that arrangements can be made to pay off the outstanding balances or transfer the liability for them to the MSO/PPMC.

WHAT TO EXPECT AFTER SIGNING AN AGREEMENT WITH A PPMC

Here are the major first steps a good PPMC will take immediately after acquiring a physician practice:

- Conduct an audit of the sources of the practice's revenues and the basis of its expenses.
- Replace the practice administrators with the PPMC's own management people.
- Trim overhead by eliminating some support staff at the same time.
- Transfer all other nonphysician practice staff to the PPMC's payroll.
- Combine as much of the practice's purchasing (supplies, equipment, insurance) with that of other practices in order to realize volume savings of 10 to 15 percent.
- Make significant investments in system improvements for the practice—such as tele-

communications, information gathering, and general computer technology.
- Try to bring the practice into existing and new managed care contracts.

An aggressive PPMC might also pursue the following strategies:

- Financially assist the practice in recruiting new physicians in desired specialties.
- Open satellite clinics to be staffed by the practice's physicians.
- Negotiate additional managed care contracts.
- Invest in staff and equipment necessary to deliver lucrative ancillary services.

THE RISKS YOU TAKE WHEN SELLING OUT TO A PPMC

There is a lot of appeal to physicians for selling their practices to a PPMC. However, do not lose sight of the several ways that the deal and the relationship can go very bad. Here are some of the risks you assume in affiliating with a PPMC:

- Until the PPMC is able to increase the profits of your practice to cover its management fees, those payments must come out of your compensation.
- The PPMC may show a profit to its investors (by constantly acquiring new practices) without improving the revenues or profits of your practice.
- If the PPMC you join merges or is acquired, you may find yourself affiliated with an unacceptable PPMC or other organization.
- You will have to surrender most of the control over the business operations of your practice.
- Increasing competitive pressure in the health care marketplace may persuade the PPMC to intervene in aspects of clinical decision making originally reserved to physicians.
- The PPMC may turn out to be more adept at raising capital and acquiring practices than efficiently managing physician practices.

- The primary goal of the dominant investors in the PPMC may be to take the organization public, continue to acquire new practices until the stock price peaks, then pull their cash out, and leave the physicians with an uncompetitive entity running their practices.

- The 20- to 40-year term of the agreement with a PPMC means that the decision to sign is for the life of the physician.

- Noncompete language in the physician's employment contract with the PPMC makes it almost impossible for him later to withdraw and resume an independent practice without moving out of the market area.

- Few PPMCs have demonstrated an ability to generate "same-clinic revenue growth." PhyCor may be one of the exceptions.

- If the PPMC's stock is publicly traded and appreciates in value, you will wish you were paid primarily in stock for your practice. If the stock never goes public or performs poorly, you will wish you had been paid in cash. Keep in mind that, if you take payment mostly in cash, you can use it to purchase stock in the PPMC or any other company you want.

For Physicians Stuck in a Failing PPMC: Some physicians may already be affiliated with a PPMC whose performance is making them nervous. There are four basic avenues for a bail out.

- Use the exit provisions that you had the foresight to negotiate into the contract.
- Try to diplomatically arrange with PPMC management for your friendly departure.
- Search for contract clauses that would render the entire agreement unenforceable.
- Determine whether any of the PPMC's actions constitute fatal breaches of the contract.

WARNING! As this book was in the final stages of preparation, it became apparent that the option of partnering with a PPMC had

changed so dramatically that an update was necessary. Do not sell your assets to or otherwise affiliate with a PPMC before reading this warning![1-4]

Since reaching a peak in stock price and market popularity in October 1997, the PPMC industry has crashed. Many of the leading publicly-traded companies have declared bankruptcy, been delisted by a stock exchange, withdrawn from the practice management business, sold out, or gone private. Here are some specifics.

In October 1997, MedPartners and PhyCor, the two largest PPMCs announced their merger. Three months later, they called it off. Since then, the price of a share of MedPartners stock has gone from $35 to $3. PhyCor's stock went from $35 to $5 a share. In November 1998, MedPartners decided to pull out of the practice management business entirely, leaving 238 clinics and 13,000 physicians without support or affiliation.

In July 1998, FPA Medical Management filed for Chapter 11 bankruptcy. Its stock price fell from a high of $40 to zero. In August 1998, PhyMatrix announced plans to cease its practice management operations. One of the more stable PPMCs, ProMedCo, saw its share price cut from $16 to $5. Physicians Resource Group faces class-action lawsuits from its physicians and defaulted on a $10 million bank loan. Meanwhile, its stock price has dropped from a high of $32 in 1996 to a low of $ .50. In November 1998, Advanced Health reported that it was laying off 60 percent of its staff and scaling back its PPM operations in order to concentrate on electronic commerce. Also in November, Doctors Health filed for Chapter 11 bankruptcy protection after its largest managed care client pulled its Medicare HMO out of the region. Still in November, the stock price of AmeriPath plummeted 45 percent to $5 after it received a three million dollar refund request from Medicare for billing errors.

Overall, the prices of PPMC stocks have fallen about 60 percent during 1998. Some analysts and investors believe that the industry may disappear within five years. The savvy PPMCs are changing their business models and strategies to reflect the lessons learned about managing physicians and their practices.

In addition to following the other recommendations in this chapter for dealing with PPMCs, physicians should take these precautions:

- Obtain from an analyst at an investment banking firm an assessment of the PPMC's general creditworthiness and its prospects for future growth.
- Obtain from a credit rating organization like Dun & Bradstreet a technical assessment of the PPMC's creditworthiness and financial solidity.
- Interview a cross-section of physicians currently affiliated with the PPMC.
- Do not sign a contract that runs for more than five years with a PPMC. Two years would be ideal. In the past, some PPMCs have required 40-year contracts with their physicians.
- Insist on contract provisions that will allow a graceful exit if the PPMC encounters financial difficulty or fails completely. This might include nullification of any non-compete agreement and the option of buying back the practice assets for a percentage of the original purchase price.
- Do not agree to pay management fees as a percentage of revenues, if some of those revenues have been earned solely by the physician's efforts and without PPMC support (i.e. independent medical research).
- Ask the PPMC to pay for malpractice insurance coverage for any claims filed after the physician has left the PPMC for care provided while the physician was still with the PPMC.
- Give very close attention to issues that might lead to later disillusionment with the PPMC: more PPMC control over practice decisions than the physician can accept, a compensation formula that does not address the physician's concerns for income security or income maximization, or PPMC authority to dictate the physical location of the physician's practice.
- Think twice about partnering with a PPMC owned by profit-driven investors whom you do not know at all.

QUICK LOOK AT THE PPMC INDUSTRY

The PPMC model for building physician networks has become a significant enough force in health care delivery to be considered an "industry" in itself. It is worth having some background information about the competitors in that industry to which you may commit your professional life.

- Approximately 35 PPMCs are publicly traded.
- There are about 250 privately owned PPMCs, dozens of which are waiting to launch their IPOs.
- Almost 10 percent of the 527,000 practicing physicians are affiliated with a PPMC (either through sale of their assets or membership in a PPMC-managed IPA).
- If present trends hold up, half the nation's doctors could be connected with a PPMC within five years.
- The physician services market for which all PPMCs are vying is worth nearly $200 billion.
- Technically, it is usually a local corporate subsidiary of a national PPMC that actually purchases the physicians' practice assets.
- Normally, a PPMC purchases the assets of significant group practices (20 to as many as 200 physicians) rather than solo or very small group practices.
- Most PPMCs may be classified by the types of physicians they plan to recruit.
  - a full complement of specialties for a multispecialty network
  - single specialty concentration (e.g., oncology, cardiology, ophthalmology, neonatology)
  - exclusively primary care physicians
  - hospital-based physicians (emergency room)

SUMMARY DATA ON PUBLICLY TRADED PPMCs

Tables 16–1 and 16–2 detail a few key pieces of financial data about the publicly traded PPMCs.* The "annual revenue" figure is the company's total annual revenues, for the calendar year 1996 or a fiscal year ending a month or two before or after December 31, 1996. The "net income" figure is for the same period. The numbers on "annual revenue per physician" are obtained by dividing the annual revenues by the number of physicians affiliated with the PPMC. This is a rough indicator of the productivity of each physician in a PPMC. It is an approximate figure since the actual number of affiliated physicians varies throughout a year.

The two ratios are indicators of how well the PPMC is managing its operations. The "health expenses as percent of patient revenues" show how much of a patient's dollar the PPMC must spend providing him with health care. As long as quality of care is not affected, a lower percentage suggests greater efficiency in care management. The "administrative expenses as percent of total revenues" is a measure of the PPMC's managerial efficiency—how large an administrative overhead it must carry to operate its network.

The immaturity of the PPMC industry shows up in the wide variation in operating efficiency figures among individual PPMCs. The ratio of health expenses to patient revenues varies from 44.4 percent to 102.5 percent. The ratio of administrative expenses to total revenues ranges from 4.6 percent to 75.9 percent. Clearly, some PPMCs cannot continue for very long operating at such inefficient levels and will drop out of the competition.

The market shares of the top publicly traded PPMCs are shown in Table 16–2. Use these data in your analysis of the PPMCs offering to buy your practice. Be cautious in selling your practice assets to one of these publicly traded entities. Be even more wary of a PPMC that has not had sufficient history to warrant its first public stock offering.

Exhibit 16–2 lists the 10 largest publicly traded PPMCs, measured by the number of physicians in the practices they have acquired. The data provided for each include its number of affiliated physicians (in early 1998), the specialty concentration of the PPMC, the states in which it operates, its annual revenues in 1996, and a contact person. (Note: The number of affiliated physicians does not include physicians in IPAs that have contracted with the PPMC solely for practice management services.)

CASE STUDY OF A FOR-PROFIT INVESTOR-OWNED PPMC: PHYCOR, INC.*

PhyCor, Inc. was formed in 1988 as the first real investor-owned PPMC, before anyone was using that term. Its revenues come from three sources: (1) the acquisition and operation of primary care–focused multispecialty medical clinics, (2) the development and management of independent practice associations (IPAs), and (3) the provision of health care decision support services for consumers. It first public stock offering was in 1992.

The company purchases the assets (including accounts receivable and liabilities) of medical clinics and a number of smaller medical practices. It is significant that PhyCor is willing to pay something for the goodwill that a physician has built up in her practice. In payment for the assets, PhyCor typically gives shares of its stock, some immediate cash, and additional cash paid over a period of time as the physicians achieve agreed upon performance goals. The use of PhyCor stock is a small part of the transaction. The performance-based payment or "earn-out" is not included in all deals. The PhyCor acquisition

---

*These data, and a great many more, are available at the Web site of Sherlock Company, a financial advisor to health plans, medical groups, and investors. Go to http://www.sherlockco.com/samp-ppme/finppmc.html

*Courtesy of PhyCor, Nashville, Tennessee.

Table 16–1 Key Financial Data on Publicly Traded PPMCs (for Calendar Year 1996 in Most Cases)

	Annual Revenue[a]	Annual Revenue per Physician[b]	Net Income[c]
Hospital Based			
Coastal Physician Group (DR)[a]	$552,109 (−31.9%)	NA	($186,262)
EmCare Holdings (EMCR)	$196,257 (25.1%)	$396,733	$10,973
InPhyNet Medical Management (IMMI)	$408,520 (25.6%)	$328,217	$17,104
MedCath (MCTH)	$66,191 (65.0%)	NA	$5,202
Pediatrix Medical Group (PDX)	$80,833 (84.3%)	$491,138	$13,120
Sheridan Healthcare (SHCR)	$92,767 (43.5%)	$458,100	$5,509
Multispecialty			
Advanced Health Corporation (ADVH)	$19,136 (NA)	$231,376	($1,465)
Complete Management (CMI)	$45,491 (39.4%)	$792,984	$5,414
Medical Asset Management (MAMT)	$13,076 (245.6%)	$334,133	$883
MedPartners (MDM)	$4,813,499 (34.3%)	$1,383,818	$201,675
Metropolitan Health Networks (MDPA)	$13,432 (NA)	$1,716,121	(S113)
PhyCor (PHYC)	$1,530,247 (78.7%)	$600,386	$36,380
PhyMatrix (PHMX)	$189,961 (168.6%)	$954,531	$12,057
Primary Care			
American Healthchoice (AHIC)	$10,187 (65.2%)	$896,538	($1,988)
FPA Medical Management (FPAM)	$683,077 (32.2%)	NA	($41,297)
PHP Healthcare Corporation (PPH)	$203,360 (−0.4%)	NA	$7,568
ProMedCo Management (PMCO)	$64,386 (NA)	NA	$765
Talbert Medical Mgmt. Holdings (TMMC)	$421,256 (NA)	NA	($56,259)
UCI Medical Affiliates (UCIA)	$23,254 (29.3%)	$383,694	$466
Single Specialty			
American Oncology Resources (AORI)	$268,880 (107.3%)	$1,474,192	$17,650
Apogee (APGG)	$78,727 (15.3%)	$760,396	$633
The Company Doctor (CDOC)	$8,479 (33.4%)	$505,715	$710
EquiMed (EQMDE)	$99,115 (68.3%)	NA	$7,900
IntegraMed America (INMD)	$18,343 (9.8%)	$473,302	($1,622)
Integrated Orthopaedics (IOI)	$14,313 (−7.9%)	$2,501,534	($1,272)
OccuSystems (OSYS)	$170,035 (24.1%)	$923,045	$11,654
Omega Health Systems (OHSI)	$42,612 (29.4%)	$1,332,649	$1,303
Physician Reliance Network (PHYN)	$310,733 (56.4%)	$1,228,077	$20,496
Physicians Resource Group (PRG)	$248,293 (176.0%)	$951,758	$13,116
Physicians' Specialty Corp. (ENTS)	$23,225 (90.9%)	$904,785	$1,903
Response Oncology (ROIX)	$67,353 (52.0%)	NA	$2,207
Specialty Care Network (SCNI)	$4,392 (NA)	NA	($1,771)

[a] These figures are in thousands.
[b] These figures are accurate as they stand; they are not in thousands.
[c] These figures are in thousands.
[d] These are the stock market ticker tape symbols. Use them when checking a company's stock price.
[e] Figures in parentheses represent change from the previous year.

continues

Table 16–1 continued

	Health Expenses as % of Patient Revenues	Administrative Expenses as % of Total Revenues
Hospital Based		
Coastal Physician Group	86.6%	20.1%
EmCare Holdings	80.1%	10.5%
InPhyNet Medical Management	85.2%	10.5%
MedCath	66.7%	18.7%
Pediatrix Medical Group	59.4%	16.5%
Sheridan Healthcare	69.8%	19.4%
Multispecialty		
Advanced Health Corporation	64.0%	30.8%
Complete Management	63.7%	24.0%
Medical Asset Management	NA	NA
MedPartners	89.6%	4.6%
Metropolitan Health Networks	44.4%	55.1%
PhyCor	85.6%	8.7%
PhyMatrix	47.5%	43.1%
Primary Care		
American Healthchoice	NA	NA
FPA Medical Management	84.4%	16.2%
PHP Healthcare Corporation	90.3%	6.1%
ProMedCo Management	102.5%	7.7%
Talbert Medical Mgmt. Holdings	91.5%	5.2%
UCI Medical Affiliates	91.5%	5.2%
Single Specialty		
American Oncology Resources	81.4%	7.8%
Apogee	80.7%	19.9%
The Company Doctor	48.8%	55.5%
EquiMed (EQMDE)	NA	NA
IntegraMed America	78.8%	21.9%
Integrated Orthopaedics	78.0%	75.9%
OccuSystems	74.7%	13.0%
Omega Health Systems	85.1%	13.1%
Physician Reliance Network	73.6%	21.2%
Physicians Resource Group	61.8%	28.1%
Physicians' Specialty Corp.	NA	NA
Response Oncology	NA	NA
Specialty Care Network	NA	NA

Courtesy of Sherlock Company's PPMC. Telephone: 215-628-2289; www.sherlockco.com; Gwynedd, Pennsylvania.

Table 16–2 Market Shares of Publicly Traded Physician Practice Management Companies, 1996–1998[a]

	Percent Market Share		
	1996	*1997*	*1998*
MedPartners	1.27	2.62	3.02
PhyCor	0.68	0.95	1.18
FPA Medical	0.56	0.76	0.95
Talbert Medical Group	0.23	--[b]	--[b]
Physicians Resource Group	0.20	0.21	0.28
PhyMatrix	0.08	0.19	0.23
Physician Reliance Group	0.11	0.15	0.21
ProMedCo	0.02	0.06	0.13
American Oncology	0.10	0.15	0.20
Occusystems	0.08	0.09	0.11
MedCath	0.04	0.06	0.09
Coastal Physician Group	0.29	0.25	0.21
InPhyNet	0.21	--[b]	--[b]
PHP Healthcare	0.12	0.14	0.16
EmCare	0.10	0.13	0.14
Sheridan Healthcare	0.05	0.05	0.07
Pediatrix	0.04	0.06	0.08
Industry Total	4.18	5.87	7.06

[a]From Salomon Smith Barney and HCFA.
[b]Included in MedPartners.

Source: Adapted with permission from L. Marsh, The Doctor's Bottom Line, Wall Street Evaluates the Physician Practice Management Industry, *Health Affairs 17*, no. 4, p. 77, Copyright © 1998, The People-to-People Health Foundation, Inc., All Rights Reserved.

strategy focuses on physician groups that are considered leaders in their markets with reputations for practicing quality medicine.

When it buys up the assets of a physician group or clinic, it enters into a long-term (often 40 years) service agreement with the physicians' group. The physicians agree to practice exclusively through the now PhyCor-owned clinics, and sign noncompete agreements to that effect. PhyCor provides administrative and technical support for the professional services delivered by the physicians through the group. In particular, it provides the equipment and facilities used in the

medical practice, manages the clinic operations, and employs most of the clinic's nonphysician personnel.

During the mid-1990s, it was customary for many PPMCs to pay a share of compensation for good will. PhyCor found that this practice was not beneficial; in fact, it was detrimental to the economics of the entire enterprise moving forward. PhyCor is currently committed to underwriting the growth of the clinic or group's operation for the first several years without burdening the physicians. That is, the investments it makes are interest-free.

Exhibit 16–2 Key Data on the Leading PPMCs

1. *MedPartners, Inc.*
   Number of affiliated physicians: 5,865
   Specialty concentration: multispecialty
   States of operation: AL, AK, AZ, AR, DE,
   CA, CT, FL, GA, IL, KY, MD, MA, MS, NJ,
   NV, NC, OH, OK, OR, PA, SC, TN, TX, VA,
   WA
   Annual revenues: $4,800,000,000
   Contact person:
     Tom Bartels
     Investor Relations
     MedPartners, Inc.
     3000 Galleria Tower, Suite 1000
     Birmingham, AL 35244
     (205) 733-8996

2. *PhyCor, Inc.*
   Number of affiliated physicians: 3,860
   Specialty concentration: multispecialty
   States of operation: AL, AZ, AR, CA, CO,
   FL, GA, IL, IN, KY, LA, MI, MS, NC, ND,
   NH, NY, OH, OK, PA, SC, TN, TX, UT, VA,
   WA
   Annual revenues: $766,300,000
   Contact person:
     Shawn Carder
     PhyCor, Inc.
     30 Burton Hills Blvd., Suite 400
     Nashville, TN 37215
     (615) 665-9066

3. *FPA Medical Management, Inc.*
   Number of affiliated physicians: 2,134
   Specialty concentration: primary care
   States of operation: AL, AK, AZ, CA, DE,
   FL, GA, HI, IL, IN, KY, LA, MD, MI, MO,
   NC, NJ, NY, OH, PA, SC, TN, TX, VA, WV
   Annual revenues: $560,000,000
   Contact person:
     Angela Rivera
     FPA Medical Management, Inc.
     3636 Nobel Dr., Suite 200
     San Diego, CA 92122
     (619) 453-1000
     arivera@fpamm.com

4. *PHP Healthcare Corp.*
   Number of affiliated physicians: 500
   Specialty concentration: primary care
   States of operation: DC, DE, MD, VA

   Annual revenues: $203,400,000
   Contact person:
     Mary Lou Schropp
     Investor Relations
     PHP Healthcare Corp.
     11440 Commerce Park Dr.
     Reston, VA 22091
     (703) 758-3600

5. *Physicians Resource Group, Inc.*
   Number of affiliated physicians: 431
   Specialty concentration: ophthalmology
   States of operation: AL, AZ, AR, CA, FL,
   IA, IL, KS, KY, LA, MA, MS, MO, NV, NJ,
   NY, NC, OH, OK, OR, PA, SC, TN, TX, WA
   Annual revenues: $248,293,000
   Contact person:
     Cristina Ingle
     Physicians Resource Group, Inc.
     Three Lincoln Center, Suite 1540
     5430 LBJ Freeway
     Dallas, TX 75240
     (972) 982-8200

6. *PhyMatrix Corp.*
   Number of affiliated physicians: 372
   Specialty concentration: multispecialty
   States of operation: FL
   Annual revenues: $189,961,000
   Contact person:
     PhyMatrix Corp.
     777 S. Flagler Dr., Suite 1000 E.
     West Palm Beach, FL 33401
     (561) 655-3500

7. *ProMedCo Management Co.*
   Number of affiliated physicians: 359
   Specialty concentration: primary care
   States of operation: AL, KY, TX
   Annual revenues: $32,890,349
   Contact person:
     Robert Smith
     ProMedCo Management Co.
     801 Cherry St., Suite 1450
     Fort Worth, TX 76102
     (817) 335-5035

8. *Physician Reliance Network, Inc.*
   Number of affiliated physicians: 326
   Specialty concentration: oncology
   States of operation: AR, IL, IA, MD, MI,

continues

Exhibit 16–2 continued

MN, NM, NY, OR, TX, WA
Annual revenues: $238,800,000
Contact person:
  Merrick Reese, M.D.
  President and CEO
  Physician Reliance Network, Inc.
  5420 LBJ Freeway, Suite 900
  Dallas, TX 75240
  (972) 392-8700

9. *American Oncology Resources, Inc.*
  Number of affiliated physicians: 311
  Specialty concentration: oncology
  States of operation: CO, FL, IN, KS, MO, NV, NY, NC, OK, OR, PA, SC, TX, VA
  Annual revenues: $205,000,000
  Contact person:
    Marc Kerlin
    Vice President of Managed Care

American Oncology Resources, Inc.
16825 Northchase Dr., Suite 1300
Houston, TX 77060
(281) 873-2674

10. *Advanced Health Corp*
  Number of affiliated physicians: 280
  Specialty concentration: multispecialty
  States of operation: DE, GA, NJ, NY, PA, TN
  Annual revenues: $18,900,000
  Contact person:
    Victoria Feder
    Advanced Health Corp.
    555 White Plains Road
    Tarrytown, NY 10591
    (914) 524-4200
    vfeder@advhealth.com
    www.advhealth.com

Note: Most of the data in this exhibit are from an article entitled "Physician Practice Management Companies: Too Good To Be True?" in the April 1998 issue of *Family Practice Management.* The annual revenue data are from a detailed listing of publicly traded PPMCs entitled "PPMC Profiles," published by Atlantic Information Services, Inc.

PhyCor manages all aspects of the clinic operations other than the delivery of medical services. The physicians maintain full professional control over their medical practices, determine which physicians to hire or dismiss, and set their own standards of practice in promoting high-quality health care.

There is established at each clinic a joint policy board comprised of equal numbers of physicians and PhyCor personnel. This board makes decisions on strategic and operational planning, marketing, managed care arrangements, and other major issues facing the clinic.

PhyCor first began managing and then developing IPAs in 1995. By the end of 1997, it had management agreements with IPAs in 28 markets, encompassing roughly 19,000 physicians providing capitated medical services to approximately 519,000 members.

PhyCor is giving more emphasis to IPA development in order to

• Provide services to a broader range of physician organizations
• Enhance the operating performance of existing clinics by giving those physicians more affiliation options
• Further develop its relationships with physicians

In late 1997, PhyCor moved its activities to a new level by agreeing with New York and Presbyterian Hospitals Care Network, Inc. to create and operate a regional managed care contracting network that will include hospitals and IPAs in New York City, northern New Jersey, and southern Connecticut.

PhyCor claims to offer the following advantages to the medical groups who join with it:

Table 16–3 Summary Data on Phycor, Inc. Clinic and IPA Operations, 1994–1997

	1997	1996	1995	1994
# of affiliated clinics	55	44	31	22
# of affiliated physicians	3,863	3,050	1,955	1,143
IPA operations:				
# of markets	28	17	13	7
# of physicians	19,000	8,700	5,300	3,600
# of commercial patients	420,000	306,000	180,000	105,000
# of Medicare patients	99,000	69,000	38,000	24,000

Courtesy of PhyCor, Nashville, Tennessee.

- a new level of strategic capability
- national strength and expertise in managed care contracting
- access to capital
- access to needed management resources and systems
- ability to develop strategic alliances in each market
- cost efficiencies through operating systems and national contracting
- access to essential medical management information systems
- education and training to empower physicians
- a physician-led alternative for nonaligned physicians through the PhyCor/medical group affiliation
- ability of the medical group to assume market leadership

Table 16–3 is a summary of PhyCor clinic and IPA operations for the last four years.

Two-thirds of the way through 1998, PhyCor claimed the following operating statistics for its clinics and IPAs:

- 60 affiliated clinics staffed by 4,045 physicians, of whom 53 percent were primary care
- 620 service sites
- 36 IPA markets with 26,000 affiliated physicians

- overall operations in 70 markets—26 metropolitan, 36 regional, and 8 rural—spread across 29 states
- managing a total of 3,450,000 managed care lives, of which 1,517,000 were capitated

Table 16–4 shows the payer mix of the total net clinic revenue earned by the clinics and the IPAs in each of the last five years. Note the steadily growing predominance of revenues from managed care contracts.

PhyCor's revenues come from several sources. Under most of its service agreements, PhyCor receives a service fee equal to the expenses it incurs in operating the clinics, plus a percentage of the clinic's operating income (net clinic revenue after clinic expenses have been paid and before physician distributions). The actual share going to PhyCor depends on the arrangement negotiated with the physician group. Usually, PhyCor gets between 12 and 17 percent of the excess and the physicians keep the remainder. As clinic operating income improves, whether as a result of increased revenues or lower expenses, PhyCor's service fee income increases. Its percentage stays the same.

To increase clinic revenue, PhyCor works with the physician groups to recruit additional physicians, merges other physicians practicing in the area into the affiliated groups, negotiates contracts with MCOs, and provides additional ancil-

Table 16–4 Payer Mix of Net Clinic Revenue of PhyCor, Inc., 1993–1997

	1997	*1996*	*1995*	*1994*	*1993*
Managed care[a]	41%	42%	37%	25%	24%
Medicare	22%	20%	20%	29%	32%
Medicaid	4%	3%	3%	3%	4%
Insurance and private payer	33%	35%	40%	43%	40%
Total	100%	100%	100%	100%	100%

[a]"Managed care" includes HMO, PPO, Medicare risk contracts, and direct employer contracts. About two-thirds of the managed care revenues in 1997 were capitated.

Courtesy of PhyCor, Nashville, Tennessee.

lary services. To lower or control expenses, PhyCor uses national purchasing contracts for common, high-volume items, reviews clinic staffing levels to make sure they are appropriate, and assists the physicians in developing more cost-effective clinical practice patterns.

PhyCor's compensation for managing an IPA is a combination of a management fee (calculated on a per member-per month basis) of the net surplus from the IPA's capitated revenues. In 1997, six percent of PhyCor's revenues were earned through IPA management agreements.

Table 16–5 shows a breakdown of PhyCor's revenues for the past three years.

During 1997, revenues at the 31 clinics and 13 IPAs that were under management for both 1996 and 1997 grew 12.8 percent. This "same market growth" is a better indicator of PhyCor's effectiveness in growing the practices its acquires. It is largely the result of the recruitment and merger of additional physicians into existing groups, increased enrollments in existing IPAs, and expansion of ancillary services. Total net revenues increased 46 percent from 1996 to 1997 ($766 million to $1.12 billion). This much larger overall growth rate is due primarily to the acquisition of new multispecialty physician groups.

The company states that its long-term strategy is "to position its affiliated primary care–oriented multispecialty medical clinics and IPAs as the physician component of competitive networks that are developing as the health system reforms." PhyCor has chosen to emphasize the physician component

in its belief that the dominant physician control over the cost and quality of health care empowers them to create value for such networks.

ACTION STEPS IN THINKING ABOUT JOINING AN MSO/PPMC

Adopting the strategy described in this chapter requires a physician to take what may be the boldest, high-risk decision in his career—selling the medical practice he spent years building. Such a step will not be taken casually. Here are a few suggestions for thinking about this dramatic move.

1. *Review your attitudes about managing the business aspects of your practice.* Some physicians very much enjoy the administrative duties of their practice and may be destined for a physician-manager role in the new U.S. health care system. For other physicians, these responsibilities are an unpleasant prerequisite to their most satisfying work—clinical practice. Decide where you stand on this issue. If you conclude that you would rather be free of these responsibilities, start thinking about the terms under which you would turn them over to someone else.

2. *Think about how important it is to you to be the owner and controller of every aspect of your practice, particularly the physical assets.* If you have been practic-

Table 16–5 Gross and Net Revenues of PhyCor, Inc. for 1995, 1996, and 1997 (in thousands)

	1997	*1996*	*1995*
Gross physician group revenue	$2,849,646	$1,928,045	$1,069,033
Less: Contractual adjustments	−1,090,329	−699,186	−359,653
Net physician group revenue	$1,759,317	$1,228,859	$709,380
IPA revenue	411,912	255,181	146,975
Net physician group and IPA revenue	$2,171,229	$1,484,040	$856,355
Less: Physician group retention	−634,983	−459,179	−266,725
Less: IPA retention	−341,937	−208,141	−118,599
Less: Clinic technical employee compensation	−74,715	−50,395	−29,435
Net PhyCor revenue	$1,119,594	$766,325	$441,596

Courtesy of PhyCor, Nashville, Tennessee.

ing solo or in a small group for a number of years, your independence and control over your work life is probably quite valuable to you. One solid expression of that independence and control is your legal ownership of the equipment, furniture, supplies, and perhaps even the building that support the practice. You also are the owner of the legal entity that constitutes the practice. It may be a partnership, a professional corporation, a limited liability corporation, or simply a sole proprietorship.

The point is that you can steer that practice in any direction you want. You can work longer or shorter hours. You can change locations. You can focus on a new category of patients. You can choose which support staff to employ.

You do not have quite the same freedom if you no longer possess the hard assets that underpin a medical practice.

3. *Learn how different kinds of MSOs work and what they have to offer a physician in your position.* All MSOs are not the same. They have different owners and they can have different motivations for forming and operating the MSO. Their leaders and executives may have different levels of experience in running physician practices and competing under managed care. This chapter gives you a good introduction to the different kinds of MSOs you are likely to encounter and some guidelines for analyzing them. Do some further research before you make any final decisions. Read some of the books or articles in the resource lists at the end of each chapter in this book. Talk with colleagues in your area and elsewhere around the country about their experiences with MSOs. Consult an experienced health lawyer or practice strategy consultant. Browse the Internet.

4. *Determine if there are any MSOs in operation or planned for your area.* It costs nothing to learn what MSO-type organizations are already in operation or planned for the near future. They should be easy to identify. Ask colleagues and administrators at local hospitals. Check with the local medical society. If there are MSOs already in the works, they probably are the choices you will have to work with. Focus your research and analysis on them.

5. *If there are no MSOs in the area or none that appeal to you, begin thinking about forming a physician-run or "physician*

equity" model MSO. As you study the MSO concept, you may become convinced that it is exactly the answer to the practice management and strategy questions you have been facing. And yet, there may be no MSOs existing or planned for your area. Consider the possibility of joining with other physicians in the same situation to initiate the formation of an MSO.

Share your information and knowledge of MSOs with the other doctors. Bring them up to speed on the benefits available to them by working with an MSO. Sketch an outline of the kind of MSO that would meet your needs—range of services offered, financial arrangements for asset purchase, source and expertise of its executives, ownership and governance, types of physician practices to be bought, long-term plans for further

integration and joint contracting, and potential relationships with other providers. Determine the approximate amount of start-up capital that will be needed. On the basis of that figure, decide whether the participating physicians can fund the MSO themselves or need to look for capital resources in a cosponsor of the MSO—a hospital, MCO, insurance company, or private investors. Contact existing MSOs in other areas to see if they might be interested in expanding into your area.

Taking the lead in forming an MSO or any other new business venture is a bold, risky move. Not every physician is cut out to fill such a role. However, these are times that call for boldness and risk taking. The rewards are commensurately great—exactly the organization you want, controlled by the people you want. It is the difference between actively creating your future and letting someone else create it for you.

REFERENCES

1. "Fighting for Survival, Many Disillusioned Doctors and Investors Look for a Way Out," *Dallas Business Journal,* 9 November, 1998, appearing on the website of the American City Business Journals, http://www.amcity.com/journals/health_care/dallas/1998-11-09/story4.html.

2. "Physicians Must Act Fast To Counter PPMC Failures," appearing on December 5, 1998 on the website of the Business Wire, http://www.businesswire.com/healthlink/.

3. M.C. Jaklevic, "MedPartners Fallout: PPM's Decision To Exit May Propel Docs toward Hospitals," *Modern Healthcare,* 16 November, 1998, 2

4. M.C. Jaklevic, "More PPMs Hit by Financial Bad News," *Modern Healthcare,* 30 November, 1998, 6.

RESOURCE LIST

"Doctors Inc.—Physician Practice Management Groups Are Revolutionizing Health Care, while Wall Street Cheers," *Business Week,* 24 March, 1997.

"The Future of Physician Practice Management Companies," *Healthcare Financial Management,* August 1997.

B. Hirsh and D. Wilcox, *How To Negotiate a Physician's Employment Contract,* (Chicago: American Medical Association, 1995).

Inside the Physician Practice Management Companies: Profiles of Top Players, Capitol Publications, (800) 655-5597.

Investor Owned Physician Practice Management Companies, Super Search Packet #4844 (Englewood, CO: Medical Group Management Association).

Key Strategies and Trends Shaping the Growth of PPMCs, Atlantic Information Services, (800) 521-4323.

Management Services Organizations, Book #4580 (Englewood, CO: Medical Group Management Association).

"Now the Nation's #2 Practice Manager, FPA Aims To Bulk Up Even More," *Hospitals & Health Networks,* 5 January, 1998.

"Physician Practice Management Companies: Too Good To Be True?" *Family Practice Management*, April 1998.

"Physician Practice-Management Company Buyouts: Is Taking the Leap Worth the Risk?" *Medical Economics,* 28 April, 1997.

"PPM Profitability Update," newsletter on PPMC industry, Fulcrum Information Services, (800) 869-4302.

"When a Physician Practice Management Company Comes Calling," *Family Practice Management,* June 1998.

## CHAPTER 17

Step Eight: Forming a Medical Foundation

INTRODUCTION

One way to view a medical foundation (MF) is as a nonprofit, charitable version of the physician practice management company (PPMC). Although they originated in California as a way to circumvent that state's strict prohibition of the corporate practice of medicine, the MF concept has spread rapidly to other states. It offers the advantage of nonprofit, tax-exempt status and, after directly employing or just contracting with physicians, enters into managed care contracts on their behalf. The Mayo Clinic has been an MF for many years.

A group practice, usually multispecialty, transfers all of its assets and practice management functions to the MF and concentrates on providing patient care and quality assurance. This chapter introduces physicians and groups to this concept as the natural next strategic step for them, summarizes the advantages and disadvantages, explains how MFs work, and suggests how they most likely will be formed.

WHO SHOULD READ THIS CHAPTER

Physicians who have been affiliated with a physician-hospital organization (PHO) or an independent practice association (IPA) for a couple of years and are looking for an organizational vehicle to pursue greater integration would do well to consider the MF model. This alternative should be especially appealing if they expect to continue in a close relationship with a hospital, if they need to rely on capital investment from the hospital, and if they prefer an organizational form that is not so clearly profit driven. The charitable, nonprofit aspect of an MF, alone, may be attraction enough for those physicians alienated by the growing commercialization of health care delivery.

In states with strictly enforced laws against the "corporate practice" of medicine, the MF may be the only type of organization available to physicians wishing to consolidate and integrate their medical practices. Physicians residing in such states should read this chapter closely.

The MF option probably is of little value to physicians on a direct course to creating a large multispecialty group practice that will eventually become a key component of an integrated multiprovider delivery system. This is especially true where the group's capital needs cannot be met by the charitable donations and tax advantages available to nonprofit organizations. Those physicians who are inclined to sell their practice assets to a PPMC or other managing entity and to concentrate on the clinical side of health care delivery should also pass this chapter by.

DESCRIPTION OF THE MOST COMMON MEDICAL FOUNDATIONS

The term *medical foundation* refers to a nonprofit organization created to provide health care services and that has qualified for federal tax-exempt status. It is often owned and controlled by a not-for-profit hospital. There are two basic foundation models. One directly employs the participating physicians. The Mayo Clinic and the Cleveland Clinic are examples of this model. The other model has an independent contractual relationship with one or more physician groups. The Santa Barbara (California) Medical Foundation operates this way.[*]

The medical foundation form was created originally in California to take advantage of a statutory exception to that state's prohibition against the corporate practice of medicine and to allow nonphysician organizations, such as hospitals, to indirectly own or manage physician practices.

A medical foundation typically operates one or more outpatient clinics and may own, be owned by, or be affiliated with one or more hospitals. The clinics may be free-standing or connected outpatient departments of the hospital. The medical foundation often acquires the assets of individual and group physician practices and provides them with capital, equipment, office space, nonphysician staff, and management services.

---

*The Internal Revenue Service (IRS) defines a medical foundation as follows:

Under the foundation model, a single corporation (the foundation), typically a nonprofit corporation under state law, is created to obtain all assets needed to operate clinics and physician offices, and possibly one or more hospitals. Assets may be acquired by purchases, leases, licenses, stock transfers, gifts or a combination of these methods. The foundation acquires the services of physicians who will provide professional medical care within the system, either through direct employment or independent contract. The foundation then becomes the provider of health care services, both medical and hospital, inpatient and outpatient. It enters into all payer contracts, provides all nonprofessional personnel for the system, maintains all assets, and collects all revenues for the services provided.[1(p.214)]

The medical foundation becomes the direct provider of medical care. It has its own Medicare provider number and bills, and it collects under that number for physician, diagnostic, and other health care services. The foundation contracts with managed care organizations (MCOs), preferred provider organizations (PPOs), insurance companies, employers, and other payers. It owns all patient medical records and accounts receivable.

REASONS THAT PHYSICIANS MIGHT FORM OR JOIN A MEDICAL FOUNDATION

The participating physicians and hospitals may have different motives for coming together to form a medical foundation. Here is why a doctor might consider this strategic option:

- Larger groups tend to be more attractive to payers; it is easier to market and administer the relationship. They also like the greater stability and visibility in the community.
- Greater size allows them to afford a medical director, professional managers, data collection systems, and staffing to support utilization and quality management.
- MFs provide access to two unique sources of investment capital: tax-exempt bond markets (to the extent that the combined financial strength of the hospital and the physician group will allow it) and contributions from the founding tax-exempt hospitals.
- The foundation can solicit and accept tax-deductible donations for worthy functions such as medical research and charity care. Some foundations have raised millions of dollars this way.
- Once the assets of the physician group are sold to the foundation, it becomes easier to recruit new physicians into the group because their required buy-in is much lower.
- The greater financial base of a hospital-backed medical foundation can more easily support fair market income guarantees for physicians.

- The transfer of the groups' practice assets to the medical foundation produces an often substantial one-time investment gain that can be distributed to the physicians or applied against the group's debt.
- The foundation model pays no income or property taxes, leaving more money to invest in operations or facilities, or to pay out in physician incomes.
- Like several other integration models, MFs take over the practice management duties and leave the physicians free to practice medicine.
- Because of its nonprofit status and ownership of all required assets, an MF usually has greater long-term stability than a does physician group.
- The foundation model facilitates joint contracting between the participating hospital and physician group with MCOs, as well as giving the physicians access to the managed care contracts that the hospital already has.
- Common participation in the MF forces the hospital and physicians to cooperate and align their goals, to the benefit of both.

ADVANTAGES AND DISADVANTAGES OF THE MF ORGANIZATIONAL FORM

This is a summary of the pros and cons of the MF as an organizational option for physicians.

Advantages

Tax benefits are the primary attraction of medical foundations, in the form of

- exemption from federal income tax,
- exemption from some state income and property taxes,
- access to tax-exempt bond financing, and
- opportunity to raise funds through tax-deductible charitable contributions.[*]

Because of the integral involvement of both physicians and hospitals, the medical foundation is often a step away from functioning as full-blown integrated delivery systems (IDSs).

- Benefits to participating physicians from the opportunity to focus more on managed care, use the capital received to enhance their practices, or sell their practices assets and retire.
- The not-for-profit nature of the MF, along with its required substantial community representation on the board, can be used to good marketing advantage.
- MFs may address corporate practice of medicine issues that exist in some states by allowing physicians to be employed by an institution not run by physicians.
- Certain MF models may be more acceptable to participating physicians than are alternatives such as management services organizations (MSOs) or physician-hospital organizations (PHOs).
- Because physician compensation occurs in the context of an employer-employee relationship, private inurement problems may be avoided.
- By qualifying for the in-office ancillary services or group practice exceptions to Stark II, physicians may gain fair access to ancillary service revenues.

Disadvantages

- Formation of an MF requires large capital investment, usually by a hospital, to purchase physician practices and to finance initial operations.
- Due to dominance of the sponsoring hospital, physicians may feel a distinct loss of control.
- To obtain and maintain its tax-exempt status, the MF must comply with numerous IRS-

---

[*]In some cases, it may also be possible to structure the transfer of a physician practice to the medical foundation as a "bargain sale," in which the foundation pays less than fair market value for the practice and the physician takes the difference as a charitable contribution deduction.

imposed restrictions on its organizational structure and operations (not true of the typically for-profit MSOs). For instance:

– Physicians may not have an equity interest in the MF (it has no equity!).
– Physicians may have only limited role in MF governance (which may lead to less commitment to the organization's goals or passion for the practice of medicine).
– There may be restrictions on the amount and type of incentive compensation for physicians.

• Formation of an MF is a complex, costly, and time-consuming process, particularly the quest for tax-exempt status from the IRS.
• MFs require ongoing annual information reporting and exposure to IRS scrutiny and potential audits.

LIMITATIONS OF TAX-EXEMPT STATUS

An organization agrees to substantial limitations on its range of operational freedom when it seeks and accepts tax-exempt status. For clarity purposes, remember that an organization is set up initially as a nonprofit corporation or foundation under state law. In most states, incorporation as a nonprofit entity gains you very little. To secure the benefits of tax-exempt, tax-deductible status, it is necessary to satisfy the requirements imposed by the IRS under federal law. In granting exemptions from their own taxes or allowing use of tax-exempt bond financing authorities, most states rely on evidence that the organization has satisfied the federal requirements.

WHAT AN MF OR ANY OTHER TAX-EXEMPT HEALTH CARE ORGANIZATION MUST AND MUST NOT DO

It must organize itself exclusively for a range of tax-exempt purposes defined in the *Internal Revenue Code* (IRC) §501(c)(3) to include "religious, charitable, scientific, testing for public safety, literary, or educational purposes." The

promotion of health is recognized as a charitable purpose. In addition to serving those purposes, the MF must be able to show that it is providing a "community benefit."

The IRS views an MF as a type of IDS and requires that an IDS do the following things to satisfy the community benefit standard:

• Integrate its medical functions in a way that benefits the general public as well as individual patients.
• Increase access by Medicare and charity patients by
  – operating an open medical staff
  – offering emergency medical services to all patients without regard for their ability to pay
  – participating in the Medicare and Medicaid programs without discriminating against their patients
  – delivering a minimum volume of charity care each year
• Conduct research and education programs designed to benefit the public.
• Assemble a community-oriented board of trustees without excessive physician representation.

The MF must not allow its operations to benefit private individuals, nor may it allow its assets to inure to the benefit of "insiders." Physicians with a financial relationship to the foundation are considered insiders.

What do these restrictions mean in practical terms?

1. The MF should create a medical records system that combines and unifies patients from inpatient and outpatient settings.
2. The MF should be prepared to guarantee a minimum level of charity care. The actual amount will depend on the foundation's financial condition and performance, the demographics of the population it serves, and the competitive pressure it faces. Recent IRS determination letters granting tax-exempt status to several MFs referred

to charity commitments of $400,000 (Facey Medical Foundation),[2] $750,000 (Harriman Jones Medical Foundation),[3] and $3.6 million (Rockford Memorial Health Services Corp.).[4]

3. The MF should conduct substantial research and educational programs in health care.

4. The MF foundation should keep the number of physicians currently or formerly employed by the foundation or under contract to it on its governing board below 50 percent of the total. If the number is held to 20 percent or less, the organization will be absolutely safe, without further precautions, under the IRS safe harbor that has existed since 1993. The closer the physician representation gets to 49 percent, the more procedural safeguards against conflict of interest the IRS wants to see.[*] These ratios also apply to committees of the board. However, it is permissible for physicians to make up all or most of the members of committees dealing with clinical issues.

5. The MF should make sure that the purchase price it pays to acquire physician practices does not exceed fair market value and is determined through arm's-length negotiations with the sellers. The best way of demonstrating fair market value is through an appraisal by a professional valuation accountant familiar with IRS concerns about practice valuation methodology. In addition, it often is better to avoid buying any intangible assets unless some firm valuation basis can be established. Chapter 15, "Step Six: Forming a PHO—An Affiliation between Your Group Practice and a Hospital" details how to structure the sale of a physician practice to a provider organization.

6. The MF should consider paying for the physician practices it acquires in a single lump sum to avoid even the argument that payments over a period of time are buying referrals from the physician. A lump sum payment puts the acquisition within the "isolated transaction" exception of the Stark law.

7. The MF should be extremely cautious about purchasing the intangible assets of a physician's practice, that is, things such as goodwill, covenants not to compete, exclusive dealing arrangements, patient lists, and patient records. This is to avoid creating the impression that these hard-to-measure payments are really inducements for physician referrals—in violation of the antikickback laws.

8. The MF should document that the compensation it pays to physicians, either employees or independent contractors, is the product of arm's-length negotiations and is close to fair market value. Compensation levels should be set by a board compensation committee that does not include physicians. Back them up with rigorous studies or surveys of comparable compensation levels, such as those offered by the Medical Group Management Association. Chapter 23, "Selection and Deselection of Physicians by Managed Care Organizations and Physician Groups," provides more detailed information on acceptable methods for compensating physicians, including financial incentives.

9. The MF should avoid physician incentive compensation plans so directly tied to revenues that a physician might be encour-

---

*These safeguards should include a formal, written conflict-of-interest policy (defining the board's decision-making process for all transactions involving interested members of the board and its committees, as well as its officers), periodic review of board activities and decisions to ensure that all are in pursuit of exempt purposes and not for the benefit of interested persons, express prohibition of compensated physicians from serving on the compensation committee, detailed records of compliance with the policy, and the regular collection of conflict-of-interest information from all board members and officers.

aged to increase referrals to the foundation in order to increase her compensation.

10. The MF should periodically conduct a self-audit to ensure that each of its activities serves primarily to benefit the general public and only incidentally to benefit individual physicians or other private individuals.

11. The MF should avoid supporting or opposing any candidate for public office and should devote no more than an insignificant portion of its resources to attempts to influence legislation.

GUIDELINES FOR FORMING AN MF

The typical founder of an MF is a not-for-profit hospital or health care system. However, there is no reason that the formation of a foundation cannot be initiated by a physician group. The problem lies in the need for two things: a charitable purpose and capital for acquiring physician practice assets.

A group of physicians trying to practice medicine together does not qualify as a sufficiently charitable purpose to deserve tax-exempt status. However, a subsidiary of a hospital that is already tax-exempt, a subsidiary that maintains an open medical staff and emergency department and engages in significant medical research and education, and a subsidiary that maintains an arm's-length relationship with its participating physicians (if not employing them directly) looks a lot more attractive to the IRS as a tax-exemption candidate.

Physicians, even those gathered into group practices, have not traditionally accumulated capital for growth and investment purposes. As a result, few of them are in a position to help fund the start-up of an MF, one of whose first tasks will be the purchase of physician practice assets. In fact, most physicians will want to participate in an MF to reap the reward of the sale of their practice assets. Therefore, a funding source separate from the doctors is necessary, and many hospitals meet the requirement very well.[*]

If you, as physicians—preferably a substantial group of physicians—take the lead in approaching an appropriate hospital and proposing joint creation of an MF, you stand a much better chance of shaping a deal and a subsequent organization that best serves your needs, as well as the needs of the hospital and the community. Here are the steps to follow in taking that route.

Decide on the Founding Participants and Sketch Out the Basic Organizational Structure

Make a preliminary decision about who the founding partners of the MF will be. You will need the advice of an attorney almost from the start to make sure that all the participants fit together in a way that will please the IRS. In addition to you and your physician colleagues, you will need a moneyed, tax-exempt partner to bring capital and charitable purpose to the venture. This will likely be a hospital, but it could also be several unrelated hospitals, a small chain of hospitals, or a tax-exempt integrated system. In small markets, you may not have a choice of partners. Where you do, look for an organization that will be a real "partner," willing to acknowledge and protect physician prerogatives in the new foundation arrangement.

Select or Organize an Appropriate Physician Group

Choose the local physicians who will be members of the founding group and, if necessary, organize them into a formal group. Your success in forming the MF and building an equitable rela-

---

*Two of the more publicized medical foundations had the following affiliations: the Friendly Hills HealthCare Network is connected to Loma Linda University Medical Center, and the Facey Medical Foundation is tied to UniHealth America, a California tax-exempt organization serving as the parent organization for a health care system consisting of 11 acute care hospitals and one acute psychiatric hospital.

tionship with your partners will depend greatly on the size and cohesiveness of the physician component. Choose them well. (Chapter 24, "Choosing the Best Strategic Partners for Your Group Practice, Physician-Hospital Affiliation, or Integrated Delivery System," has more details on this crucial step.) Be prepared for peer pressure, political pressure, and pressure from the hospital to accept all interested physicians from the hospital medical staff. You may not be able to avoid this. Minimize the problem by setting strict, fair, and relevant criteria for physician participation in the group. Accept the fact that, in the coming years, you will have to cull the physician ranks for those best suited for managed care practice.

Appraise the Market Value of the Practices in the Physician Group

Hire a professional appraiser to place dollar values on the physician practice assets to be purchased by the foundation. The appraiser should have specific experience in these kinds of assessments. Your attorney will work with the appraiser to focus on those assets that the foundation can legitimately acquire. The valuations produced by the appraiser will be a significant factor in determining how much capital the foundation will need to get started.

Draft a Formal Business Plan

Prepare a carefully considered, comprehensive business plan describing the first three to five years of the MF's operations. Although changing circumstances may call for frequent amendment of the plan, it should guide most of your early operational decisions. Give it the serious attention it deserves.

Design an Acceptable Governance Structure

Agree with all partners on the governance structure for the MF and the role each will have. This includes the size of the board of trustees and the number of seats reserved for various constituents; the number, responsibility, size, and membership of the board committees; and the special issues that will require supermajority votes or be

subject to the veto power of certain participant groups. These may be the most important questions in the entire planning process. They also are likely to generate the greatest political charge.

The answers they receive will powerfully affect the rights and interests of you and your physician colleagues. The balance of power struck among the participating groups (physicians, hospitals, community representatives) will also influence the ultimate success of the venture. Keep in mind the new opportunity for physicians to fill as many as 49 percent of the seats on a tax-exempt board. Do not grab power for its own sake, but do seek more than the traditional 20 percent representation.

Review the Compensation Currently Paid to the Participating Physicians

Once you have identified the physicians and groups likely to join the MF, gather data on the compensation and benefits each is currently receiving. Find out also whether they have radically different expectations for future compensation. These numbers are important inputs to the business plan. They indicate the revenues that will be necessary to support the physicians—the contract fees (capitation or fee-for-service)—that the foundation will have to charge and, therefore, how competitive the organization will be in the local market.

Draw Up the Necessary Legal Organizational Documents

Your lawyer will prepare the legal documentation required to bring the nonprofit MF corporation into existence and set the stage for the application to the IRS for tax-exempt status.

Decide Whether the Physicians Will Be Employees or Independent Contractors of the MF

The physicians must decide whether they wish to be employees of the MF or to have an independent contractual relationship with it. The decision will be driven by several factors:

- the kind of relationship with its physicians necessary for the foundation to avoid violation of a state "corporate practice of medicine" doctrine[*]
- the physicians' feelings about retaining some degree of autonomy and control over what is left of their practice styles
- the physicians' desires to maintain some independence from its hospital partner
- the physicians' desires for control over their own compensation levels
- the trade-off under the Stark law between qualifying for the "bona fide employment relationship" or the "personal services arrangement" exceptions

Draw Up the Professional Services Agreement or Employment Agreement That Will Be Used

On the basis of the decision of whether the physicians will be employees or independent contractors, your lawyer will draw up the appropriate agreement between them and the MF. If you are to be employees, it will be an employment agreement that will define your compensation and the circumstances under which the agreement can be terminated. A noncompete covenant probably will be included. If you are to be independent contractors, the document will be a professional services agreement. It may be with you individually, but it is more likely to be a contract between the foundation and a physician group. It should be much more detailed than an employment agreement, something like the managed care contracts you may have signed. It will describe the services that you or your group promise to provide, as well as other commitments

---

[*]Some states allow only nonprofit corporations to employ physicians, whereas others (such as California) permit a nonprofit organization to work with physicians as independent contractors.

you are making (access, quality assurance, utilization management, data reporting). The agreement will set out the terms of your compensation, including any incentives.

Draw Up the Agreement by Which the Foundation Will Purchase the Physicians' Practice Assets

Your lawyer will prepare a common asset purchase agreement by which the foundation will acquire the physicians' practice assets. This document is likely to mention the specific assets to be acquired, warranties or indemnities given by the physicians for the condition of the assets, the liabilities connected to those assets that the foundation will assume, and the method by which the foundation will pay the physicians.

The purchase agreement must address some sensitive and critical issues. First and foremost, most physicians will be interested in maximizing the payout they receive for their practice assets. This is especially true for an older physician who may be retiring in a few years or who cannot contemplate restarting an independent practice if the MF does not work out. Nonetheless, the purchase price really must be somewhere close to fair market value of the assets or it will appear to be a payment for referrals. These antikickback concerns may also preclude including soft assets (such as goodwill) in the transaction or spreading the payments out over a period of years. There also will be some complex tax issues. The price paid for the assets may create capital gains that might be avoided through careful planning. Some physicians may find it advantageous to actually sell their assets for less than their appraised value (in a so-called bargain sale) to reap tax deduction benefits.

Conduct a "Due Diligence" Review of the Transaction

It is a standard procedure in substantial legal transactions, particularly sales, to conduct a "due diligence" review of the items being sold and their legal status. This is to make sure that the buyer is getting the objects he bargained for and that they are not legally encumbered. The review begins with a physical inspection of the basic condition, structural integrity, environmental impact, and similar conditions. This is followed by a thorough examination of legal and financial issues such as legal title, contracts, leases, bond and loan agreements, outstanding debts of and to the practice, medical records, personnel records, pension and other benefit plans, and union contracts.

Decide How the Medical Foundation Will Be Financed

All participants must agree on the sources of the financing to acquire the physician practice assets and begin implementing the business plan. The possible sources are straightforward. If some of the physicians are willing to take a loss on the sale of their assets (which they recoup through a tax write-off), they are in effect making a donation to the foundation. The result is that less capital is required to buy those assets. The primary funding sources are likely to be contributions from the participating hospital and the proceeds of a tax-exempt bond financing. Because a tax-exempt hospital may contribute only to another tax-exempt venture, and it will take some time for the foundation to receive its tax-exempt status, it may make sense to configure the contribution initially as a loan. Anticipate taking at least six months to negotiate a new tax-exempt bond financing.

File the Necessary Legal Incorporation Documents

Your lawyer will handle the formality of filing the articles of incorporation and bylaws with the appropriate state government offices. This will bring the MF into existence.

File the Application for Tax-Exempt Status

Your lawyer than will file an application with the IRS seeking tax-exempt status for the founda-

tion. It will take a few months for the IRS to grant an initial tax-exempt certification. If all of your previous planning steps have been guided by an attorney experienced in the tax law of health care institutions, there should be no problems.

Obtain a Medicare Provider Number for the Foundation

The next step normally is to apply to the Health Care Financing Administration (HCFA) for a Medicare provider number for the foundation. This is done in the interest of developing the foundation as a unified delivery system through which all provider revenues are channeled. There are a couple of hitches in this phase of process. As a general rule, a physician who delivers Medicare services may not reassign her claim to another party. An MF may directly bill Medicare

- for services delivered by employee-physicians
- for services delivered by nonemployee physicians in a facility (such as a hospital) owned by the foundation
- for services delivered by nonemployee physicians with whom the foundation has a contractual arrangement authorizing the billing
- as a billing agent for nonemployee physicians

This issue should be given close attention when structuring the MF and deciding whether the participating physicians will be employees or independent contractors.

Inform Existing Contract Payers of the Organizational Change

It is important to notify the payers with which the physicians and the hospital have significant dealings about your intentions to form an MF. This should be done before the organization takes final shape to ensure the payers' willingness to continue dealing with the providers in their new affiliation. It would be best if you could obtain the payers' assent in writing. The foundation's business plan is likely to be premised on a continued flow of prior revenues.

Carry Out the Closing of the Asset Purchase Agreement

The last step in the formation process is the closing on the transfer of the physician practice assets to the new foundation entity. It will look a lot like a real estate closing.

CASE STUDY: MERCY MEDICAL FOUNDATION OF SACRAMENTO

One of the first endeavors to use an MF to work around the California prohibition of the corporate practice of medicine was the Mercy Medical Foundation of Sacramento.[5] It was formed in 1990 by the Medical Clinic of Sacramento ("Clinic") and Mercy Healthcare Sacramento ("Mercy").

The Clinic is an integrated multispecialty group practice founded in 1948. At the time the foundation was created, it was composed of 57 physicians, half of whom were in primary care and 27 of whom were shareholders. Roughly half of its patient population was covered by capitated managed care contracts. It operated a modern clinic in downtown Sacramento and five satellite facilities in the surrounding areas.

Mercy is a subsidiary of Catholic Healthcare West, responsible for running five hospitals in its Sacramento region. It already had some relationship with the Clinic, in the form of part ownership of its clinic and collaboration with its physicians under a contract with TakeCare, a major health maintenance organization (HMO) in the Sacramento area.

There were several forces pushing the Clinic and Mercy into a closer affiliation.

- There was a serious shortage of primary care physicians (PCPs) in the area; however, Mercy was restricted by its tax-exempt status and the antikickback laws from doing aggressive recruitment.
- The Clinic was experiencing serious financial difficulties as a result of the cost of

opening the new clinic, some poor investment decisions, downward pressure on revenues from the shift to managed care, and unrealistically high physician compensation.
- The Clinic recognized a need to secure additional capital to compete in the expanding managed care market in Sacramento.
- The Clinic was concerned about its ability to retain existing medical staff as their employment contracts expired.
- Mercy developed and provided management services to an IPA that, by its nature, was unable to integrate physician practices and implement effective utilization and quality management programs.
- The Clinic and Mercy, through cooperation on managed care contracts, development of the clinic facility, and restructuring of the Clinic's debt, had begun building a working relationship based on shared values, goals, and a vision of the future.
- Both parties saw long-term benefits, as well solutions to short-term problems, in a closer affiliation.

There was little disagreement between the Clinic and Mercy about the value of structuring themselves as an integrated hospital-physician provider organization. The only question concerned the form of that organization.

The first model considered was an MSO, a for-profit collaboration alternative. Several problems became immediately evident with this form. First, because California has a strong doctrine against the corporate practice of medicine, the MSO could not directly deliver physician care and would be limited to carrying out management functions. This would make it difficult to align the financial goals and incentives of the physicians and the hospital. Second, the MSO was legally prevented from acquiring the intangible assets of the Clinic, such as goodwill, medical records, and trade names. This meant that the purchase price for the Clinic's assets would be limited to the fair market value of tangible assets—an inadequate amount to pay off the Clinic's substantial debt or to induce the physicians to participate. It also wasted the Clinic's primary asset—its value as an ongoing, leading multispecialty group practice. Third, the hospital would be investing substantial funds to develop the Clinic as a modern managed care provider and to cover operating losses during the development/turnaround period. There would be a risk that the injection of substantial funds by the tax-exempt Mercy into a for-profit MSO would be viewed by the IRS as "private inurement," thus compromising Mercy's tax-exempt status.

Some research revealed a California state licensing option allowing nonprofit, tax-exempt organizations to own and operate clinics—as long as they satisfied several prerequisites

- had contracts with at least 40 physicians (covering at least 10 board-certified specialties),
- two-thirds of whom worked full time delivering care for the organization, and
- carried out education and research in health services.[*]

There were no apparent reasons that a tax-exempt hospital could not sponsor the organization set up under that law.

The Clinic and Mercy used this law in the following manner. The Mercy Medical Foundation ("Foundation") of Sacramento was established under the law as a nonprofit subsidiary of Mercy Healthcare Sacramento. As such, it qualified for exemption from California's licensing requirements. The Foundation then acquired the Clinic's assets (tangible and intangible), obtained a Medicare provider number, and began operating the clinic facility in its own name. It entered into a professional services agreement with the Clinic, which employed the physicians who provided professional medical services to the Foundation's patients.

Because the Foundation was able to purchase the Clinic's intangible assets, the Clinic received enough money to retire almost all of its existing debt. The Foundation also acquired the tangible assets, employed the support staff, took over the property leases, and assumed the payer contracts. With the backing of the larger, better-endowed Mercy, the Foundation was able to negotiate a line of credit to finance further investment in operating systems, physician recruitment, and creation of new facilities. The private inurement issue was reduced to assuring the IRS that the asset acquisition price and the compensation for the physicians' professional services was close to fair market value.

Mercy was the dominant partner in this relationship and served as the sole corporate member of the Foundation. As such, it appointed the entire board of directors and the chief executive officer (CEO), approved budgets and capital expenditures, and strongly influenced the strategic direction of the new system. Commensurate with IRS rules at the time, the Clinic's physicians were limited to 20 percent representation on the Foundation's board. Through the Foundation, the Clinic physicians agreed to provide a certain amount of charity care and to pursue certain educational and research activities.

A special feature of the collaboration was the position, under Catholic Canon Law, that the Foundation was a Catholic health care provider and, therefore, subject to the ethical and religious constraints governing Catholic health care facilities. This did not impede the progress of the affiliation.

The formation of the Foundation was a groundbreaking event in the California health care marketplace. Both the doctors and the hospital had some apprehension about working together in such an arrangement. The Clinic physicians feared losing the independence necessary to practice quality medicine; Mercy had no previous experience in managing group practices. They took certain steps to adapt themselves to each other.

---

[*]You may wonder how such a narrowly written law was ever enacted. It was adopted in 1980 to accommodate the desires for tax exemption of two large multispecialty group practices that were then converting to nonprofit status: the Palo Alto Medical Foundation and the Santa Barbara Medical Clinic.

They decided that the necessary structural and operational changes would be carried out in an evolutionary fashion, as the trust and cooperation between them grew naturally. This was particularly true in the sensitive areas of physician credentialing, utilization management, and quality assurance.

The Clinic board of directors continued to function, retaining control over matters directly connected to the physician group, such as scheduling of physicians, physician compensation, hiring and firing of physicians, and out-of-group referrals. The Clinic hired and paid a formal medical director, who acted as the liaison to the Foundation's management. They shared responsibility with the Foundation for physician recruitment and payer contracting strategies. As time has passed and the parties have become more comfortable with each other, more and more responsibilities are being shared.

There were political ramifications to the decision to establish the Foundation. The Clinic included only a fraction of the physicians on the medical staffs of Mercy's hospitals. The others felt left out, and some—especially the specialists—viewed the Foundation as direct competition. Mercy assuaged these fears somewhat by promising a "pluralistic" approach to medical staff development. It would continue to support a prior-existing IPA, to develop specialty "centers of excellence," and would contemplate the possibility of similar foundation relationships with other physician groups.

Because of the tensions within the medical community over the new foundation, publicity of developments was kept low-key. A simple press interview was held, without any further media events.

The Foundation has made rapid progress since its creation. In fact, it has not had the capacity to take advantage of all the opportunities for growth and expansion. It has moved deliberately to maintain consensus between the leadership of the Clinic and Mercy.

The Clinic has retained financial responsibility for out-of-group medical services. With such an incentive to control those expenditures, it has subcapitated as many of those services as possible, negotiated reduced fees for others, and tightly managed their use without compromising quality of care. To meet the increased demand for its services, the Clinic more than doubled in size—mainly through the addition of PCPs.

Rather than affiliating primarily with a single HMO, the Foundation has entered into managed care contracts with multiple payers. The Clinic and Mercy have been able coordinate their negotiations for these contracts, an advantage that has persuaded a couple of HMOs to trade exclusive arrangements with other area hospitals for contracts with the Foundation. It also has embarked on Medicare risk contracting.

At the beginning, the management structure of the Clinic simply moved over to the Foundation. Since then, it has become more specialized and sophisticated, adding capabilities in operating systems, financial accounting, contract analysis and negotiation, and utilization management. The management information system has been upgraded, with the long-range goal of integrating the financial and clinical information systems with those at the hospitals. Employee benefits have been improved, and support staff morale has increased.

Despite the clear success of the Foundation, the Clinic's physicians still have some worries. They are the rapid rate of growth, the loss of physician autonomy, competitive compensation for physicians, the development of managed care systems, and the strategic direction of the Mercy hospitals, as well as the larger Catholic Healthcare West.

CASE STUDY: SUTTER MEDICAL FOUNDATION (SACRAMENTO, CALIFORNIA)

The Sutter Medical Foundation (SMF)[6–8] emerged from a fairly typical background in 1992. It was originally established as the Sacramento Sierra Medical Group (SSMG) in 1984 by 25 PCPs and three specialists. Some described it at that time as a "group practice without walls"[9(p.114)]; an affiliated hospital executive called it a "subsidized IPA."[10(p.116)] It combined centralized business operations with decentralized delivery of care. One of the founders described the SSMG's vision to "organize an effective single business entity to maximize economic clout and yet preserve some traditional values of autonomy."[11(p.114)]

Participating physicians maintained their separate offices and employed their own staff. The SSMG central office employed 65 people who provided a variety of support services, including purchasing, personnel, payroll and benefits, accounts payable, patient billing, malpractice insurance, contract administration, financial reporting, and patient placement. In return, each physician paid a monthly fee of $1,000 plus a percentage of net revenues.

Financial problems began to develop in the late 1980s and reached a crescendo in 1991. The SSMG was investing significant sums in growth projects such as new information systems; it failed in its efforts to establish regular sources of ancillary income; it was not delivering health care at competitive costs; and the physician incomes were lower than those available elsewhere. It became clear that SSMG was seriously undercapitalized.

The SSMG's strategic vision was revised to become a multispecialty clinic, provide reasonable incomes to its physicians, and offer competitive costs to its payers and patients. It estimated that it would require $20 million over five years to realize this vision.

The SSMG set out to find a suitable capital partner. It sent out a request for proposals (RFPs) to several area PPMCs and health systems. Negotiations quickly focused on Sutter Health, a nonprofit integrated health system of hospitals, medical groups, health plans, ambulatory centers, nursing homes, and other facilities covering most of Northern California. In a very painful decision-making process, the physicians decided to affiliate with Sutter. There was great concern about a perceived loss of control, but a capital partner was essential, and Sutter seemed to be the best choice.

The SMF was established in 1992 as a nonprofit organization that owned and operated outpatient medical care facilities. It employed most of the nonphysician personnel, contracted with third party payers, leased facilities, owned all the assets, incurred all the liabilities, and provided a range of business, administrative, and financial services to the physicians. The SSMG continued as a physician-owned, for-profit professional corporation.

The SSMG entered into a professional services agreement with the SMF under which the SMF compensated the SSMG for the medical services it provided. The agreement also covered the costs of physician staff, physician benefits, quality assurance and utilization review, physician recruiting, and credentialing. A premise of the compensation arrangement was that each PCP would receive $20,000 over the volume of revenue personally generated.

Sutter Health made some immediate moves to improve the operating efficiency of the physician group. The total number of participating physicians was reduced from 140 to 100, with most of those who left being specialists. As a result, the group became very much oriented toward primary care. The original 70 physician offices were consolidated into a much smaller number of "medical plazas."

As part of Sutter Health, the SMF now has become four separate MFs. The SSMG is now the Sutter Medical Group, composed of 139 physicians.

QUESTIONS TO ASK WHEN YOU ARE INVITED TO JOIN A HOSPITAL-SPONSORED MF

Selling your practice assets to an MF should be approached with the same caution as selling to a PPMC. Here are some questions to ask yourself and the MF officials.

1. Where will the management of the new organization come from? What is their experience in running organizations of this sort? Does their prior history or affiliation suggest a bias toward one partner or another in the venture (i.e., the hospital)?
2. Which of your practice assets will be acquired by the foundation? Will the intangible value of your practice as an ongoing

business be included? How will the value of the assets to be acquired be determined?

3. What will be the composition of the foundation's board of trustees? What proportion of the board members will be physicians? How will those physician members be chosen? Despite the composition of the entire board, what will be the makeup of the several committees under the board? Will physicians dominate the clinical committees and have leading roles on the committees addressing physician compensation?

4. Are you part of a group of physicians who will participate, as a group, in the foundation? If not, would it make sense to first organize such a group, even informally, to present a stronger, united front in negotiating with the hospital?

5. Which area hospital(s) will be your partner in the foundation? If there is a choice of potentially interested hospitals, is this hospital the best one for what will be a permanent relationship? What is its reputation for dealing with physicians? What is its experience in managing physician practices and providing services under managed care contracts? What proportion of its medical staff are physicians who will participate in the foundation? If a significant number of the medical staff will be excluded from this new affiliation, how are they likely to react?

6. Will the foundation act as the agent and conduit for all managed care contracts entered into by the physicians and the hospital(s) or will the hospital continue to receive significant revenues outside the scope of the foundation?

7. Has a comprehensive business plan been prepared for the new organization, including projections of income statements, balance sheets, and cash flow statements for the first three to five years? How much capital is the foundation projected to need, both to get started and to carry it through two or three years of possible operating losses? Where will this capital come from? What will the foundation be giving up in return for the capital?

8. What is the strategic vision of original participants for the future of the foundation? What are the specific strategic objectives set out in the business plan? Do they fit with what you know is going on in the local health care marketplace?

9. What is the historical relationship between the physicians and the hospital(s) joining in the foundation? How would you describe the culture and values of the physicians and the hospital(s)? Do they appear to be compatible? Is there a sufficient foundation of trust upon which to build a close and permanent working relationship?

REFERENCES

1. *1994 Exempt Organizations Continuing Professional Education Technical Instruction Program* (Washington, DC: Government Printing Office, 1993), 214.

2. "Facey Medical Foundation" (Release Date 31 March, 1993, Doc. 93-4212), *Tax Notes Today*, 6 April, 1993, Cite 93, 76–102.

3. "Harriman Jones Medical Foundation" (Release Date 3 February, 1994, Doc. 94 '-1574), *Tax Notes Today*, 15 February, 1994, Cite 94, 31–103.

4. Rockford Memorial Health Services" Corporation (Release Date 4 April, 1994, Doc. 94-3802), *Tax Notes Today*, 19 April, 1994, Cite 94, 63–75.

5. D.F. Covert, "Mercy Medical Foundation of Sacramento: A Case Study," *Topics in Health Care Financing 20*, no. 3 (1994): 70–79.

6. D.C. Coddington and B.J. Bendrick, *Integrated Health Care: Case Studies* (Englewood, CO: Center for Research in Ambulatory Health Care Administration, 1994).

7. Sutter Health. http://www.sutterhealth.org

8. "Old Sutter Rivals Forge Alliance," *Sacramento Business Journal*, 3 February, 1997, http://www.amcity.com/sacramento/stories/020397/story1.html

9. Coddington and Bendrick, *Integrated Health Care*, 114.

10. Coddington and Bendrick, *Integrated Health Care*, 116.

11. Coddington and Bendrick, *Integrated Health Care*, 114.

CHAPTER 18

Step Nine: Selling Your Practice to a Hospital, Managed Care Organization, or Physician Practice Management Company

INTRODUCTION

A couple of the strategic steps already covered—physician practice management companies (PPMCs) and medical foundations (MFs)—have involved the acquisition by a new outside organization of the assets of the physicians and the groups. There are several other scenarios under which this asset transfer will be required. In the end, when virtually all care in the United States is delivered by large, multistate integrated delivery systems (IDSs), there are likely to be few physicians or group practices still in legal possession of their practice assets.

This chapter discusses all of the key issues that must be considered by the physician or group wishing to participate in such a transaction. It will review the circumstances under which a physician may want to sell his practice or, in some cases, purchase another physician's practice. The different ways in which the transaction can be carried out will be explained, with the pros and cons of each laid out. It also will explore the key structural, economic, and legal issues on which the selling or buying physician should focus.

WHO SHOULD READ THIS CHAPTER

If you are under the age of 50 and engaged in the private practice of medicine, it is almost certain that, at some point in your career, you will be involved in the sale of your practice or, as an individual or member of a group practice, in the purchase of another physician's practice.

Rapidly growing numbers of physicians are selling their practices to hospitals, PPMCs, MFs, hospitals, and physician group practices. The selling physician's motives usually are to pass on the responsibilities of day-to-day management of the practice in order to concentrate on delivering care. Organizations are buying practices to lock in that physician and her skills toward a goal of becoming more competitive in the managed care marketplace. The most serious potential problem is a transaction that looks as if it is compensating the selling physician for future referrals to the buying entity. Both sides will learn in this chapter how to avoid this legal outcome and still produce a win-win transaction.

WHY YOU MIGHT BE SELLING A MEDICAL PRACTICE

If you are thoroughly engaged in conducting a thriving solo or group practice, you might have trouble imagining the circumstances under which you might want to sell your practice. The pressures of managed care and increased competition make this possibility much more likely.

The traditional reasons for selling your practice still pertain. Through illness or other calamity, you may become incapable of practicing medicine at an acceptable level of quality. Eventually, you will choose to retire from medical practice. Family or personal motives may push you to relocate to a new geographic area—requiring that you dispose of your present practice and acquire or establish a new practice in your new community.

Of course, the move to a new geographic area may be caused by market or competitive pressures. Other physicians in your specialty may have organized so early and so quickly that you have been squeezed out and can no longer get patients. You didn't get on the managed care bandwagon soon enough and now the managed care organizations (MCOs) that dominate the local market have all the physicians in your specialty that they need. Perhaps, you are just trying to find some place in the country still untouched by the move to integration and managed care—such as Alaska or southern Mississippi.

More likely, you will choose to sell your practice and continue practicing medicine in the same area. Here are some of the possible scenarios:

- The management requirements of claims processing with multiple payers, as well as the practice demands of utilization review, ask for more responsibility and competence than the physician has available.
- Local market competition threatens the survival of the practice in its present form, and its market value is dwindling. Without a clear idea of what he will do next, the physician simply wants to get out while the price is high.
- A new strategic organizational option has become available that offers the physician a way to negotiate on better terms with managed care companies entering the local market. Examples are PPMCs, MFs, and multispecialty group practices. Participation in that option requires selling the physician's practice.
- Economic survival in the future requires participation in an IDS. Frequently, that participation requires that the physician yield legal ownership of her practice.
- By selling to and taking a leading role in a larger physician-run organization, the physician may see an opportunity to acquire suffi-

cient capital resources and management expertise in order to offer managed care services directly to purchasers. In other words, he sees the opportunity to compete directly with the MCOs.
- Younger physicians are more sympathetic to managed care and willing to practice in large multispecialty groups, with the result that small groups have difficulty recruiting new physicians as either employees or owners.

To put it more bluntly, under the coming new order in health care delivery, there will be no solo or small group practices. They all will have been absorbed into larger entities. The only exceptions will be in specialties not covered by managed care contracts (e.g., cosmetic surgery) or practices that cater to the very wealthy.

WHY YOU MIGHT BE BUYING A MEDICAL PRACTICE

If the solo or small group practice doctor needs to become part of a larger, more influential group of providers, that "grouping" can occur in two basic ways. The doctor can be bought up by one of the developing larger groups or, perhaps in collaboration with colleagues, the doctor may be the catalyst for building the large group. In the latter case, the doctor will be buying other practices rather than selling her own practice (Exhibit 18–1).

Let's look at some scenarios.

- If you live and practice in a small community and have the necessary capital, you may start from scratch in acquiring the practices of other physicians in town. You will almost certainly continue to employ the affected physicians. You might begin with practices in your own specialty. Then you could turn to other related specialties (e.g., family medicine, obstetrics/gynecology, pediatrics). Eventually, the group will reach a critical mass, at which point development of a full-blown multispecialty group practice will seem the

EXHIBIT 18–1 Special Note on Integration through Acquisition

The word *integration* keeps coming up in discussions of the American health care industry. It is an important term. It refers to the deliberate combining—through contract, purchase, or affiliation—of different providers and different kinds of providers. This is being done with the intent of creating larger delivery organizations offering a full spectrum of health care services through a group of providers that share common goals.

By working together under the same organizational umbrella, they are able to minimize inefficiencies, utilization, and costs, while maintaining high-quality levels.

Integration is not a new term. It has been used for decades to describe the way that the industry evolves over time. Integration can take place in horizontal and vertical directions. Both trends are apparent in the health care industry.

Look at the creation of a product for delivery to a consumer in terms of a long chain, beginning with raw materials, which are refined into basic manufacturing elements, which are transformed into product parts, which are assembled into finished products, which are sold to a wholesaler, who sells them to a retailer, who passes them on to the final customer. Each of these steps can be performed by a separate business.

For instance, a company may decide to be the assembler of product "A." It buys the necessary parts from parts manufacturer "B" and sells the finished products to wholesaler "C." *Vertical* integration for company "A" would be to buy companies "B" and "C," and perhaps to go even further backward and forward in the chain of manufacturing and distribution. There is nothing to prevent one organization from owning every link in the chain, from an iron ore mining company to the retail stores selling to the customer. *Horizontal* integration occurs when a business acquires or merges with other organizations just like itself (e.g., product assembler "A "buys product assembler "D").

These same concepts exist in the health care industry. The pieces of the chain look different, perhaps including these entities:

Free-standing emergency center
↓
Free-standing ambulatory, outpatient, or walk-in clinic
↓
Primary care physicians (solo practice)
↓
Specialist physicians (solo practice)
↓
Small, single-specialty group practice
↓
Large, multispecialty group practice
↓
In-patient hospital
↓
Subacute medical facility
↓
Rehabilitation facility
↓
Skilled/long-term care facility
↓
Home health service

If you are a physician in a small, single-specialty group practice, the development of your group into a larger practice comprising several specialties or the purchase or establishment of an outpatient clinic would be considered vertical integration. Simply purchasing or merging with other practices in the same specialty would be considered horizontal integration.

It is important to understand the concept of integration as it will be a major part of the long-term strategy for a successful physician practice.

obvious next step. This is the most ambitious scenario.

- To secure contracts or business with any new payer that comes into town—MCO, insurance company, or employer—you prefer that

all the physicians in your specialty form a unified group and speak with one voice. Toward that end, you commit to building, through acquisition, a single specialty group practice that simply cannot be ignored by any purchasers of health care in your market area.

- You are proficient at managing your practice and feel comfortable performing that kind of work, along with delivering patient care. It would be a source of accomplishment and income for you to take over (that is, purchase) and run the practices of other physicians in the area.

Horizontal Integration

- You are generally concerned about the competition from other medical practices in your area. They are negotiating attractive managed care contracts, entering into affiliations with a variety of other providers, and becoming more formidable in size and competitive acumen. Before it is too late, you decide to start buying up the competition, getting bigger than the competition, and enjoying the economies of scale that come with greater size.
- To become a more professional and efficient medical care delivery organization, you realize that substantial capital resources and sophisticated management expertise are necessary. These assets are more readily available to a larger organization. So you decide to build the size of your practice through the acquisition of other practices.

Vertical Integration

- You are confident that you could compete as well as the next physician for managed care contracts, if only you had a tighter rein on the costs of care delivery. You could achieve better cost control if you had some say over what happened to your patients before they came to you and after you passed them on to other physicians. To obtain that control, you elect to purchase practices that typically refer patients to you or to whom you refer patients.
- Instead of cost control, you conclude that better quality control is the key to your competitive success. The solution is similar—extend your control over the delivery process

backward and forward in the referral continuum. Buy up practices above and below you on the feeding chain.

- In contract negotiations with MCOs, you have noticed their preference for "one-stop shopping," the opportunity to execute one contract or a very few contracts with provider organizations that offer several, if not all, of the health care services promised to their members. The negotiations are easier, less costly, and less time-consuming than trying to deal with a much larger number of solo or group practice doctors. Your patients also are likely to be happier if they can obtain all the services they need from the same organization, probably in the same facility. The best way of building this capability seems to be the creation of a larger multispecialty group practice. You will begin acquiring numerous practices in the specialties needed to compete for comprehensive coverage managed care contracts.
- The physicians who will do best under capitated managed care are those with the greatest capacity to accept and manage risk. Managed care payers seek such providers. It probably will be easier to learn risk management skills if you are part of a larger group of like-minded physicians. The peer interaction will catch problem practice styles and reinforce cost-effective practice techniques. Experimentation with internal utilization review may be possible. The larger number of patients or lives covered by a larger group of physicians will permit spreading the risk over a larger population. Acquiring practices is a dynamic way of gathering around you such a group of physician colleagues.
- You have a strong entrepreneurial spirit and, after careful market analysis, have determined that you and some colleagues have the ability, resources, and determination to create an IDS offering comprehensive enough services to compete directly with any MCO that comes into town. You embark on an active strategy of acquiring the practices and other providers necessary to form an IDS.

FROM WHOM YOU MIGHT BE BUYING A MEDICAL PRACTICE

The sellers of medical practices are likely to be physicians with the same motives for selling as you might have, as explained earlier. They will be doctors who are unable to practice any longer, who are retiring, who are moving away, or who are simply giving up trying to practice medicine in the new health care industry. However, you also may find sale candidates among colleagues who are dismayed and confounded by the managed care/integration revolution and realize that they do not have the entrepreneurial spirit to respond on their own. They see that they must become part of something bigger and will leap at the opportunity to ally themselves with a physician-run organization. As a physician, you have a real advantage in persuading other doctors to sell their practices to you and become employees under your enlightened management.

TO WHOM YOU MIGHT BE SELLING A MEDICAL PRACTICE

If you have good reasons for getting rid of your practice, you might then wonder who would have a good reason for buying it from you. There are a number of candidates, best classified as (a) physician-run entities and (b) non–physician-run organizations such as hospitals and for-profit MSOs. The nature of the buyer and the motives for seeking your practice are factors you will consider in deciding whether to sell to them, not to mention whether to be employed by them.

Here are some typical situations in which physicians, hospitals, and other may be motivated to purchase your practice.

Physician Buyers

- A younger physician wishing to take over your patients or quickly establish a practice without taking the time to slowly build it up.
- Another physician or small group wishing to eliminate the direct competition you offer.

- A larger multispecialty group practice that requires a practitioner in your specialty in order to offer a full range of medical services to managed care purchasers and patients.
- A large and growing group of physicians planning to acquire sufficient physician mass to bargain more effectively with MCOs and insurance companies.

Nonphysician Buyers

- The local hospital, at which you have admitting privileges, wants to secure more tightly the patient referrals or hospital admissions you generate. By purchasing your practice and employing you directly, it virtually guarantees that all your patients will be sent to that hospital.
- In certain hospital-based specialties (e.g., radiology and anesthesiology), the local hospital prefers to have more direct, unified control over the practicing physicians. Toward that end, it wishes to acquire the assets of several doctors in your hospital-based specialty and to employ the selling physicians as a somewhat integrated group.
- The local hospital recognizes the advantage of being able to offer an MCO something close to a full package of the medical services required by the MCO's members. To accomplish that, it takes steps to affiliate the hospital with all the other providers needed to deliver those services. Some of the affiliations with physicians involve outright purchase of their practices and subsequent employment of the doctors.
- An entrepreneurial individual or group sees the opportunity to earn a profit by offering a needed service in your area. To meet the desires of physicians to avoid practice management headaches and to concentrate on clinical work, they set up a simple corporation to buy practices, manage the business of the practices, and employ the previous physician owners.

In surveying the range of potential buyers, you will encounter different kinds of organizations created primarily for the purpose of buying physician practices. These are some of the most common types, along with their key advantages and disadvantages.

Management Services Organization— Hospital-Owned

- provides administrative and practice management services (billing, purchasing, space rental, equipment rental, information systems, marketing, etc.)
- purchases, then owns the assets of the physician's practice, though some do not get involved in practice acquisition
- is not at all involved in the delivery of clinical services
- is owned by a hospital or a subsidiary of a hospital created specifically for this purpose
- hospital's goal is to influence the physician's referral patterns, without literally paying for them
- has further advantage to managed care negotiations from greater efficiency through tighter integration between hospital and physician
- PLUS: may enter into relationships with almost any kind of physician practice entity—solo practices, group practices, independent provider organizations (IPAs), or physician-hospital organizations (PHOs)
- PLUS: can become the cornerstone for strategic movement in any direction, to take advantage of competitive changes
- MINUS: economic incentives for participating physicians may clash with those of hospital owner, making further affiliation and integration harder

Physician Practice Management Company— For-Profit Business

- provides administrative and practice management services (billing, purchasing, space rental, equipment rental, information systems, marketing, etc.)
- purchases, then owns the assets of the physician's practice
- negotiates managed care contracts on behalf of the participating physicians
- is not at all involved in the delivery of clinical services
- might be created by almost anybody with an entrepreneurial urge
- has a strategic goal of building a physician network, if not an IDS
- has primary motive of earning profits
- PLUS: professional management of business aspects of medical practice
- PLUS: substantial infusion of new capital
- PLUS: opportunity for physicians to realize great gain on PPMC stock when it goes public
- MINUS: some PPMC entrepreneurs are in for the quick kill
- MINUS: profit motivation may impinge on physician autonomy

Medical Foundation

- this is particularly appealing, and virtually necessary, in states that prohibit the corporate practice of medicine
- the purchasing organization is a charitable, nonprofit, tax-exempt foundation
- the foundation purchases the practice assets of individual physicians or groups of physicians
- the physicians continue to deliver medicine through a physician group that has a professional services contract with the foundation
- this model also may employ physicians directly
- PLUS: access to lower-cost, tax-deductible capital financing
- PLUS: common goals shared by physician and hospital components facilitate MCO contracting
- MINUS: more expensive to gain federal tax-exempt status
- MINUS: rules affecting tax-exempt organizations limit possible physician compensation arrangements and amounts

Physician-Owned Integrated Delivery System

- ultimate purchaser and owner is a large physician group practice
- long-term goal is formation of an IDS that competes directly with and beats non–physician-owned MCOs at their own game, while keeping overall control in the hands of physicians
- "system" is probably composed of many interconnected pieces, one of which may be the entity that legally purchases and owns the practice assets
- participating physician is usually required to become a member of the controlling group practice, to make a substantial capital investment in the system, and to sell assets to the system
- selling physician may also have option to join the IPA that is another component of the system or to be employed directly by a component hospital or the physician-run parent corporation
- PLUS: attracts as owners/founders/investors, physicians desiring to invest in a direct service delivery organization
- PLUS: attracts as practice sellers, physicians preferring to yield control of their practice assets only to an organization run by other physicians
- MINUS: high capital costs as there are no tax-deductible advantages
- MINUS: many physicians simply cannot afford the high initial investment threshold

EXACTLY WHAT YOU MIGHT BE BUYING OR SELLING

Generally, "buying a business" means one of two things. On one hand, you may simply purchase the identified assets of the business—as they might be listed on the balance sheet. On the other hand, you may purchase the business as an ongoing commercial entity that synergistically combines its assets to produce, and promises to produce in the future, an outcome greater than the sum of the sale prices of the assets separately.

The value of a medical practice to a purchaser is the sum of its tangible and intangible assets. These include:

Tangible Assets

- furniture and equipment
- supplies
- accounts receivable
- real estate
- balance sheet items (cash, investments)

Intangible Assets

- use of practice name
- patient lists
- patient information (included in medical records)
- location
- advantageous lease arrangement
- noncompete agreement
- patient care contracts (particularly managed care and capitation)
- employee contracts
- reputation of the physician and the practice for a certain kind of care

Although *intangible assets* are often defined collectively as "goodwill," it probably is more accurate to say that the value of a business that is left after you subtract the worth of the tangible assets and of the intangible assets that can be specifically identified is the goodwill of the business. It is the mysterious value that results when an entrepreneur combines just the right mix of resources in a way that produces a commercial outcome that exceeds the sale value of the individual resources. It is the value of the collection of tangible and intangible assets as a "going business enterprise."

The buyer usually decides what it wants to buy. A hospital or management services organization (MSO) buyer is interested in binding the physicians to the hospital without alienating them. They accomplish this by purchasing the tangible assets of the physicians' practices, leasing them back to the physicians, providing practice management services, and otherwise letting the physicians continue to operate their individual practices under their original practice names. Modest size group practices, aiming to diversify and grow larger, may follow this same strategy. It is the least threatening approach to physicians.

Larger, heavily capitated multispecialty groups in more mature markets are after one thing: covered lives and warm bodies to treat them. They are primarily interested in physicians who will enhance their ability to deliver capitated care. Their preferred targets are physicians with large populations of capitated patients. They also will pursue those who fill specialty gaps or practice in geographic areas consistent with their expansion strategies.

These large purchasers prefer to pay for the business enterprise value of a practice. Unless the practice will continue in its present location, the tangible assets are not worth much to the purchaser. Money will be paid for those assets, but only to placate the selling physician or as a more legally acceptable way of paying for goodwill. *

The price that you will receive for your practice is a function of both the type of assets purchased and the value at which they are purchased. If you believe that some worthwhile assets are being ignored, the difference often can be made up in the value placed on the assets actually purchased, and vice versa. Different buyers employ different methodologies to arrive a final purchase price. Focus on the overall price you are being offered.

BASIC OUTLINE OF A PRACTICE ACQUISITION PROCESS

It is a good idea to understand practice acquisition as a detailed multistep process that must be followed religiously. If you try to improvise as

you go along, you will miss something and probably commit serious blunders.

A. The initial purchase decision emerges from a long-term strategic plan. The process of buying a medical practice should be a logical part of your own personal, or your organization's, long-term plan. Because many individuals and group practices lack such plans, the first step in this process often is to develop one. Strategic plans have to do with overall missions, measurable long-term goals, and tactical actions for achieving them. There is a multitude of articles, books, and consultants prepared to assist with the planning. Do not prepare the plan to justify your intuitive decision to purchase another's medical practice. If created objectively, the plan may indicate that you should not purchase a medical practice.

B. Test the purchase decision against the alternatives. You should purchase another practice only to achieve a strategic objective. Make sure that a purchase is best way of reaching that objective. If you have concluded that survival depends on being part of a larger multispecialty physician group, perhaps it makes more sense to sell out to an existing group than to buy enough practices to create your own. Do some brainstorming on alternatives and evaluate them with an open mind.

C. Prepare a tactical business plan for carrying out the acquisition. Do not start down the road toward purchasing a practice or selling your own without a game plan prepared in advance. Without one, you are very likely to miss a step or make an ill-informed decision. You may regret it for years. Start with this outline now. Then fill in the smaller tasks as you explore the different directions your strategy might take. Set timelines for completing the steps and the tasks.

D. If you are a solo or small group practitioner and will have to conduct the purchase or sale transaction yourself, set aside sufficient time for carrying out all the related tasks. Then double that time. If you are a member of a larger group planning such a transaction, delegate one or more of your colleagues to handle the duties. Choose them because of their business and negotiating skills. If a team has been selected, assign clearly defined roles to each person.

*The Office of the Inspector General (OIG) of the federal Department of Health and Human Services has informally called into question the legality of payment for intangible assets, particularly "goodwill." This is discussed later in this chapter.

E. Review the regulatory and other legal implications of the proposed transaction. This chapter lays out most of the important ones. Do this with the assistance of a health lawyer. Be prepared to restructure the transaction to take into account the legal constraints.

F. Prepare three-year financial projections that include the practice's requirements for capital investment, working capital, human resources, and other inventory purchases.

G. Study thoroughly the market in which your practice competes. Come to an understanding of the influence and role that you are playing. How do other providers view you? Who are your primary competitors? How large are they and what are their strategic intentions? Where does your practice fit into the market equation? Write all this down. Most of this information is available from the physicians, hospitals, insurance companies, and MCOs you already deal with. Begin politely "debriefing" every health care provider and payer you encounter. Perhaps you can use some assistance in this important data-gathering and evaluation—such as a local business school student or a full-blown marketing consultant.

H. Specify the criteria that you would like to satisfy in choosing the practice or practices you will acquire—or in choosing by whom you will be acquired. Look at it this way: You are choosing a practice partner for life. Before you speak with any prospects, sit down with your practice colleagues and list the benefits you want to obtain through this transaction. Here is what one group came up with:

- Offer an improvement in lifestyle (more vacation time, continuing medical education [CME] reimbursement, less stressful working conditions, improved benefits, more time for teaching and research, more time for personal life).
- Protect employment status of current staff.
- Increase access to capital resources for physician recruitment, equipment purchase, facility growth, and new ventures.
- Exhibit interest and willingness to invest in certain community-based programs (neonatal, geriatric).

- Continue physician control of routine practice management issues.
- Share control with physicians over long-term strategic practice matters.
- Maintain existing specialist referral patterns to avoid antagonizing specialty physicians who feel threatened by the purchase/sale.
- Take prompt action (by the purchaser) on physician concerns and requests for decisions.
- Continue the practice name and identity.
- Have a bail-out plan for either party in the event that the partnership proves unworkable during the first year or two.
- Offer a fair purchase price. This is not the sole criterion!

I. Start scouting for potential buyers or sellers. Go through this phase even if you think you know who the other party to the transaction will be. You may come up with a better candidate than you already have.

J. Identify, evaluate, and prioritize—according to your predetermined criteria—potential practices to purchase or potential purchasers of your practice. This can be done quantitatively by rating each prospect for each of the criteria, weighting each of the criteria, and multiplying the numbers. The result is a numerical assessment of your purchase options. Do not be lulled by a false sense of objectivity. Feel free to adjust the ratings according to your gut feelings about a person or organization.

K. Open a dialogue with your top three sale or acquisition candidates. The first approach can be tricky, and there are several recommended strategies. The easiest and, usually, the most effective is respectful and uncontrived candor about what you are proposing. Have all your facts and opinions assembled. More than ever, try to present your proposal in terms of the benefits it offers the candidate person or organization. Keep in mind that, depending on how you answered the question about continued involvement, you may be working and practicing with this person for several years into the future. View this step as the beginning of a long-term relationship, rather than the opening of negotiations. Insist on dealing with key people who have the knowledge and authority to answer your questions.

Execute a confidentiality agreement between you and the other party. If the proposed purchase or sale is revealed prematurely, many interests can be compromised. Patients and payers that you serve may be confused by the rumors and may limit their contacts with your practice. Colleagues in the medical community, including referral sources and targets, may feel threatened enough by what they hear to cut off referrals. Even if they do not go that far, there is no point in antagonizing them unnecessarily. Other potential partners may be alienated or given a negotiating advantage if they hear of your current deal too soon. Signing a confidentiality agreement with any serious prospective buyers or sellers is an essential formality. Even with such protection, be prepared for possible leaks.

M. Collect basic information needed to assess the practice. This is less rigorous than the due diligence check, which comes later. This information will include historical financial statements, as well as data on the routine operations of the practice. Learn about the demographics of the patient population, the mix of payers, and the reputation of the participating physicians.

N. Preliminary negotiations. This is the period running from the opening of a dialogue with the prospective partner through the signing of a letter of intent. During this stage, the goal should be to work out the major terms of what the buyer wants or is willing to give and what the seller wants or is willing to accept. The parties also will be feeling each other out as potential long-term partners. This may be the beginning of a close and enduring business relationship. Approach that prospect with awareness and sensitivity.

O. Make or receive an initial offer, including a price for the assets, an employment agreement for the selling physician, and a noncompete agreement.

P. Carry out the process that lawyers call *due diligence*. This is an extremely thorough and detailed check of all the background information about the buyer or seller that a reasonably responsible person would want to know. Your lawyer will have a very clear idea of the kinds of facts and documents to ask for. Some of it may seem to be nit-picking; get it and review it anyway. A fuller listing of the items in a good due diligence audit appears later in this chapter.

Q. If you have gotten this far without any major problems, reach an informal agreement with the buyer or seller on the critical issues, commit it to a letter of intent, negotiate the remaining small (but sometimes deal-breaking) details, and consummate the transaction. This letter represents an explicit moral obligation of the parties to continue negotiating in good faith until a final agreement is reached. It also is a documentation of the basic terms of the understanding so far. However, until the final agreement is concluded, neither party is legally bound.

R. Determine a value for the practice components to be sold or purchased. This is a very sensitive phase of the transaction. The resulting figures have the potential for displeasing either the buyer or the seller and sometimes both at the same time. The legal implications of an inaccurate or biased valuation of inappropriate assets may doom the deal and subject some participants to criminal or civil penalties. The entire valuation is covered more thoroughly below.

S. Conclude the purchase agreement, the employment agreement, the noncompete agreement, and other related legal documents.

T. If an outgoing relationship between you and the buyer/seller is contemplated, now is when it officially begins.

KEY STEP: UNDERSTANDING THE LEGAL RAMIFICATIONS

If buying and selling a medical practice were like buying an automobile, the health care industry would be much further along the road toward integration and consolidation. One of the primary barriers has been the legal constraints on these transactions. They are not a cause for great anxiety, but they must be recognized and observed, and—in some cases—the transaction must be restructured to account for them.

Here is what to be worried about. These are the issues your attorney should be discussing with you.

A. Corporate Practice of Medicine

A few states still prohibit what is called the *corporate practice of medicine*. In fact, this is a prohibition against corporations directly employing physicians or exercising significant control over their clinical practice of medicine. The legal doctrine was created several decades ago to protect the practice autonomy of physicians. This doctrine presents four problems in connection with buying and selling medical practices.

First, many types of organizations simply cannot become involved in practice acquisitions if the net result gives them any noticeable control over a physician's clinical practice. At the very least, a traditional for-profit hospital or MSO may not directly employ a physician whose practice assets it just has purchased. Even without actual employment, the hospital or MSO may not retain enough control over the physician to influence her practice behavior. Of course, this usually obviates the purchase in the first place.

It normally is not enough simply to execute a contract that states that the physician is an independent contractor who controls all aspects of her practice if the actual relationship between the buyer and the physician appears to be that of employer and employee. The most common solution to this problem is to create a charitable nonprofit foundation to purchase the practice assets and employ the physician. An even better solution is to let the foundation own the assets and require the selling physician to join a single, large medical group that provides professional services under contract to the foundation.

Medical foundations and allied group practices are very popular in California because that state's law both dictates that "Corporations and other artificial legal entities shall have no professional rights, privileges, or powers." and permits "charitable institutions, foundations, or clinics"[1] to employ physicians.

Second, corporate entities in "corporate practice of medicine" states may not own the "goodwill" of a medical practice. Therefore, even if they do not attempt to employ the physician after the purchase, the acquisition must be limited to tangible assets.

Third, the "corporate practice" doctrine may inhibit compensation to an MSO based on a percentage of the practice's net revenues. Such an arrangement gives the impression that the MSO has an ownership interest in the practice.

Fourth, it might be argued that the MSO is managing certain practice issues that have the effect of interfering with the physician's clinical autonomy.

B. Federal Antikickback Law

If the purchaser of a physician's practice is another provider (e.g., hospital-owned MSO) to whom the physician might refer patients, the federal antikickback or fraud and abuse law forbids any part of the practice purchase price from being reimbursement, current or prospective, for such referrals. This requires a transaction in which the final price is not a vague number subject to misinterpretation, but rather one tied to specific assets for which solid fair market values have been established.

Furthermore, the ongoing fees paid for the MSO's practice management services must also reflect fair market values. This is necessary to avoid the charge that fees are set artificially low to reward the physician for referrals.

Finally, this legal pitfall becomes very dangerous when the selling physician is subsequently employed by the hospital-buyer. There must be no connection between the physician's compensation and the flow of patients the physician directs to the hospital.

C. Federal Income Tax: Purchase by a Nonprofit, Tax-Exempt Organization

If the purchaser of a practice is a nonprofit, tax-exempt organization, it may not pay more than fair market value for the assets it acquires, nor may it receive less than fair market value for the practice management services it provides. To do otherwise would violate the Internal Revenue Service (IRS) bans on "private benefit" and "private inurement" out of tax-exempt funds.

To put it another way, an organization functioning solely as an MSO, providing practice management services to physicians, would not qualify for tax-exempt status. However, a larger, tax-exempt parent organization, such as a hospital, normally can own and operate a for-profit MSO. The net revenues from the MSO are "unrelated business income" to the hospital and may not be excessive in amount—compared with the total income of the hospital.

The same tax exemption restrictions apply to the compensation paid to the selling physician subsequently employed by the purchasing organization. Compensation arrangements must be reasonable, arrived at through arm's-length negotiation, be within the range of compensation for other physicians in the same specialty in similar markets, and be somewhere close to what the physician earned in private practice.

D. Covenants Not To Compete—When the Physician Is Not Employed by the Buyer and Continues To Practice

Noncompete covenants are a legitimate device for restricting the freedom of another person to compete against you or your organization. To be effective, the person who promises not to compete must receive something of value in return for his promise. Such covenants are requested by hospitals from physicians who either (a) sell their practices to the hospital but do not accept employment with the hospital, or (b) sell their practices to the hospital, accept employment, but someday may leave and return to private practice. The law is concerned that the covenants are not unduly restrictive and that payment for them is not disguised reimbursement for patient referrals.

Noncompete covenants have three dimensions: the type of competitive activity restricted, the geographic area in which it is restricted, and the time period for which it is restricted. If any one of these elements is excessively restrictive, the entire covenant could be thrown out by a court. A covenant that keeps you from practicing a specialty that the purchaser does not offer or practicing for an organization (e.g., neighborhood health center) with which the purchaser does not compete is unacceptable. The health care industry is in such turmoil that a noncompete agreement extending for more than two years is probably unacceptable. A hospital that services patients in a metropolitan area cannot prevent a physician from practicing anywhere in the state.

The value of noncompete provisions depends on the loss the purchaser could be expected to suffer if the selling physician went into competition with it. Computation of this loss involves estimates of the volume of patients and revenues that would move from the purchaser to the physician. Clearly, any value placed on a noncompete agreement is a very fuzzy number. The OIG will accept some payment for this highly intangible asset, as long as there are plausible facts and calculations to back it up.

E. Federal and State Antitrust Laws

One or a small number of physicians acquiring a few physician practices are not likely to create a violation of the federal or state antitrust laws. Legal problems may arise when the number of physicians in the group approaches a significant proportion of all those in a particular market area. Certainly anything over 50 percent will attract attention. Antitrust law enforcement authorities define the market for physician services by specialty. If a single group absorbs 7 of the 10 cardiologists in the area, it may be seen as a threat to monopolize the market for cardiology services.

There also are certain practices that are deemed to be anticompetitive and a violation of the antitrust laws. These are discussed in greater detail in Chapter 28, "Collaborating with Other Physicians without Legal Risk."

KEY STEP: INFORMATION GATHERING ABOUT THE MOTIVES OF THE PROSPECTIVE PURCHASER OF YOUR PRACTICE

One of the best ways to determine whether a prospective purchaser meets your criteria is to get answers to some basic strategic questions like these:

- What is the mission of your organization?
- What are your short- and long-term goals in this transaction and how do you see our practice helping you achieve those goals?
- How will our physicians, administrator, and current staff be utilized if this transaction is concluded? Will there be guarantees for current physician-employee relationships?
- How will you make decisions to invest further capital in growth or new programs for our practice?
- What governance structure and procedures will be applied to our practice? What role will our physicians and administrator have in decisions affecting our practice, such as the hiring of new physicians or the selection of new payer contracts?
- How much control will our physicians have over the routine clinical decision making, quality assurance programs, and utilization management mechanisms?
- Will our present practice name and identity be preserved?
- Who are the key decision makers in your organization and what is their previous experience in acquiring practices like ours?
- How will your acquisition of our practice benefit the local community?
- What exactly will be the responsibilities and authorities of the physicians in our group after the acquisition? How will their ongoing performance be evaluated?
- What assistance will you give us in announcing and explaining this transaction to anxious and suspicious members of the area medical community?

Note the substance of the answers you receive. In addition, grade the thoroughness, accuracy, and promptness of the answers from "A" to "E." Compile report cards on each candidate.

KEY STEP: CARRYING OUT DUE DILIGENCE

This means gathering a standard collection of documents and information relating to the legal status and financial condition of the people and organizations involved in the transaction. If things later go wrong, a court is more likely to find that you or your lawyer were as diligent as any reasonable person could be if you have looked at these documents. Incidentally, the volume of information you amass will help you decide whether owning this other practice will be as advantageous as you hope. It also will help you conclude whether these are people you want to work with on a long-term basis.

The list of appropriate documents is long and detailed; most of them fall in the following categories:

- organization and standing of the corporation
- financial statements
- accounts receivable
- condition and value of all key assets
- current and long-term liabilities
- corporate operating policies and budgets
- long-range strategic plans
- contractual and other legal commitments
- all insurance agreements
- federal and state tax status and returns
- all pending litigation and threatened claims (especially medical malpractice)
- real estate leases
- employment policies, contracts, and documents
- employee benefit plans
- environmental compliance actions and reports
- agreements with health care providers and payers

Unless you are selling your practice to retire, you will not be able to give this task the time it deserves. Pay a lawyer to have one of her paralegals do this.

KEY DECISION: HOW MUCH TO PAY FOR THE PRACTICE

There are two issues here—how much you want to pay and how much the law will allow you to pay. Your price preference should depend on two considerations. You want to pay as little as possible to bring a desirable practice into your organization. You also want to pay the physicians enough to entice them to sell and to leave them feeling good about it. If they are going to continue practicing—productively—for your group, they must not start off feeling bitter at being forced to sell at an unfair price.

Get a general idea of an appropriate price by obtaining valuations on the tangible and identifiable intangible assets of the practice. Those numbers, however, will not tell you much about how effectively the physicians have mobilized and managed those assets. If the practice is dying (older physicians, no managed care contracts, poor location), the book value, replacement value, or fair market value of the assets may really overstate its worth. If the practice is thriving (substantial capitation experience, modern information systems, open-minded physicians), simple asset values will understate its true worth.

Add or subtract from the asset valuation to account for the worth of the practice as an ongoing business. It also is possible to obtain a scientific valuation of the entire practice on an enterprise basis.

With those numbers in hand, you can proceed to negotiate a price mutually satisfactory to the buyer and seller. If the agreed-upon price is higher than any of the valuations that were obtained, it normally is possible to inflate, carefully, the prices paid for certain of those assets. The intangibles are most amenable to this kind of adjustment, such as a noncompete agreement that the selling physicians are willing to sign.

Warning!: This is an area of great concern to the law, particularly the OIG of the Department of Health and Human Services. In 1993, the Associate General Counsel of that office, D. McCarty Thornton, said, "Our concern is where the payment for intangibles is used as a disguise for the intention of the parties to recompense the practice for the future flow of patients from to the hospital. That would be illegal."[2] He is absolutely right. The question is whether his statement applies to any payments made for the worth of a practice as an ongoing business—for its "goodwill." The best answer right now is "probably not."

Hospitals are continuing to pay extra for the goodwill inherent in a practice, and none have been challenged by the OIG for doing so. The IRS regularly allows tax-exempt organizations to base part of their purchase price for practices on the goodwill of the practices.

To avoid liability in this area, do these things. Be clear in your own mind that you are not paying for or receiving money for an implicit promise from the selling physician to refer patients to the purchasing organization. State this verbally during the negotiations and repeat it in the purchase/sale agreement and the contract or employment agreement for continued services with the selling physician. Obtain valuations for the assets, tangible and intangible, and for the practice as an ongoing business from professionally trained, independent third parties. If goodwill appears to be a significant factor in the purchase, obtain a professional valuation of it, as well. Formulate a clear, convincing explanation for every aspect of the price that is being paid.

KEY STEP: VALUATION OF THE PRACTICE

The first step in determining a sale price for the practice is listing and valuing its assets, tangible and intangible. The broad categories of assets listed earlier must all be valued. The best valuation experts will use the following methodologies.

Tangible Assets

- furniture and equipment—fair market value on a going concern basis
- supplies—estimated by multiplying the average cost of supplies over the last several years by the weeks or months of supplies kept on hand
- accounts receivable—aged into 30-day categories and multiplied by adjusted collection percentages for each category
- real estate—conducted by a certified real estate appraiser or a local Realtor
- balance sheet items (cash, investments)—face value or market value

Intangible Assets

For solo and small group practices, the preferred valuation method for the entire package of intangible assets is the *comparative sales model*. This involves obtaining standard average data on the value of such assets (broken down by specialty, state, and urban/rural location of practice), adjusting them for the reputation of the practice and the quality of its management, and adding them to the valuations for the tangible assets. Such data are available from the Goodwill Registry, maintained by the Healthcare Group in Plymouth Meeting, Pennsylvania.

The *business enterprise model* calculates a discounted present value for five or more years of projected cash flows for the practice. A third approach compares the recent sale prices or income-earning characteristics of similar practices within the same geographic market to the practice in question. The problem there is that it is difficult to find two practices that are truly similar.

The IRS currently requires that a valuation or appraisal report be prepared and filed in connection with the purchase of a medical practice. It expects to see the following content in the report:

- executive summary
- description of the type of business and its history since it was founded

- analysis of the overall economic outlook for the region where the practice is located, as well as for the market in which the practice competes
- book value of the tangible assets of the practice
- overall financial condition of the practice
- earning capacity of the practice
- estimated value of the intangible assets
- discussion of comparable practices and their market value

Note: The valuation report serves two critical legal purposes—to demonstrate that a tax-exempt purchaser (i.e., a hospital) has paid no more than fair market value for the practice and to show that no portion of the purchase price is payment for patient referrals in violation of fraud and abuse laws.

It is in everyone's interest to have the valuation report prepared by independent third parties. It often makes sense to employ a health care consultant who is an expert in practice valuation to coordinate the several accountants, attorneys, and other specialists who may be needed to complete the report.

KEY DECISION: HOW MUCH TO PAY THE AFTER-EMPLOYED PHYSICIAN (WHEN THE BUYER AGREES TO EMPLOY THE PHYSICIAN SELLING THE PRACTICE)

Hospitals and other organizations most interested in acquiring physician practices very much want the physician to continue in practice. They have little use for equipment, supplies, leases, or even lists of patients primarily loyal to a departing physician. The physician will be invited to enter into a relationship with the acquiring organization as either an employee or an independent contractor.

The question arises, How much should that physician be paid? The answer is, as much as the buyer thinks he or she is worth—within limits set by the IRS and the OIG.

> **Note:** A miscue on this issue can affect the physician selling a practice as well. If the compensation is excessive or improper, the employment arrangement may fall apart. The physician may earn a salary lower than anticipated or may be without a job at all. If the antikickback law is implicated, the physician can be held liable for having received the excessive payments.

The IRS becomes interested in physician compensation, as it does with the purchase price for practice goodwill, only when the purchaser and subsequent employer of the physician is a tax-exempt hospital. It is concerned about preventing private inurement and excessive private benefit. It accomplishes this by requiring that the total compensation package for the physician, including base salary, incentive payments, benefits, and other gifts or gestures of value not exceed a "reasonable compensation" for the services actually provided by the physician.

The compensation level must be determined on the basis of arm's-length negotiations that result in rates competitive with what the market is paying for similar medical services. The compensation arrangement should be comparable to those used by other hospitals or medical groups of similar size and composition in the same market area. The rates paid must take into account that an employed physician does not have to cover the usual operating expenses of a private practice. The IRS Hospital Audit Guidelines[3] list the following factors as determinants of the "reasonableness" of physician compensation:

- duties performed and amount of responsibility
- time devoted to those duties
- special knowledge and experience
- individual ability
- previous training
- physician's salary history
- working conditions

- general economic conditions in the area (wages and prices)
- available living conditions in the area

In establishing the comparability of a particular compensation level, it is a good idea to obtain the baseline data from independent sources. Their objectivity will make your compensation arrangements more defensible. Look to the physician compensation surveys conducted by the American Medical Association and the Medical Group Management Association.

The OIG enforces both the antikickback provision of the Medicare/Medicaid laws and the so-called Stark I and II prohibitions on physician self-referrals. Compensation plans run into problems with these laws when they appear, in any way, to reward referrals made by the physician to the hospital or to any entity in which the physician has a financial interest. The best defense against such charges is objective justification for every piece of the physician's compensation package. Be able to explain how every dollar of his salary and benefits is directly related to specific services that he personally has provided.

The practical and legal issues surrounding physician compensation arise whenever a physician is being paid for her medical services. There is no real difference between a physician newly recruited onto an MCO panel, an established partner in a large group practice, and a physician who has just sold her practice to a hospital and has become one of its employees. A more extensive discussion of physician compensation matters can be found in Chapter 25, "The Kinds of Physician Reimbursement Systems You Can Expect under Managed Care."

KEY CIRCUMSTANCE: SELLING YOUR PRACTICE TO A HOSPITAL

The most frequent purchasers of medical practices are hospitals. If you might consider selling your practice, it makes sense to know how to evaluate your most likely purchaser. These are the questions you should raise in negotiations with a hospital:

Strategic Plans

Does the hospital have a strategic plan, one reaching out at least five years? It should be in writing. Ask for a copy. Look for contingency elements to it, in case unforeseen events occur or assumptions prove unfounded (state health reform enacted, new large MCO enters the market).

Managed Care Expertise

Does the hospital employ at least one high-level executive with solid expertise in managed care? Do not be satisfied with claims that consultants are advising the hospital on managed care strategies.

Primary Care Emphasis

Does the hospital understand the preeminent role of primary care under managed care delivery? This is important, whether you are a specialist or a primary care doctor. Try this acid test question: What percentage of capitation revenues do you think should be devoted to primary care services? A good answer exceeds 10 percent and approaches 20 percent. If the hospital official has no idea, that tells you a great deal.

Financial Strength

Carry out a standard analysis of the hospital's finances. Look at key numbers such as revenue growth, market share, net earnings, age of accounts receivable, liquidity ratios, and debt service coverage ratio. To put the numbers in perspective, compare them with those of other competing hospitals.

Patient and Payer Mix

Ask the hospital for figures on the revenue shares that it gets from different types of patients and payers. Make a comparison with competing hospitals and with national averages. A good source of these kinds of data is *The Comparative Performance of U.S. Hospitals: The Sourcebook*,

prepared by HCIA. Look particularly at the predominance of Medicare and Medicaid patients; a disproportionately high percentage could portend some fiscal weakness. However, the most important revenue number is the share coming from managed care contracts. If this ratio is well behind that of other hospitals in the area, the hospital is not well positioned for the future. Think twice about selling out to a competitive laggard.

Managed Care Contracts

Besides managed care revenues, ask to see a list of the hospital's individual managed care contracts. Think about the number of such contracts and the covered lives each represents. Two extremes to be avoided are a lot of managed care contracts (anything over 20) that each account for a relatively few covered lives, and just two or three contracts representing a substantial number of lives. Many small contracts are more expensive to administer and suggest a lack of enthusiasm for managed care. If one of a couple of large contracts is canceled, hospital revenues may take a serious hit.

Physical Location

Look to see whether the hospital operates any satellite clinics or ambulatory centers that may give prospective managed care patients more immediate access. Geographic dispersion of facilities is appealing to MCOs.

Hospital Network Participation

Hospitals increasingly are joining together in networks or systems designed to attract managed care contracts covering very large numbers of patients. It is part of the trend toward consolidation into fewer, larger health care delivery systems. Find out whether your prospective purchaser belongs to such a network. If it does not, what are the reasons, and does it have plans to do so in the future? Notice whether the hospital officials are able even to talk intelligently about this issue. If the hospital is part of a network, you need to evaluate the other network members almost as carefully as you do the purchasing hospital itself.

Medical Research and Teaching

If your prospective purchaser is a teaching hospital, it probably has a substantial infrastructure supporting medical research and education. With the questions about continued support for such activities through MCO and Medicare reimbursement contracts, you might ask the hospital how it expects to stay competitive and deliver cost-effective care.

Purchase Price Considerations

Some hospitals have used the vague threat of IRS and OIG law enforcement as an excuse for offering unfairly low prices for physician practices. The best rejoinder is for you and your attorney to be familiar with the true positions of the IRS and OIG on practice acquisitions and to reject the hospital's rationalizations.

Most hospital payments for physician practices are made in installments over a period of time. Insist on some guarantee arrangement so that you do not go unpaid if the hospital falls on financial hard times.

Some hospitals may offer shares in a new for-profit medical group subsidiary in return for a physician practice. This usually is not a good idea. To ever see your money, the entire group must be successful, and that may take years. If the relationship does not work out and you want to back out, you may lose everything in the process. If you want to make risky investments, insist on payment in cash, then put the money into the stock market.

Physician Employment Considerations

The compensation you receive from the hospital for subsequently employing you may take a variety of forms. Some will give a salary guarantee equal to your income for the last two or three years. This is desirable; get it if you can. Some-times your compensation will be tied to productivity. Just make sure that it is your productivity and not that of the larger group.

Frequently, certain overhead costs will be deducted from your compensation. Make sure you know in advance what those items are and how you can control them.

Out of concern that you will set up a competing practice if you leave its employment, the hospital may ask that you sign a noncompete covenant. Unless you are confident that you will spend the rest of your career with this hospital, try to avoid such covenants. If the hospital demands it, negotiate the least restrictive terms and additional compensation for giving up the right to compete.

It probably is a good idea to have the hospital write into the employment contract what it expects of you in terms of hours worked and patients seen. Include any significant administrative responsibilities as well, such as work on quality assurance committees.

Regular performance reviews are a part of employment relationships that will be new to physicians coming from private practice. The reviews should be conducted in adherence to written employment policies designed specifically for physicians. The conditions under which discipline may be meted out should also be described.

Physician Role in Governance

A question just as important as the level of compensation is the role that physicians will have in the governance of the physician division of the hospital organization. The ideal situation is where the physicians are employed by a free-standing subsidiary of the hospital organization that is governed by a board of physician and hospital representatives. The physicians should have an equal or majority position on that board. If the hospital can make all decisions in its favor, the physicians will be helpless. Be sure that the board includes a physician knowledgeable about managed care. The hospital's appreciation of the need for some degree of physician control and its willingness to negotiate the matter is an acid test of its intentions to enter into a long-term "partner-ship" with the doctors.

STEPS YOU CAN TAKE TO ENHANCE THE VALUE OF A PRACTICE YOU PLAN TO SELL

If you can anticipate that you will be selling your practice at some time in the near future, there are some steps you can take now to enhance its value later. Work on these areas:

Build the Patient Base

The patients who come to you regularly for care are your most valuable asset. If you are a primary care physician, develop an image with your patients as their portal of entry to the entire health care system. Then they will come to you whenever they have a medical problem. Do this through call-back procedures, patient reminders about checkups and follow-ups, preventive health programs, and health information literature.

If you are a specialist, certainly try to ingratiate yourself socially with your referral sources. However, the most effective action is establishing a name for returning patients to their primary care source for treatment and keeping him or her informed.

Gain Managed Care Experience

Sign at least one contract with an MCO; several contracts would be better. Gain experience in negotiating those contracts, dealing with problems that come up under them, responding to the utilization management and quality assurance requirements of the MCO, and generally practicing a more managed form of medicine.

Combine with Other Physicians

Recruit even one additional physician into your practice, either as a partner or as an employee. More would be better. The larger numbers will make you more attractive to a prospective buyer. They imply your ability to work with others and

to minimize the costs of acquiring practices. Even a small physician group will carry more weight in negotiating a sale of the practice.

Depersonalize the Practice Name

Give your practice a more generic name that is not personally identified with you. That helps establish a market presence that has value and continues after you leave the practice.

Install Information-Gathering Systems

Start to spend money, even modest amounts, on computerized systems for gathering data on the cost and quality implications of your practice style. On a small budget, this may mean nothing more than buying an additional computer and some software for entering, tabulating, and analyzing the data already available in your practice. It may also involve allocating a staff person's time to studying these issues.

Bond Staff with Patients

Work with your staff to develop skills that will enable them to build a rapport with the patients who come into the practice. This kind of personal connection will immediately enhance patient satisfaction with the treatment experience at your practice. Over time, it will build loyalty in patients to you and your practice, making it more likely that they will follow you when you join another organization.

Repair and Modernize Equipment

Look around your office. Identify pieces of equipment that are obsolete, not functioning well, or simply appear to be worn out. Replace or repair them. Within budget constraints, all your equipment should function as efficiently as possible. This includes computers, lab equipment, and furniture—almost any asset that may affect your practice productivity or present an impression of obsolescence or inefficiency.

Improve the Physical Appearance

This suggestion is similar to the one above. It concerns the more superficial appearance of the office setting, the style of furniture, the wall décor and decoration, the arrangement of the office, the outside signage, the magazines and other distractions offered in the waiting room, and even the practice's stationery. All these features work together to create impressions in the minds of patients and prospective buyers who visit the office. The goal is to be modern, appealing, tasteful, and in good condition.

Put Medical Records in Order

Any organization interested in acquiring your practice will inspect the medical records. Make sure that they are properly organized so that specific records can be found quickly. The folders and forms used should present a neat, accessible appearance. Most important, the records content should be complete and legible. It is difficult to go back and rewrite poorly written record entries. It is possible to begin now in keeping better records.

Build a Strong Financial Track Record

You may feel that you have been trying to do this all along. Try some things like tightening up on your claims processing, getting claims in sooner, and following up on collection more promptly. Keep closer track of your operating expenses and look for ways to cut costs, even marginally. Switch from a cash to an accrual basis for your accounting. Start reinvesting net earnings in the practice, rather than withdrawing them all as personal income at the end of the year.

WHAT YOU NEED TO WORRY ABOUT WHEN SELLING YOUR PRACTICE

When selling your practice to another organization, and perhaps then accepting employment with it, there are issues of primary sensitivity to a physician. Here is what to worry about most:

- how much money you will receive for your practice
- what form the purchase money will take: immediate cash, delayed cash, cash contin-

gent on subsequent performance, stock in a private company, stock in a publicly traded company
- if you will be employed by the purchaser:
  - the amounts of your employment compensation
  - the long-term assurance of your continued employment
  - the purchaser's reputation within the medical community and the public at large
  - the purchaser's competence in practice management
  - the purchaser's potential interference in your clinical autonomy
  - the purchaser's plans for improving and growing your practice
  - how your practice fits into the purchaser's strategic plans
  - opportunities for personal growth under the purchaser's employment
- fraud and abuse and Stark legal implications of all compensation arrangements with the purchaser

WHAT YOU NEED TO WORRY ABOUT WHEN BUYING ANOTHER PHYSICIAN'S PRACTICE

The risks present when acquiring another physician's practice are not quite as serious as when selling your own. If it does not turn out to be a wise investment, you will lose the purchase price. However, it is not likely to compromise your own practice and career. To prevent the deal from turning out badly, consider these critical issues:

- the continued market viability of the practice
- the reputation in the community and with other physicians of both the selling physician and his practice
- the amount of money you will have to pay to get the practice
- the amount of cash you will have to pay immediately for the practice

- the proportion of current patients who will stay with the practice when it changes hands
- if you will employ the selling physician:
  - his fit with your strategic plans and his reputation with patients, other physicians, and payers
  - his reputation for practicing quality medicine
  - his proven ability to deliver managed medical care

- his responsiveness to your reasonable initiatives in utilization management, quality control, and patient satisfaction
- his compatibility with other physicians whose practices are being acquired
- fraud and abuse and Stark legal implications of all compensation arrangements with the selling physician

---

REFERENCES

1. California Business and Professional Code §2400 (1997).
2. D.M. Thornton, "Impact of the Anti-Kickback Statute and the Stark Amendment on Vertically Integrated Delivery Systems in the Health Care Industry," in *Health Care Fraud 1994* (Chicago, IL: American Bar Association, 1994).
3. *IRS Hospital Audit Guidelines: Exempt Organizations Examination Guidelines* (Washington, DC: U.S. Government Printing Office), 7(10)69-27-7(10)60-30.7.

RESOURCE LIST

Assessing the Value of the Medical Practice. (Chicago, IL: American Medical Association, 1996).

Bodenger et al., *A Guide to Buying Physician Practices* (Washington, DC: Atlantic Information Services, 1995).

J.E. Bolinger and D.E. Hough, "Making Acquired Physician Practices Profitable," *Healthcare Financial Management*, February 1997.

Buying, Selling, and Owning the Medical Practice (Chicago, IL: American Medical Association, 1996).

Buying, Selling and Valuing a Practice, Super Search Packet #1018 (Englewood, CO: Medical Group Management Association, updated annually).

The Comparative Performance of U.S. Hospitals: The Sourcebook (Baltimore, MD: HCIA, Inc., published annually).

K.M. Hekman, *Buying, Selling and Merging A Medical Practice, Proven Valuation and Negotiation Strategies* (Burr Ridge, IL: McGraw-Hill Healthcare Education Group and Healthcare Financial Management Association, 1997).

T. Hudson, "Necessary Losses? Medical Practices Owned by Hospitals Are Swamped by Red Ink," *Hospitals & Health Networks 71*, no. 24 (1997): 67.

## CHAPTER 19

Step Ten: Increasing the Level of Integration in Your Provider Organization

INTRODUCTION

Beginning with the large multispecialty group practice and continuing through most of the other practice forms discussed in the book, there are many degrees of integration that can be tried and implemented without radically altering the organization or literally becoming an integrated delivery system (IDS). Indeed, acquiring experience in integration and managing care at an early stage will make a physician and her group more attractive candidates for the kinds of affiliations that are an ingredient of the later stages.

The term *integration* has at least three different meanings for ambitious, foresightful physicians. It is the combination of separate, usually small physician practices into larger entities. In classical economic vocabulary, this is called *horizontal integration*. It can be seen in organizational structures such as independent practice associations (IPAs), management services organizations (MSOs), group practices without walls (GPWWs), medical foundations (MFs), and large group practices.

Integration also refers to the combination of physician groups with other kinds of provider entities, such as hospitals, outpatient clinics, laboratories, long-term care facilities, and home health agencies. Economists describe this as *vertical integration*. It takes the shape of physician-hospital organizations (PHOs) and other full-blown IDSs.

Both of these versions of integration involve structural or strategic changes for the participating physician practices. The bulk of this book examines those traditional forms of structural integration. There are chapters recommending ways to consolidate with other physicians like yourself and with other types of providers, with the intention of ultimately becoming a prominent component of an IDS.

This chapter is about a third form of integration—the wide variety of operational modifications that must be made within physician organizations to permit them to function in a managed care–friendly manner. These are the adaptations that can and should be started now by any group or practice, whether or not it has current plans to pursue the other forms of integration.

The kinds of operational integration needed to be competitive under managed care include utilization review (UR), sophisticated information systems, selective physician recruitment, and quality assurance, among many others.

WHO SHOULD READ THIS CHAPTER

This is a must-read chapter for any physician who has picked up this book with the intention of preparing for managed care. Even if someone else in your group is handling the negotiations for various strategic affiliations, you will learn from this chapter the internal changes you must make in the way you practice medicine. It will provide an introduction to the steps in implementing the changes; and you will get a feel for how the changes will affect you personally.

A physician who is looking for a quick introduction to the basic programs, principles, and systems of integration required by managed care will benefit from this chapter. It does not provide the detailed descriptions and guidelines necessary to implement each of the programs. Articles and entire books have been written to give practical instructions in doing this. The resource list at the end of the chapter is a good place to start when you want to learn much more about any of these recommendations.

PURPOSES OF OPERATIONAL INTEGRATION IN THE PRACTICE OF MEDICINE

Operational integration is carried out to serve the interests of the managed care marketplace. The most important of those interests are

- minimizing the utilization of all resources (to minimize costs)
- minimizing all the costs of operation (to permit the practice to break even at lower and lower capitation fee levels, and to earn the maximum profit above break-even)
- maintaining, if not maximizing, the quality of care provided (to please both the employer paying for the care and the patient receiving it)
- maximizing patient satisfaction—to the extent that it is based on factors in addition to care quality (to please the payers and the patients)

From the viewpoint of the physician, these initiatives offer the following benefits:

- Make the physician, and his practice, group or network as attractive as possible to the marketplace.
- Tools to compete successfully against similar provider organizations.

- Assurance of the long-term survival of the physician's organization.
- Optimization of the revenue and income of the organization and its individual physicians.

These are the primary operational integration programs or procedures that will exist in the competitive physician organization of the twenty-first century.

DEVELOPING A COMMON STRATEGIC VISION

There is a saying that "If you don't know where you are going, you'll never know when you get there" or "You could wind up anywhere." This is a catchy way of emphasizing the importance for any organization of having some vision of the future toward which it is moving. Naturally, when an organization is the product of the combination of several previously independent businesses (i.e., medical practices), it is equally important that they each do not pursue different visions.

Every physician considering joining with others in any sort of joint venture needs first to have fleshed out an image of the medical practice setting she desires 3, or 5, or 10 years from now. What must she have? What would she like, but can do without? What does she want to avoid?

Then, when the discussions about consolidation begin (whether one physician is considering joining an existing group or several physicians are planning to form a new physician organization), each physician needs to reveal, in detail, her or his expectations for the future.

All participating physicians should have a candid discussion about what they want the organization to be. There is a variety of vehicles for accomplishing this. A strategic planning retreat at a comfortable, remote location, facilitated by a professional, is used by many organizations. The process will consume time. It may take several meetings, stretching over several months. Expect much emotional outpouring as doctors argue passionately for or against various future scenarios. Sometimes, painful compromises will be made as the physicians, together, negotiate common strategic visions and goals to which all can commit themselves. It is better not to settle for a plan that the physicians have decided they can "live with." In the current health care marketplace, it is necessary to define the best possible future and to work aggressively to achieve it. Physicians who cannot adapt their attitudes and desires may have to drop out of the group.

Once agreement is reached, the resulting strategic vision will become a unifying, motivating force for the participating doctors. That vision lays the foundation for the centralized planning and decision making that will follow at the operational level (see "Establish Consistent Medical Direction and Organizational Leadership," below). It will be supported by various incentives that align the motivations of everyone in the organization (see "Align Incentives among Physicians, Ancillary Staff, and Other Employees," below).

HIRING A MANAGER TO INSTALL AND OPERATE THE OTHER INTEGRATION PROGRAMS

It is no small undertaking to implement the variety of integration measures described in this chapter. It requires time and expertise normally not available to physicians who also are trying to practice medicine.

At the very least, you must hire a full-time business manager. This person will not be a physician and is not likely to have an MBA. Both these credentials would probably be overkill for the job, though the MBA eventually might be a useful qualification.

Initially, the business manager will symbolize the movement of all the providers participating in the organization away from small, physician-run, physiciancentric medical practices to a larger, professionally run, patientcentric health care delivery organization. Eventually, the manager will assume more and more administrative duties,

performing them more efficiently and freeing the physicians to concentrate on clinical work.

The Best Candidate for this Position Will Have the Following Skills

- practice management expertise
- experience in working with physicians
- grasp of latest technology as it is applied to the management of health care delivery
- understanding of trends sweeping health care delivery and changes necessary for physician practices to survive
- ability to think in system and information terms
- skill at negotiating with vendors of all sorts
- the respect and trust of the integrating group of physicians

This manager's effectiveness will depend to an important degree on the willingness of the physicians to delegate authority to her, to cooperate with her, and, in some cases, to take direction from her.

Many of these physicians will have managed the business aspects of their individual practices for some years. They would be reluctant to turn over those responsibilities to other physicians. Now their survival may depend on allowing a nonphysician to take over these tasks.

This Person's Primary Duties Will Be To

- Hire and supervise the nonclinical employees of the organization.
- Oversee the day-to-day operations of the organization.
- Direct the clerical aspects of physician credentialing, utilization management, quality assurance, and other managed care–friendly programs.
- Negotiate with vendors for the design and installation of necessary integrated information systems.
- Arrange for capital financing and manage the operating finances of the organization.

- Oversee the claims processing, risk-sharing, and physician compensation functions.
- Negotiate and manage the organization's relationships with managed care organizations (MCOs), employers, affiliated providers, and regulatory agencies.
- Deliver appropriate reports on these activities to the governing body of physicians and to all participating physicians.
- Help resolve conflicts among physicians and staff of the organization.

As the organization grows in size, establishes affiliations with more and more other entities, and evolves toward a fully integrated delivery system, this role of the business manager will expand. Eventually, this person will need to function as a true chief executive officer (CEO), with appropriate training and experience, supported by a team of vice-presidents in key functional areas (operations, finance, marketing, human resources, etc.). This person will be no different, in most respects, than the CEO of any large business organization in any sector of the economy.

> **Think about This**: Much of the debate about the direction of market-driven health care reform concerns the role and influence of clinicians at all levels of the new system. A window of opportunity has opened—before profit-motivated executives and entrepreneurs achieve dominance—for physicians themselves to own, control, and manage the emerging delivery entities. They will do this as members of boards of directors and as CEOs or other top-level executives.

These duties cannot be handled as in the past, with little formal preparation; nor can they fit into a schedule filled with medical practice, research, and teaching. There is evolving a new model of physician leader. This person will be a top-flight practitioner of medical arts. He will have solid and ongoing experience in patient treatment. A physician leader also will have formal training and growing experience in business functions and decision making, probably including an MBA.

If this person aspires to major management responsibility, he will devote the vast majority of his time to that activity—at least 80 to 90 percent. Running a regional IDS or even a large multispecialty group practice demands no less.

The question for physicians today is whether they have the ambition for such responsibility. The time is approaching when physicians must choose deliberately either to build a career as a physician executive or to work primarily as a caregiver, researcher, or teacher. These will become mutually exclusive career paths.

The physician seeking a role in top management of a delivery organization might take the following steps:

- Attend shorter-term management training workshops designed for physicians.
- Enroll in longer-term management degree programs, typically an MBA aimed at health managers or at future business managers in general.
- Begin to allocate time to acquisition of management skills and acceptance of some management duties.
- Seek and accept increasing management responsibilities within the current organization.
- Prepare mentally for the eventuality of directing the activities of more and more people and larger and larger organizations.

SYSTEMS AND PROCEDURES FOR MANAGING AND LIMITING THE UTILIZATION OF ALL RESOURCES

Provider organizations succeed in the managed care game by delivering the same (or better) quality of care at a lower cost than do competing provider organizations. The greater net revenues that result from lower costs can be used to accept lower capitation rates than does the competition or to reward the providers more handsomely than does the competition.

Costs are lowered in two ways: by paying less for each unit of the resources used to deliver the care or by using fewer resource units to deliver a given level of care. The purpose of utilization management is to minimize the volume of resources consumed. It accomplishes this through systems like these:

Discriminating Selection of Physicians

Accept into the organization only physicians with demonstrably efficient utilization practices. To identify those practices, look at claims data, hospital discharge data, and actual medical records. Because it is often too time-consuming and expensive to conduct this data gathering when an organization is first forming, use provisional physician membership status to manage and adjust practice habits and, if necessary, deselect high utilizers.

Reeducation of Physicians

Educate all participating physicians in the most cost-effective treatment practices. To maximize its impact, combine this training with several other initiatives.

- Show that cost savings are achieved without any diminution in quality of care for patients.
- Enlist the visible support of clinical authority figures.
- Ensure that practicing physicians are actively involved in patient care decision making.
- Offer participating physicians concrete evidence of excessive resource utilization.
- Continually reinforce the newly learned practice techniques in all available ways.

Financial Incentives to Physicians

Financial incentives are one of the best complementary reinforcements to new practice techniques. Physicians will respond to such incentives if they are carefully designed, well explained, large enough to attract their attention, and directly related to their own practice behav-

iors. There must also be rigorous, independent, simultaneous monitoring of quality of care. Experience suggests that the incentive must be a significant percentage of the fee or charges involved (certainly more than 10 percent) and must apply to a significant proportion of each physician's caseload (probably at least 40 percent).

Review of Individual Physician Clinical Utilization Decisions

This is the mechanism traditionally employed by MCOs to restrain the utilization rates and costs of their providers. It is roundly resented by many physicians as blatant interference in their clinical decision making. The difference in a physician group or organization is that the utilization review (UR) is under the direct control of physicians.

This form of utilization management encompasses prospective review (before treatment starts), concurrent review (during treatment), retrospective review (after treatment is completed), second-opinion consultation, and case management. If your organization is operating under substantial capitation or other risk-sharing contracts, it has the choice of the kind of UR to implement or whether to use UR at all. It is free to decide the severity or laxness of the procedures. It may carry out the procedures in house or farm them out to a third party. In either case, it may control every aspect of their impact on the physicians.

Physician Profiling for Large Numbers of Patients

Prepare profiles for the resources utilized and costs incurred by individual physicians. Initially, simply provide comparative practice profiles to all the group's physicians. Make clear where each one stands in relation to other doctors within a geographic area, medical specialty, or demographic patient group. Adjust for severity of illness of each physician's patient load. To heighten a physician's concern over an outlier profile, combine it with the threat of a medical record review.

Ingredients of a Good Utilization Management Program

- Track utilization rates by physician, subspecialty, geographic area, payer, and patient.
- Make severity adjustments to the figures.
- Get out from under MCO-directed UR.
- Conduct in-house URs at frequent intervals and give prompt feedback to individual physicians.
- At the least, disclose utilization data to similarly situated physicians so that they may compare themselves to each other.
- Keep physicians informed of the unit costs of the resources they use or prescribe.
- If outcomes data are available, correlate them with utilization rates to make cost-benefit analyses of practice styles and procedures.
- Through this mechanism, discover the techniques that result in desirable outcomes and lower costs.
- Catalog these superior clinical procedures and teach them to other physicians.
- Educate all physicians in proven strategies and tactics for truly "managing" the care they deliver (provide in-house workshops, send them to outside seminars, offer one-on-one advice and mentoring).

SYSTEMS AND PROCEDURES FOR MAINTAINING AND IMPROVING THE QUALITY OF CARE PROVIDED

Since the emergence of managed care, thoughtful physicians have been concerned that utilization control measures would inhibit the quality of care they could provide. They can find great satisfaction in the growing variety of quality management initiatives that are being developed to prevent decline and actually promote improvement. Many of these are necessary pieces of a forward-looking integration strategy. The physician organization should either implement these systems and procedures or be prepared to operate under them at the insistence of an IDS or MSO with which it is affiliated.

Formal, Regular Evaluations of Physician Performance

At regular intervals, at least annually and perhaps quarterly, prepare written evaluations of each physician's practice-related performance. The evaluation should include issues like these:

- productivity measured in terms of patients seen or a similar criterion not related to resource utilization
- demonstrated clinical competence and ability to deliver quality care, measured in terms of clinical outcomes
- compliance with agreed-upon treatment protocols, clinical pathways, and other scientifically determined guidelines
- compliance with established rules on accuracy, thoroughness, and timeliness of medical record documentation and reporting
- effectiveness in working constructively with patients, physician colleagues, and ancillary personnel
- results of patient satisfaction surveys

The writeup is used as the basis for a conversation with the physician about performance shortcomings and steps that will be taken for improvement.

To prepare a performance evaluation like this, other quality-related systems must be in place.

Patient Satisfaction Surveys

Clinical outcomes and patient satisfaction do not always coincide. It is important that the organization regularly measure the levels of patients' satisfaction with every aspect of their contacts with the organization—from scheduling of appointments through length of wait to see a clinician, demeanor of the physician and ancillary personnel encountered, as well as specific treatments administered and the perceived results in level of health. Collect the data in a scientifically rigorous manner and report it promptly in an accessible form to the affected physicians. If the data are reliable enough (i.e., the sample sizes are large enough), tabulate the results by individual physician.

Outcome Measurement Results

Clinical outcomes are what physicians traditionally consider to be an indicator of quality of care. The organization must tailor its information system to gather or calculate outcome variables such as

- low birth weights
- deaths per 100 bypass surgeries
- appendicitis with rupture
- Caesarian sections per 100 births
- infections following treatment
- unexpected deaths
- allergic reactions
- adverse reactions
- readmissions to facility
- patients progressing according to treatment plan
- treatments discontinued before completion
- patient complaints

The goal of these measurements is to determine which treatments and physicians provide positive outcomes for patients.

Development of Treatment Pathways and Protocols

The data on clinical outcomes, patient satisfaction, and utilization rates are combined to develop treatment pathways or protocols. These protocols serve as ideal standards of treatment— given particular diagnoses. Carefully conceived and implemented, they have the potential to improve quality, decrease variability, and decrease cost.

Only the largest physician organizations have the resources to develop treatment protocols internally on their own. It is more likely that they will be acquired from a third party. Several thousands of such protocols have been created by physician panels assembled by federal agencies, medical subspecialty societies, hospitals, MCOs,

insurance companies, and utilization management firms. The scientific integrity of these guidelines varies considerably, and they must be approached with caution.

Whether developed by the physician organization or acquired from a third party, the protocols will be based on either a thorough and rigorous review of current medical literature on the particular condition or the consensus views of numerous expert physicians in the appropriate specialty. The optimal process for protocol development— and an expensive and time-consuming one, at that—was described by the Institute of Medicine (IOM) in 1990.[1]

Do not expect every good protocol to have followed the IOM development model. Likewise, do not accept a protocol that is based on the opinions of a handful of physicians hired by an insurance company. Always inquire into the origins of the protocol's development.

Plan carefully how you will employ the protocols. View them as tools for improving the quality of care delivered by the organization. Protocols have been criticized as "cookbook medicine." Just remember that good cooks frequently stray from their recipes when it is warranted in their judgment. Similarly, protocols are not used as rigid rules from which no deviation is tolerated.

Keep track of individual physician deviations from protocols. Correlate these data with the clinical outcomes achieved by each physician. In some cases, this will reveal inappropriate treatment by a physician. Communicate this information to the physician, seek explanation or justification, agree on changes and improvements in practice style, provide continuing education to support the changes, and, only if they are not forthcoming, consider disciplinary action.

In other cases, it will be apparent that the physician's deviant treatment results in better outcomes. The correct response here may be to upgrade or refine the protocol.

Of course, even good protocols are not static. As medical technology and science progress and as physicians all over the country test the protocols, they will naturally evolve. Stay up-to-date on the changes that occur regularly.

Medical Record Reviews (Regular, Random, and in Response to Other Indicators)

The review of medical records of patients treated by particular physicians is a traditional method of quality management. In a patient-centered managed care environment, it becomes an even more versatile tool.

It still is possible to conduct records reviews at regular, predictable intervals or to pull random samples of records for inspection. This approach may help keep all physicians "on their toes" regarding quality, and it will occasionally discover treatment deficiencies. In general, however, record reviews are less effective at initially discovering quality problems than they are at determining the nature, severity, and causes of problems identified by the other measures described here.

For instance, poor results on patient satisfaction surveys or a pattern of undesirable clinical outcomes might prompt a close look at the medical records involved. That review could lead to several different conclusions.

- The patient's condition was unusually severe, and the treatment followed was the best under the circumstances.
- The patient's condition was unusual and demanding; the physician's treatment was innovative and groundbreaking. The treatment protocol for that condition can be upgraded and quality improved.
- The physician's treatment was inappropriate and inadequate. Remedial action is taken with the physician.

MCO Member Transfer and Termination Rates

If the organization does not ask patients about their levels of satisfaction with the care they receive, they often will express their opinions anyway by transferring to another physician within the MCO or by leaving the MCO (and the physician organization) entirely. It is worth keeping track of the patients who leave in this fashion and trying to learn the reasons. The best course is to ask the patient directly, if that is permitted, or to seek an explanation from the MCO. In the absence of a clear reason, check with the physician, and review the medical record to see whether any causes stand out. In the last resort, simply follow the transfers and terminations by individual physician. Excessively high raw numbers likely indicate some problem.

MCO Member Complaints and Grievances

The best way to gauge patients' satisfaction with the quality of care they have received is to let them tell you. In addition to the periodic satisfaction surveys, implement a formal complaint or grievance procedure. Make it as easy to understand and use as possible. Give it wide publicity. The goal is to encourage patients to communicate any disagreement, discomfort, or upset they have with the provider organization. Many will be frivolous or insignificant and can be screened out. The more serious complaints can be addressed and probably defused. This is an opportunity to learn what features of the organization are not working for the patients, take corrective action, and frequently keep them from reaching the patients' MCOs or the courts.

Those complaints that implicate physician behavior should be discussed with the doctor responsible. Appropriate adjustments to behavior are then negotiated. The complaint log, properly interpreted, is another indicator of the quality of care provided by the entire organization and by individual physicians.

Keep in mind that, if your organization does not offer an avenue of redress for unhappy patients, their MCOs surely will. It is preferable to catch the complaints before they come to the MCO's attention. Nonetheless, some patients will take their grievances directly to their MCOs. Request from all MCO contract partners regular reports on complaints they have received about the physician organization.

Patient Malpractice Suits

This is the ultimate indicator of possible poor quality. Not all medical malpractice lawsuits are the product of physician treatment errors. The circumstances surrounding each need to be investigated to determine physician responsibility. Interviews with the physician, as well as medical record reviews, are mandatory follow-ups. Repeated malpractice actions against a single physician are strong signs of a quality problem requiring prompt, decisive attention.

SELECTING PHYSICIANS WHO BEST MEET THE GROUP'S OBJECTIVE REQUIREMENTS

Physician organizations competing for managed care contracts must apply the most rigorous standards in choosing their physician members. Their degree of success, and perhaps even survival, will depend on it.

In the modern integrated practice, participating physicians must be selected for three broad qualities: ability to provide competent, quality medical care; to utilize just the right amount of resources in doing so (no more, no less); and to work collaboratively with clinical and nonclinical personnel in different disciplines to meet all the patient's needs.

First are the more traditional credentialing criteria concerned with the physician's basic competence to practice medicine. They include

- confirming licensing to practice medicine
- determining levels of training—medical education, specialization, board certification
- checking references from previous practice settings
- consulting the National Practitioners Data Bank
- following up on any hints of problems revealed by the above checks

Second are the more modern qualifications demanded by payers and competitive pressures in a managed care marketplace.

- expressed willingness (with some past experience) to participate in multidisciplinary clinical teams
- expressed willingness (with some past experience) to practice within a system of treatment protocols and guidelines
- proven/documented ability to minimize utilization of key resources without compromising quality (in comparison with benchmark utilization and quality figures)
- expressed willingness (with some past experience) to practice/work under a system that profiles each physician's performance and expects her or him to respond appropriately to the data reported, working constantly to improve her or his performance
- expressed willingness (with some past experience) to cooperate with programs for managing both utilization and quality by providing data required by the programs, reading and responding to their output, heeding recommendations for changes in practice patterns, and accepting continuing education in new practice styles
- demonstrated ability to satisfy patients, regardless of utilization and quality levels

Third are the more subjective qualifications relating to interpersonal skills. The physician of the future can no longer be an independent free spirit. Increasingly, the physician must be an eager, open-minded member of small and large teams—composed of physicians in the same and different specialties, nonphysician clinicians, clerical, and administrative personnel—working together toward common goals. The physician must be able to collaborate amicably and productively with these disparate people and not always from a position of leadership. When the modern physician is leading, she needs to direct others through rational, respectful discourse, rather than peremptory commands. These credentials will be discovered (or not) through thoughtful interview questioning and conversations with the physician's former supervisors and coworkers.

There are a couple of points to keep in mind about these credentialing requirements, even the less traditional ones that are obviously concerned with reducing costs. The least desirable state of affairs is to have these requirements imposed and enforced by a third party, such as an MCO. The MCO or any other payer will want to see all of these controls in place.

If the physician organization is large enough, has the necessary resources, systems and expertise, and can negotiate successfully with the payer, it can and should assume responsibility for these credentialing functions. The payer may still insist on periodic audits of the credentialing activities, but the physicians will have the satisfaction of knowing that they are being judged by professional peers. In addition, they are more likely to accept recommendations, demands, and, perhaps, even deselection, coming from other physicians. The entire issue of credentialing in a managed care environment is discussed in greater detail in Chapter 23, "Selection and Deselection of Physicians by Managed Care Organizations and Physician Groups."

MANAGING ALL HUMAN RESOURCES OBJECTIVELY AND SYSTEMATICALLY

Physicians in solo or small group practice rarely have the time or the ability to manage effectively the people who support them in delivering health care. When physicians consolidate in larger and larger organizations, integration of human resource management means several things.

- Standards are established for all aspects of employee relations (hiring, payroll structure, performance management, benefits, disciplinary matters, termination, etc.) across all physician practices in the organization.
- Resources are available to carry out valuable new functions, such as writing an employee manual, drafting up-to-date job descriptions, conducting regular performance appraisals, training supervisors, documenting disciplin-

ary steps taken, and seeking legal advice on sensitive employment decisions.
- Human resource professionals are employed to advise managers and supervisors; design necessary policies, procedures, and systems; and generally promote the fair, effective employment of all personnel.
- Formal systems (in terms of computer and organizational technologies) are designed or acquired, then implemented, for routinizing human resource management tasks, ensuring that employees throughout the organization are treated uniformly and predictably, and accomplishing this in the most cost-effective way.
- Human resource management tasks from many separate practices are aggregated to exploit the economies of scale that come from purchasing the same goods or services in larger volumes and from simply centralizing the performance of the tasks.
- Redundancies in staffing, if not outright excesses, often demonstrate that significant savings may be achieved through layoffs.

These changes in the way that the people in physician practices are managed are one of the first, most obvious, and simplest benefits to be achieved through integration.

EMPHASIZE MANAGEMENT OF PATIENT DEMAND FOR HEALTH CARE SERVICES

Until recently, managed care has been concerned with providing the care demanded by patients as efficiently as possible. A new facet has been added to modern medical practice—demand management. Instead of waiting until a patient develops a medical problem and comes to an outpatient clinic, physician's office, or emergency department, the goal now is to preclude the demand for medical care in the first place. This is accomplished through a variety of devices.

The first step is a *preventive health program*. This begins with a lifestyle profile and health risk appraisal for each patient. These will identify factors in the patient's behaviors and lifestyle that are increasing the likelihood of trauma or illness that will require medical treatment, such as smoking, poor nutrition, overweight, high stress, and high-risk activities, including sex practices. Education through different media is then provided to the patient with the intention of reducing or eliminating those factors. Specific remedial programs may be offered: smoking cessation, weight reduction, improved eating, and stress reduction. If the program achieves its aim, the patient will demand fewer medical services than were actuarially calculated for someone of her demographic characteristics. As a result, the group will make more money under the capitation rate, based on those calculations.

The next step may be to *educate and train* the patient to self-diagnose and treat medical problems that do arise—without needing to consult a caregiver at all. This strategy can be applied to only certain kinds of ailments, normally those less severe in nature, perhaps recurring and, therefore, familiar to the patient and amenable to treatment by a lay person. It also is workable only for patients with necessary intelligence, confidence, and discipline. Once again, the goal is to prevent the patient from seeking care from the group.

In those cases where the patient does need to speak to a medical professional, set up a mechanism for initially trying to meet her needs over the phone. This is one of several variations of *telemedicine*. With proper preparation of the patient and provider (at either end of the phone line), it is possible in a significant number of cases to gather necessary information and to give adequate instructions to resolve the matter without a face-to-face meeting—and the attendant costs.

Demand management is a concept in the early stages of implementation. It has not been established that money spent on such programs is more cost-effective than simply treating patient ailments when they occur. Research is in progress. Your organization should pay close attention to evaluating the economic feasibility of demand initiatives that it takes.

CONSOLIDATE SERVICES TO ACHIEVE ECONOMIES OF SCALE AND OPTIMIZE RESOURCE UTILIZATION (PERSONNEL, SUPPLIES, EQUIPMENT, AND FACILITIES)

One of the easiest and most immediate benefits from integration comes through combining the purchase decisions of the previously separate provider units. Within the first six months of beginning integration, the operations of all participating practices should be scrutinized to determine

- which services can be performed at a central location
- which services can be purchased from a single vendor
- which products can be purchased in more economic large lots from a single vendor
- which equipment could be located at one or more centralized sites to facilitate joint use
- which facilities are underutilized, inappropriately located, or otherwise would benefit from being closed, relocated, or centralized
- which personnel positions have become redundant, would be better combined into fewer, more comprehensive positions, or relocated more centrally

There are considerable savings available through these traditional methods of consolidating and integrating previously separate business units. However, do not rush to centralize every possible function. There may be benefits, particularly in terms of patient satisfaction, to leaving certain functions at dispersed locations. Some examples might be scheduling appointments, small-scale local purchases, and simple bookkeeping tasks. Each activity and each expenditure should be evaluated on its own merits for potential gains through integration.

TERMINATE UNPRODUCTIVE ACTIVITIES, SERVICES, AND PROGRAMS

Small practices rarely have the luxury of pausing to assess the usefulness of all the activities they perform and services they provide. When consolidation occurs is an ideal time to go through all the practices with a fine-toothed comb to remove any features that are not necessary to the mission of the new, larger provider organization. What sorts of features might be found unnecessary?

1. Services that do not justify their expense—in terms of cost savings, quality enhancements, revenue generated, or patient satisfaction. They may have made sense in the context of the solo physician's small, more idiosyncratic practice but not in a larger, professionally managed, efficiency-maximizing physician organization.
2. Expenditures required by the physician's previous style of practice, geographic location, revenue sources, or type of patients. When these change, the need for the expenditures may disappear.
3. Programs or activities that are still important but that will be provided at a central location or contracted out to a third-party vendor.

Integration of physician practices means becoming very rational about which operational features to keep and which to drop.

ESTABLISH CONSISTENT MEDICAL DIRECTION AND ORGANIZATIONAL LEADERSHIP

The combination of 20 individual physician practices into a single organization brings together 20 separate leaders with 20 different notions of appropriate medical practice. The new organization must move quickly to unify them under one vision of medical direction and organizational leadership. Accomplish this through several steps.

Hire or designate a medical director for the entire organization. Give this person authority, with input from appropriate physician committees, to determine physician credentialing criteria, adopt treatment guidelines, frame utilization management programs, resolve physician disciplinary issues, and negotiate with MCOs on other issues impacting clinical decision making. He or she will be primarily responsible for speaking on the physicians' behalf and assuring that uniform clinical policies prevail throughout the organization.

Hire a professional business manager to direct all of the nonclinical activities of the organization. This person will have formal training in management and is not likely to be a physician. He or she will be responsible for managing the finances, facilities, purchasing, human resources, practice operations, contract negotiations, claims processing, marketing, compensation, and similar operational matters. In consultation with the medical director and the board of directors, the business manager will help plan the strategic direction of the organization.

Formulate and enforce organizationwide policies and procedures on all aspects of operations management—both clinical and nonclinical—to ensure uniformity and predictability. This will mean that some long-standing habits of individual physicians will have to change—in some cases, to their distress. Do not pursue standardization for its own sake, but only where it serves the interests of efficiency and equality of treatment. Idiosyncrasies can be tolerated in specific practices to accommodate unique circumstances or interests.

Assemble a board of directors composed, to the extent permitted by law, of respected business-experienced physician leaders. They will be the primary unifying and harmonizing force in the organization. They will be the leaders in steering the organization and all its components on a coherent, fruitful strategic path. If the board members are generally trusted by the mass of participating physicians, their decisions and pronouncements are more likely to be accepted and followed.

Prepare and implement a market-sensitive long-range strategic plan for the organization. Once this plan, its mission, values, and objectives have been acknowledged by the organization's doctors, it will serve as the reference point and lodestar for all the policies and procedures they are asked to carry out.

An organization made up of providers and business units that are pursuing their own aims is a contradiction of the purposes of "integration." Its activities will be disjointed, inefficient, and sometimes at odds with each other. The organization that thinks with one mind and speaks with one voice is more likely to succeed that one that does not.

COORDINATE ACQUISITION AND DEVELOPMENT OF NEW TECHNOLOGY

The modern, competitive provider organization employs a wide variety of constantly evolving technology. It includes sophisticated laboratory testing equipment, medical diagnosis and therapeutic equipment, computerized systems for gathering, analyzing, and reporting information on cost, quality, patient satisfaction, resource utilization, practice patterns, and claims processing—to mention the most obvious. Technology may also include nonhardware proprietary procedural/analytical systems purchased from vendors. If an organization does not possess these technologies now, it will have to acquire or develop them in the near future. They are expensive and constantly changing, requiring regular upgrading and new investment.

Plan the acquisition or development of new technology in a synchronized, organizationwide fashion. Set limits on the amounts that individual business units can spend on capital assets. When deciding whether to purchase a significant new technology, prepare a thorough business plan that looks at the benefits it will provide (throughout the organization), any disadvantages it presents,

alternative technologies or methods serving the same function, all costs related to its acquisition (including support equipment and operator training), and the financial returns expected. Ideally, the investment in the technology should occur within the framework of an organizational capital budget.

ALIGN INCENTIVES AMONG PHYSICIANS, ANCILLARY STAFF, AND OTHER EMPLOYEES

People are motivated in their actions by a variety of concerns, only one of which is money. To ensure that everyone in a new provider organization is working synergistically toward the same goals, pay attention to exactly what incentives are driving each person and adjust them so that they fit with the organization's goals.

The first step is communicating clearly to each physician and other staff members the higher-level goals of the full organization, as well as those of the department or unit in which that person works. Then ensure that monetary awards are tied in some manner to each person's contribution toward achievement of those goals. Next, to the extent that individuals may seek other kinds of satisfaction in their work (e.g., promotion, skill development, symbolic recognition), try to provide them in some proportion to desired goal achievement. It also is possible to work more closely with specific staff people to help them define their personal goals, then to demonstrate to them how those goals coincide with those of the organization.

CREATE COMPUTERIZED INFORMATION SYSTEMS FOR MANAGING COSTS AND CLINICAL DECISION MAKING

It is an understatement to say that health care delivery is more and more shaped by a growing volume of information about the inputs, processes, and outputs of that delivery. Incidentally, the collection and dissemination of that information on an enterprisewide basis tends to unify the people and business units that comprise it. The net result is to integrate and align all their efforts.

The organization should implement computerized systems that receive and analyze data in the following areas, among others:

- resource utilization by physician (tests, drugs, hospitalizations, ancillary personnel time)
- tracking of clinical outcomes by diagnosis and procedure, with a view toward definition of treatment guidelines
- attention to clinical pathways and treatment guidelines, by physician
- combination of these physician-specific data into "profiles" of each physician's practice behaviors
- measurement of clinical outcomes, by physician
- measurement of patient satisfaction, by physician and patient origins (MCO membership, demographic group)
- reporting of total costs by diagnosis, by treatment, and by physician
- reporting of net earnings, by MCO contract

This is all in addition to the typical functions expected of a management information system: general cost accounting, financial management and analysis, claims coding, processing and filing, compensation and benefits administration, inventory control, etc.

The systems required to gather all these data will not be installed at once. The cost is probably too great for even the largest organization; the effect would likely be too disruptive. Lay out a multistage plan for installation of the information system components. Assign priorities to them. Obtain best estimates of their cost and time to completion. Proceed prudently and aggressively.

CENTRALIZE PROCESSING OF REIMBURSEMENT CLAIMS

This task may have one of the highest priorities for computerization and centralization. There is no logic for allowing individual practices to con-

tinue preparing and filing their own claims. There are great efficiencies and savings to be realized by carrying out this function at a single location through trained personnel using modern systems and equipment.

SHAPE PHYSICIAN COMPENSATION TO PRODUCE DESIRED BEHAVIOR

The compensation formula is a powerful tool for steering physician behavior in directions that satisfy organizational goals. It is fairly well established that compensation on a fee-for-service (FFS) basis encourages physicians to deliver more services and utilize more resources. On the other hand, capitated compensation pushes them to minimize resource utilization by providing fewer services. There have been natural complaints that FFS increases costs, whereas capitation degrades quality.

It is possible to devise more sophisticated compensation formulas for individual doctors that inspire a more acceptable mix of physician behaviors. For example, a primary care physician in a largely capitated multispecialty group practice might be paid on the following terms:

- 10 percent of total compensation withheld until the year's end, to be offset against excessive utilization of inpatient and specialist resources
- base salary paid, regardless of any variations in physician practice behavior
- additional fixed amounts (per hour or per day) paid for time spent in managerial, administrative (e.g., committee participation), supervisory, teaching, and research activities
- incentive payments for utilization of nonhospital, nonphysician resources (such as pharmaceuticals, laboratory tests, ancillary services) at less than a predetermined target rate
- incentive payments for clinical quality performance (as measured by reliable outcomes data) greater than a predetermined target figure

- incentive payments for creating patient satisfaction (as measured by reliable surveys) greater than a predetermined target figure
- general performance bonus awarded at year's end by the physician's supervisor on the basis of more subjective factors such as the physician's relations with coworkers and subordinates and her or his effective participation in clinical teams

It is easy to devise a complex system that looks good in theory but that does not really produce the desired results. There are at least two prerequisites to an effective incentive compensation scheme.

1. The formula must be comprehensible to the physicians affected by it. If they do not understand clearly what rewards they will receive by engaging in certain behaviors, the scheme will not work.

2. The size of the withholds, bonuses, or incentives must be large enough to have meaning for the physicians. For instance, it is a rule of thumb that a withhold of less than 10 percent of base salary will not be an effective motivator. Likewise, a $5,000 performance bonus may not make much difference to a physician earning $200,000 a year.

Businesses in all industries, not just health care, are still refining the design and implementation of their incentive compensation programs. A physician organization should expect to spend a few years making adjustments to its compensation formula. Closely track the operating variables that the incentives are meant to affect. As you make adjustments, look for correlations between monetary reward and physician behavior. Keep in mind, too, that people are not all motivated in the same way by rewards of any kind. Aim for a compensation package that inspires as many physicians as possible, while recognizing that it will not make sense to a minority of them.

PHYSICIANS INVEST IN CAPITALIZING AND GROWING THE ORGANIZATION

From the initial planning of a physician organization, require capital investments from the participating physicians. This will serve several vital purposes.

1. At the very outset, there will be no other source of funds to cover the organization's planning and startup costs.

2. Even a modest initial contribution will be an important expression of interest and commitment by the physicians.

3. Their investment in the organization will bind the physicians and their actions to the success of the organization.

4. It will move them to place the organization's long-term welfare above their own short-term gain.

5. Because the organization will always be straining to find enough capital, the more that is contributed by the physicians, the less needs to be sought from third parties who will want a share of control in return.

6. If the investment takes the form of publicly traded stock and the organization thrives, the physician's interest will grow.

The physician investments may take different forms: dues, stock purchases (in for-profit corporations), outright contributions (to nonprofit entities), and loans.

PHYSICIANS DOMINATE THE GOVERNANCE OF THE ORGANIZATION

A significant role for participating physicians on the governing body of the organization—usually the board of directors—goes a long way toward persuading them that the organization is theirs. It helps physicians to believe that it is worth joining cooperatively with colleagues to build the organization and to help it grow, contributing personally to its capital needs and subordinating their immediate desires to the overall welfare of the organization.

With a few exceptions, there is no reason that all the members of the board of directors should not be drawn from the ranks of participating physicians. However, those exceptions can be critical. Three good reasons for choosing a nonphysician as a director are

- The person brings a unique expertise, usually managerial or fund-raising, to the organization.
- Board representation is necessary for a third party (i.e., hospital or MCO) that has made a substantial capital investment in the organization.
- As a charitable entity, the organization is required by the Internal Revenue Service (IRS) to restrict physician board membership to less than 50 percent and to grant majority community representation.

PREPARE SYSTEMATICALLY TO ASSUME FINANCIAL RISK

The organization's contracting partners, MCOs primarily, will want it to assume increasing amounts of financial risk. By assuming and effectively managing higher levels of risk, the organization can increase its net earnings.

There are several steps that must be taken to prepare the organization's people and operating systems to handle risk effectively. The sooner these measures are in place, the better.

- Design the compensation systems for all employees, particularly physicians, to promote behavior that optimizes performance under risk sharing.
- Install systems that report to all employees, particularly physicians, the quantitative results of their work performance in key areas such as utilization, cost, quality, and patient satisfaction.
- Set performance standards in the areas of utilization, cost, quality, and patient satisfaction.

- Through outcomes research and patient satisfaction surveys, constantly look for new ways to provide higher quality of care at lower cost. Wherever appropriate, translate the findings into treatment protocols, guidelines, or pathways that staff members are encouraged to follow.
- Continually experiment with new concepts in health care delivery, such as disease management and demand management.
- Provide training and continuing education to all staff, including physicians, on practice and work techniques suited to a risk-sharing environment.
- Through ongoing education and appropriate data reporting, begin to change the organizational culture to be more supportive of a focus on patients and entire communities within a risk-sharing milieu.

Chapter 26, "Managing Risk in the Practice of Medicine," examines this topic in a little greater detail.

UNIFY MANAGED CARE CONTRACTING UNDER A SINGLE PROVIDER NUMBER

Unless the organization's doctors are still very hesitant about embracing managed care (as they might be in looser forms of IPAs and PHOs), one of the first steps is to execute all future managed care contracts in the name of the organization under its single provider number. This is a good dramatic demonstration that it is no longer a tentative collection of autonomous practices, but rather a unified, integrated enterprise comprised of the physicians from those practices now pursuing a common goal.

CONTROL DRUG PRESCRIPTION PATTERNS THROUGH A FORMULARY

Do not allow individual physicians to have uninformed discretion to prescribe any pharmaceutical they wish. At a minimum, establish a formulary of drugs that are recommended for use.

For a particular condition, determine (internally and from outside sources) which of several alternative medications best balances cost and efficacy. Eventually, consider making the formulary mandatory: Except in extraordinary cases, the organization will not pay for drugs outside the formulary that are prescribed by one of its physicians. As the value of certain medications becomes well established, incorporate them into treatment protocols.

LIMIT SPECIALIST REFERRALS TO A SELECT PANEL

If the organization is large and multidisciplinary enough and moving close to being a true IDS, it should be possible to require that participating primary care physicians restrict their referrals to specialists who are also members of the group or a separate panel selected for their ability to provide managed care.

At first, physicians will be reluctant to change old referral patterns. The transition should be handled with tact. Start out by merely recommending that referrals go to designated specialists. Follow up with data on cost and quality profiles for the physicians most often used. Explain the connection between referrals to high-cost specialists and the organization's ability to prosper under risk-sharing contracts. Show how the referring physicians' individual income may be affected. Gradually, make the "recommendations" more and more mandatory. This gradual, educational approach is just as applicable to the introduction of the drug formulary.

TIPS ON WORKING WITH OTHER PHYSICIANS TO IMPLEMENT OPERATIONAL INTEGRATION

If you come from a solo practice background, you may not have much experience in working with others toward a common goal. When it came to decisions about your medical practice, you had all the responsibility and authority. Simply participating in a joint discussion among physician group colleagues about how to proceed with operational integration may not come easily. It is even more difficult when the issues being considered involve affiliations with other organizations. These are some basic concepts to employ in those meetings and discussions.

Set Up a Planning Committee

Unless the group is so small that all the physicians can meet to discuss and resolve every issue, appoint a subset of them as a planning committee. It should be comprised of people with the greatest expertise and interest in the integration project being planned. They must be willing to act in the group's best interest, not necessarily their own. Delegate to the group the authority it needs to do its job. This may be where you first begin to trust in the decisions of others. Hold the committee members accountable for the results they achieve.

Meet Regularly with a Preset Agenda

The committee should meet at regular intervals, with time between meetings for reflection, information gathering, and consultation with noncommittee members. Prepare a specific agenda for each meeting. Identify and prioritize the key issues and steps necessary to get the project off the ground. It may help to distinguish between those issues of personal attitude and preference, and the action steps that make the project an operating reality. Allocate specific time periods to each topic. Describe the outcome expected at the end of each topic discussion. Provide the agenda, with appropriate backup material, to the committee members well in advance of the meeting.

Use a Chairperson or Facilitator To Guide the Meeting

A chairperson calls on people to speak and makes sure that the agenda is being followed. A facilitator does the same thing, as well as making personal comments or suggestions designed to move the group toward its desired outcome. One or the other is essential if the meetings are to be productive and the participants are to feel that their time is well spent.

Take Thorough Minutes of the Meetings

This usually means including a nonparticipant in the meetings for the sole purpose of taking notes. Detailed minutes immediately satisfy both participants and nonparticipants that a rational decision-making process was followed. Well

after the meeting, they are useful in resolving questions about what was actually decided.

Proceed in an Orderly Fashion

The discussion, planning, and implementation of a project should follow a rational, systematic path. It should be comprehensible to all group members, whether they are participating on the committee or not. It should be clear that the process has addressed all key issues and alternatives, and has heard all interested views. These measures will go a long way toward minimizing the uncertainty and doubt of those physicians not on the committee.

REFERENCE

1. Institute of Medicine, Committee to Advise the Public Health Service on Clinical Practice Guidelines, *Clinical* *Practice Guidelines: Directions for a New Program* (Washington DC: National Academy Press, 1990).

RESOURCE LIST

D.C. Coddington et al., "Making Integrated Health Care Work," *Physician Executive 22*, no. 5 (1996): 24.

K.J. Devers et al., "Implementing Organized Delivery Systems: An Integration Scorecard," *Health Care Management Review 19*, no. 3 (1994): 7.

Integration Strategies for the Medical Practice (Chicago, IL: American Medical Association, 1996).

S.S. Meighan, "Managing Conflict in an Integrated System," *Topics in Health Care Financing 20*, no. 4 (1994): 39.

M.W. Peregrine, "Creative Alliances Offer Alternatives to Corporate Mergers," *Healthcare Financial Management 51*, no. 1 (1997): 52.

B.J. Ryan and D.J. Daugherty, "Degree of Integration Can Influence Organizational Economic Decisions," *Healthcare Financial Management 51*, no. 8 (1997): 46.

L. Scanlan, Jr., "Building Consensus for Integration," *Healthcare Financial Management 49*, no. 1 (1995): 33.

D.V. Schultz, "The Importance of Primary Care Providers in Integrated Systems," *Healthcare Financial Management 49*, no. 1 (1995): 58.

CHAPTER 20

Negotiating and Practicing under a Capitation Contract

INTRODUCTION

It is one thing to deliver medical care under a managed care contract; it is quite another to practice under a capitated managed care contract. In the former case, the physician is likely to be reimbursed according to some form of fee schedule, probably discounted. She may be subjected to a fairly limited range of utilization management and quality control procedures directed by the managed care organization (MCO) issuing the contract. In a capitated arrangement, the physician assumes the much greater responsibility of implementing the practice measures required to provide quality health care within the agreed-upon capitation fee.

In this chapter, the physician-reader learns about what to look for and negotiate for in a capitation contract. A couple of methods are suggested for calculating whether she can make money under a particular capitation rate. There are tips on adapting one's practice to optimize productivity and success in a capitated environment. If capitation is the world of the future, you might as well get good at it.

WHO SHOULD READ THIS CHAPTER

The material in this chapter is most useful for physicians who have yet to enter into their first capitation contract. It explains, in some detail,

how capitation works and how it affects the way physicians must deliver care. There is a healthy discussion of the key provisions in a capitated contract. Recommendations are provided for analyzing and changing the contract language. The chapter includes some good tips on adjusting your practice style and management to thrive under a capitation arrangement.

Even if you already are party to one or two capitation contracts that account for a modest share of your total revenues, you probably will gain new insights from reading this chapter. If capitation becomes the dominant, or universal, form of medical care reimbursement by the twenty-first century, you would be smart to learn all you can now about the concept and how to accommodate it. There is a sound rule of thumb for medical practice under capitation: It is much easier to make the necessary changes in your attitudes, your style of delivery, and the business aspects of your practice when capitation fees are a small or nonexistent part of your income than when you are largely dependent on capitation revenues.

Only if you have been practicing successfully under capitation for three or four years and it accounts for a majority of your practice income might you consider passing this chapter by. That probably also means that you are practicing in California or Minnesota. If you live in any of the other 48 states, you will benefit from this discussion.

WHAT IT IS LIKE TO BE REIMBURSED THROUGH CAPITATION FEES

Under a capitation contract, a physician agrees to provide a defined package of services to the members of an MCO who select him as their primary provider. In return, the MCO agrees to pay the physician a fixed amount of money every month for every one of those members. That fixed amount is called the *capitation rate* (from the Latin *caput*, meaning "head") and abbreviated as the PMPM (per member per month) payment. The group of members for whom you are responsible is referred to as *covered lives*. In the future, when your practice is almost entirely capitated, you will describe the size of the practice by saying "I am responsible for 785 covered lives."

> **Note**: The term *covered lives* might remind you of the concept of insurance coverage. It would be an appropriate reminder. Under capitation, you are agreeing to provide a form of insurance coverage for the unpredictable possibility that your member-patients will become ill and require an unpredictable level of medical services.

The physician receives the fixed monthly payment for each MCO member he sees—regardless of how sick the patient may or may not be, regardless of what volume of services he may or may not require. If a particular member has no medical problems during a particular month and perhaps never comes in to the doctor's office, the doctor still receives the predetermined payment. If the member is extremely ill during that month and requires health care costing twice the monthly amount, the doctor still receives the predetermined payment.

If money is a primary motivator for most people, how would you expect a physician to respond to such a reimbursement arrangement? Capitation gives doctors an incentive to keep patients as healthy as possible, minimizing the number of medical services that they demand. When a patient does truly need medical care, capitation also spurs physicians to deliver those services as efficiently as possible.

This is the essence of what a physician must do to succeed under capitation:

- Deliver care differently than he does under fee for service.
- Manage his practice differently than he does under fee for service.

If this seems daunting to you, it should. What is required is no less than a re-creation of your medical training and practice. It is necessary that you revise attitudes and habits that were impressed upon you during your years as a medical student and during subsequent years in your own medical practice. You can begin the revision here.

HOW CAPITATION RATES ARE CALCULATED BY AN MCO

The capitation rate you receive is the "premium" paid you for the health care coverage you are providing to all your covered lives. To decide whether the capitation rate you are offered is adequate and whether you want to try to negotiate an increase, it helps to know how the rate was calculated. There are four pieces to the premium paid for any kind of insurance.

Cost of Claims

The bulk of a health insurance premium dollar—70 to 90 percent—pays for the cost of the claims brought under the insurance policy. In your case, this includes your salary, the salaries of your clinical assistants, and the out-of-pocket costs of services and goods directly related to the delivery of care.

Insurance companies use statistical specialists called *actuaries* to try to predict just how sick a group of members will be and how much medical care they will require. One of their primary sources of data is the information contained in millions of health insurance claims that have been filed over the years. The result is projected rates of utilization of every kind of medical service. The utilization rates are multiplied by the fees the companies must pay to providers for those services to come up with the total cost of claims from that group of members.

The actuarial projections are so complex and time-consuming that they generally are prepared only for very large populations, such as all the inhabitants of the United States. However, there are great variations in medical service utilization among subgroups in the U.S. population. Insurance companies have a natural impulse to highlight those variations in order to make appropriate adjustments to their premiums. They do that through a process called *risk rating*.

Risk rating is an actuarial procedure for adjusting a global premium for the unique characteristics of the smaller group being insured. At an initial level, risk rating takes into account broad demographic variables, such as

- Age—very young and very old people consume far more medical care than do people of other ages.
- Gender—at different ages, men and women vary in the amount of medical care they require.
- Income—people with more money buy more medical care.
- Education—people with more education use more health care services.
- Employment—employed people tend to be healthier than do unemployed people.
- Industry—employees in certain industries use more medical services than do those in other industries.
- Geography—health care utilization rates vary from state to state, among cities of different sizes, and between rural and urban areas.
- Coverage—the details of a person's health insurance coverage (deductibles and copayments) will influence how often she makes a claim under that coverage.

At the next level, risk rating attempts to predict the utilization rates for the particular group of people enrolling in an MCO—for instance, the employees of single large company. Ideally, the actuary wants to know the actual health care claims experience of that group. These data are readily available if the MCO has had an ongoing relationship with the employer. They will show utilization rates by current procedural terminology (CPT) code. Taking into account that experience, as well as the demographic idiosyncrasies of the group, the actuary will adjust the global premium up or down.

There is a final, hypothetical level of risk rating. The insurer could try to predict the health care utilization rates of individual enrollees and adjust their premiums accordingly. This is not done because it would be too expensive, too inaccurate to be worth the effort, and probably politically unacceptable. Furthermore, this approach would almost completely erode the notion that insurance spreads the risk of claims awards over many people.

Cost of Administration

Between 10 and 20 percent of the premium dollar pays the insurer's or MCO's cost of administering the capitation arrangement. The cost includes contracting with employers, contracting with providers (such as you), marketing the managed care plan, calculating the capitation rates, and managing the program on a continuing basis.

The equivalent in your practice is the nonclinical cost of managing the practice. This includes the salaries of nonclinical personnel, rent for administrative office space, office equipment, claims filing and follow-up, and similar items.

Cost of Risk

Calculating a capitation rate involves an attempt at predicting future events—the likelihood that enrollees will require certain types of medical services. Even the best actuaries are not soothsayers. They are making only very informed guesses. There is a very good chance that the incidence of illness and utilization of services among the designated enrollees will be higher or lower than the actuary's prediction.

If they have overestimated utilization, that should be fine with you. You will receive your fixed capitation rate and spend it on fewer services. The problem arises if your managed care enrollees require more services than the capitation rate assumed, perhaps considerably more. There is a definite "risk" of that happening. There are several ways to reduce that risk. In setting the capitation rate, a certain amount—rarely more than 5 percent or 10 percent—is added to pay you for accepting that risk.

Cost of Market Advantage

Sometimes, it is possible for the insurer (whether an insurance company or a physician) to charge a slightly higher premium because it has a competitive advantage in the marketplace. In the case of a physician entering into a capitated contract, this advantage may take the following forms:

- superior reputation among patients
- specialty shared by few other physicians in the area
- highly unique procedures or services
- office located in an area especially convenient to enrollees
- exceptionally accessible office hours
- demonstrably higher-quality care

These are factors that you may be able to use to negotiate a higher capitation rate.

THE "RISK" YOU ASSUME UNDER A CAPITATED ARRANGEMENT

One of the key elements of the movement toward provider integration is the concept of "risk sharing." Whereas the sharing of risk can occur at different levels in the health care delivery chain,

capitation contracts are the primary device for carrying it out. *Risk* sounds like a scary word and, if you are going to be assuming more risk than ever before, it pays to understand what you are getting yourself into.

Risk is the possibility of suffering harm or loss. Each person lives constantly with the risk that he may become ill and require medical care. The person is concerned that he will not have enough money to buy the medical care he needs, so he purchases a health insurance policy that will pay for the medical care if he needs it. The person's risk has been shifted to the insurance company. That is where the risk stayed for several decades while the insurance companies paid providers on a fee-for-service basis to deliver medical care to its policyholders.

The insurance companies began to realize that a lot of judgment went into providers' decisions about how much care to deliver. In an attempt to influence those decisions, the insurance companies started to contract with managed care companies to arrange for providers and to manage the way they deliver care. Some of the risk was now shifted to the MCO.

Neither the MCOs nor the providers that they were trying to manage were satisfied with the traditional utilization control procedures. As a result, the MCOs contracted with providers and groups to manage their own utilization. The MCOs simply say, "Let's agree on a pot of money we will give you to meet the health care needs of this bunch of enrollees. Then you can do whatever you want, as long as those needs are met. If you are able to meet them more efficiently than we both thought, you get to keep the difference." A big piece of the risk is now shifted to physicians.

These are the dimensions of the risk. If the capitation rate underestimates the actual utilization by your enrolled patient population, you will not have sufficient revenues to cover the cost of the services you must provide. Your practice will lose money, which probably translates into lower take-home income for you.

There are two fundamental causes of higher-than-expected utilization.

1. The demographics of the MCO members who selected you as their physician were different than the demographics of the total MCO enrollment group upon which the capitation rate was based. People with more serious health care problems chose you to be their doctor. This phenomenon is called *adverse selection*. Your patients may be older than usual, more likely to be smokers, generally less fit or less educated. They may earn less or live in a less healthy section of town. Sometimes you influence these unpropitious choices through your office location or your reputation for treating certain kinds of patients. Often, you will never know why these patients came to you.

2. Health care problems are not planned. They occur randomly, accidentally, sometimes beyond the ability of even actuaries to predict. If misfortune causes your patients to utilize considerably more medical services than expected, your capitation revenues again will prove to be inadequate. Randomly unanticipated medical problems are more likely with a smaller population of patients under capitation. The probabilities behind the capitation rate work better with larger groups of patients.

HOW CAPITATED REIMBURSEMENT CHANGES THE WAY YOU PRACTICE MEDICINE

When you begin practicing under capitation, you will deliver care differently and more efficiently. You do this to optimize your productivity and income under that reimbursement scheme. This is exactly the behavior response that the MCOs want to see from you. Here are more specific changes that will take place.

Changes in Practice Style

1. *Your primary focus is on meeting the health care needs of the collective commu-*nity of lives that you have agreed to cover for the MCO. This is in contrast to the traditional emphasis, under fee for service, on the needs of each patient separately. If one of your covered lives has minimal health care needs in a given month or year, you do not count her PMPM payment as profit. Instead, you apply it to another covered life that has greater health care needs than predicted. In addition, you may choose to allocate from your total capitation budget funds to install a preventive care program that will benefit an undefined large number of your covered lives.

2. *You develop a new style of practice that involves lower utilization of all medical services and more cost-effective versions of the services you do utilize.* You look for less-intensive or less-costly therapies that produce the same health outcomes.

3. *You offer preventive health services that keep your patients healthier and less likely to require medical care.* The preventive services cost less than the treatment of the health problems they prevent.

4. *You implement measures to ensure that you do not underutilize medical services and that you maintain the quality of your medical care in the face of the other practice changes you have made.* The concern has switched from providing too much care to providing too little care.

Changes in Practice Management

The extent of these changes will depend to a degree on the contractual demands of each MCO.

1. *You spend more time, money, and energy in managing your practice.*

2. *You become a professional manager, as well as a professional clinician, or you hire a professional manager.*

3. *You invest significant amounts of capital in new systems for your practice.*

4. *You gather varieties of information about your practice style that you have never*

gathered before. You do some of this because an MCO demands it; you do some of it because you decide you need the data to better operate and market your practice.

5. *You install sophisticated information collection and management systems, probably computerized.*

6. *You establish computerized electronic links with MCOs and other providers in your group or network.*

7. *You keep track of every patient encounter and the services provided during that encounter, recorded by CPT code.* You normally do this because an MCO requests the information to protect against underutilization.

8. *You track utilization patterns by patient and MCO, and constantly compare the costs you are incurring with the capitation revenues you are earning.* On the basis of these data, you identify high-cost procedures that may be replaced by lower-cost variations. You single out high-utilization patients for special case management and preventive measures.

9. *You scientifically document the quality of the medical care you provide.* You do this by measuring clinical outcomes and surveying patient satisfaction. You use these data to continually refine your clinical decision making, focusing increasingly on the most efficacious treatments. Ultimately, practice guidelines may emerge from this knowledge. You use the data also to demonstrate to MCOs your high-quality, cost-effective practice techniques. They may be the basis for negotiating a more attractive capitation rate.

IMPACT OF CAPITATION RATES ON SPECIALIST PHYSICIANS

MCOs negotiate capitation rates first and predominantly with primary care physicians (PCPs). This is because these doctors are increasingly being placed in the role of medical care gatekeepers, making most of the decisions that trigger utilization of health care resources. To a large degree, specialist physicians still are reimbursed on a fee-for-service basis, albeit a discounted one. Nonetheless, the movement toward capitation contracts impacts specialists in several ways.

Specialists do not receive as many referrals from PCPs. One of the ways that primary care gatekeepers practice more cost-effective medicine is by making fewer specialist referrals. They either find ways to provide the necessary treatment themselves or decide that the patient can do without. This happens, however, only if the primary care capitation rate covers all physician services or the primary doctors are placed at risk for specialist utilization through a risk-withholding pool. If this is not the case, if the gatekeepers are not in any way responsible for the costs of specialist referrals, they have an incentive to use specialists whenever possible to minimize the utilization of their own services.

Specialists are reimbursed less for the referrals they do receive. Whether it is the MCO or the PCPs who contract with the specialty doctors and bear the risk of their utilization, they will exact the deepest possible discounts in their fee schedules.

Specialists increasingly are subjected to capitation. The basic principles that support primary care capitation make it just as feasible for specialists—as long as the enrollee population is large enough. Physician groups and MCOs are realizing this and increasingly entering into subcapitation contracts with a variety of specialist groups.

> **Note:** There are a few complications with specialty capitation. Specialty medical services are required less often, so it is harder to predict their utilization unless the covered patient group is rather large. Also, errors in actuarial prediction are generally more costly when they involve more expensive specialty services. The necessary mass of patients is usually ensured through exclusive contracts with a specialist or specialty group.

The exclusivity creates its own problems. Your practice may not have the current capability to handle all the patients referred to you. Because you are the only physician in that particular MCO offering that kind of medical service, you cannot turn anyone away. To accommodate them, you may have to hire additional professional and ancillary personnel, and turn down referrals from outside the MCO. By allowing one MCO's patients to dominate your practice, you are putting all your eggs in one basket. If the MCO fails, so will your practice. Of course, when the MCO thrives, your monopoly over their patients guarantees your success.

GOOD REASONS FOR WELCOMING MANAGED CARE CONTRACTS THAT PAY CAPITATED RATES

Many physicians enter into capitation agreements with great reluctance and apprehension—then discover that their practice life has improved. Here are some of the advantages you can look forward to in a capitation arrangement with an MCO:

- *Less outside scrutiny*—Managed care plans have greatly eroded physician practice autonomy in the last decade through oppressive utilization review procedures, often at the hands of nonphysicians. They have done this in the interest of controlling utilization and, thereby, costs. With capitated contracts, the MCOs are turning over responsibility for utilization control to the physicians themselves. Accordingly, the physicians absolutely must implement the necessary review and control systems. The difference is that physicians govern those systems and make the final clinical decisions.
- *Potential for greater revenue*—Particularly if you are a PCP, a capitated contract makes you responsible for how a larger portion of MCO premium dollars are spent. If you develop skill at cost-effective practice under capitation, you can enjoy the savings not only from your own reduced utilization but also from the lower utilization of other health care services (hospital care, specialty care, ancillary services, lab tests, and medication). The potential for substantially increased income is great.
- *Steady, predictable cash flow*—Because you know for a certainty what your revenues will be each month, it is much easier to plan and meet your working capital needs.
- *Better cost control*—The improved cash flow and increased practice autonomy allows you to budget and control your costs much more effectively than under utilization-reviewed fee-for-service arrangements.
- *Facilitated long-range planning*—Your improved ability to project your finances into the future and to control your own fiscal destiny gives you the freedom to carry out some valuable long-range planning. You know what funds will be coming in and going out. As a result, you can make more confident decisions about expanding your practice, affiliating with other providers, purchasing equipment, and hiring new personnel.
- *Improved quality of care*—Capitation affords providers an incentive to improve health care quality. They can play an important role in prevention, early detection, and medical management of disease in an effort to prevent catastrophic problems—and costs—from developing.

ANALYTICAL TOOLS FOR REVIEWING A CAPITATION CONTRACT

Not all capitation contracts work to the benefit of the participating physicians. A few MCOs are simply so cutthroat that they will execute win-lose contracts with physicians if they can get away with it. Most MCOs have good intentions. There are simply honest misperceptions between them and physicians about appropriate terms for a good win-win capitation contract. It behooves physicians to analyze proposed capitation contracts and to prepare themselves to negotiate changes. Here are some tools for conducting that analysis.

Read every word of the contract. Even better, do it with another physician who has the acuity to ask "What does that mean?"

Categorize every provision of the contract into one of the following groups:

- "I do not understand what this language means or how it will affect me, and I must get an explanation from the MCO." (Designate with a question mark ["?"] in the margin.)
- "I am not clear about the financial impact of this language on my practice. I need to get more information from the MCO and study the finances of my practice more closely." (Designate with a dollar sign ["$"] in the margin.)
- "This is a provision I absolutely cannot accept. I must persuade the MCO to change it or I will not enter into the contract." (Designate with "NO" in the margin.)
- "This is a provision that will make my life much more difficult or uncomfortable. I can live with it if the rest of the contract is worthwhile, but I would prefer that the MCO change it." (Designate with "BAD" in the margin.)
- "This provision is a minor nuisance to me and otherwise pretty tolerable. However, I will use it as a bargaining chip in negotiations with the MCO if I cannot get some of the other changes I want." (Designate with "CHIP" in the margin.)
- "I like this provision a lot; it works very much to my advantage. I will definitely not give this up during a negotiation with the MCO." (Designate with "GOOD" in the margin.)
- "This language does not affect me one way or the other. I do not see it as a topic of negotiation." (Designate with "OK" in the margin.)

Put one of these labels in the margin next to every provision of the contract.

Prepare a list of the provisions with space for three items next to each one.

- The first item is the label, followed by a brief description of what is positive or negative about the provision for your practice.
- The second item is a statement of the desired action in a negotiation with the MCO.
- The third item explains how the matter was, in fact, resolved in the negotiations.

Use this list to plan your negotiation strategy with the MCO and to assess your progress in coming up with a contract that is acceptable to you.

CAPITATION CONTRACT PROVISIONS THAT WILL AFFECT YOUR PRACTICE INCOME

There are certain provisions you can expect to find in nearly all capitation contracts. These are the provisions that will have the most direct impact on your practice income and deserve your closest attention. That may mean raising them as issues in negotiations with the MCO.

Covered Services

The MCO is going to pay you a monthly capitation fee. In return, you are going to provide to its enrollees a defined package of covered services. That package can vary from MCO to MCO, from contract to contract, and from provider to provider. To decide whether you can make money under a given capitation rate, you must know the services you are promising to provide.

Insist that the contract include, even as an incorporated document, a list of the covered services, defined by CPT code.

Examine that list closely. Compare it with the services you normally provide to patients and see what is included and what is left out. The best services for capitation inclusion cost relatively little and are delivered frequently in large volumes. The utilization of these is easier to predict, and unanticipated overutilization is not so expensive a calamity.

Carve-Outs

Certain more expensive, less common services will be completely "carved out" of the capitation contract. They will not be among your covered services. Their unpredictability and high cost significantly increase your risk of inadvertent over-utilization, resulting in costs exceeding the capitation rate. Typical carve-out services are emergency care, trauma, epidemic infectious diseases, and mental health ailments. Some MCOs also carve out a few services that have preventive value or special appeal to patients—such as immunizations.

If you have the capability to provide the carved-out services, you normally will be reimbursed for them on a discounted fee-for-service basis. However, some of the services are so specialized that the MCO will contract separately with other caregivers to provide them. For instance, all mental health cases may be directed to a group of psychologists under exclusive contract with the MCO.

Usually, it is in your interest to see more services carved out of the package covered by the capitation rate. This reduces the range of services for which you are at risk. On the other hand, if you become proficient at the cost-effective delivery of the services for which you are responsible, you might prefer to be at risk for more services.

Risk Pools

Capitation contracts typically include another utilization control feature—the "risk pool." This pool consists of money that the MCO holds back from your capitation payment and from its payments to other providers, such as hospitals. The withhold you are most likely to see is 10 to 15 percent of your capitation fee. The MCO itself often makes a contribution to the pool as well. The pool funds are used to pay for services whose utilization you control, but which you do not directly provide. They usually include

- hospital care
- prescription drugs
- laboratory tests

- specialty physician care
- radiology and pathology services

The MCO budgets a sum of money intended to cover all these services. If utilization of the services comes in under budget, most of the excess stays with the MCO. A portion of the excess will go to you. The entire withhold risk pool also is returned to you, as it was not needed. If the utilization of these services is more than the basic budgeted amount, the deficit is paid for out of the risk pool. If the utilization is so out of control that even the risk pool is used up, the MCO makes up the difference. If only part of the risk pool is consumed, a share of the remainder comes back to you.

The risk pool serves as an incentive for you to be as cautious and cost-sensitive in utilizing these other services as the capitation rate encourages you to be with your own services.

Look most closely at six aspects of the risk pool language in the contract.

1. How large is the risk pool? Determine this in absolute dollar terms and as a percentage of your capitation rate. You want to know what proportion of your expected compensation from the MCO is a direct function of your utilization management abilities.

2. To whom does the pool apply? Your preference is for a pool that covers you individually or the members of your physician group. You then are in the best position to influence the utilization covered by the pool and to earn an efficiency bonus for yourself. Less desirable is a global risk pool that encompasses all the physicians on the MCO's panel. You and your colleagues can practice great, cost-effective medicine and see no reward if the other MCO doctors are less disciplined in their practice patterns. With whom are you sharing risk?

3. When are risk pool surpluses paid back to you? Some MCOs track physician utilization performance on an ongoing basis and make these payments quarterly. It should

not be necessary to wait until a fiscal year has been completed for the MCO to calculate the risk pool allocations and return any surpluses to you.

4. What range of services are covered by the risk pool? Your preferences about this issue will depend on your confidence in your ability to manage tightly the utilization of these other at-risk services. If your confidence is high, you will want to be held responsible for the utilization of as many services as are within your reasonable control. The size of the risk pool will be greater and so will your opportunities for additional reward for cost-effective practice methods.

5. How are funds remaining in the risk pool distributed? A well-designed risk pool is not very useful if your payments are not made on a rational basis or on time. Pay attention to the formula for dividing risk pool surpluses. It may be a fixed percentage allocation between you and the MCO—for example, 50–50. Alternatively, the portion that you receive may be tied to the achievement of targets for utilization of key services (such as inpatient hospital days, office visits, or specialty referrals) or goals for the clinical outcomes, patient satisfaction, or quality of care. Your share of the risk pool surplus rises as the utilization rate falls or as the quality measures improve. It is important to understand exactly what you have to do to earn a risk pool payment and to increase the amount of that payment. It is equally important that the variables that determine your payments are within your sphere of control or influence.

6. What is your liability if the risk pool funds are inadequate? Most risk pool arrangements call for the MCO to bear the entire amount of any overrun due to excessive utilization. However, be alert for the occasional contract that requires the physicians to chip in to meet these unrestrained service costs.

Payment Procedures

This section of the contract describes your capitation rates and the steps the MCO will follow in paying them to you.

In the simplest arrangement, the contract will give a single rate, expressed as a payment in dollar terms for each month that each MCO member is a patient of yours. There also may be several versions of that rate, depending on the exact benefit package the member has chosen and sometimes even on her demographics (age or gender). They will appear as a rate schedule. Small and growing MCOs may wish to set their capitation rates as a percentage of the premium they receive from payers. Accept such rate formulas only if you are confident that the MCO is efficient and well managed, that its payers are reliable, and that its premiums will remain steady or even increase.

The section will tell you *how often* the capitation rates will be made—usually monthly, occasionally quarterly. Look for an *exact date* each month when you can expect to see the payment. A conscientious MCO will also indicate the *penalty it will pay* you if the regular capitation is late. This is important because any payer organization has an incentive to delay payments as long as possible in order to use and enjoy interest on the money.

> **Caution:** Even with a late payment penalty clause, be wary of consistently or increasingly late payments from the MCO. This often is a sign of developing financial troubles.

Reinsurance or Stop-Loss Insurance

We discussed earlier just how unpredictable patient illness and need for medical services can be, even for the most skilled actuary. There is a possibility that an individual MCO member will suffer a catastrophic health problem and consume a hugely disproportionate share of your capitation revenues, inhibiting your ability to treat properly other patients. Better MCO capitation contracts protect against this eventuality by offering a reinsurance or stop-loss insurance option. The two terms mean essentially the same thing. They work this way.

A stop-loss insurance provision covers annual treatment costs that exceed a predetermined threshold. The threshold may be defined for each individual patient—for example, $10,000 per year—or as an aggregate amount for all capitated patients from the MCO. The treatment costs over the threshold are paid according to a discounted fee-for-service schedule. The MCO may pay all the excess costs or may divide them with the physician (for example, the MCO may cover three-fourths and the physician one-fourth of the amount). The cost or premium for the MCO assuming this added risk is deducted from the capitation rate.

Look closely at the following features of a stop-loss insurance clause:

- the treatment cost threshold that triggers the insurance
- the method of calculating those treatment costs
- the treatment services for which the costs are calculated
- the division of costs above the threshold, between you and the MCO
- the cost to you of the stop-loss insurance
- the personal professional liability insurance coverage

Examine the contract to determine whether the MCO pays the premiums for your professional liability insurance coverage or the purchase is left up to you. Also notice whether the MCO requires that you maintain certain levels of coverage. There is general agreement on responsible coverage limits, so there should be little controversy with the MCO.

Physician Extenders as Caregivers

To manage your clinical costs, you may have a strong desire to use physician extenders (nurse practitioners, physician assistants, and the like).

In the interests of maintaining quality of care, the MCO may prefer that most care be delivered by physicians. This may limit your ability to prosper under the capitation rate offered you. If you use extenders extensively now, a requirement such as this raises your operating costs significantly. Check this provision closely.

Access to Care Requirements

The MCO may insert language in the contract requiring you to provide patients with certain levels of access. Typical obligations are

- maintaining a minimum number of office hours
- providing for after-hours patient visits
- serving on-call duty for other physicians

Measure these demands against your current practice habits. They may require radical changes in your personal and professional life.

Patient Copayments

Find out whether your MCO patients will be subject to copayment requirements. If so, check to see whether you have the responsibility to bill them and collect the copayments. You may have contracted with the MCO to avoid just this kind of billing headache. Determine also whether you keep the copayment proceeds or must remit them to the MCO.

Quality Assurance Reporting and Responsibilities

Responsible MCOs have become more and more sensitive to concerns that quality of care is being compromised by their emphasis on cost management and reduction. The capitation contract is likely to define physician obligations for quality assurance activities. For instance, you may be asked to

- Sit on peer review panels.
- Meet MCO-specified credentialing criteria for new physicians or other personnel added to your practice.
- Maintain your patient records in a new MCO-defined format.
- Participate in regular quality assurance training sessions.
- Collect and provide to the MCO new levels of detail on all patient encounters.

Study these commitments to make sure that you are willing to live up to them.

Required Practice Operating Policies

The MCO contract may also bind you to comply with an entire range of other practice operating policies and procedures. These may be in areas such as employee relations, hazardous waste disposal, or infectious disease precautions. Compliance may add noticeably to your operating expenses. Decide whether you want to practice according to these new guidelines and whether you can afford to.

"Most-Favored-Nation" Physician Fees

This contract language requires that you charge the MCO the lowest fees that you charge any other payer. MCOs hate to feel that some other payer has struck a better bargain with you than they have. If all your payer contracts include a "most-favored-nation" clause, then you must unavoidably charge everyone the same fees.

This clause applies only to any fee-for-service components of your reimbursement under the contract. Payments for your "carve-out" services are a good example. The capitation rate is set through negotiations between you and the MCO.

Contract Termination

If you have had no substantial experience practicing under capitation, you are going to be nervous about your ability to adjust your practice style and continue to do well financially. You may not be sure that you can trust the MCO. You probably do not want to make any long-term commitments just yet. Also, if things go terribly wrong, you might want to be able to bail out.

These are legitimate concerns. They are the reasons for paying close attention to the termination provision in the contract. This is the language that defines when and how you and the MCO can break off your relationship.

The contract will state the exact date on which it becomes effective. It will state the term of the contract (in months or years), perhaps also giving the exact date on which it ceases to be effective. The contract may also provide for automatic renewal unless one party or the other declines.

An *automatic renewal clause* can present problems in the future. If you find that you are unhappy under the capitation contract, you may wish to renegotiate some terms before renewing or simply to not renew at all. However, if you are preoccupied when the term expires, you could be automatically recommitted for another term without being aware of it. At the very least, insist that the MCO give you advance notice that automatic renewal is coming up. Also, get an explanation of how key contract terms (such as the capitation rate!) will be updated upon renewal. The contract would be even better without automatic renewal language. It usually is preferable to make a conscious decision to continue a relationship as important as the one with an MCO.

It is worth thinking about the term or *duration of the contract*. If you are just starting out in practice under capitation, you may prefer to test the waters with a shorter-term contract. On the other hand, if you are confident of your cost-effective practice skills and feel that the MCO has offered you a great deal, you might want to lock yourself in with them for a longer period. Think carefully about this.

This section will also explain how the relationship might be aborted in midterm. It will distinguish between contract *terminations with and without cause*. Scrutinize this language because it can make the difference between life and death for your practice.

When an MCO ends its working relationship with you, its member-patients leave, too. If you have become heavily dependent on the MCO for patients—if MCO revenues make up a substantial portion of your income—a contract termination could devastate your practice.

You have two primary concerns with termination language. First, must the MCO have a good reason—a cause—for terminating? Second, must the MCO give some amount of notice that it intends to terminate?

Recommendation: Seek a contract that does not include a "termination without cause" provision. If the provision is unavoidable, negotiate the longest possible advance notice requirement you can. Try for 30 days; anything less than two weeks is almost worthless.

When it comes to terminations with cause, the contract should describe the circumstances that constitute a sufficient basis for breaking off the relationship. They will include things such as loss of credentialing, failure to meet MCO reporting requirements, unprofessional behavior, and unwillingness to cooperate with quality assurance programs. Try to negotiate added language permitting you a period during which you can remedy the infraction.

Bear in mind that these provisions work both ways: Though they do allow the MCO certain freedoms to end the contract, you enjoy the same discretion.

> **Note:** There is a special kind of termination right you should seek, separate from the basic termination clause. During the life of the contract, the MCO will have the occasional need to make changes in the terms and language of the contract. In most cases, it will do this more or less unilaterally, because it simply cannot negotiate every change individually with each of its participating providers. However, you should request, in return, that the MCO notify you in advance (anywhere from 30 to 90 days would be fair, depending on the type of change) and give you the opportunity to withdraw from the contract if you find the changes intolerable.

There are several other important matters related to termination. The contract should make clear your responsibilities if either you or the MCO calls it quits. You will have certain obligations to continue providing care to your current patients until a replacement provider is found. You will be liable for outstanding debts to the MCO, for example, risk pool deficiencies.

The contract may also impose a continuation of care duty on you in the event that the MCO should go out of business. This is an unlikely event (especially if you have done your homework in checking out the MCO before you signed the contract) but, without the MCO around, you are the only one left to look after the patients until they can be transferred to other care.

ASSESSING THE PRACTICABILITY OF A PARTICULAR CAPITATION RATE

An employer, an MCO, or a provider network of which you are a member will offer you a capitation rate for assuming the responsibility of meeting the health care needs of a given population of people. Your long-term success depends on being able to practice within that capitation rate.

The rate offered to you may not be fair or reasonable. The MCO may be inexperienced at calculating accurate capitation rates and may set the rate too low. (Note: The MCO might also set the rate too high. Though that might be attractive to you in the short run, it is no good for either one of you if it causes the MCO to go out of business in the long run.) The MCO may know the reasonable rate but simply be trying to push you to accept an unreasonably low rate to maximize its short-term earnings but ignoring its effect on your long-term survivability. The rate may be quite reasonable for an average practice but not applicable to yours because of unique circumstances. You may offer special services or practice under special hardships that drive up your costs. Or, you may simply not practice in a modern, cost-effective manner.

It makes sense to figure out whether there is a good match between the capitation rate and your practice style and cost structure. You will find this out very quickly if you just accept the rate and immediately begin losing money under it. Within a year, your practice will have failed or the MCO will have deselected you. It would be better to discover this incompatibility in advance. The following are steps for assessing whether a capitation rate fits your practice.

Risk-Sharing Experience of Providers

- Gather, review, and analyze data for all treatment that current and prospective patients have received.
- Examine the prior managed care experience of the providers in your group or system.
- Learn how many of them have assumed risk before.
- Determine what degree of risk was assumed and the providers' performance under it.
- Wherever possible, quantify that experience—size and type of population served, over- or underperformance with the capitation rate, satisfaction levels of the patients and their payers, etc.

Health Care Utilization of Prospective Patients

- Obtain from the MCO information on the demographics, epidemiology, and treatment intensity of the patient population you will be responsible for under capitation.

Utilization Habits of Providers

- Gather the best data available about the utilization patterns of providers in your group or system.
- Examine the data for evidence of medically unnecessary tests or procedures.
- Examine the data for evidence of outside specialist referrals for services that could

have been provided as well and for lower cost by an in-group specialist or a PCP.
- From the data, learn each provider's incidence of hospitalization, length of hospital stays, and bed-days per 1,000 patients for various specialty services.
- From the data, learn each provider's utilization of outpatient care (i.e., outpatient visits per 1,000 patients).
- Determine the incidence of emergency department usage by each provider's patients.
- Compare each provider's utilization rates with the averages for your group, for the medical community in your region, and nationally. If you can obtain data on the utilization rates of the MCO's present physicians, compare with them as well.
- If you have the time and the ability (you may need an accountant for this task), project the costs of your group of providers—practicing with their existing utilization rates—in treating the population of MCO enrollees likely to become your patients.
- Compare the hypothetical costs of treating that population with the capitation revenues that the MCO is offering you (Exhibit 20-1).

Provider Resources within the Group

- Look closely at the PCP/specialty care physician ratio in the group or network to ensure a proper balance. (Note: A ratio of 50 percent to 60 percent PCPs is a good target.)
- Regardless of their specialties, examine the range of medical services offered by these physicians. Too limited a range means that there will be more referrals to nongroup specialists over whom there is less cost control.
- Review the practice patterns and utilization experiences of all outside physicians to whom the group might be referring. Get a sense of their commitment to risk-bearing and cost-effective health care. Create relationships with those outside physicians who emphasize the same high-quality, cost-sensi-

Exhibit 20–1 Calculating Your Profit or Loss under a Particular Capitation Rate

There are several established methodologies for calculating more accurately whether a practice will make or lose money at a particular capitation rate. Here are two of the easiest to understand and carry out.

Methodology #1: *Cost per service analysis*

Your goal under capitation is to earn revenues that at least cover your practice costs (including your salary) and to earn even more by practicing more effectively. This analytical approach estimates your practice costs under the capitation while factoring in improvements in your practice effectiveness. Carry out the following calculations for your most recent complete fiscal year:

1. Determine the number of times you delivered each service per 1,000 patients, by CPT code. This should be available from your financial records. This is the utilization rate you achieved using your current practice style with your current patients.
2. Determine the number of Relative Value Units (RVUs) for each CPT code service.
3. For each CPT code, multiply the utilization rate by the number of RVUs. The result is the number of RVUs of that service that you delivered to each 1,000 patients.
4. Add up the number of RVUs per 1,000 patients for all the services you performed. The result is the total number of RVUs you delivered to each 1,000 patients.
5. Determine the total of all your practice costs for the year. Include every cost item related to the delivery of care to your patients—salaries, overhead, supplies, purchased services.
6. Divide your total practice costs (from step 5) by the total number of RVUs per 1,000 patients (from step 4). The result is your cost per RVU.
7. Multiply your cost per RVU (from step 6) by the number of RVUs for each type of service you deliver. The latter figures are available through the Resource-Based Relative Value System (RBRVS). The result of the multiplication is your cost per service typically delivered in your practice.

8. Determine or estimate your expected utilization rates for each service under the capitation contract. This figure may be based on several sources: your own historical utilization rates, the utilization rates or projections for the MCO's current physicians, consultants with access to actuarial data, and the American Medical Association's Center for Health Policy Research.
9. Multiply your expected utilization rates by service (from step 8) times your cost for that service (from step 7). The result is your expected practice cost by service per 1,000 members. Add the costs for all the services you promise to provide under the capitation contract to get your total practice costs under that contract.
10. Divide your expected total practice costs (from step 9) by 1,000 patients. Then divide by 12 months. The result is your expected total practice costs for 1 patient for 1 month.
11. Compare the figure in step 10 with the per member–per month (PMPM) capitation rate offered by the MCO in its contract. If the capitation rate exceeds the step 10 figure, you are in good shape, on the road to turning a profit under the contract.

These calculations are based on a lot of estimates and predictions. The margin of error is considerable. When you are first starting out in capitation, you need not worry if your projected costs actually exceed the capitation rate by a small margin. As you gain experience with capitation, you will accumulate more accurate data about your costs and utilization rates, and you will practice more efficiently.

Methodology #2: *Cost per member analysis*

This method is a little less precise but has the advantage of showing general ways to improve the efficiency of your practice. It determines the number of patients who can be seen by each physician. The various practice costs per physician are identified and then allocated per member per month. The calculations go like this:

continues

Exhibit 20–1 continued

1. Estimate the number of patients each physician will be able to accept and treat under the capitation contract. The figure will be somewhat related to the number of regular patients each physician has now. Because increased productivity is expected under capitation, the figure will probably be higher.

2. Break down all the practice costs into monthly per-physician equivalents. For instance, each physician is paid a salary and benefits that are directly attributable to her. In addition, she is supported by a certain number of clinical staff, let us say 2.35 FTEs (full-time equivalents). There are salaries and benefits associated with them. Each physician also consumes a certain volume of supplies and services. The cost of these can be allocated by physician. The same approach can be taken with other cost categories such as administrative staff, professional liability insurance premiums, and several types of overhead.

    All practice costs will be divided up among the physicians who are directly responsible for seeing the capitated patients. When you have a fairly accurate fix on the costs attributable to each physician (e.g., one physician has a larger private office and therefore can be assigned rent costs on a per-square-foot basis, or your accounting system tracks the supplies requested and consumed by each physician), use them. Otherwise, you will probably just divide the total cost figure (e.g., cost of utilities) by the number of physicians.

3. For each cost category, divide each physician's allocated cost (from step 2) by the number of patients she is expected to see under the capitation contract (from step 1). The result is the estimated cost to treat one patient for one month. When the figures for each category are added together, they show the total estimated cost to treat one patient for one month.

4. Compare the final figure in step 3 with the PMPM capitation rate offered by the MCO in its contract.

5. If the capitation rate exceeds your estimated total PMPM cost, you can examine the costs per category to decide where to cut back or be more efficient. For instance, if you need to save $0.53 PMPM, you might plan to reduce each doctor's consumption of supplies by $0.17, usage of staff personnel by $0.22, and consumption of overhead by $0.04, while increasing her efficiency by $0.10.

Source: Methodology #1 data from E.S. Holzberg, Tracking Costs of Providing Care under Managed Care, *American Medical News*, p. 17, © 1997.

tive care that you demand of your group physician colleagues.

Allocation of Risk among All Providers

- If the services covered by your capitation rate include hospital care, see whether the hospital(s) you use will assume its share of the risk.
- Consider whether it is appropriate to subcapitate the specialist physicians in your group or network who will be providing specialty care. This decision will depend largely on how much authority the PCPs are given over the full spectrum of medical care. The more authority they have, the more risk they must assume.

CONTRACTUAL STRATEGIES FOR REDUCING RISK UNDER CAPITATION

You already know that you are bearing considerable financial risk in practicing under a capitation contract. You will practice as efficiently and effectively as possible to minimize your costs of delivering care to the MCO's member-patients. This will somewhat reduce the chances of your exceeding your capitation revenues. Still, you have no control over the possibility of a randomly high proportion of catastrophic illnesses among your patients or the unanticipated demand for certain very expensive services. Also, you may find that you do not adjust to the cost-effective practice of medicine quite as quickly as you had hoped.

There are a number of strategies for reducing your risk even further. They involve options and choices built into the contract, with the complete understanding and cooperation of the MCO. The MCO is delighted to help you minimize your risk legitimately, as long as it does not involve shifting the risk back to the MCO.

Look carefully for the following provisions in the capitation contract. If you take advantage of them, they can make your practice life a lot easier. If they are not in the contract, negotiate with the MCO for their inclusion.

Stop-Loss Insurance

This contract provision was explained in some detail earlier. Keep two things in mind about this insurance alternative. The MCO offers it to you as an option. You can buy it from them or purchase it independently from a third-party insurance company. If you are contracting with several MCOs, you may find it less expensive to reject all their individual stop-loss offers and, instead, obtain from an insurance company a policy for single blanket coverage for all your MCO contracts.

> **Tip:** If you are just starting out with capitation, starting out with a new MCO, and likely to serve a fairly modest-sized patient population for the first year or two, you would be very wise to obtain stop-loss insurance coverage from someone.

Service Carve-Outs

We also examined service carve-outs earlier. Give them a lot of attention. They have the potential for completely removing from the capitation rate the most problematic services. Make sure you understand precisely which services have been carved out (CPT codes should be used) and how they will be reimbursed, if not under the capitation rate.

Minimum and Maximum Patient Population

The very number of patients sent to you by the MCO can raise or lower your risk. The actuarial predictions used to calculate the capitation rate require a rather substantial body of patients to be statistically accurate. It may take several months before the MCO patients selecting your practice reach a critical mass to justify the risk inherent in the capitation rate. Some MCOs will be willing to pay you on a fee-for-service basis until that number is reached. It is worth exploring this option with the MCO.

At the other extreme, your practice may be so attractive that more MCO patients choose you than your practice can handle. The added numbers may force you to spend a lot more hours in your professional work than you want, or it could drive you to the added expense of new personnel, space, and equipment. If you think there is any chance of this happening, talk to the MCO about contract language allowing you to stop accepting new patients when the capacity of your practice is reached.

Revenue Minimum Guaranteed by the MCO

If the MCO especially wants you and your practice and appreciates the doubts you may have about practicing profitably under capitation, it may be willing to ensure you a minimum level of income. It will do this by promising to pay you at least the amount you would have earned if the MCO patients were under fee for service. In fact, it will be at discounted fee for service rates. The key question for you is the depth of the "discount" of the fee for service. Too deep a discount renders this kind of provision almost meaningless.

Contracted revenue guarantees will be available only when you are new to capitation and new to a particular MCO. Even if the terms of the provision do not seem to offer much, you have nothing to lose. Accept such a guarantee.

> **Note:** This is a good example of a contract point on which you may have some negotiating leverage. If you are a desirable practitioner to the MCO, there is a good chance you can persuade them to assuage your capitation anxieties with a clause like this.

Trial Participation in the MCO

A generous MCO that wants you on its panel badly enough might offer to let you treat its patients on a limited trial basis with reimbursement figured on a discounted fee-for-service schedule. The trial period could be from six months to a year. During that time, you find out how you like practicing under capitation and whether you can do it profitably.

REENGINEERING STRATEGIES FOR PRACTICING SUCCESSFULLY UNDER CAPITATION

If your practice management paradigm still reflects a fee-for-service tradition, it will be necessary to make changes so substantial that they are tantamount to re-creating the practice from scratch. Capitation demands an entirely new range of administrative systems. These are the most important ones:

Patient MCO Membership and Eligibility

- Gather up-to-date information from related MCOs on who their enrollees are and which of them have selected you or your group as their primary caregivers. This process is best handled through an electronic link with the MCOs.
- Obtain from each patient the identity of her or his MCO.
- Install procedures for quickly reconciling these data to confirm membership and eligi-

bility—to ensure that you understand what services the patient has contracted for and the capitation fee you are entitled to, and to guarantee that you are paid that fee.

Cost Management

- Track carefully every service and product provided to a patient, as well as its cost, to compare the aggregating cost of the services and products with the capitation fee.
- At least until you are well experienced with capitated medical care delivery, also compare the capitation revenues you are receiving with the fee-for-service revenues you might previously have been receiving. You may be surprised at the positive difference.
- For services and products not covered by the capitation fee, establish a claims-reporting and payment-receiving channel with the MCO. Electronic means would be best—and fastest.

> **Note:** The need for systems like these should be taken into account as you are assembling the participants in your group or network. It is desirable that each component practice in the network have data collection and claims reporting systems that are compatible with each other and with the relevant MCO's systems. This will save money, speed data and claims transmission, and allow you to collect your capitation revenues more quickly.

Utilization Management

- Specify as clearly as possible the circumstances when a referral may be made and the prior authorization that must be obtained.
- Implement a computerized system to monitor the utilization rates of individual providers in the network.
- Devise a procedure for employing the utilization data to modify inappropriate utilization rates. The procedure should be

graduated, starting with gentle, conscious-ness-raising measures (e.g., showing physicians how their rates compare with those of their peers) and moving to more coercive actions only as a last resort.

- To ensure cost-effective handling of catastrophic and chronic cases, install a case management system.
- To ensure that quality is not compromised by any of the utilization management or other efficiency measures, put into place a quality assurance system.

Operational Analysis

- Gather comprehensive data on patient encounters, utilization rates, related costs, and revenues earned. The goal is to evaluate how well individuals and the group or network as a whole is managing the risk they have assumed.
- Analyze deviations (surpluses or deficits) from the overall capitation rate, determine their causes or sources, and be prepared to take immediate appropriate action to correct.
- Generate detailed utilization reports for individual patients, for individual physicians, for all in-group physicians, for all outside physicians, and for all patients from each MCO. Use these reports to identify and correct developing problems.
- Install the best mechanism available to provide quickly to the MCO the information it needs to pay the monthly capitation fee and to receive that fee from the MCO. It always is advantageous to obtain money you are owed sooner rather than later.
- Develop a system for allocating capitation revenues among the participating physicians, preferably in proportion to the amount of risk each is bearing and her influence over the degree of medical care delivered.

EVALUATING AND NEGOTIATING A CAPITATION CONTRACT

What follows is a summation of the steps you ought to follow in evaluating, negotiating, and deciding whether to sign a capitation contract. It addresses most of the issues already discussed in this chapter.

Step 1. Review Your Practice

- Think long and hard about your attitudes toward practice under capitation.
- Assemble every bit of historical data you have on the operating costs of your practice. To the degree possible, break it down by broad or narrow category of service, preferably CPT code.
- Gather the best available data on the demographics of your current patient population.
- Examine the prior managed care experience of the providers in your group or system.
- Learn how many of them have assumed risk before.
- Determine what degree of risk was assumed and the provider's performance under it.
- Wherever possible, quantify that experience—size and type of population served, over- or underperformance with the capitation rate, satisfaction levels of the patients and their payers. etc.
- Gather the best data available about the utilization patterns of providers in your group or system.
- Examine the data for evidence of medically unnecessary tests or procedures.
- Examine the data for evidence of outside specialist referrals for services that could have been provided as well and at lower cost by an in-group specialist or a PCP.
- From the data, learn each provider's incidence of hospitalization, length of hospital stays, and bed-days per 1,000 patients for various specialty services.
- From the data, learn each provider's utilization of outpatient care (i.e., outpatient visits per 1,000 patients).
- Determine the incidence of emergency department usage by each provider's patients.
- Compare each provider's utilization rates with the averages for your group, for the

medical community in your region, and nationally. If you can obtain data on the utilization rates of the MCO's present physicians, compare with them as well.

- If you have the time and the ability (you may need an accountant for this task), project the costs of your group of providers—practicing with their existing utilization rates—in treating the population of MCO enrollees likely to become your patients.
- Look closely at the PCP/specialty care physician ratio in the group or network to ensure a proper balance. (Note: A ratio of 50 percent to 60 percent PCPs is a good target.)
- Regardless of their specialties, examine the range of medical services offered by these physicians. Too limited a range means that there will be more referrals to nongroup specialists over whom there is less cost control.
- Review the practice patterns and utilization experiences of all outside physicians to whom the group might be referring. Get a sense of their commitment to risk bearing and cost-effective health care.

Step 2. Review the MCO

- Obtain from the MCO information on the demographics, epidemiologic profile, and treatment intensity of the patient population you will be responsible for under capitation.
- Gather the best information you can on the MCO's finances and recent financial performance.
- Obtain the names of some or all of the other physicians already on the MCO's panel of providers.
- Check the names for the mix of specialties, for the locations of their practices, and for their reputations within the medical community. Decide whether this is a group with which you wish to be associated.
- Contact some of them to learn their experiences working with the MCO. In other words, use them as you would references for a job applicant.

Step 3. Review the Contract

- Obtain a complete copy of the contract the MCO is asking you to sign, including all exhibits, appendixes, and other documents included by incorporation.
- Read the contract through, slowly, from beginning to end.
- Review the contract language in detail, using the analytical tools described earlier.
- Annotate every section, paragraph, and separate concept in the contract, using the labels described earlier.
- Prepare separate lists of the parts of the contract that you find intolerable, seriously discomforting, or mildly discomforting, and list those parts that appear that they will impact your income or for which you need clarifying information.

Step 4. Ask the MCO for Data Elaborating on the Contract

- Ask for a list of the CPT codes for the services that you will be required to provide under the capitation rate.
- Ask for a description of the actuarial process by which the capitation rate was calculated.
- Ask for a copy of the actuarial projections that are the foundation of the capitation rate.
- Ask for a list of the employers from whom the MCO enrolls its members.
- Ask for a statement of the demographics and geographic locations of the members currently enrolled in the plan.
- Ask for a list of the other physicians on the MCO panel, particularly physicians to whom you may be required to refer.
- Ask for additional information or clarifying statements regarding contract provisions that you do not understand.

Step 5. Plan Your Negotiation Strategy

- Candidly assess the importance of your practice to the MCO and, thereby, your likely bargaining power in a negotiation with the MCO.

- List and describe the characteristics of you and your practice that would make you especially valuable to the MCO.
- List the uncomplimentary features of you and your practice that might make you less attractive to the MCO and prepare explanations, rationalizations, or work-arounds for each one.
- Learn from other physicians currently participating in the MCO what their negotiation experiences were and what strategies worked best. (Note: Do not try to coordinate negotiation strategies with other physicians outside your practice, particularly on matters of compensation or reimbursement.)
- Using the lists prepared during your review of the contract, decide on the order in which you will raise contract issues that you would like to change. Begin with trivial, nonmonumental issues on which you believe you and the MCO can reach agreement fairly quickly.
- Get very clear on the issues that are "deal-breakers" for you.

Step 6. Negotiate with the MCO

- Be prepared for an MCO with a "take-it-or-leave-it" attitude and decide whether you want to work with such an organization under any circumstances.
- Do not approach the negotiation as an adversarial encounter with a win-lose outcome.
- In most cases, assume that you and the MCO will be working together as partners for many years to come. Also assume that the MCO will be responsive to reasonable requests.
- Understand that the MCO needs uniformity on certain issues among all its participating physicians. It may not be in a position to negotiate separate and different language with each physician.
- During a negotiating session, if you are surprised by a proposal of the MCO or otherwise are uncertain about how to proceed on a particular issue, say that you would like to postpone it and move on to other issues. Do not agree to something in haste or confusion.

- Realize that negotiating or bargaining involves trades—if you ask the MCO to give up something it wants, you may have to give up something you want in return.
- Through early agreement on some issues, build the MCO's investment in a relationship with you, so that the MCO is more inclined to also agree on later, tougher issues to sustain the relationship.
- Put off discussion of financial matters, such as the capitation rate, fee-for-service schedules, stop-loss insurance, and the like, until all nonmonetary issues have been resolved.
- As you are negotiating, keep in mind that, for both you and the MCO, there often are (and should be) direct trade-offs between financial benefit and risk assumption. For example, if you want the MCO to pay you a slightly higher capitation rate, you may have to assume a slightly higher level of risk.

Step 7. Adapt Your Practice to Capitation

- Begin making these changes right now, even if your first capitated contract is six months away. Capitation is the future of health care reimbursement, and you cannot start adapting too soon.
- Accept the fact that the sweeping changes necessary will continue for a long time into the future.
- If you possibly can, do not make these changes grudgingly. Embrace them. The changes and your practice will be more likely to succeed.
- Allow yourself to be surprised by how much more comfortable you are practicing under capitation than you thought you would be.
- Look at the next section of this chapter for the specific changes in practice management and style you should consider.

Note: This process of adjustment will be much easier if you make the transition while capitation revenues are a relatively small part of your total income—no higher than 20 percent. The mistakes you are bound to make will be less far-reaching and expensive.

PRACTICE CHANGES TO IMPLEMENT AFTER SIGNING A CAPITATION CONTRACT

Your practice will never be the same again. Spend as much time as you need (not to exceed one week) venting your anger and disappointment at this fact. Then get down to the business of re-creating your medical practice.

If it helps, imagine that you have just finished medical school and your residency, and you are taking steps to set up a new practice that will permit you to prosper in a largely capitated health care system, as you see it developing.

This is what those steps should be:

- Reconcile yourself to practice under capitation and commit yourself to becoming the most competent capitated practitioner possible.
- Do not harbor hopes that someday you will be able to return to your previous style of practice.
- View the MCO as a partner.
- Provide the same level of cost-effective, high-quality care to both capitated and fee-for-service patients, as long as you are treating the latter.
- Emphasize patient education, lifestyle changes, prevention, screening, and early detection.
- Institute mechanisms for regularly measuring patient satisfaction. Pay attention to the findings and take immediate corrective action when problems emerge. You will also use this information to promote your practice to the MCO.

- Implement procedures for measuring the clinical outcomes of your practice decisions. Notice the treatments and therapies that are more efficacious and tend to employ them more often. You will also use this information to promote your practice to the MCO.
- Create an information system that tracks utilization rates by provider in your practice, by patient, and by payer. You will use these data to manage and adjust your practice style.
- Install an accounting system that enables you to follow direct and indirect costs on a continuing basis, broken down by procedure, patient, and provider. You will use these data to measure your cost-effectiveness and to evaluate the capitation rate.
- Consult with your colleagues already practicing under capitation to learn which treatments have produced the best outcomes for them.
- Look for less expensive treatments or procedures to accomplish the same purpose as your traditional approach.
- Be receptive to suggestions from the MCO's medical director on more cost-effective treatments.
- Commit yourself to any kind of change in your practice that makes you more attractive to your MCO partner.

If all of this sounds daunting and yours is a healthy-sized group, think seriously about hiring a consultant in one or all of the practice aspects you are trying to change (e.g., management information systems, revenue and cost accounting systems, utilization tracking, claims management, or overall practice management).

RESOURCE LIST

D. Azevedo, "Preparing Your Practice for Capitation," *Medical Economics 74*, no. 7 (1997): 48.

P.L. Beard, *How To Negotiate Capitation (Without Losing Your Head)* (Shawnee Mission, KS: ProSTAT Resource Group, 1994).

P. Boland, ed., *The Capitation Sourcebook: A Practical Guide to Managing At-Risk Arrangements* (Chicago, IL: Health Administration Press, 1997).

Capitation: The Physician's Guide (Chicago: American Medical Association, 1995).

A. Cherney, *The Capitation and Risk Sharing Guidebook: A Manual for Physicians and Alternate Site Providers* (copublished, Burr Ridge, IL: McGraw-Hill Healthcare Education Group, and Westchester, IL: Healthcare Financial Management Association, 1996).

K.M. Kennedy, "Evaluating and Negotiating a Profitable Capitation Contract," *Healthcare Financial Management 51*, no. 2 (1997): 44.

"Know What To Do in Getting Started with Managing Capitation Contracts," *Managed Care Week 7,* no. 16 (1997).

J. Lechtman, *Physician Capitation Strategies* (Washington, DC: St. Anthony Publishing, 1996).

"Looking for Hidden Health Plan Costs before Signing Capitation Agreements," *Physician Manager 7*, no. 22 (1996).

Managing under Capitation: Critical Success Factors for Group Practices (Publication #4988, Proceedings from select sessions at the 70th Annual Conference of the Medical Group Management Association, Minneapolis, MN, October 1996).

J.F. McCally, *Capitation for Physicians: Understanding and Negotiating Contracts To Maximize Reimbursement, Increase Financial Viability and Manage Financial Risk,* Publication #4907 (copublished, Englewood, CO: Medical Group Management Association, and Westchester: IL: Healthcare Financial Management Association, 1996).

H. Mondschein, "Get Ready for Capitation," *Independent Living Provider 11*, no. 2 (1996): 14.

D. Murray, "This Group's Motto: Don't Duck Capitation, Embrace It," *Medical Economics 74*, no. 15 (1997): 79.

D. Samuels, *Capitation, New Opportunities in Healthcare Delivery* (copublished, Burr Ridge, IL: McGraw-Hill Healthcare Education Group, and Westchester, IL: Healthcare Financial Management Association, 1996).

S.L. Schramm, *Global Capitation: Strategies and Techniques for Assuming Full Risk* (copublished, Burr Ridge, IL: McGraw-Hill Healthcare Education Group, and Westchester, IL: Healthcare Financial Management Association, 1998).

CHAPTER 21

Step Eleven: The Final Step–Evolving into a Regionwide Vertically Integrated Delivery System

INTRODUCTION

The process of growing an organization steadily larger as it integrates an ever-wider variety of health care providers culminates in the integrated delivery system (IDS). Once an IDS covers a reasonably broad geographic region (as determined by community demographics and market conditions), there is really nowhere else to go. The system may spread itself over an even wider area or link up with other IDSs, but this will not produce dramatic competitive advantages. The system can take on a financing function, becoming a managed care organization (MCO), but that step is not necessary to physician survival or prosperity. Few will have the desire to take it.

This chapter defines the IDS form, in its several variations, and summarizes its good and bad features. It explores the reasons physicians choose to affiliate with an IDS. There is a step-by-step methodology for planning and creating an IDS. The prerequisites to success for an IDS are laid out. Overall, it helps a physician decide whether he wants to be part of forming or even joining an IDS.

WHO SHOULD READ THIS CHAPTER

Every physician attracted by the title of this book should read this chapter. It describes the ultimate form of delivery organization—the IDS. If you are ambitious and entrepreneurial, it is the form to which you should aspire. Otherwise, you should come to understand the IDS as your eventual source of income and, possibly, your direct employer.

Some physicians reading this book may already be active members of a large, integrated physician group, probably combining primary care physicians (PCPs) and specialist physicians. The topic of this chapter should represent the next stage in their strategic ambitions. It provides numerous suggestions and guidelines for moving into that stage successfully. Other readers are not so far along the evolutionary path; they are still practicing in smaller-scale, less-integrated environments such as independent practice associations (IPAs) or physician-hospital organizations (PHOs). They will likely want to first implement the organizational structures described in other chapters—such as the management services organization (MSO) in Chapter 16, "Step Seven: Partnering with a Management Services Organization or Physician Practice Management Company," or the large, integrated multispecialty group practice in Chapter 13, "Step Five: Growing into a Larger, Multispecialty Group Practice." Eventually, however, the most ambitious of them will want to wind up in a position of influence with an IDS.

BASIC DEFINITION OF AN IDS

An IDS is a network of legally affiliated organizations (ambulatory care clinics, physician groups, diagnostic centers, hospitals, nursing homes, home health care units, rehabilitation facilities) that combine their resources and efforts to provide, or arrange to provide, a coordinated continuum of services to a defined population and are willing to be held clinically and fiscally responsible for the health status of that population.

The "umbrella" IDS entity performs all strategic planning and payer contracting for the providers, and allocates economic rewards and capital among the various participating interests. Typically, one organization owns and operates the hospital or hospitals, and a separate organization operates the medical practices. Frequently, the medical practices component is organized as a "medical foundation," an IPA, or simply a large multispecialty group practice. There is nothing to prevent a single large organization from owning all the delivery facilities, including hospitals, and employing all the necessary clinical personnel, including physicians. Increasingly, however, IDSs are based on various forms of "virtual integration" through contracts and other legal agreements.

After structural consolidation into an IDS, the parties typically focus on unified governance, the implementation of integrated management, clinical and information systems, and the use of consolidated budgets for the entire network system. The economic interests of the parties are aligned, and the provider participants do not maintain separate economic businesses that might potentially compete with each other.

An IDS often owns or is closely allied with an insurance product, such as a health maintenance organization (HMO) or other health plan.

An IDS primarily pursues a vertical integration strategy (often in a discrete geographic region), as opposed to the more horizontal strategies of multihospital systems or chains providing services at a single stage of the delivery process (inpatient care, psychiatric care, laboratory tests).

An IDS is based on the premise that such systems can provide care more efficiently and effectively than if individual operating units carry out

tasks independently or are linked through contracts in a loose confederation.

REASONS PHYSICIANS CHOOSE TO FORM OR PARTICIPATE IN AN IDS

You may be wondering why exactly you should feel motivated to become part of an IDS—as either a founder or a participant. As a guide, these are some of the reasons other physicians have mentioned for their involvement:

- to be owners, or at least participants, in the health care delivery systems of the future, not simply vendors to someone else's system or—even worse—left out entirely
- to maintain and increase their competitiveness and attractiveness to payers
- to increase their negotiating strength with payers
- to increase the future value of their medical practices and facilities
- to strengthen their primary care referral channels (if they are specialists)
- to position themselves with hospitals as a unified entity seeking to achieve common goals and speaking with a single, more powerful voice
- to reduce costs and create economies of scale
- to gain access to capital for expansion
- to secure future financial viability
- to increase operating efficiency and probability
- to gain freedom from the administrative hassles of current payment systems
- to improve their information systems to better respond to payer needs
- to integrate in order to reduce legal risk (because in a large multispecialty group practice or an IDS, there is only a single actor and a decreased possibility for improper conspiratorial or collective behavior)

BASIC PRECEPTS OF "INTEGRATING" YOUR DELIVERY SYSTEM

It is important to understand the characteristics of the truly integrated delivery system that you are attempting to create or evolve. These are the features you will want to implement in order to reap the benefits of this wonder, "integration."

Integration in a health care organization can occur along at least four different scales: physician, clinical, functional, and delivery process. All are essential elements of a genuine IDS.

Clinical integration concerns the coordination of patient care services across the departments, component organizations, services, units, and functions of the IDS. Physician integration reflects the degree of their involvement with and commitment to the IDS. Functional integration has to do with the coordination of business functions and activities across the component operating units. Delivery process integration is a measure of how many of the traditionally separate delivery organizations (which, together, provide the full range of health care services a patient might need) are integral parts of the IDS. These are the characteristics of each type of integration.[1]

Clinical Integration

Clinical Protocol Development

Begin the development of standard treatment protocols or clinical practice guidelines within as many IDS operating units as are receptive to them. Move aggressively to increase the number of working protocols and guidelines, and the number of units in which they are applied. As appropriate, work for the acceptance of the same protocols and guidelines in as many comparable operating units as possible.

Medical Records Uniformity and Accessibility

Take steps to increase the proportion of medical records features that are available to or shared by other operating units in the IDS—typically through electronic access to the records among operating units. Over time, expand the number of operating units tied into the unified medical records access system. Improve the time required to obtain medical record information from another operating unit. Add to the number of operating units a common numbering system and an integrated record with a problem-oriented flowsheet.

Clinical Outcomes Data Collection and Utilization

Increase the categories of outcomes data that are collected and shared within individual operating units, then steadily draw other units into the collection and sharing through the same methodology.

Clinical Programming and Planning

Start with the implementation of key programs and assessment tools, such as medical staff planning and common patient satisfaction indicators, throughout individual operating units. Then standardize and introduce these same tools across multiple units. Look for physician groups and PHOs (if any are included) whose members span more than one operating unit. This makes it easier to spread these and other innovative ideas across operating unit boundaries.

Shared Clinical Support Services

These are the various key support services that all direct providers need to enable their delivery of hands-on care—services such as laboratory, pharmacy, and rehabilitation. Push each operating unit to share in these services offered across the IDS, rather than developing them internally. Simultaneously, keep increasing the number of such services available on a systemwide basis.

Shared Clinical Service Lines

Keep track of the number of key clinical service lines, such as behavioral health, oncology, and cardiology, which each operating unit shares with one or more other units. Pay attention as well to the proportion of service lines shared by all relevant operating units. The goal is to continually increase these levels of sharing until all units are contributors to seamless service lines that run through the entire IDS.

Physician Integration

Physician integration into the IDS is a critical factor affecting the other three forms of integration, particularly the clinical integration. Physician input is needed to determine where and how clinical integration efforts will be most successful. Physicians also are best suited to striking an appropriate balance between cost saving and medical necessity. These are mechanisms for tying physician interests and behavior more closely to the mission and goals of the IDS.

Practice Commitment

In this area, the practice activity of the participating physicians is increasingly concentrated within the IDS. This is accomplished by persuading more active staff physicians in all operating units to do several things.

- to admit a minimum number of patients to IDS facilities
- to admit a minimum number of patients through two or more operating units
- to see a minimum number of patients per time period (month, year) in an outpatient facility of the IDS

Act to encourage more physicians in individual operating units to accept responsibility for larger and larger percentages of its admissions or outpatient visits.

Practice commitment will also be reflected in the number of active staff physicians who have offices in IDS-owned or -affiliated medical office facilities or who have their practices managed by or closely affiliated with the IDS. The ultimate goal is to move the physicians with highest IDS admissions and outpatient visits into offices in IDS-owned or -affiliated medical office facilities or practices managed by or closely affiliated with the IDS. The final result is the bulk of IDS physicians seeing the bulk of their patients in IDS facilities through practices based in or managed by the IDS.

Economic Involvement

A small integration measure that can have great appeal to some physicians is the opportunity to be involved in joint venture activity with the IDS. Push to get as many physicians at each operating unit connected in this way, particularly those who account for a high proportion of their operating unit's admissions or outpatient visits.

Physician Benefits from IDSs

Another powerful sign of physician integration with the system is the extent of benefits they receive from the IDS. This shows up in the percentage of total active staff physicians in all IDS operating units receiving benefits (health care insurance, disability insurance, pension) from the IDS for themselves or their employees or receiving practice management support services (e.g., billing, recruiting, marketing). The higher these percentages, the more the physicians' practices are tied to the IDS. It is even better when the physicians who are responsible for a high proportion of their unit's admissions or outpatient visits have tied their futures to the IDS in these ways. One other benefit that can be given to physicians to connect them literally to the IDS is a computerized electronic link to their operating unit and to other units in the system.

Contract Participation

One of the primary functions of an IDS is to negotiate global capitation contracts to provide the full spectrum of health care services to an MCO's members. At the same time, many of the providers participating in the IDS may have separate subcapitation or even fee-for-service (FFS) contracts with some MCOs. Move steadily to pull active staff physicians into the IDS's managed care contracts so that more and more of their revenues come through the IDS rather than from external relationships.

Administrative Involvement

Physicians who become involved in the governance, management, and administration of the IDS feel an investment in its success and an empowerment to influence its direction. There are several avenues for enabling this involvement. Within each operating unit, take steps to increase the

- number of physicians elected to the unit's governing board
- number of board committees with physician members
- number of physicians serving as senior managers
- number of physicians invited to participate in strategic planning retreats
- number of physicians serving on system-wide committees or task forces

Make sure that active staff physicians are paid for the time they spend on administrative duties. Look for opportunities to give active staff physicians administrative responsibilities that cross boundaries between operating units.

Group Cohesion

Interestingly enough, a system's integration is enhanced when its physicians are organized into groups, rather than participating as individuals. For one thing, when a group commits to partnership with the IDS based on its own tight integration, it will take steps to ensure compliance by its member physicians. Desirable characteristics include a high percentage of active staff physicians practicing in groups, especially those physicians responsible for a predominant share of their operating unit's admissions or outpatient visits. Pay attention to the percentage of physicians

practicing in primary care, single specialty, or multispecialty groups. Each group type has advantages and disadvantages; most important is maintaining an appropriate balance between PCPs and specialist doctors.

Physician Oversight

Physicians are subject to a variety of oversight mechanisms in any health care setting. The interests of integration and maintaining uniform physician standards are served by bringing as many physicians as possible within individual operating units and throughout the system under unified oversight programs. Concentrate first on developing these programs within each unit to cover all physicians within that unit—organizing the medical staff, physician credentialing, quality assurance and improvement, and formulating of patient care diagnostic and treatment protocols. Then build links among the programs of different units, with the goal of eventually of creating unified systemwide programs with responsibility for all clinical providers.

Functional Integration

Beyond the integration of clinical and physician activities, the IDS must start to unify the business functions throughout its system. As the IDS takes form, push for the coordination across operating units of key support functions and activities (i.e., financial management, human resources, information management, managed care contracting, administrative practices, new product and service development, quality assurance/improvement, strategic planning, marketing). One of the intermediate steps in carrying out this coordination is encouraging the operating units to adopt the same standards for the policies and procedures governing these functions.

Delivery Process Integration

When economists talk about integration, they usually refer to *horizontal* and *vertical* integration. An organization integrates horizontally when it acquires, merges, or affiliates with another organization pretty much like itself. For instance, a primary care group practice might combine with another primary care group practice. Vertical integration involves an expansion up or down the "chain of production" of a product service. The primary care group practice would be vertically integrating if it joined with a specialty care group practice or a hospital.

An aggressively growing IDS engages in both forms of functional integration. To provide medical care to a larger number of patients spread over a broader geographic area, the system may choose to acquire additional PCP practices or another hospital. To deliver a full spectrum of medical care services (from ambulatory care to nursing care), the system may choose to acquire provider entities not already part of the system—such as emergency care centers, rehabilitation facilities, home health agencies, and the like.

In contrast with the other forms of health care integration, which involve the unification of policies, procedures, and programs, functional integration is based on the amalgamation of entire organizations. This amalgamation may begin with contractual affiliations that grow steadily to bind the organizations more and more closely to each other. Ultimately, one organization will acquire or merge with the other. Full legal ownership and control is the ultimate form of delivery process integration.

The first phase of this integration is sometimes referred to as *virtual integration*. The IDS establishes links and relationships with provider organizations, which, together, offer the full range of services in a complete health care delivery process (i.e., emergency care, outpatient care, acute care, primary physician care, specialty physician care, diagnostic testing, laboratories, pharmaceuticals, rehabilitation care, home health care, nursing care, long-term care). The provider organizations maintain legal independence. Some systems and many providers would like to see the integration stop at this point. As long as the IDS can compete successfully, that strategy is acceptable. In many health care markets, however, the IDS will need the efficiencies and benefits that

accrue only when all these services are provided by operating units owned and controlled by the IDS. It probably is necessary to aim for the ultimate goal.

This aspect of integration is discussed more thoroughly in Chapter 5, "A Step-by-Step Strategy To Take You From Solo Practice to an Integrated Delivery System, Chapter 18, "Step Nine: Selling Your Practice to a Hospital, Managed Care Organization, or Physician Practice Management Company, and Chapter 19, "Step Ten: Increasing the Level of Integration in Your Provider Organization."

AVOID INTEGRATION FOR ITS OWN SAKE

In the effort to restrain escalating health care costs, providers and payers have pursued a variety of strategies as though each was a complete solution to the problem. What usually happens is that some useful elements are taken from each strategy, absorbed into regular operations, and the rest are discarded. At various times, we have gotten excited about prepayment, utilization review, capitation, disease prevention, and gatekeepers. One of the current popular cure-alls is "integration." Evidence is gathering that the mere fact of structural integration, particularly vertical integration, is not producing all of the expected benefits.

It is not sufficient to bring together just the right mix of providers and facilities to create an IDS. The mere size and bulk of such a system certainly catches the attention of payers, employers, and patients. It probably enables the IDS to negotiate a better contract with payers than its participating providers could have done separately. However, much more must be expected of health care delivery institutions.

- They must provide greater satisfaction to their patients. Is patient satisfaction higher in IDSs than in competing delivery models?
- They must create a work environment that is rewarding and stimulating to the physicians who practice there. Are IDS physicians hap-

pier and more motivated than physicians practicing in other settings?

- They must produce earnings and returns on investment (ROI) that are equal or superior to those available in other industries. How do the earnings and ROI in health care compare to the alternative uses of those funds?
- They must deliver health care of higher quality than that available from other delivery models. Does an IDS provide a better quality of care than do preferred provider organizations (PPOs) or separate FFS providers?
- They must deliver health care at a lower cost than that available from other delivery models. How does the cost of IDS care compare with that from less integrated providers?
- They must combine providers in a way that enhances productivity for the entire system. Is productivity in IDSs any higher than it is in less integrated models?

If the IDS is a superior delivery model, it must give superior value to all its stakeholders—patients, health plans, employers, physicians, employees, and investors. Do IDSs provide superior value?

On most of the scores, the best that can be said is that there may not be enough data to conclude that IDSs are a better form. In one very important area, earnings and ROI, the flagging interest of capital investors suggests that IDSs are not the best performers.*

Throwing together some PCPs, some specialists, a hospital or two, a long-term care facility, a rehabilitation facility, and some ancillary service entities, then building some clinics and calling it an IDS is just not enough. Each of those providers and facilities must be the best of their kind available. Then they must be truly integrated in a thoughtful, artful way. Most of all, the IDS leaders must constantly measure their strategies and

efforts against the available alternatives—because that is what their customers are doing.

If the best cardiologists in town are part of a group that has chosen to remain independent, perhaps the IDS is better off contracting with them than relying on the inferior cardiologists it has employed.

Remember always that the U.S. health care system is in transition. The way it looks today is not the way it will look tomorrow. The delivery models that seem to work in the 1990s are not the models that will work in the 2010s.

It may be helpful to take the attitude that your delivery structure, whatever it is, must be re-created every day until the market has settled on an ideal model or until you have beaten out all the competition. Because neither of these outcomes is very likely, look forward to an organization that is constantly evolving.

According to Jeff Goldsmith, PhD, President of Health Futures, Inc., as far as integration is concerned, "The most important integration that needs to occur is integration people notice when they use the product or services."[2(p.7)]

CRITICAL EARLY CHOICES IN CREATING AN IDS

There are almost endless decisions to be made in the process of forming an IDS. These are the most basic, the ones that create the framework on which the other decisions will hang.

1. Profit and Tax Status

The IDS can be set up as a for-profit or not-for-profit (NFP) organization. If NFP status is chosen, the founders may or may not seek tax-exempt/deductible status. These choices should be made after careful analysis of the benefits and penalties of each alternative—in light of the physicians' strategic objectives. The options available will also be affected by the profit and tax status of the component organizations of the IDS. The help and advice of a consultant or attorney will facilitate the decision.

---

*There is a strong argument that the success of a nation's health care system should not be measured by the standards of the capital markets.

2. Ownership and Control

The question of who owns and controls the IDS entity will be very important to the participants, and should especially concern the physicians. The available options are:

- If the IDS is for-profit, it could be owned and controlled by participating physicians, participating hospitals, nonparticipating physicians, other outside investors, or any combination of these.
- If the IDS is not-for-profit, no one will own it, and control will reside with those authorized to appoint and remove directors or members (member rights may be issued to one or more of the participants).

The goal of the participating physicians should be to retain as much control as possible—consistent with the dedicated participation of the other, nonphysician providers and the possible need to raise equity capital.

3. Single or Multiple Organizations

The IDS will consist of either a single unitary organization that owns all necessary assets and employs all necessary personnel, or multiple organizations (representing different types of providers) tied together by contractual agreements. There are definite pros and cons to each approach. These are discussed further in the section below dealing with organizational forms of an IDS.

4. Business and Clinical Functions

Decisions must be made about exactly which business and clinical functions will be performed by the IDS. The answers may seem obvious once you commit to provide a defined package of health services to a defined patient population. Just keep in mind that these functions can be performed at different levels in the organization and may even be contracted out to third-party vendors and providers.

5. Levels of Integration

The participating providers must agree on how far they will integrate their business and clinical operations. Their decision will determine how cost-efficient they will be, how seamless the delivery of care will be perceived by patients, and how competitive they will be as service providers. Adequate integration minimizes legal problems with antitrust, fraud, and abuse. Integration that moves too far, too fast, can disturb providers who are not accustomed to working with others, in teams, or in large unified organizations. The major forms of integration are described above.

6. Legal Forms of Organization

As part of the decisions about profit status, tax status, number of organizations, and the ownership and control of them, it will be necessary to choose the legal forms of organization that will be used. The following options are available in most states: for-profit business corporation, nonprofit corporation (membership and nonmembership), professional corporation, limited liability company, general partnership, and limited partnership. Professional legal advice is essential to making an informed decision.

7. Role of Nonphysicians

If physicians are dominant in the IDS, there remains the question of how to treat nonphysician participants. What role will they be given in governance and management? The physicians must decide how much power they are willing to share with nonphysician providers such as hospitals and how much authority they are willing to delegate to lay professional managers. Lower-priority decisions must also be made about whether to treat participating physicians as employees or independent contractors and how participating physicians will interact with nonparticipating physicians on the medical staff of a participating hospital.

ORGANIZATIONAL FORMS OF AN IDS

There are several organizational variations of the IDS. It can be set up as a single unitary legal entity that encompasses all the necessary provider components. Alternatively, the IDS can be created as a combination of organizations, a kind of holding company that owns and controls separate physician and hospital entities. The critical question is, Who controls the single-organization or the multiple-organization holding company? The goal is for physicians to be in charge.

"Single-Organization" IDS

The single-organization model is the easiest to understand and may ultimately be the most effective and competitive. It owns or leases all the assets and employs or contracts with all of the people required to provide all the services it has promised to its payers. As a result, it has direct control over them and is better able to determine their deployment and behavior. This form also encourages participating providers to align their economic interests and to work for the common good of the overall organization.

The single-organization IDS could come about through the merger of a hospital and a physician group, the acquisition of a hospital by a physician group, or the purchase by a hospital of numerous physician practices. When combining physicians with hospitals and other providers, the goal always is an arrangement in which the physicians have a dominant or equal power position.

This single-organization model is probably the tightest form of health care consolidation and integration possible. It operates in the following fashion:

- A single for-profit corporation owns the medical practices and the hospitals.
- The corporation enters into all payer contracts for physician and hospital services and collects all the revenues for those services.
- A single board of directors governs all the organization's operations, with physicians and nonphysicians sitting on the board and playing roles in the governance.
- A single management team is responsible for orchestrating the delivery of the combined health care services.
- Physicians are directly employed by the corporation or serve as independent contractors if state law requires.
- Consolidated capital and operating budgets are prepared for the entire corporation.
- A single computerized information system is implemented to serve the needs of all the organization's components.
- A primary purpose of the corporate consolidation is to deemphasize the adversarial mentality that often exists between hospital managers and physicians, replacing it with an acceptance of the interdependency of all the participants.
- The participants acknowledge that they are in the business of delivering a seamless package of health care services, not separate hospital and physician services.

"Multiple-Organization" IDS

The multiple-organization approach typically consists of a parent holding company that owns or controls two or more subsidiary organizations. One of the subsidiaries owns and operates hospitals. The other subsidiary handles the medical practices. If several hospitals are involved, each may be located in a separate subsidiary. The participating physicians may be separated into more than one organization, each in its own subsidiary. For instance, some physicians may be grouped into a multispecialty group practice, others into an IPA, and still others into an MSO.

The several organizations that make up this model may be nonprofit, tax-exempt entities or for-profit enterprises owned by physicians or private investors. With certain limitations, the profit status of the organizations can be mixed.

There are several variants of this basic multiple-organization model.

1. The holding company may be owned by its participating physicians, its participating hospitals, an MCO or insurance company, private investors, or any combination of them in a shared arrangement.

2. The holding company may be a nonprofit membership organization operated for the public welfare.

3. The holding company may own the entire hospital subsidiary and may share ownership of the physician subsidiary with the physicians.

4. The IDS is composed of a hospital organization and a physician organization, both owned entirely by the physicians. There is no holding company. Two organizations are used to insulate the physician organization from any liabilities the hospital may incur. This physician-dominated system is sometimes referred to as an *equity* model.

5. The IDS is composed of a hospital organization and a physician organization, and the former owns the latter. This arrangement often is not acceptable to physicians and should be avoided unless they can be actively included in the governance and management of the entire system.

6. The tangible assets that the system needs to function are transferred to, and owned and controlled by, a separate proprietary organization such as an MSO. The system leases the assets in return for payments that help generate revenues and profits for the MSO. Physicians and other investors capitalize and have equity shares in the MSO. This arrangement allows physicians to have an indirect equity interest in the system, even if it is nonprofit and tax-exempt. They will see their investment grow as the IDS thrives. The outside investors provide capital for expanding the IDS operation without taking direct control. The separation also ensures that nonphysician owners of the assets will have no influence over the IDS practice and clinical operations.

Caution: Do not fixate on one of these models or another. An organizational structure that works well in one marketplace for one group of providers may be a disaster elsewhere. Every IDS should be custom designed to meet the needs of its founders and owners and the demands of the local competitive and regulatory environment. Think in terms of what you want to accomplish with the IDS and what kinds of relationships you want to have among the participants. Explain this to a good health-knowledgeable corporate attorney; she will find the best forms, instruments, and structures to make your dreams a reality. Just about anything you can imagine is possible.

Virtual Delivery Systems

The above discussion of organizational forms is misleading in another way. It emphasizes the combination of existing traditional entities (hospitals and physician practices) into new networks or systems that maintain the traditional attitudes and biases toward acute care hospitals and specialist physicians. The mainstream business model of hierarchy, control, and detailed reporting has been imported without question. This is particularly likely to happen when the IDS is sponsored primarily by a hospital, insurance company, or outside investors.

There is evolving in the health care industry a new paradigm of service delivery. It may be 10 or 15 years before the current turmoil settles down and new market equilibrium is reached. We are clearly in a phase of transition from the way things were to the way they will be. It is impossible to predict what kind of health care delivery infrastructures and organizations will emerge, but there are some signs of what may be coming.

- flatter, less hierarchical organization
- organizations are not necessarily owned and controlled by a single party
- intensive collaboration among different kinds and sizes of organizations and among people with different skills and disciplines

- focus on pleasing the purchaser (employer) and the customer (employee-patient)
- a hospital is just a building, a replaceable asset
- the key resource is people (and not just physicians), an asset not as easily replaced
- a primary goal is keeping patients out of the system
- work occurs in fluid, self-directed, multi-skilled, multidisciplinary teams
- separate legal entities that compose a system are invisible, the boundaries between them transparent
- system leaders "coach" and "facilitate" members, rather than "manage" or "direct" them
- efforts of the system members are harmonized through common values, shared risks, and aligned incentives
- resources are redeployed from cure and correction to wellness, prevention, and early detection through total quality management (TQM), reengineering, and similar initiatives; organizations constantly probe their environments and reinvent themselves to adapt
- multimedia communications systems are critical assets by which actions throughout the system are coordinated
- participation in the system is highly discriminating—only the best of everything, including people, are employed
- system participation is exclusive; once in the system, work efforts are inclusive
- systems continually experiment with new theories and concepts of health care delivery—many of which fail

Imagine a "virtual system" of separate but indistinguishable legal entities linked more by a shared vision and values than by written contracts and lines on an organizational chart.

The virtual system is designed from scratch. That design largely ignores the existing organizations, operating units, departments, and even functions that may have been assembled to form the system. Instead, it looks at the important care delivery processes that cut across all of these traditional divisions. The result often is to downsize or eliminate traditional organizational components or functions, thereby lowering costs while improving service quality. Think of an IDS as a living organism, with an anatomy and a physiology. The new paradigm is more interested in the physiology than the anatomy.

This should be a very appealing prospect for physicians. There is a potential for you to assume almost any role you want in a virtual organization—practitioner, innovator, supervisor, or leader. You probably cannot replicate an independent solo practice operating out of a home office. However, you should be able to avoid having to ask a faceless voice on the phone for permission to perform a procedure. You should not have to feel like a commodity to be used and discarded like an obsolete computer. If you can commit yourself to the principles and values of the organization and are willing to concentrate entirely on what is best for the health of the patient and the community, you should enjoy a considerable degree of personal freedom. Also, you will not have to worry about arbitrary deselection.

FACTORS TO CONSIDER IN CHOOSING AN ORGANIZATIONAL FORM

As you are choosing between single and multiple-organization forms, in all their variations, take these issues into account.

1. Participants' Prior Experience with Integration

If you are part of a large (for example, 200 physicians) multidisciplinary group practice with several years' history of integrating individual physician practices and if your prospective IDS partner is a hospital with which you have been collaborating for several years to reduce utilization and costs while maintaining quality, you can afford to be more aggressive in forming an IDS. You can move faster and implement more advanced forms of integration. You will not have to be as concerned with resistance to change from physicians inexperienced in working with others toward common goals.

On the other hand, if the founding members of the IDS are 200 physicians in an IPA who have done little more than sign managed care contracts together and a hospital that, until recently, concentrated on protecting its inpatient revenues, you should allow more time for those participants to become familiar and comfortable with the principles of managed care and with each other. It will be challenge enough for the physicians to adjust to each other, not to mention the hospital's executives.

It might be better for inexperienced participants to start off in a looser multiple-organization IDS. Within their all-physician subgroup (the IPA, for instance), the doctors may develop their integration skills more painlessly. Once they have become adept at teamwork and delivering managed care, the physicians might be more willing to accept a tightly integrated role in a single organization IDS.

2. Participants' History of Working with Each Other

If there is a history of acrimony and distrust between the physicians and the hospital, it probably will be smarter to start them out in separate organizations. If they can learn to work amicably with each other, the system might later be shifted to a single organization. Sometimes, there will be outright political resistance from physicians, which is more smoothly managed through separate system components. In addition, the physicians might be better able to develop their own group values and culture.

3. Separation Perpetuates Historical Biases

Keeping physicians and hospitals in their own separate organizations allows them to maintain their old self-centered attitudes—which are at odds with the group consciousness that needs to develop. It will take longer to overcome the "us-and-them" mindset between doctors and hospital administrators. Perhaps it is easier to endure a

relatively short but highly tumultuous period of adjustment at the very beginning than to risk continued bickering that distracts the entire organization for years.

4. Board and Management Complexity

Multiple organizations mean multiple boards of directors and management staffs. Such arrangements can complicate and delay decision making. Things move more smoothly in a single organization.

5. Separation of Assets and Control

By locating most of the system assets in one organization and the responsibility for most decision making in another, it often is possible to raise capital without giving up substantial control of the most important parts of the organization.

6. Isolation of Liabilities

By carefully designing the component organizations of the IDS, it may be possible to isolate the greatest risk of liability in one organization so that providers in other operating units are not exposed to it. This may be important in encouraging some physicians to participate in the system.

7. Corporate Practice of Medicine

In a number of states, the prevailing legal doctrine against the corporate practice of medicine requires that physicians be the sole owners of the entity delivering medical care. This normally is handled by locating the physicians in their own separate organization and establishing appropriate contractual links between it and the rest of the IDS.

8. Duplication of Management and Administrative Staff

It is inevitable that a multiple-organization IDS will entail some duplication of managerial and administrative personnel, which translates into extra expense. It can be acceptable if kept to a minimum and more than offset by the benefits gained.

9. Organizational Barriers to Operational Integration

Common wisdom says that the daunting task of implementing operational integration (both business and clinical) should go more smoothly if everyone involved is an employee of the same organization. This also seems to avoid having to push new policies and procedures through the governance and decision-making bureaucracies of several organizations. The common wisdom may not be correct. It remains to be seen whether a virtual system of multiple entities cannot be made to function just as synergistically as a single organization under tight control.

10. Allocation of Costs and Revenues

It is somewhat more complex to allocate costs and revenues among several component organizations than within a single organization. The complexity may be a fair trade-off for the gains realized.

11. "Putting All the Eggs in One Basket"

If IDS operations, assets, and personnel are concentrated in one organization and that organization fails, everything goes down with it. A multiple-organization arrangement allows parts of the system—such as the physician component—to survive when the primary IDS entity suffers major losses and becomes bankrupt.

BUSINESS ISSUES THAT MUST BE ADDRESSED IN FORMING AN IDS

If the physicians joining in the formation of the IDS have followed something like the progression described in this book, they should already be members of a professionally managed, collaborative physician group. They should have wrestled with many of the issues they will face in

putting the IDS together. These are the issues likely to attract the most attention.

1. Culture Conflicts between Physicians and Hospital Administrators

The largest groups of participants in a new IDS will almost always be physicians and managers from the hospitals in the system. They will certainly bring with them the cultural differences that have caused clashes between them in the past (when the physicians served on the medical staffs of the hospitals). These differences stem from the different training, responsibilities, values, and regular routines of these two groups, as well as from the variances in the missions and policies of the institutions they represent—solo or small group practices versus large bureaucratic acute care hospitals.

The characteristics of the two groups could be roughly generalized this way. Physicians tend to be individualistic, self-reliant, quick to decide and act, disdainful of bureaucracies and hierarchies, and biased toward personal autonomy and democracy when working in groups. Their prior experience gives them much greater patient contact; their practice settings usually place their personal assets at risk. Hospital administrators are more accustomed to hierarchical organizations, formal planning, chains of command with unrestricted authority in individual managers, and teamwork. They rarely have a personal investment in the success or failure of their organizations. The two groups generally disagree on which of them is the more efficient manager of health care delivery.

In forming an IDS, physicians and hospital administrators may for the first time be thrown into peer working relationships that demand consensus on common goals. If the physicians have been part of a large integrated group practice for several years, they should have a greater appreciation for the importance of trained, full-time professional managers. The administrators must come to understand that the fate of their hospitals depends on the creation and operation of infrastructures that support the work of physicians.

The coming together of these two historical adversaries does not have to cause prolonged controversy and disruption. Anticipate the potential conflict and prevent it through programs of education and communication. Create frequent opportunities for all participating parties to meet, to learn each other's viewpoints, and to explain their own. If possible, bring in as guest speakers physicians and managers from another successful IDSs. Be as patient as necessary for everyone to reach a consensus on the purpose and direction for the new system, and his or her role in it. The time spent now will prevent future disagreements that could cripple the IDS.

2. Control and Governance of the New System

The combination of disparate groups of providers and managers into an IDS quickly raises the question of how the entity will be controlled and governed. The goal for physicians is to retain as much authority as possible over this venture, bearing in mind that holding "authority" does not prevent them from deferring to the informed judgments of professional managers employed by the IDS.

Control and governance is manifested primarily through two mechanisms: the ownership of the organization via stock or membership and positions on the board of directors. These issues are discussed in greater detail in Chapter 22, "Creating an Effective Governance Structure for an Affiliated or Integrated Physician Group."

Ownership is the ultimate determinant of control. Dominant owners appoint the board of directors. Ownership interests are usually directly related to the amount of money a person or organization invests in the business. Also, investment capital is a critical need in forming an IDS. As a general rule, physicians, even in large groups, do not accumulate the volume of funds necessary. It is their partners in the IDS—hospitals and health plans—that bring the most money to the table. If they receive proportionate shares in the IDS, they are bound to control. This is why physicians have

had minority interests in most of their joint ventures with other health care providers or payers.

There are numerous ways to work around this problem, involving loans, different classes of stock, and more than one corporation in the IDS system. For example, if the participating physicians contribute as much capital as they are able and the participating hospital (and any other institutions) matches that amount, then the institutions loan to the IDS any additional funds[*] necessary, the doctors and the hospital will each hold a 50 percent interest in the entity.

Control can also be achieved through membership on the board of directors. Some hospitals have been the primary sponsors of PHOs, yet allowed the participating physicians to have a 50 percent or greater position on the board. Other devices, such as reserved seats or supermajorities, can help protect the interests of minority participants. The problem with these mechanisms is that they are "gifts" from the dominant investor—the hospital—which it can take back at any time.

There may be something fundamentally wrong with such attempts to make sure that different parties have enough "control" over the IDS and its operations. The logic usually has been that physicians need the control to ensure that adequate attention is given to clinical matters (as opposed to financial ones) and the role of physicians in them to prevent unreasonable restraints on physicians' clinical decision making and to keep the organization focused on community, not parochial, needs.

Initially, where there is some mistrust between the parties, it may be necessary to recognize and protect specific constituencies. In the long run, however, this recognition perpetuates the divisions between these groups. As quickly as possible in the development of the IDS, build an atmosphere in which everyone naturally is working for the overall good of the organization, and it

---

[*]To be repaid before any net income is recognized or any dividends paid.

becomes irrelevant to talk about "physician interests" or "hospital interests."

3. Physician Compensation

How the physicians are compensated will determine how satisfied they are in working for the IDS and what physician behavior will be encouraged through monetary incentives. This entire topic is examined more thoroughly in Chapter 25, "The Kinds of Physician Reimbursement Systems You Can Expect under Managed Care."

If the physicians participating in the IDS are members of a large group practice that has been working under managed care contracts for several years, their compensation should be well adapted to managed care by now. If they are members of an IPA or PHO, with little integration or managed care experience, it will take more time to shape an appropriate compensation program. These are some of the questions likely to come up along the way:

- Will the physicians be expected to put some of their personal wealth at risk in establishing the IDS? If nothing else, remember the powerful effect on physician behavior of a direct investment in the business.
- Will physician incomes be guaranteed? For how long? What physician performance must be maintained to earn the guaranteed income?
- What compensation will be made for non-clinical work—supervision of personnel, other managerial or administrative work, service on quality review and other committees, research on clinical outcomes instruments, and so on?
- What part of a physician's income will be ensured and what part will be tied to performance?
- What exactly are the measurable performance variables you want physicians to emphasize? What formula will connect compensation to the achievement of those variables? To the degree that it is an incentive,

compensation should stimulate behavior that benefits the entire organization.
- How will ancillary service revenues, honorariums, and deferred compensation amounts be treated by the IDS? Bear in mind how much these items might have accounted for physician incomes prior to joining the IDS.

4. Later Reversal of the Integration Deal

It usually is a good idea to anticipate the disassembling of the integration arrangement if the parties find that they cannot work together. This will be of greatest concern to the physicians and perhaps necessary to get them to commit in the first place.

A common device is to allow physicians to repurchase the assets they have sold to the IDS venture if certain conditions occur within a certain number of years. In framing such an option, it is necessary to define

- within what time period the option may be exercised
- what conditions must occur before the option may be exercised or whether a physician can choose to opt out at any time
- at what price the assets can be repurchased by the physician

Once a clause such as this has been written, it should be forgotten. All energies must be focused on making the venture a success and not on worrying about whether it is time to make an exit.

5. Dealing with the Psychologic Effects

The formation of an IDS will have a dramatic competitive impact on the local marketplace. There also may be traumatic psychologic effects on the people involved—and on some of those not involved. As the final date for creation of the IDS approaches, implement a plan for communicating with current employees of the several component organizations of the IDS: the physician group, any individual physician practices, the hospital, and any ancillary service businesses.

Inform them of the progress in the formation process, the positive reasons for creating the IDS, their important roles in making it a success, and possible effects on their job security. Do not let them learn of developments through rumor and gossip.

The people to be most concerned about are the area physicians who will not be part of the IDS. They are going to feel rejection, anger, resentment, and fear. In small ways, they may attempt to sabotage the IDS project. At the very least, they may want to shun both the organization and the physicians practicing with it. This is undesirable in the event that the IDS wants to work with some of them in the future.

If the physicians joining the IDS come as members of a large group practice, a lot of the backlash from excluded physicians may already have occurred when the group was first established. Nonetheless, be prepared for the feelings that may show up now.

Implement a program for communicating with these physicians. Explain to them the nature of the IDS being formed, the positive reasons for forming it, the benefits it will bring to the community and to the physicians practicing there, and the negative implications of not forming the IDS. Speak candidly about the competitive effects of the IDS on the livelihoods of the excluded doctors. If there is any possibility or circumstance in which the IDS might be willing to accept them into its physician panel in the future, tell them about it. Tell them the specific criteria they will have to meet to be considered. Look for other ways in which you can involve them in the planning of the IDS without actually bringing them on board. One suggestion is to pay a nominal sum to each excluded physician for an option to purchase her practice. Even if you never exercise it, her anxieties and upset will be partially assuaged.

WHAT SORT OF PERSONS AND ORGANIZATIONS DECIDE TO CREATE AN IDS

It may be difficult for a group of physicians to imagine how they would go about assembling an IDS. It is instructive to look at the different parties that have come together, in different combinations, to form IDSs. Here are some examples of how an IDS has been or might be formed.[3] Use them to conceive your own strategy for putting together an IDS.

- Multispecialty group networks with a multihospital system.
- Hospital merges with a multispecialty group.
- Multihospital system acquires the assets of a multispecialty group.
- Independent PCPs form a group practice without walls (GPWW), which then establishes a relationship with a hospital.
- Independent PCPs form an MSO in a joint venture with a hospital.
- Independent PCPs open planning discussions with a hospital, which lead to the formation of a network composed of the hospital and a broad group of primary and specialty care physicians.
- Existing MCO contracts for hospital and physician services.
- Independent physicians in a variety of specialties seek out a hospital and then an MCO, as partners in forming an IDS.
- Hospital encourages PCP groups to merge, then join with it to form a PHO, as a transition toward an IDS.
- Hospital brings together numbers of independent PCPs in solo and small group practices, and directly employs some of them while encouraging the others to form a group for joint managed care contracting with the hospital.
- Hospital organizes a select panel of physicians (both PCPs and specialists) from its medical staff for the purpose of joint managed care contracting.
- Insurance company hand-picks a multispecialty panel of physicians around which it builds an IDS.
- Physician-owned IPA concentrates on a few select hospitals for inpatient care before contracting with a variety of MCOs.

- Insurance company purchases primary care practices and contracts with single hospital to form an IDS.

There is no one route to creating an IDS. As long as the end product is a full-service health care delivery system covering the geographic area where the prospective patients are, any party can take the initiative to get the process started. Even the scenarios that appear to be hospital based can be initiated and led by physicians. In many markets, the competitive conditions are still so fluid that a determined, savvy group of physicians can be the primary moving forces behind the emergence of a dominant IDS.

CHOOSING THE RIGHT PARTICIPANTS

The diverse characters and backgrounds of the individual and institutional participants in an IDS create a need for understanding the expectations, needs, and rights of each party and selecting them carefully for participation. One of the reasons IDSs take so many different shapes is to accommodate the divergent and even competing motivations of the groups that are trying to integrate.

Choose the participants on the basis of what the marketplace demands, not on what the founders want. Do not begin identifying prospective participants in the IDS until you have properly defined and evaluated the marketplace. The appropriate marketplace will be local and, frequently, regional. Rarely will it be statewide and not for quite a few years will even the largest IDSs be able to think in terms of national markets.

Within that marketplace, identify all the key players: competitors in key provider categories; customers among the MCO, employers, and insurance company payers; policy makers in the legislative and executive branches; law enforcement authorities; and general community leaders. For each, determine their strengths and weaknesses, current agendas, future plans (as well as you can know them), and likely responses to any moves that your group makes. Gather data for providers and payers on their financial strength and market share. Using demographic and epide-

miologic data on various population groups within the marketplace, project future demands for major categories of health care services.

Set rough goals for the share of those demands that your integrated organization might try to meet. Begin to develop a vision of the size of organization required to deliver that volume and mix of health care services—measured in terms of the numbers of different types of providers, particularly physicians in each specialty and hospital.

At an early stage, think about what parties will have to be included in the IDS governance structure for political or legal reasons. These will include trustees from participating hospitals, leaders of physician groups and ancillary providers who will be involved, representatives of important capital financing sources and major investors, and community leaders and representatives.

During the time that the IDS is forming, it is not too early to anticipate parties that you may want to affiliate with as strategic partners in the future. Consider the following possibilities:

- An IDS that starts out with minimal risk sharing and no payer component may see value in linking up eventually with MCOs or insurance companies.
- A physician-heavy IDS will want to plan for future connections with additional hospitals, ancillary providers, and general sources of managerial support.
- An IDS created as a nonprofit entity may look forward to the time when its strategies will require formation of for-profit subsidiaries or affiliation with existing for-profit corporations.
- The never-ending need for expansion capital makes it advisable to plan ahead for future liaisons with outside investors.[*]

---

*If a public offering of stock seems like a near-term possibility, it is important to establish governance structures now that support public accountability.

Here are some criteria to follow in choosing specific integration partners:

Physician Partners

- understanding of and commitment to the integration process
- acceptance, if not full embrace, of the concept of managed care
- willingness to work in a team with other providers, not necessarily all physicians
- demonstrated ability to manage personal utilization of resources or to learn the necessary skills
- compatibility with other system members, in terms of goals, culture, and work style
- ability to engender trust and to trust others
- ability to make decisions and to act expeditiously or willingness to delegate this authority to others
- willingness and ability to play leadership and administrative roles
- location and size of current practice
- reputation for quality care among colleagues and patients
- willingness and ability to contribute capital to the start-up of a physician-driven IDS venture
- if a specialist, willingness to accept a more prominent role for PCPs and to work with them accordingly; perhaps also a willingness to sacrifice some short-term income growth
- if a PCP, recognition of the primary role he or she will play as a form of gatekeeper
- apparent willingness and ability to adapt practice behavior as competitive and financial circumstances demand
- willingness to accept risk—of all kinds

Hospital Partners

- understanding of and commitment to the integration process
- acceptance, if not full embrace, of the concept of managed care
- compatibility with other system members, in terms of goals, culture, and work style

- ability to engender trust and to trust others
- ability to make decisions and to act expeditiously or willingness to delegate this authority to others
- understanding that the purpose of forming a provider-sponsored IDS is not to preserve the status quo
- understanding that the hospital is less and less the focus and centerpiece of health care delivery
- acceptance of physicians in leadership and managerial roles in the new IDS organization
- location, size, and financial strength of the hospital operation
- willingness and ability to contribute capital to the start-up of the IDS venture, perhaps without a commensurate share of control
- demonstrated ability to manage utilization of resources and to otherwise contain costs
- willingness to accept risk—of all kinds

Look also at Chapter 24, "Choosing the Best Strategic Partners for Your Group Practice, Physician-Hospital Affiliation, or Integrated Delivery System."

HOW AN INTEGRATED SYSTEM TAKES SHAPE

If you are a physician in a solo or small group practice, the very idea of playing a leading role in the development of an IDS sounds daunting. It is easier to grasp when you realize that it does not emerge overnight. The formation of an IDS is the culmination of an evolutionary multiyear strategy that can begin at a very modest level. The progression might go like this:

- Solo practice physicians clump into small group practices.
- Small group practices, along with some narrow specialty solo practitioners, merge into a partially integrated medical group.
- A hospital or an existing health care system establishes an MSO to provide capital and management services to the medical group,

with the goal of moving it as rapidly as possible to become a fully integrated medical group.

- As the medical group is moving toward full integration, the hospital initiates affiliation with it, through formation of a PHO that seeks risk-sharing managed care contracts.
- As the physicians and the hospital grow more comfortable with each other, they take the natural next step—creating an integrated delivery system. For many, this arrangement provides all the efficiencies they need to compete, and they will evolve no further.
- Seeking the benefits of even tighter integration, the system participants merge into a single organization.
- The IDS, whether a system or a unified organization, merges and integrates its operations with a payer organization—an MCO or an insurance company.

It is not inconceivable for physicians in a small group practice at the beginning of the process to wind up as prominent physician leaders and important board members in a large IDS.

PLANNING THE FINAL INTEGRATION OF THE IDS COMPONENTS

At this point, you probably can see most of the essential components of an IDS in front of or around you. You may be the member of a fully integrated group practice. It may be part of a large IPA, delivering care under several capitation contracts. You also may have an affiliation with one or more local hospitals, through a PHO or an MSO, which is the basis for additional risk-sharing contracts with MCOs. The group practice may have an agreement with numerous long-term care and rehabilitation facilities, laboratories, and specialized clinics for the provision of ancillary services. There may be further links with other smaller group practices on which you rely for specialist care.

The next step, the penultimate step in the classic strategic evolution, is to unite these components into a formal IDS.

Begin the planning process this way:

The Preplanning Stage

1. Review your organization's mission and goals. As you have proceeded to constantly redefine your role within the health care system, you should have critically examined your goals several times to see whether they still make sense, whether you are still on course, and whether they need adjustment. Do it again now.

2. Study the concept of integration as it will be implemented in a full-blown IDS. Distinguish among nonclinical operational integration, clinical operational integration, legal/structural integration, financial integration, governance integration, and facility integration. Be clear on what is contemplated in forming the IDS and the practical changes it will require.

3. Translate this understanding of integration into a listing of what you and your organization will gain and lose by joining with the other IDS components.

4. Prepare a clear statement of how participation in the IDS will serve the strategic mission and goals of your organization.

5. Determine your firm preferences regarding the ownership and governance of the IDS. Decide what share of the legal ownership of the new entity you would like your organization to have, bearing in mind that there usually is a correlation between capital contribution and level of ownership. Regardless of your ownership interest, think about the role you want to have in governing the IDS.

6. Identify the stakeholders in the IDS, at two levels. First, identify all the potential components of the newly integrated entity— hospitals, clinics, group practices, IPAs, MSOs, PHOs, ancillary facilities, and the like. Second, recognize all other organizations and parties that will have a vested interest in the formation of the IDS. Be

sure to include the competition, whose interest will be a negative one.

> **Note:** Avoid trying to choose all the IDS partners too early in the planning process. Start with a critical mass of providers sufficient to keep the planning process moving forward. A large multispecialty group practice and a well-regarded community hospital are probably the bare minimum. If you are confident of the commitment and suitability of other providers, do include them. However, be thoughtful and deliberate in selecting most of your partners; they will determine the market success of the IDS. Take time to gather adequate background information on them. They can be added at any time during the planning process, right up to the moment that the IDS is created.

7. Assess the personal and political dynamics that will determine each stakeholder's response to the IDS formation. There will not be unanimous consent of all the component organizations to join in the IDS. Within individual organizations, including yours, there will be dissenting views. Take the time now to try to anticipate them, then formulate strategies for defusing them.

8. Decide what members of your organization must sign off on the move to form and join an IDS. It may be a simple matter of executive discretion or you may need to seek board approval and the informal acquiescence of subgroups within the organization.

Working with Others To Do the Planning

1. *Form a planning task force* composed of representatives from the key component organizations. Keep it to a size that can

work quickly and effectively, without long debates. A group of between 5 and 10 members works well; more than 15 will slow progress noticeably. Within some organizations, there will be special constituencies that deserve separate representation.

> **Note:** It is especially important that the several, different physician views on the new initiative be heard. At the same time, it is necessary that a few doctors be delegated to speak and act for the entire group. However, it would be wise to talk informally and regularly with all of them, announcing plans, reporting progress, and seeking feedback.

Consider forming transitional planning subgroups to deal with hot issues. The main planning task force will have its hands full dealing with overall strategy and keeping the process moving forward.

2. *Bring everyone in the task group up to speed* on the meaning of integration with a diversity of other providers. Provide a rough outline of the form that integration will take and the detailed steps necessary to achieve it. Bear in mind that well-laid plans may change as new partners are brought on board and new problems emerge. The final shape of the IDS may differ from the original model.

3. *Thoroughly study the alternative forms that the IDS might take.* The possibilities are almost infinite. Do not focus on one or another "model" employed by existing IDSs or recommended by health care management writers. Instead, find a good lawyer or consultant experienced in working with physician groups to carry out innovative practice strategies. With his or her help, use various organizational structures and contractual interconnections to create a custom-made structure that meets

exactly your needs and those of your IDS partners.

4. *Draft a formal business plan.* Write this plan as though you were going to use it to solicit financing from a venture capitalist—because that is just what you might end up doing.

5. *Estimate the cost of implementing the business plan* and allocate the cost among the participants. The planning becomes quite challenging at this point. The first cost estimates may stun some of the participants. The figures will be in the tens of millions of dollars. Each IDS partner will see for the first time exactly how much it must contribute to the start-up capital of the IDS. Intertwined with the simple and daunting cost numbers are the issues of who will legally own the organization and who will govern it.

6. *Consider seeking financing from outside investors.* Depending on the organizational form you adopt, several forms of outside financing may be available. If you create a for-profit corporation, there is a good and improving chance of attracting the interest and money of venture capitalists. You also may be able to borrow money against the assets of the IDS partners or to sell the assets to another entity that leases them back to you. Insurance companies will probably be willing to share some of their capital with you if you will share some of your control with them. If the IDS is able to qualify for tax-exempt status, you will have the opportunity to issue tax-exempt bonds. (For a more detailed look at the possibilities, see Chapter 27, "Financing Strategies To Support Your Integration Plans.")

7. *Define the governance mechanism* for the IDS and the power shares of each partner. Get more information on this in Chapter 22, "Creating an Effective Governance Structure for an Affiliated or Integrated Physician Group."

8. *Obtain official commitment to participation* in the IDS from the governing bodies of each confirmed participant.

9. *Document thoroughly every aspect of the planning process.* Commit to writing all of the information you gather, key points in your planning discussions, and every decision you make. It will force you to think more objectively about what you are doing. If questions arise about the reasons for decisions, you will have an unassailable record. The process of documentation will lend credibility to your organizing efforts.

10. *Carry out all tasks with systematic rigor.* Whenever there is agreement on a step to be taken or a task to be performed, be sure to do the following:
    * Make one person primarily responsible for its accomplishment.
    * Make sure that she has the necessary authority and resources to accomplish it.
    * Set a specific time deadline for its accomplishment.
    * Define the accomplishment in such clear-cut, preferably measurable terms that there can be no disagreement about whether or not it has been accomplished.

    If you are not this thorough, things will not get done when needed. Deadlines will slip and opportunities will be lost. More rigorous competing groups will beat you to the goodies—the best contracts, the best specialists, the best new physicians, and the best facilities.

11. *Schedule regular meetings, according to an ambitious timetable.* The planning and execution of a strategy so complex, expensive, and risky takes a lot of work compressed into a short period of time. Act as though you are planning the rest of your life, because that is pretty close to what you are doing. Set aside time from your regular practice for IDS planning sessions (this may mean sacrificing some income in the short run). Be prepared for long, often contentious meetings. In your plan of

activities, designate dates by which key decisions must be made or on which you will hold deliberate review sessions to catch your breath and see whether you are still on course.

> **Note:** By moving ahead as quickly as you can, you will save money and gain a lead on the competition. By moving ahead as quickly as you can, you also may alienate some physicians who need more time to "get the picture," and you may simply miss some important issues. It's a trade-off.

12. *Communicate effusively and cautiously.*
Keep the people and organizations that are committed to participation in the IDS thoroughly informed about progress being made, decisions reached, problems encountered, and the expectations of them. The goal for interactions with all the participants is to avoid surprising or confusing them. If that happens, they become suspicious and begin withholding their support. Result: The process stalls.

At the same time, many of your deliberations will have great competitive market value. Maintain confidentiality for all critical items of information.

- Require all participants and other parties given access to inside information to sign nondisclosure agreements.
- Appoint an individual to hold and secure key documents.
- Consciously designate certain documents, pieces of knowledge, and meetings as confidential, with restricted access.

13. Prepare yourself for the fact that the plans for configuring the IDS will not please everyone. After making all the compromises you can, some people will still be so unhappy that they will opt out. Accept it and move on!

CASE STUDY: LOVELACE HEALTH SYSTEMS (ALBUQUERQUE, NEW MEXICO)

Lovelace Health Systems[4] is a for-profit corporation composed of the Lovelace Clinic, Lovelace Hospital Medical Center, and Lovelace Health Plan. The Clinic was founded in 1922 by two physicians with tuberculosis who moved to New Mexico for health reasons. It was modeled on the Mayo Clinic. It describes itself as "a physician-directed organization with the state's only physician CEO [chief executive officer]."

The Health Systems operates in the New Mexico marketplace, one of the most highly developed and hotly competitive in the country. It is dominated by capitated managed care, and FFS medicine has almost disappeared.

The entire IDS is a wholly owned subsidiary of CIGNA Healthcare. In 1997, it had net revenues of $343 million and a net worth of $40 million. It employs over 3,300 physicians, nurses, allied health professionals, and support staff throughout New Mexico.

The Clinic has grown to become a group practice of approximately 300 physicians in 43 specialties. They were split almost evenly between primary care and specialist doctors. Where the Clinic's physicians are not available, the Health Systems contracts with roughly 2,000 independent practitioners.

In the early 1970s, the predominately specialist Clinic saw a need to expand the number of PCPs to provide patient referrals. A deliberate effort was made to add general internists and pediatricians. Most of these new doctors were located physically at the Clinic, which did not always provide the best access for patients. This led to one of the most positive strategic moves in the Clinic's history—the creation of a series of more conveniently placed primary care centers. By the 1980s, Lovelace specialists were able to rely on their primary care colleagues for two-thirds of their patient referrals.

Just after World War II, Lovelace encouraged the construction of the Bataan Memorial Methodist Hospital next door to its clinic building. It purchased the hospital in 1969. The current Lovelace

Hospital and Medical Center was opened in 1987 with 225 acute care beds. It is located in Albuquerque.

The Health Systems also offers patient access through 12 primary care centers. Other Lovelace facilities include a behavioral health center and hospital, rehabilitation facilities, a department of occupational medicine, a birthing center, and a cosmetic and reconstructive surgery center.

The Health Plan began operation in 1973. It stumbled initially but quickly became a major patient and revenue source when a professional manager was hired in 1979. It now offers a complete range of managed health care products and traditional employee benefits to over 850 employer groups, government agencies, and small businesses. These products include a PPO, point of service (POS) plans, the Lovelace Senior Plan for Medicare beneficiaries, and the Lovelace Community Health Plan for Medicaid recipients.

In 1996, the Clinic received full, three-year accreditation from the National Committee for Quality Assurance. In that same year, it also was the first integrated health system in the nation to receive a three-year Joint Commission on Accreditation of Healthcare Organizations (Joint Commission) network accreditation for a delivery system and health plan. The Lovelace Health Plan regularly reports its performance through the Healthplan Employer Data and Information Set (HEDIS). The HEDIS report cards compare the Health Plan's performance to industrywide benchmarks in several critical areas, such as effectiveness of care, participant access and satisfaction, cost of care, and use of services.

By the late 1980s, the hospital was looking run down and needed replacement. The Health Systems was in the process of building its network of primary care centers. It was embarking on a number of quality assurance initiatives, such as continuous quality improvement (CQI), disease management (called *episodes of care* by Lovelace), practice guidelines, and care management training for its physicians. It began installing a sophisticated management information system that would tie the pieces of the system together and help in managed care.

These were expensive projects that required a major new infusion of capital. Lovelace started looking for a partner. It settled on Hospital Corporation of America (HCA) because it was headed by physicians and seemed to understand the value of a physician-run delivery organization. HCA took 80 percent of the shares in a newly formed for-profit corporation that included the clinic, the hospital, and the health plan. HCA also was willing to allow Lovelace physicians to have half the seats on the board of this corporation.

In 1986, HCA merged with Equitable Life Assurance Society to form EQUICOR, which purchased from HCA half (40 percent) of its interest in Lovelace. In 1990, CIGNA bought the combined 80 percent interest in Lovelace from EQUICOR and HCA. A year later, it acquired the remaining 20 percent from the nonprofit Lovelace Medical Foundation. This last stock sale removed the last vestiges of Lovelace and local New Mexico ownership in and control of the system's operations.

Lovelace Health Systems is governed by a nine-member board of directors. Three of the members are elected by the Lovelace Clinic doctors, three come from the Health Systems' management, and three represent CIGNA.

There is a separate medical practice board, which directs quality improvement, peer review, performance appraisals, physician compensation, and Lovelace University. It is made up of the three physicians from the main board and three other physicians.

CIGNA's oversight of Lovelace's operations seems to have increased over the last few years. Initially, they took a hands-off attitude to the Health Systems. More recently, CIGNA has imposed greater reporting requirements and has shown greater interest in Lovelace's financial performance.

The Health Systems' organizational structure does not employ profit centers. It cannot, for instance, separate the performance of the hospital from the clinic. It uses a matrix management model that allows physicians influence at every level of the organization.

Lovelace Health Systems was not the lowest cost provider in the marketplace. Because of its ownership of and heavy investment in all the components of the system, as well as facilities, it had high fixed costs. Its competitive advantages came from its reputation for quality health care, the convenience of its primary care centers, and its ability to measure and demonstrate clinical outcomes. Employers also appreciate Lovelace's ability to project future costs and, therefore, premiums with reasonable accuracy.

Traditionally, Lovelace paid its physicians a salary based on national surveys of comparable earnings for their respective specialties. Under pressure from managed care competition, it was moving quickly to place more of the physicians' income at risk. Initially, it would make 20 percent of physician compensation contingent on performance of criteria in six areas.

- *Quality of care*—eventually relying on outcomes measurements
- *Patient satisfaction*—using large-scale surveys already being conducted
- *Utilization management*—with factors such as length of hospital stay and inpatient admissions per 1,000
- *Productivity*—with factors such as numbers of office visits or patient population managed by PCPs
- *Peer satisfaction*—concerned with teamwork and the earned respect of physician colleagues
- *Good citizenship*—with factors such as committee participation, teaching responsibilities, and community involvement

It was thought that eventually the portion of at-risk physician compensation might grow to 40 percent.

Lovelace is using or developing several tools to ensure the quality of its medical care and that it is appropriate to the patient's needs.

Disease Management

Lovelace is focusing on what it calls *episodes of care*, which account for more than 80 percent of all the care that it provides. Teams of PCPs,

specialists, and other health care providers work together to study and apply the best practice patterns for chronic and high-risk health conditions. Current targets of this initiative are low back pain, childbirth, depression, diabetes, stroke, breast cancer, hypertension, pneumonia, and asthma.

Outcomes Measurement

The measurable results of health care are gathered by Episodes of Care teams in four areas: patient satisfaction, cost, clinical quality, and functional status. Medical care is continually monitored across the entire organization and data are collected on patient demographics, preventive health behaviors, comorbidity, generic health status treatment, and condition-specific variables. By feeding these data back to providers, Lovelace is better able to tailor care to the patients' needs. They also are useful in measuring the effect of a given procedure, product, or medical technology on patient health and costs.

Provider Support Reports

These quarterly reports give physicians feedback on their individual practice patterns, compared with their colleagues, along with patient-specific information on their own patient population. Patients at high risk or who appear to fall outside of Episodes of Care recommendations are listed in the report.

Practice Guidelines

The Episodes of Care programs incorporate the use of traditional physician practice guidelines and what Lovelace calls *CareLines*. Guidelines suggest the most effective course of treatment for a wide variety of patient conditions. The CareLines are concerned with inpatient care and offer an outline of the expected sequence of care to be provided during the patient's hospital stay, recovery process, and therapy.

Care Management

This program sets up a care continuum that continuously manages the chronically ill patient. Patients and family members are drawn in as partners with the Lovelace health care team. Together, they make decisions and take actions in the areas of wellness, prevention, primary care, specialty care, home care, acute hospital care, rehabilitation, skilled nursing, hospice, and alternative medicine.

Health Risk Assessments

This tool is designed to help Health Plan members take charge of their own health by becoming aware of what they can do to promote their own health. On the basis of the assessment, Lovelace sends members recommendations for lifestyle changes, self-care, and medical care.

Case Management

Lovelace uses this procedure to coordinate a patient's care into a single, long-term management plan that monitors the quality and cost of health services being delivered. The case manager's job is to coordinate care, develop treatment plans, arrange for specific services, and communicate with treatment team members and service providers.

BASIC INGREDIENTS OF SUCCESS IN OPERATING AN IDS

1. A Large Number of Highly Skilled Clinicians, Absolutely Committed to the Success of the IDS

The primary resource of an IDS is the clinicians, primarily the physicians, who deliver its medical care. The more skilled they are, the higher the quality of the care they provide. Patients want high-quality care. The more dedicated they are to the success of the organization, rather than to their own personal advancement, the more likely they are to deliver their services

efficiently and effectively. Payers want cost-effective care. The more physicians affiliated with the IDS, the more patients it can serve, the more managed care contracts it can secure, the more revenues it can earn, and the larger delivery infrastructure it can create. Large size begets even larger size, and that growth means success.

2. Optimization and Unity of Governance, Investment, Strategic Objective, Operational Management, and Information Systems

When IDSs emerge from a union of provider organizations—hospital systems, physician group practices and networks, outpatient and urgent care clinics, home health agencies, rehabilitation facilities, and nursing homes—the components try to maintain as much of their operating autonomy as they can for as long as they can. Every time a component organization exercises that autonomy, it risks making a decision that may be optimal for it but less than optimal for the overall IDS enterprise. A competitor in the cutthroat health care market needs every edge it can get. To compete as a single, aligned, and efficient organization, the ideal IDS will establish policies, procedures, and systems to ensure that strategic and operational decisions are made, capital and operating funds are expended, and equipment and systems are acquired in a way that primarily serves the interests of the IDS. It is fair to allow a unit of the IDS some independent authority, as long as you acknowledge that it may compromise your competitiveness.

3. Integration as Reflected in a Seamless Continuum of Care to the Patient

A *seamless continuum of care* means that the patient feels that the different steps in her treatment process are just part of a natural flowing stream of services (consultations, lab studies, surgery, medications, rehabilitation treatment, and home health care) created by a synergistic team of providers that is a single unified organization. The patient is hardly aware that one step ends and another one begins. Each provider (and this includes everyone from physician to receptionist) knows everything that has been done to the patient up to that point. All the providers have only one perceptible focus—the patient. This is the height of integration.

The beauty of seamless care is that it also tends to be the lowest-cost, highest-quality care. Furthermore, it is more satisfying for providers to practice within such a system.

There are several key ingredients to seamless care. The most important is an information system that gives every provider in the IDS access to all the knowledge about each patient collected anywhere within the IDS. Another element may be the physical arrangement of the facilities, equipment, and personnel with which the patient must interact. The design and implementation of clinical pathways or protocols helps avoid hitches in the patient's treatment, where someone has to stop and think about what to do next to the patient or where to send her.

4. Accumulating and Conserving Investment Capital

Conserving capital means spending as little as possible to achieve your goals and as much as you must to survive. An IDS cannot behave as a loose confederation of affiliated providers, allowing each operating unit to maintain its own governing board and budgeting process, else they will squander capital on inconsistent and incompatible purchases—particularly in the area of information and communication systems. Ultimate goal: computer-based patient records that transcend the organizational boundaries of their various operating units.

From the patient's viewpoint, integration means a sense of dealing with a single delivery entity of invisible, nonexistent boundaries between components of the system, a treatment process so smooth that movement through its seems natural, almost organic. There is no awareness that the patient may be passing from one organization or department to another. It feels as though the

entire IDS is focused on meeting the needs of this one patient.

From the physician's viewpoint, genuine integration produces two critical results. The increased efficiency reduces costs, thereby improving the likelihood that the IDS will come in under its negotiated capitation rate. It also generates additional cash, which is not automatically paid out to the participating physicians but, instead, is saved for later investment in capital projects such as practice acquisitions, physician recruitment, information technology systems, and strategically placed clinic facilities.

5. Decision Making That Is Planned and Deliberate, Rather Than Opportunistic and Disjointed

Until the managed care revolution began, there was relatively little bold decision making in the health care industry and no significant moves toward growth and expansion. Since the emergence of integrated regional systems as the delivery model of choice, there has been a lot of merger, acquisition, consolidation, and affiliation activity. In only a few cases (Columbia/HCA, some of the physician practice management groups such as Phycor) does it seem to have been as carefully thought out as traditionally done by professional business managers. Generally, the scenario has been a loose collection of physicians, perhaps organized into a good-sized group practice or an IPA, accepting an invitation to join a PHO being formed by the hospital at which most of them have privileges. The move is not part of a careful long-term strategic plan. There is no agreement on how the PHO serves the needs of the physicians, individually or collectively. No one asks whether there are better alternatives than the PHO form or this particular hospital.

The levels of managed care penetration and resulting competition now require that IDSs aiming to prosper into the next century make all decisions, strategic and operational, according to rational, agreed-upon criteria, in pursuit of a long-range strategy capsulized in a formal five-year or longer plan. This approach ensures that the decisions of separate operating units will not conflict with each other and that the minimum amount of money necessary will be spent to implement the decisions.

6. Know Your Costs and What Determines Their Levels, Then Constantly Push Them Down

There are several success-critical reasons for IDSs to be obsessed with costs. First, MCOs, employers, and other payers with whom you contract will want to see this kind of emphasis. You will be more likely to secure contracts with them in the first place. Second, your prowess at cost management will help you to assert a leadership position in any affiliation you join. Third, an ability to manage and reduce costs will permit you to operate within the capitation rates you have negotiated. Fourth, if you operate well within the rates, you will produce greater profits, which can be invested in further growth and improvement of systems.

Managing costs means defining them, gathering data that measure them, determining which activities create the costs, and adjusting the activities to minimize the costs. The hardest part is figuring out the connection between costs and what the IDS is trying to achieve. Generally, this requires studying the outcomes of all the organization's procedures and activities, particularly the patients' outcomes, to identify the most effective and efficient procedures in producing the best patient outcomes. Those procedures are then promoted and broadcasted throughout the IDS organization, including all its components. If one physician group or one facility produces much lower complication rates or much better functional status scores, the treatment procedures they use are studied and compared with what other, less effective groups or facilities are doing. When their effectiveness is substantiated, they may be translated into practice guidelines or other standards and their adoption encouraged throughout the organization.

This same methodology is applied to the managerial, as well as the clinical, processes. It is not carried out once but is an ongoing course of self-analysis and improvement. It is the essence of CQI.

7. Standardize Information Systems To Smooth Data Flow throughout the Organization

Every component of the IDS must use the same data variables and formats, collection and analysis methodologies and software, and system and network hardware, so that data are collected in the same way at multiple locations throughout the IDS and can flow smoothly among those locations. This standardization is necessary to ensure that the data used to evaluate outcomes and manage costs are useful and meaningful to everyone relying on it in the IDS. Without it, you can expect the historical problems of redundant (and expensive) data collection, unnecessary repetition of diagnostic tests, delays in treatment, omissions in treatment, difficulty in comparative analyses, inadequate bases for clinical and health services research, and general inconvenience to patients.

MISTAKES TO AVOID IN CREATING AN IDS

There is an endless variety of mistakes that can be made in trying to assemble and operate an IDS. Here are some of them. You will still make some missteps, but you can plan to avoid these:

1. The integrating parties do not realize that they are creating an entirely new kind of health care delivery enterprise, not just a clumping together of traditional delivery vehicles. They end up making decisions for the IDS out of their old hospital or physician practice mindsets. This is most likely to be a problem for the hospital component, as it requires the most radical transformation.

2. If a hospital dominates the IDS complex, it views the alliance with physicians as a mechanism for funneling patients to support its inpatient operations. Even though

it talks a good story about emphasizing primary care, the hospital ultimately expends most of the IDS capital funds on acute care operations.

3. The leaders and executives of the IDS do not fully appreciate that their primary resource is their physicians and do not act accordingly.

4. With several disparate groups coming together, trying so hard to accommodate each other's concerns while protecting their own, there may be no focused leadership for the organization. As a result, the strategies adopted are watered down, and no single person feels accountable for their implementation.

5. Because they were not part of the IDS planning process, middle-level managers are not invested in the success of the outcome. They may not be clear on their responsibilities in the new system. In fact, they may be more worried about what they may lose than what they have to contribute to the IDS.

6. Personnel in each of the component organizations do not understand the new relationships they will have with each other. In the absence of specific instructions, they fall back on the old ways of dealing with each other.

7. The IDS system eventually will take on significantly new functions as a provider of managed care. From top to bottom, in each of the component organizations, personnel are not aware of how their duties and roles will have to change. In a variety of ways, the IDS founders have not thought through how their IDS strategies will be carried out with their existing resources, human and otherwise.

8. The resources required, rewards sought, and risks presented by the IDS strategies are commensurate or synchronized with each other.

9. The planning process and early operations of the IDS stress achievement of financial goals and give inadequate attention to

building a positive community image, cultivating patient satisfaction, developing and publicizing quality measures, and fostering collaboration among the IDS partners.

10. Once the key players reach agreement on forming an IDS, they rush the project, concentrating on the structural changes and giving little attention to the process by which all the human participants come to terms with what is happening and the effect on them. Too many decisions are made unilaterally by a small group of committed visionaries. The lack of informed commitment by all the other participants snarls and delays implementation of the integration plans and goals.

11. From the start, the IDS establishes exclusive relationships with its various providers—hospitals as well as physicians. In addition to antagonizing those left out, it ties its own hands in responding quickly to the sudden changes that occur in today's health care market.

12. The IDS founders resort to old models of management, based on hierarchy and control. They do this because it is the only way they know to manage, and they believe it will protect the interests of the constituency they represent—hospital or doctors. They ignore the considerable evidence that health care is better delivered through a structure based on multidisciplinary teamwork, constant organization-wide learning, and empowerment of all employees.

13. The IDS is brought into existence; on an organizational chart, the participating parties are connected by solid lines. In reality, however, no serious steps are taken toward serious integration. Perhaps in a misguided effort to avoid offending anyone, all of the parties are allowed to continue functioning pretty much as they had before the combination.

14. In the interests of political tranquillity, the IDS accepts almost any physician onto its

provider panel, permits the physician leaders from small group practices to continue in positions of authority, automatically appoints as managers and executives of the IDS administrative officials from the participating organizations, and sets up a large (20+ people) governing board to accommodate the many divergent interests in the IDS. The result is that the IDS is staffed, at many levels, by people with less than optimal capabilities. Its decision-making processes are also impeded.

15. The founders underestimate the capital that is required to plan, start up, and operate to the point of break-even a very large, very complex entity such as an IDS. This is not surprising as there is so little history of creating IDS ventures. As the money runs out, physicians and vendors are not paid promptly, concerned payers suspend their contracts with the IDS, and eventually it collapses.

16. The IDS fails to keep visionaries in prominent positions or to remind everyone of the long-term goals they have committed themselves to. It is easy to bog down in the tedium of day-to-day operations and lose sight of the never-ending path that the IDS is traveling.

It is unclear whether any substantial IDSs have actually failed, but the hospital-sponsored ones seem to have the most problems. One of the reasons for this is their tendency to bring together physicians on their medical staffs who have never worked together before. Although the hospital may bring capital and general management skills to the enterprise, they are not especially adept at organizing physicians. Indeed, the one form of IDS that is thriving is that based on multispecialty physician groups (such as the Marshfield Clinic). Not only do such a groups have a history of physician collaboration, but also they involve physicians organizing themselves or other physicians—which is perhaps the most effective way to mobilize physicians.

The common wisdom is that 80 percent of all hospital-owned primary care practices lose money. There are several reasons for this:

- The hospitals often make the mistake of putting the physicians on higher salaries or of giving them substantial income guarantees.
- The hospitals are too eager to acquire the practices and fear offending their medical staff, so they pay too high an acquisition price.
- Executives who are effective at administering hospitals are not necessarily capable of managing physician practices.

Perhaps the lesson is to be wary of any affiliation that places hospital administrators in unfamiliar managerial positions.

REFERENCES

1. S. Shortell et al., "Implementing Organized Delivery Systems: An Integration Scorecard," *Health Care Management Review 19*, no. 3 (1994): 7.
2. *Medical Network Strategy Report 6*, no. 7 (1997): 7.
3. D. Coddington et al., *Integrated Health Care: Reorganizing the Physician, Hospital and Health Plan Relationship* (Englewood, CO: Center for Research in Ambulatory Health Care Administration, 1994).
4. D. Coddington et al., *Making Integrated Health Care Work: Case Studies* (Englewood, CO: Center for Research in Ambulatory Health Care Administration, 1996): 1–23.

RESOURCE LIST

D. Amerongen, *Networks and the Future of Medical Practice: Integrating Physician, Hospital, and Payor* (Chicago, IL: Health Administration Press, 1998).

M. Barrett, "IDSs, PSOs: Wrestling with Development and Contracting Issues," *Physician Manager 8*, no. 16 (1997).

J. Blair, M. Fottler, A. Paolino, and T. Rotarius, *Medical Group Practices Face the Uncertain Future: Challenges, Opportunities and Strategies* (Englewood, CO: Medical Group Management Association, 1995).

"Checklists Help Hospitals, MD Groups Prepare for Medicare PSO Development," *Physician Manager 8*, no. 19 (1997).

D.C. Coddington and B.J. Bendrick, *Integrated Health Care: Case Studies* (Englewood, CO: Center for Research in Ambulatory Health Care Administration, 1994).

D.C. Coddington, C. Chapman, and K. Pokoski, *Making Integrated Health Care Work: Case Studies* (Englewood, CO: Center for Research in Ambulatory Health Care Administration, 1996).

D.C. Coddington, K. Moore, and E. Fischer, "Costs and Benefits of Integrated Healthcare Systems," *Healthcare Financial Management 43*, no. 3 (1994): 20.

D.C. Coddington, K. Moore, and E. Fischer, *Integrated Health Care: Reorganizing the Physician, Hospital and Health Plan Relationship* (Englewood, CO: Center for Research in Ambulatory Health Care Administration, 1994).

D.C. Coddington, K. Moore, and E. Fischer, *Making Integrated Health Care Work* (Englewood, CO: Center for Research in Ambulatory Health Care Administration, 1996).

W. DeMarco and K. Hekman, *Physician Driven Health Plans, Innovative Strategies for Restoring Physician-Community Integration* (New York: McGraw-Hill, 1998).

Developing a Managed Care Business Plan (Chicago, IL: American Medical Association, 1997).

K. Douglass, "My Brother's Gatekeeper—When Doctors Venture into Managed Care, They Run the Business Just Like HMO Execs or Else They Learn the Hard Way," *Hospitals & Health Networks 71*, no. 19 (1997): 54.

R.N. Ehrie, "PSOs Prepare To Make Their Mark," *Medical Industry Today*, 12 January, 1998.

C. Evans, F. DePorter and R. Wilson, *Integrated Community Healthcare, Next Generation Strategies for Developing Provider Networks* (copublished, Burr Ridge: IL: McGraw-Hill Healthcare Education Group, and Westchester, IL: Healthcare Financial Management Association, 1997).

E. Fonner, Jr., "Milestones for Developing Integrated Delivery Systems," *Journal of Health Care Finance 1*, no. 23 (1996): 1.

D. Goldstein, "The Building Blocks of an Integrated Delivery System," in *Alliances: Strategies for Building Integrated Delivery Systems* (Gaithersburg, MD: Aspen Publishers, Inc., 1995).

D. Goldstein, "Moving beyond Generic Integration Models," *Healthcare Financial Management 21*, no. 9 (1995): 42.

D. Goldstein, "Physician Equity Alliances: Attractive Alternatives to PHOs," *Healthcare Financial Management 51*, no. 4 (1997): 98.

A Guide to Forming Physician-Directed Managed Care Networks (Chicago, IL: American Medical Association, 1994).

Integrated Health Systems Resource Guide: 1995 Report Based on 1994 Data (Englewood, CO: Medical Group Management Association, 1995).

G. James, *Making Managed Care Work, Strategies for Local Market Dominance* (copublished, Burr Ridge, IL: McGraw-Hill Healthcare Education Group, and Westchester, IL: Healthcare Financial Management Association, 1997).

P. Manus, "The Future of Integrated Systems: An Interview with Stephen Shortell," *Healthcare Financial Management 49*, no. 1 (1995): 24.

G. Peters, "Organizational and Business Issues Affecting Integrated Delivery Systems," *Topics in Health Care Financing 20*, no. 3 (1994): 1.

M. Ruffin, "Factors in Successful Move to Organized Care Systems," *Physician Executive 21*, no. 6 (1995): 41.

M. Ruffin, "New Governance for a New Era: Issues and Challenges for Integrating," *Physician Executive 21*, no. 8 (1995): 45.

D.K. Settlemayer and S.K. Phillips, *Provider Risk Sharing and Provider Sponsored Organizations* (Washington, DC: American Health Lawyers Association, 1998).

E. Thompson, H. Honeycull, D. Orenstein, and J. Cawley, *Medicare PSOs: Assessing the Market, Risks and Opportunities* (Washington, DC: Atlantic Information Services, 1997).

S. Walston, J. Kimberly, and L. Burns, "Owned Vertical Integration and Health Care: Promise and Performance," *Health Care Management Review 21*, no. 1 (1996): 83.

M. Woodward and K. Lindstrom, "Analyzing and Executing Mergers and Acquisitions," *Healthcare Financial Management 51*, no. 4 (1997): 62.

A. Zuckerman and H. Finarelli, Jr., "Rightsizing the Delivery System," *Healthcare Financial Management 51*, no. 5 (1997): 33.

Creating an Effective Governance Structure for an Affiliated or Integrated Physician Group

INTRODUCTION

Governance usually means influence and control. There is little difficulty with a standard model group practice—chosen representatives of the physician members are in control. In small groups, decisions may be made by a consensus of all the member physicians. However, as the group grows larger and begins to affiliate or integrate with other provider organizations—hospitals, groups of other specialists, health plans—questions arise about the ownership, governance, and ultimate control, not only of the group practice itself, but also of the other entities in which it has a stake.

An effective governance structure means that the participating physicians feel more comfortable with the decisions made that affect them. It enables the organization to act decisively and intelligently.

This chapter explains some of the basic principles underlying good governance of a physician-run organization. The key decision points in designing an effective governance structure are explained. The ways in which a poor structure can compromise the organization's decision-making effectiveness are examined. The goal of the chapter is for physicians and groups founding or joining new organizations to understand how dependent their smooth operation is on a mutu-ally acceptable governing structure and what they can do to create one.

WHO SHOULD READ THIS CHAPTER

The physician who is a founder or leader in the formation of a new provider organization must pay close attention to the design of its governance structure. Simply letting all interested parties vote for a traditional and large board of directors may result in counterproductive decisions, frequent impasses in decision making, and fatal damage to participant morale. This chapter offers guidance on the problems to anticipate and measures for avoiding them.

Even if you are simply joining an existing group, it is important to know how decision-making power is allocated. This is particularly true if you are a primary care physician (PCP) considering an organization dominated by specialists or any physician looking at an organization run by a hospital or a managed care organization (MCO). You should want to know whether your interests will be adequately represented, even if you are not the one representing them.

If you are late in your medical career or, for other reasons, have chosen to be a passive participant in the organization, you may feel that you can live with almost any decision it is likely to make. In that case, the governance structure may be of little concern. You probably have better things to do than to read this chapter.

ROLE AND SCOPE OF GOVERNANCE IN A HEALTH CARE ORGANIZATION

Governance is that business function that lies between ownership and management. *Ownership* covers those parties that legally possess the organization and its assets. The parties may be people or other organizations. The owners of a for-profit corporation are its stockholders. The owners of a partnership are its partners. Nonprofit corporations do not have owners in the strict legal sense, except to the extent that they are "owned" by the entire community on whose behalf they are operated.

The owners normally do not directly manage the organization. Professional managers and executives are hired for that purpose. In an organization with many owners, it is impractical for most of them to be directly concerned with hiring the management team and giving it the strategic direction it requires. That important responsibility is delegated to a board of directors. In a nonprofit organization, they may be called a *board of trustees*. That board and its related committees carry out the governance of the organization.

The primary duty of the board is to serve the interests of the owners. It accomplishes that by defining a long-term mission for the organization, translating the mission into a goal-oriented strategic plan, and selecting a chief executive officer (CEO) to implement the plan. For instance, the board of a multispecialty group practice may commit itself to becoming a leading component in an integrated delivery system (IDS). Toward that end, it may decide to concentrate on growing its revenues, patient load, and number of managed care contracts. It will more tightly integrate its physicians' practices, gain experience in delivering cost-effective managed care, and increase its proportion of PCPs. Alternatively, it might immediately join a physician-hospital organization (PHO) formed by a local hospital and concentrate on maintaining the incomes of its current physician membership.

There often are divergent views among the owners about which strategy to pursue. In the above scenario, primary care and specialist physicians are likely to have very different preferences between the two alternatives. The board member's role is complicated further by the sheer number of options available. Also, constant changes in the health care industry leave little time for slow deliberation of the possibilities.

The following are the typical issues decided by the board of directors of a health care organization (HCO):

- amendment of the organization's articles of incorporation and bylaws
- appointment or election and possible removal of board members
- recruitment, hiring, and dismissal of the CEO
- approval of financial budgets
- participation in networks, affiliations, joint ventures, mergers, and acquisitions
- organization or formation of an affiliate or subsidiary controlled by the organization
- development, construction, or implementation of new health care facilities, programs, products, or services
- creation of an insurance or risk-financing function within the organization
- approval of public stock offerings, bond issues, and other forms of major financing

Keep in mind that different interest groups on the board of directors (e.g., physicians versus hospital) can be allotted different levels of voting authority over each of these issues. For instance, a hospital partner that contributed a larger share of the start-up capital may be given greater voting authority over major capital expenditures.

Perhaps it is obvious from the significance of these issues that the governance structure of an organization has a major influence on its future direction and the welfare of its constituent members. You must pay attention to the governance of any entity you are considering joining. Be prepared to negotiate its shape to protect your interests.

KEY COMPONENTS OF THE GOVERNANCE STRUCTURE

In a traditional corporate organization, governance is carried out by several different components. The principal one is the board of directors. Legally, board members are the agents of the owners in choosing, directing, and overseeing the management of the organization. State incorporation laws require the board to choose officers with designated tasks, typically a president, vice-president, treasurer, and secretary. In some organizations, these individuals can wield great practical power; in others, they perform nothing more than their titular functions.

Most boards create and delegate responsibilities to a variety of specialized committees. Among these is the executive committee, which often guides the board as a whole and acts in its place when it is not assembled.

FEATURES TO NOTICE ABOUT AN ORGANIZATION'S GOVERNANCE

There are a few key variables that determine where the decision-making authority will lie in an organization's governance structure. They are summed up in these questions.

What Is the Composition of the Board?

Who are the people on the board and where do they come from? Generally, the organization bylaws provide that a certain number of seats on the board will be filled by representatives from groups or entities that founded the organization or are important to its success. For instance, a nonprofit IDS created by two hospitals might reserve spaces for executives from each of the hospitals and for the community representatives required by tax-exempt status. In addition, the IDS may wish to give a prominent role to physicians by allotting them a significant portion of board seats.

What Proportion of the Board Members Are Physicians?

This is your primary concern. Physicians must have a prominent, if not dominant, role in the governance of any organization you join. This is for your long-term benefit and for the long-term success of the organization. A standard rule of thumb is that physicians should hold at least 50 percent of the seats on the board. The only reasons to accept less than this share is when you are in a market with high managed care penetration or excess physicians and there are few alternatives to the organization in question, or when a major contributor of start-up capital demands a controlling board interest. On the other hand, the physician proportion may exceed 50 percent where the organization founders recognize that, politically and economically, they will do better if physicians drive most of the board decisions.

What Proportion of the Board Members Are Primary Care Physicians?

A modern, ambitious provider organization is not satisfied with placing a substantial number of physicians on the board. It will make sure that a preponderance of them practice in primary care specialties. The same rule of thumb for primary care representation on the total physician panel—50/50 or even 60/40—should be applied to the governing board.

Just as hospitals are challenged to allow physicians to have prominent roles in joint ventures with them, so, too, will specialist physicians be tested to acknowledge the growing preeminence of PCPs. Think twice about affiliating with a physician group that is not on this track.

What Proportion of the Board Members Are Hospital Representatives?

The only reason that board seats are reserved for hospital representatives is that the hospital often is the major initial funding source and because it comes into the organization as a separate and historically dominant entity. The hospital is nothing but "bricks and mortar" and, 10 years from now, the idea of allocating seats for hospital managers will seem anomalous.

In the near future, you can expect to have to guarantee the hospital some representation on the board. The wisest hospitals, however, will see the value in giving away control to the doctors. Its willingness to cede this control may be a litmus test of the hospital's commitment to the new paradigm of physician-driven health care delivery.

If the hospital is the primary capital investor in a new organization, it will be effectively giving the money to the doctors by granting them a disproportionately large role in its governance. There is no problem with the hospital (or any other nonphysician investor) doing this with a for-profit corporation. It cannot be done when the organization is a nonprofit tax-exempt entity. The "gift" of control would be viewed as private inurement. The Internal Revenue Service (IRS) has made clear that physician board representation should not exceed 20 percent.

What Proportion of the Board Members Are Private Investors?

Most of the arguments related to hospitals participating in the organization also apply to private investors. Smart ones will allow physicians a prominent position on the board; less forward-looking investors may demand control for themselves.

There is an added concern here. Hospital managers at least have working experience with physicians and in the health care field. They are likely to have some appreciation for the critical role physicians play in clinical and managerial decision making. They will be more receptive to substantial physician participation in governance.

Many of the private investors now coming into health care have backgrounds in other industrial sectors quite unlike this one. They are not sensitive to the subtle dynamics among providers in delivering quality medical services in a variety of settings. They usually are motivated exclusively by a desire to make as much money as possible.

There are serious questions about the role of profit motive in health care delivery. Caution is warranted when it appears that private investors will have a significant position on the organization board (Exhibit 22–1).

What Proportion of the Board Members Are Public Representatives from the Community?

There are generally two reasons for having community representatives on an HCO board. If it desires tax-exempt status, it will be required to have such representation as evidence of its commitment to community welfare. Even for-profit organizations often see a public relations and marketing advantage in placing some community leaders on their boards.

How Are the Board Members Selected?

As a practical matter, the board members representing certain organizations often are appointed by the CEO of the organization—if she herself does not fill the seat. In the case of physician entities, particularly when the organization encompasses many of them (perhaps through an independent practice association, (IPA)), the method of selecting representatives for the governing board may deserve more attention. For instance, it might be inadvisable to allow each participating physician group to put forward its own board representative. That could result in voting solely on the basis of self-interest—not especially desirable if integration and goal alignment are the objectives. Instead, some organizations arrange for all physician board members to be elected at large from the entire body of physicians.

Sometimes, the method of choosing board members from a certain constituency can be as important as the choice of constituencies to be represented.

What Qualifications Are Expected of Board Members?

The effectiveness of the board and the power that it exercises will be further determined by the qualifications that are demanded of any candidate

Exhibit 22–1 A Party's Capital Contribution vs. Its Share of Control

A critical turning point in the development of provider organizations comes when the need for growth capital requires the invitation of a well-heeled strategic partner into the organization. Increasingly, a variety of for-profit organizations and investors are eager to allow the use of their money by organizations in the health care industry with high growth potential. In return, they want to share in the growth and the profits it generates. They usually accomplish this by asking for and getting an ownership interest in the organization. Generally, an owner of 20 percent of a business will be entitled to 20 percent of the profits or 20 percent of the appreciation in the value of the stock.

This may seem like fair recompense for the use of much-needed capital. There are two problems with it. Ownership of a significant percentage of a company's stock also translates into seats on the board of directors and a share in the decision making. This may confound the desire to keep physicians in control of the organization. In addition, once a percentage of company stock has been traded for capital at one stage of its evolution, it is no longer available to be traded for still more capital at a later stage.

The group's physician leaders must perform a delicate balancing act, giving away the least amount of control for the greatest amount of capital at just the right times along the organization's growth path. Sometimes, enlightened partners, understanding the competitive strength of physician-dominated organizations, will accept a smaller percentage of an organization's stock than its capital investment warrants. For instance, it might put up 50 percent of the start-up capital for a physician-led management services organization (MSO) in return for 30 percent of the stock. Unfortunately, the parties most likely to see the value in such an arrangement, such as a local hospital, would be inhibited from doing so by both the fraud and abuse law and the tax laws (if they are charitable entities).

There are legal and imaginative ways of enabling a physician group to accept investment capital without giving away too much control. For instance, the investor may be given a special class of nonvoting stock with full rights to a share of the profits. Consult a corporate attorney experienced in capital financing for health care organizations for more ideas.

for a board seat. The disadvantages of allowing private investors or hospital executives may be offset by a requirement that they display a minimal amount of direct working experience with physicians. A reasonable package of prerequisites for membership on an HCO board might include

- experience as a high-level executive in any industry
- experience as a high-level executive in the health care industry
- experience working in an organization that provides managed care
- experience practicing medicine under capitation or other form of managed care
- experience practicing medicine in a large group practice setting or as part of a multidisciplinary team

- demonstrated leadership or managerial skills
- grasp of the trends that are transforming the health care industry
- comprehension of health care financial matters and the ability to analyze financial statements
- willingness to make decisions for the benefit of the entire organization rather than the component that the director represents
- embrace of the need to evolve rapidly and radically to thrive in the constantly changing health care marketplace

Board seats should not necessarily go to the persons with the greatest seniority or popularity within their respective component organizations. Directors need to be sufficiently respected by their constituents to engender their trust in board decisions.

What Specific Decision-Making Powers Will Be Granted to the Board, Rather Than to Its Parent Organizations?

When two independent organizations come together (through merger or joint venture) to form a third entity, they can cede as much or as little authority to the new organization as they wish. Initially, the parents may be reluctant to give up control to an unproven enterprise. Their tentativeness may doom its success.

One of the primary purposes for forming new, larger provider organizations from several smaller ones is to more tightly integrate their care delivery and administration activities. It also is a key to any future success. Integration requires a surrender of some autonomy. If there is not significant surrender at the outset, there should be rapid progress in that direction. One strong measure of the transfer of control is the amount of authority given to the board of the new organization.

Start by giving the new board as much nonclinical administrative responsibility as possible—covering matters like financial management, billing and claims, purchasing, marketing, and nonclinical human resource management. Lay out a firm schedule for steadily transferring more and more responsibilities from the parent organizations. The most sensitive will be the clinical functions, such as credentialing, quality assurance, utilization management, and clinical human resource management. As physicians gain confidence in the new organization and their incentives become increasingly aligned with the organization's, they will feel more comfortable with these functions being managed through the organization.

There are three other ways to assuage the anxieties of new participants about turning over decision-making power on issues they care about to the new organization: reserved powers, special voting requirements, and delegation to board committees.

What Powers Are Reserved to Specific Interest Groups on the Board?

It is possible to implement corporate bylaws that reserve decision-making power on certain issues to subgroups of the board uniquely concerned with those issues. For instance, it is reasonable that the physicians on a board should either make the final decisions or have veto power over those decisions regarding physician selection and credentialing, physician services to be provided under managed care contracts, quality assurance, utilization management, and all aspects of clinical decision making.

In any event, notice exactly where the authority over these matters lies. Be skeptical of any arrangement that gives nonphysicians great influence or complete control over them. The result may be decisions that you cannot live or practice with. At the very least, excluding physicians from a prominent role here is a sign of an organization insensitive to the importance of physician involvement in appropriate areas of management.

Are Special or Supermajority Voting Requirements in Effect for Certain Issues?

The bylaws also may be written to require that special voting requirements must be satisfied to approve proposals on certain topics. Such measures are another mechanism for ensuring that physicians have strong influence in decisions affecting clinical practice and quality assurance. A classic example is a board equally divided between physician members and nonphysician administrative members, with a majority of each half required to pass any initiative. Alternatively, a majority of the physicians must approve decisions on clinical matters or a two-thirds or three-fourths majority of all board members must okay proposals on issues of great significance, such as capital expenditures over a certain dollar amount, affiliation with a major new strategic partner, offering of a substantial new managed care product, or institution of a much more rigorous form of utilization management.

Train yourself to notice bylaw language that creates these kinds of subtle distinctions. Some may operate to your great benefit, and others may pose a serious detriment.

What Are the Composition and the Duties of the Committees Created by the Board?

Careful design of the board's committee structure can be used to allocate power among key interest groups on the board and within the organization. Although the board of directors always retains the legal responsibility for all decisions made on the organization's behalf, it can, as a practical matter, delegate large pieces of authority to board committees or other subordinate deliberative bodies. Indeed, it is common for boards to accept without a lot of question the action recommendations of committees on credentialing, physician discipline, quality assurance, and so on. Look for such transfers of power as a form of protection of physician rights and interests.

GIVING DISPROPORTIONATE GOVERNANCE POWER TO PRIMARY CARE PHYSICIANS

You already understand the strategic value of placing physicians in positions of authority in any integrated health care delivery organization. Physicians are better able than any nonphysician professional manager to balance market-driven cost-effectiveness initiatives with solid quality maintenance and improvement. No one but a physician can appreciate whether an excluded diagnostic test, an alternative medication, or an abbreviated hospital stay will have a seriously detrimental effect on quality of care. The wisest organizations increasingly acknowledge this by granting physicians power in governance beyond what their capital contributions may warrant.

Similar attitudes have developed toward the role of PCPs. Whether they are referred to as *gatekeepers* or something else, there is no denying that PCPs are the primary decision makers in the allocation of health care resources. In recog-

nition of this influential role in delivery operations, many organizations are delegating disproportionately large shares in governance to their primary care participants. This may present a major challenge to the specialist doctors in the organization (Exhibit 22–2). Nonetheless, they must accept this new imperative.

The "ideal" composition of the board of directors of a physician/hospital coventure might be nine members, broken down in this way:

- three primary care physicians
- two specialist physicians
- four hospital administrators

Keep in mind the opportunity to move gradually toward the board makeup you desire. You might start out with a board that is larger and more heavily weighted, for political and psychologic reasons, toward nonphysicians or less qualified but currently influential physicians. Then set a definite timetable for reducing board size and readjusting the background and qualifications of board members, and stick to it.

CREATION OF A SINGLE GOVERNANCE STRUCTURE

When a new delivery entity is formed through the combination of two or more relatively powerful organizations (such as a hospital and a large physician group), there may be a temptation to reconcile the inevitable control conflicts by retaining substantial authority in the two organizations' existing boards and delegating little of it to the new board. This would be a mistake.

The reason for a unified governance body is that provider organizations need to make difficult strategic decisions, often in response to suddenly emerging competitive conditions, within short periods of time. Provider systems that try to maintain multiple boards and CEOs often have trouble defining a single shared vision, resulting in competing interests and internal power struggles.

Exhibit 22–2 Do Specialists Subsidize Primary Care Physicians?

As physicians in all specialties are integrating their practices into unified organizations, there is some discomfort over the fact that the compensation and influence of PCPs is going up while that of specialists seems to be declining. There is a tendency to say that the specialists are "subsidizing" the PCPs.

Such a claim is based on assumptions about what the two groups of physicians could earn in solo or small group practice. That model is no longer viable. The current and evolving delivery system is based on a symbiosis between primary care and specialist physicians. It makes no sense to reference a fading system of medical practice when assessing the relative value of different specialties.

In the future, surgeons will not have the option of earning $400,000 a year in private practice, while PCPs pull down only $150,000. In fact, the surgeons will see virtually no patients without the cooperation and referral of a PCP.

Stop thinking about how much specialists could earn if they could practice in a setting that is no longer available to them. Start thinking about how much specialists and PCPs can earn together if they synchronize the delivery of their respective specialty services.

PLAN FOR A CONSTANTLY EVOLVING GOVERNANCE STRUCTURE

You might think that the governance structure carefully and painfully devised for a new provider entity would suffice for some years to come. In fact, there is a good chance that the board configuration will go through several iterations as the entity grows in size and retunes its strategic direction.

Consider This: Many physician groups, even rather large ones, govern themselves through a model based on pure democracy. All physicians in the group vote for all the board members and, often, also vote in referenda on key decisions. When the group first joins with other parties (whether a hospital, an existing health system, or simply other physician groups) to form a new entity, it probably will have to give up this governance structure. For the reasons stated earlier, decision-making authority must be delegated to a small number of people who will be guided by what is in the best interests of the entire group.

Initially, the composition of that new board may be artificially shaped to accommodate the unique circumstances surrounding start-up—anxieties of the constituent groups, general politics among the group members, and the need to acknowledge and ensure large capital contributors. As time passes and the new entity matures and evolves, those initial concerns fade and new ones emerge. New partners in the entity, new contributors of capital, and a need to centralize decision-making power even further may compel more restructuring of the governance body. Board seat reservations for some groups will be canceled and transferred to later participants who require at least temporary seats at the governance table.

When planning the form of a new organization, acknowledge up front that the governance structure will have to adapt, perhaps several times, to new combinations of participants and new market pressures.

DETERMINING THE RIGHT NUMBER OF BOARD MEMBERS

The size of the board is a major determinant of its decision-making effectiveness. Sometimes, in a desire to accommodate a wide variety of interests and viewpoints, boards are created with 20, 30, or more members. This is seen frequently in nonprofit organizations trying to give a board presence to a multitude of community groups.

At various points in an organization's development, it may have to operate with a larger board than it prefers. Nonetheless, the goal always must be to push the size of the board toward a smaller, more workable number. A good target is five to seven people. More than seven complicates and slows the decision-making process at a time when organizations must react quickly and efficiently to the changing health care environment. Few multiprovider organizations are mature enough yet to have achieved this target.

If you must start with a larger board, obtain a commitment from everyone involved to gradually reduce the board size. Set size benchmarks for points in the future.

COMMITTEE STRUCTURE MAY BE AS IMPORTANT AS BOARD COMPOSITION

Active governing boards almost always rely on an infrastructure of committees to lighten their load and streamline their decision making. There are standing committees (which are in continuous existence) and ad hoc committees (which exist for the duration of a discrete task). Typical standing committees for a physician/hospital entity are

- executive matters
- credentialing and membership
- quality assurance
- utilization management
- managed care contracting
- clinical operations
- finance

These committees are made up of subsets of board members and some regular employees of the organization.

The executive committee is the most important of these. Its members are empowered to make urgent decisions on the board's behalf in the times between full board meetings. They also prepare the board's agenda, largely determining which matters will be brought to the full body's attention. A small, efficient executive committee

given substantial authority can go a long way toward offsetting a large, ponderous full board.

A board's committees must be managed with care. The right people must be assigned to the right committees. Physicians must have dominant roles on the credentialing, utilization management, quality assurance, and clinical operations committees. Those physicians must be leaders who have won the respect of their colleagues—the people who will have to accept their decisions.

Duties must be delegated to the committees in a way that enhances, not impedes, the board's functioning. Committee responsibility for preparing or reviewing action proposals must facilitate faster, wiser decisions. If the committees do not meet regularly or are not staffed competently, they can actually slow down decision making. Avoid establishing a committee report and review procedure that looks good on paper but delays critical decisions by months.

SELECTING THE OFFICERS OF A NEW ORGANIZATION

The traditional positions of president, vice-president, treasurer, and clerk may be created in response to statutory mandates, but they should not be taken lightly. These officers can play pivotal roles in governance. The president, in particular, who should not be confused with the CEO and serves as something closer to a chairman of the board, often emerges as the leader of the board. If she is a physician, she will likely be recognized as the leader of the physician participants in the organization. Also, if it is a physician-sponsored or -dominated organization, the president may appear as the strategic guiding force of the entire operation.

When selecting a president, keep in mind the role you expect her to play. In most organizations, she will have to be a person who will be respected and followed by the factions on the board and in the organization. If her background is in hospital management, she must be able to inspire the confidence of physicians—and vice versa. It will help tremendously if she has prior experience in governance.

BUILDING PHYSICIAN LEADERSHIP AND GOVERNANCE EXPERTISE

As physicians claim leading roles in the governance and management of new health care delivery organizations, a major challenge for physician groups and the medical community as a whole is to develop appropriate skills among their members. The tradition of successful physicians slipping into key positions as department heads and medical directors, without any serious managerial training and while maintaining significant practices, research, and teaching activities will no longer suffice. The demands of managing large, complex, competition-threatened health care systems require full-time attention by professionals.

It is in the interests of physician groups, existing and planned, to promote systematically the cultivation of physician leaders. This means instituting a development program with the following pieces:

- consideration of prior management training or experience in admitting new physicians to the group
- early in their tenure with the group, identification of physicians with potential and interest for future leadership
- for those designated physicians, plotting of a career path of increasing management responsibilities
- sponsoring of continuing management education for interested physicians (through in-house workshops and attendance in public training and degree programs)
- requirements for demonstrated management experience of all persons, physician and otherwise, hired into leadership positions

COMMUNICATING GOVERNANCE ISSUES TO OTHER STAKEHOLDERS

In designing a responsive and responsible governance structure, make provision for communicating what it does to the stakeholders of the organization. That is *stakeholders*, not just *shareholders*. Stakeholders are all those people or parties with an interest in the activities of the organization. They include shareholders, as well as employees, affiliated strategic partners, patient/members, and the public. Technically, the competition and government regulatory agencies are stakeholders, though you will probably want to communicate much less to them.

If you have a board of directors and its members are chosen by election of all the participating physicians, they must be fully informed of the election process and the candidates. When the board makes important policy or strategy decisions, it usually is a good idea to pass detailed information on to shareholders, participating physicians, and all the employees who will have to implement the decisions. On those matters that directly affect them, you will want to communicate board decisions to health plan members and other patients of the group.

EXAMPLES OF GOVERNANCE STRUCTURES EMPLOYED IN MAJOR HEALTH SYSTEMS

Presbyterian Healthcare Services (Albuquerque, New Mexico)

Presbyterian Healthcare Services (PHS) is composed of 3 acute care hospitals (with 628 beds) in Albuquerque, 13 hospitals in smaller communities throughout New Mexico and Colorado, 11 primary care facilities around Albuquerque, and a medical panel of 600 physicians, of whom 120 are PCPs. It operates a multiproduct financing subsidiary, HealthPlus, Inc.

PHS was formed five years ago on the initiative of 17 primary care doctors on the Presbyterian Hospital staff, with the goal of linking physician practices and the three Presbyterian hospitals into an integrated health care delivery organization.

The PHS board is composed of 27 community representatives who oversee all operations of the nonprofit Presbyterian hospitals. They perform traditional tasks of the directors of a multihospital system: credentialing for the hospital medical staffs, strategic planning, financial planning, CEO hiring, and overall performance evaluation.

Reporting to the PHS board is a network board, which is more directly responsible for the integrated provider activities. It is made up of seven primary care physicians, nine specialty physicians, two hospital administrators, and one PHS board member. A two-month questionnaire and interview process was used to select the original board from among 60 physician volunteers. Key criteria were an ability to think strategically and to put personal interests aside.

There also is a physician management board (PMB), subordinate to the network board, whose primary responsibility is policy making for the economically integrated physicians on the network panel. Its specific duties include development of new health plan products and contracting guidelines, participation in the network budgeting process, and physician compensation and performance evaluation.

There are 14 physicians and 1 hospital administrator on this board. Nonphysician practice managers are nonvoting members of the PMB. The physician board members are elected by their respective medical groups for two-year terms. They meet biweekly and are compensated for one-fourth of their total work time.

The health maintenance organization/preferred provider organization (HMO/PPO)/indemnity subsidiary, HealthPlus, Inc. is governed by a board of six physicians and three administrators.

Carle Clinic (Urbana, Illinois)

The Carle Clinic Association is a 240-physician multispecialty group practice clinic with an arm's-length affiliation with the 288-bed Carle Foundation acute care hospital. The nonprofit Foundation owns all of the real estate of both organizations, including the clinic building. The for-profit Clinic owns and operates the Health Alliance Medical Plans (a for-profit stock insurance company) which offers, HMO and PPO products.

The origins of the clinic go back to 1931, when it was formed by physicians from the Mayo clinic hoping to emulate the model. The Carle system has continued to be a physician-dominated one.

The Foundation board is composed of six community representatives, five physicians from the Carle Clinic and the CEO of the Foundation.

The Clinic is led by a six-physician board of governors whose members are elected by its shareholders to staggered three-year terms. There are nearly 200 physician shareholders currently. New physicians may become shareholders after they have been with the Clinic for two years and receive the approval of three-fourths of the existing shareholders.

The governing boards of the Clinic and the Foundation act independently of each other. They collaborate on strategic issues affecting the entire system through the joint policy council. It is composed of the entire Clinic board and the executive committee of the Foundation. It has no independent legal authority.

The Clinic board also serves as the governing board of the Health Alliance Medical Plans entity.

Scott & White (Temple, Texas)

The Scott & White system consists of three entities—a 450-physician for-profit multispecialty group and clinic, a 390-bed nonprofit hospital, and a health plan (the seventh largest in Texas). The system originated in 1897 through a partnership formed by its namesakes.

The clinic is organized as a for-profit professional association of physicians, reflecting state laws against the corporate practice of medicine. It is governed by a board of seven physicians elected to seven-year terms, with one term expiring each year. The current board is composed of six specialists and one PCP. The executive director and medical director of the clinic also attend the weekly board meetings.

The nonprofit hospital is steered by 5 physicians and 12 community leaders from the surrounding area. The health plan, which also is nonprofit, has a board of 15 directors. In accordance with IRS guidelines, 80 percent of them are not affiliated in any way with the Scott & White system.

These formal governance structures are supplemented by weekly meetings of what is referred to as the "Big Six"—which includes the top physician and top administrative person from each of the clinic, hospital, and health plan. Their deliberations provide the necessary level of strategic integration among the three components.

Oregon Medical Group (Eugene, Oregon)

The Oregon Medical Group (OMG) was organized in 1988 by 24 PCPs. In partnership with 450-bed Sacred Heart Hospital, the group formed a management services organization (MSO) to purchase many of its tangible assets and to manage their physician practices. The group currently consists of over 50 PCPs providing care at seven locations in the Eugene area. The OMG is also part of the physician component of the Sacred Heart Health System, along with the Eugene Clinic, the Sacred Heart Hospital, and an HMO component, SelectCare.

The Medical Group is governed by a board of seven physicians. They are elected by the shareholders to staggered three-year terms. New physicians to the group may become shareholders after a one-year waiting period. The board meets once a month.

The MSO entity is headed by an eight-person board composed of four OMG doctors, two administrators from the hospital, and two non-physician hospital board members. All eight are elected for three-year terms. Board decisions require the approval of three of the physician directors and three of the hospital directors (i.e., a majority of each half of the board). The board chairperson rotates between representatives from the medical group and the hospital.

The OMG is affiliated with the Sacred Heart Health System through the system's physician practice board. This board reports directly to the System CEO, as do the hospital and the HMO. The board is composed of seven physicians appointed by the System board of directors. It is a powerful body whose responsibilities include making recommendations to the System board, maintaining the physician panel for managed care purposes, determining the formulas for distributing funds from risk pools, quality improvement programs, product development, marketing, and sales.

Nearly all the hospital's specialist physicians are on the panel. Primary care doctors must meet specific prerequisites to participate: organized into a group, information system in place, ability to perform quality assurance and utilization management, and willingness to accept risk. Only OMG and the Eugene Clinic have been able to saisfy these criteria.

ACTION GUIDELINES FOR CREATING OR ASSESSING A GOVERNANCE STRUCTURE

1. *Whenever you join or form a provider organization, scrutinize the governance structure*—the board of directors, criteria for board membership, method of selection of board members, decision-making powers held by the board, board decision-making procedures, and the role of subordinate committees.

2. *Make a strong request for giving physicians a prominent role on the board of directors.* Push for at least 50 percent physician representation among the directors and preferably for a majority position.

3. Insist that physicians be given complete authority or at least veto power over the issues of physician selection and credentialing, physician discipline, quality assurance and improvement, utilization management, and other areas of clinical decision making.

4. *Walk away from any organization that leaves authority over those issues largely in the hands of nonphysicians.*

5. *Strongly urge that at least 50 percent of the physicians in the governance structure be PCPs.*

6. *Be open to creative governance mechanisms that will protect and assert the inter-*

ests *of physicians*: empowered board committees, special or supermajority voting requirements on certain issues.

7. *Aim for the smallest size board that will fairly represent the interests of the organi-* zation's stakeholders. *Seven to nine members is a good target.*

8. *Establish a formal program for identifying and developing leaders among the physician participants in the organization.*

RESOURCE LIST

E. Gallup, *How Physicians Can Avoid Surrender and Lead Change* (Chicago, IL: American Medical Association, 1998).

Organizational Structure and Governance in Group Practices (Englewood, CO: Medical Group Management Association, updated annually).

J. Pollard, *The Physician Manager in Group Practice* (Englewood, CO: Medical Group Management Association, 1993).

## CHAPTER 23

Selection and Deselection of Physicians by Managed Care Organizations and Physician Groups

INTRODUCTION

Through the application of one legal doctrine or another, every organization that delivers health care is responsible for checking the qualifications of or "credentialing" the physicians who actually administer the care. Traditionally, this has been an issue for hospitals trying to make sure their medical staffs deliver quality care without malpractice. Managed care organizations (MCOs) have that same burden plus a desire to use only physicians who practice cost-effective medicine. That kind of screening is sometimes called "economic credentialing."

This chapter explains how and why these decisions are being made. It defines the legal authority MCOs and groups have to exclude or reject physicians. It also describes the legal rights of the excluded physicians, what procedures they can demand from the group, and tactics for challenging the decision. There are suggestions on how to make yourself or your group so attractive that you will be last on the exclusion list. The chapter lays out some surprisingly effective strategies deselected physicians have used to hang on to their patients.

If you are a leader or manager in a physician group that may have to reduce its physician panel, you will learn here the due process procedures to follow to minimize legal exposure. This is accompanied by a full explanation of those legal risks—particularly in the areas of antitrust

and contracts. The chapter explores the legitimate use of exclusive contracting and economic credentialing in configuring a physician panel. Finally, the implications of state "any willing provider" statutes and the federal Health Care Quality Improvement Act for physician exclusion are examined.

WHO SHOULD READ THIS CHAPTER

This chapter will be most valuable to physicians who are about to have their first experiences with MCOs. It will prepare them for the criteria and procedures that will likely be used to determine their initial acceptance and continued participation with the MCO. Other physicians may have had several managed care contracts for some time, without noticing or encountering the credentialing systems to which they are exposed. Reading this chapter may help them understand contract language on renewal and termination. All physicians in relationships with MCOs will learn how to protect themselves before and after deselection.

On the other hand, some physicians may be in leadership positions in physician-run organizations. They might be wondering how they can, discretely and fairly, assemble a physician panel that serves the economic interests of those organizations. In this chapter, they will find a description of a balanced credentialing program and the legal constraints on their selection and deselection of doctors.

Under a predominantly managed care system, the threat of deselection goes to the heart of every physician's pursuit of her profession. The only doctors who can afford to skip this chapter are those that are such competent managed care practitioners that deselection is nearly inconceivable. These also are physicians who are not involved or interested in how their organization handles physician dismissals. Everyone else will benefit from reading what follows.

VARIETIES OF CREDENTIALING

An easy way to understand the credentialing that physicians are encountering in the health care industry of the 1990s is to separate it into categories based on the criteria used and the point in the contract relationship when it occurs.

In terms of credentialing criteria, there are two broad groups. The first is the quality and competence-based credentialing traditionally conducted by hospitals on their medical staff members. This form of credentialing is mandated by common law—unless the hospital wants to be held vicariously liable for a physician's negligence. It is focused entirely on the physician's qualifications and ability to practice medicine of reasonable quality and function harmoniously in a clinical setting. It does not attempt to determine how "good" the physician is. It aims only to make sure that her competence does not fall below certain minimal levels.

If the hospital carries out its credentialing duty adequately, when a physician on its medical staff commits malpractice, the hospital is able to argue in court that "We did everything a reasonable hospital would do in these circumstances to screen this physician. There is nothing more we reasonably could have done to determine that he had a potential to malpractice." If that argument succeeds, the hospital escapes liability for the physician's negligence, even though he himself may be held liable.

The second category of criteria is concerned with the physician's ability to practice cost-effective medicine and otherwise meet the business and economic performance expectations of his employer or contract partner. This credentialing hurdle is imposed entirely by the organization through which the physician is treating patients—whether a hospital, clinic, MCO, or group practice. The physician becomes legally subject to the requirement because it is written into the contract he signs with the organization. These kinds of demands are being made of physicians because health care has become a hotly competitive cost-conscious business. In all fairness, companies in the rest of American industry have held their employees to such performance-based standards for decades.

This second group of requirements is sometimes referred to as "economic credentialing." That term has been defined by the American Medical Association (AMA) as "the use of economic criteria unrelated to quality of care or professional competency in determining an individual's qualifications for initial or continuing medical staff membership or privileges."[1] A more mundane definition reads simply "the evaluation of a medical staff member based on resource utilization."

When some hospitals and MCOs first began to evaluate physician performance, they did concentrate on resource utilization. Recently, however, the scope of the credentialing has been expanded to include factors like patient satisfaction, relations with support staff, and an ability to work in teams. In other words, they are looking for a well-rounded physician, with a variety of staff- and patient-oriented abilities, in addition to good technical clinical talent.

There are four points in a physician's relationship with a MCO where the credentialing process and data have an impact. First is the initial selection (or rejection) of the physician to join the MCO's provider panel. Second is at the expiration of the contract term, when the MCO decides whether to renew or not. Third is any time during the term that the MCO chooses to deselect the physician, for whatever reason. The fourth point occurs at those times during the contract term when the MCO carries out a scheduled recredentialing of the physician.

At each of these points, the relevant law and the physician's opportunity to prevent or remedy the rejection are different.

LEGAL DUTY OF HEALTH CARE ORGANIZATIONS TO CREDENTIAL

It was just over 30 years ago that the courts first held a hospital directly responsible for the quality of care delivered by independent medical staff doctors, accompanied by a duty to exercise ordinary care in selecting those doctors. Credentialing has been the primary tool used by hospitals to assess the clinical skills of their physicians. The legal doctrine upon which this holding was based is Corporate Negligence. The case was *Darling v. Charleston Community Memorial Hospital.*[2]

The same legal reasoning applies to MCOs and large group practices that are as intimately involved in delivering medical care as hospitals. For example, in the case of *McClellan v. HMO of Pennsylvania,*[3] the court held that an independent practice association (IPA)-model health maintenance organization (HMO) had a nondelegable duty to select and retain competent providers. "Nondelegable" means that the HMO could not avoid this responsibility by turning it over to someone else, such as the members of its physician panel.

There are two other possible grounds for the legal duty of MCOs to exercise reasonable care in selecting the physicians who will treat its enrollees. Under the doctrine of *Respondeat Superior,* the employer is responsible for damages caused by one of its employees, acting within the scope of her employment. For example, if a physician-employee of an MCO accidentally injured a patient in the course of treating him, the MCO could be held liable. There would be no liability for the MCO if the physician shot a patient in the waiting room with a gun. He would not have been acting within the scope of his employment.

The application of *Respondeat Superior* is complicated by the question of who is an employee and who is an independent contractor. The way that the parties characterize the relationship, say in a contract between them, is irrelevant.

The key distinction is the degree of control the organization has over the physician and the way she does her work.

The other legal basis for holding an MCO liable is called *Ostensible Agency.* This doctrine comes into play when the MCO engages in conduct that leads a patient to reasonably believe that it, rather than the physician, is the ultimate provider of care. This might occur if a patient chose a physician from a picture book of physicians published by the MCO, with its name on the cover, and was seen by the physician in a clinic building with the MCO's name on the front and on all the stationery, brochures, and signage inside.

Worried about all these legal risks, it is not surprising that most MCOs devote significant attention to the clinical abilities of their physicians. Some go even further. When contracting with a group of physicians, the MCO may insist on screening any new physicians who join the group, even to replace a departing member. A few MCOs have inserted themselves into the process by which the group hires ancillary clinical personnel.

TYPICAL MCO CREDENTIALING PROCEDURES AND CRITERIA

The credentialing procedures and criteria used with physicians vary depending on the integrity of the MCO and the dynamics of the managed care marketplace.

In an all too common scenario, an MCO may be one of the first health plans to enter an immature managed care market. To get in with a minimum of fuss and offer enrollees the widest selection, it signs up as many physicians as will join. It asks relatively few questions, just enough to make sure none of the doctors pose a serious malpractice risk. The doctors are inexperienced in such contract negotiations, so fail to notice missing and imprecise language in the contract. Because the physicians have no history with managed care, they are unable to provide any evidence of the ability to provide cost-effective quality care.

Two or three years later, several things have changed. The market has become more competitive; other MCOs have come into town. The first entrant feels pressure to reduce its costs in order to keep premiums down. It has enrolled a significant share of the potential patient population and does not feel as great a need to offer a wide choice of physicians. It has at least a couple years of utilization and quality data on its physician panel. The next step is obvious—it uses the data to begin thinning the ranks of its physicians. In most cases, the MCO makes rational decisions to deselect the physicians who consume too many resources or deliver substandard care.

Frequently, however, the MCO does not give a physician the reason for her deselection. It is concerned that the physician will find some basis for challenging the decision in a lawsuit. Deselected physicians often argue that their utilization rates were higher because they were treating higher-risk patients. Even if the MCO were confident that it could back up its deselection decision with data, it would rather not go to the expense of a court trial. So, it uses one of the provisions in the contract that the physician may have skipped over, the one that allows either party to cancel the contract "without cause." The MCO tells the physician that she is no longer on its panel, gives her no reason, and leaves her with nothing to grab on to and complain about.

Once the size of an MCO physician panel has been reduced to numbers that better match the patient population they must serve, the MCO conducts ongoing monitoring and evaluation of each physician's performance. When problems are observed, the MCO (through its medical director) will usually work with the physician to try to figure out the causes. If the problems seem to be the result of the physician's behavior, corrective steps are taken. The physician is allowed a reasonable period of time to bring her performance back in line with group norms. Failure to make necessary adjustments will lead to deselection or nonrenewal of the contract.

There are other, more benign reasons why an MCO may decide to shrink its physician network. It may have lost contracts with employers, result-ing in lower enrollments. Even if enrollments remain steady, the MCO may restructure the way it serves them, perhaps placing greater emphasis on primary care physicians as gatekeepers or negotiating carve-outs for certain specialties or diseases.

A good physician does not want to be deselected and looks for ways to prevent it. Several issues come up, such as:

- What are the criteria used by the MCO to evaluate its doctors?
- What procedure does the MCO follow in deciding to deselect a physician?
- What are the facts upon which the deselection decision is based?
- What can he do before signing with the MCO to prevent deselection?
- What can he do after signing to prevent it?
- How can he respond to a notice that he has been deselected?

When they are simply cutting the absolute number of physicians, MCOs tend employ the following criteria:

Board Certification

One of the first steps an MCO is likely to take to begin shrinking its physician force is requiring them to be board certified, rather than just board eligible. When the new standard goes into effect, the MCO will either immediately terminate the contract of uncertified physicians (if it has reserved that authority in the contract) or will fail to continue the contract when it comes up for renewal.

The problem with the sudden imposition of a requirement like this is that certification cannot be earned on short notice by taking a few continuing medical education (CME) courses. In fact, some physicians well along in their careers would have trouble winning certification at all. In cases where the requirement applied to only a fraction of the physician's patients, she has had to arrange with a board-certified specialist to treat them.

Utilization Management

From the moment you begin treating the MCO's members, it will monitor your cost of care and evaluate your practice style. The deselection process will focus on high-cost practitioners who achieve no better results than their lower-cost peers do.

The process begins with a review of the services you provide in your office—usually reflected in professional fees and ancillary services. The scrutiny then moves to your utilization patterns outside the office. This will include items like number of hospitalizations and length of stay, referrals to specialists, drug and test prescriptions, ancillary services, and overall quantity of services provided per patient—all compared with similar physicians on the panel and in the community.

Another facet of utilization management concerns patient access to care. This will be measured by timeliness of appointment scheduling, response to clinical phone calls, appropriate and timely referrals to specialists, and interactions with ancillary service providers.

The affected physicians often argue that they were let go because a computer printout indicated that they had ordered more tests or performed more procedures than their colleagues had.

Patient Satisfaction

Responsible MCOs are concerned that cost-cutting efforts may lead to lower quality care and patient unhappiness. They begin controlling these factors by conducting random surveys of patients and then using the findings to determine your future value to the organization.

> **Practice Tip:** Carry out your own patient surveys. Do them at regular intervals (at least once a year, perhaps every six months), note the problems and suggestions that come up, and take immediate action to correct and implement solutions. Get to new patients as soon after their first visit as possible.

Be sure to use a valid survey instrument. You might want to get the advice of a consultant on this. The questions must be designed properly, the sample selected carefully, and the results interpreted accurately. The survey might be conducted by mail, by phone, or in person when patients are in the waiting room.

Well-planned and well-executed patient satisfaction surveys serve several valuable purposes.

1. They may contradict negative survey results presented to you by the MCO.
2. The very act of seeking patients' opinions will increase their satisfaction with your care.
3. They will tell you what areas of your practice need improvement.
4. They provide powerful support when negotiating a new contract with an MCO, perhaps justifying an exclusive arrangement with it.

Clinical Quality

The clinical results of a patient's care are the other side of the coin to patient satisfaction. Most MCOs are just beginning to examine the effectiveness of clinical decision making by individual physicians in a rigorous way. They are using criteria like these:

- The crudest measure of care quality is the incidence of *malpractice claims*. Regardless of the basis for them, if you experience too many such incidents—particularly if they involve the MCO in litigation, your deselection may be imminent.
- The traditional indicators of findings by various *peer review and credentialing committees* will also be watched closely by the MCO. Although the infractions may be minor, they may be more than other comparable physicians have and, therefore, sufficient basis for dropping you from the physician panel.
- Within the last five years, there has been a dramatic increase in research on the actual

clinical outcomes of different courses of treatment. Much of this winds up guiding the development of practice guidelines and clinical protocols. However, where the research methodology is refined enough to identify individual physicians, it can be used to screen out poorly performing physicians.

- The indicators of utilization, patient satisfaction, and clinical outcome, applied to individual physicians, sometimes are lumped under the term "*physician profiling.*"
- Within your lifetime, MCOs will begin using the ultimate physician evaluation tool—*functional status surveys*. These are questionnaires that measure how your patients feel and function before, during, and after treatment.[*] It is uncertain whether health status can be correlated with the quality of treatment. Other variables like patient compliance, health behavior, morbidity, and mental attitude all affect functional ability. Currently, functional status works best as a gross measure of how well a group of physicians is treating common diseases. It is not a statistically accurate way to distinguish among individual physicians. Because a few large employers are pushing the development of these surveys, wise physicians might begin collecting the necessary data voluntarily.

---

[*]There are two basic kinds of functional status surveys: generic and condition specific. Generic questionnaires measure a patient's overall health status. They are ideal for population screening and monitoring, comparing data across diagnoses, and measuring changes in patients with certain conditions. The most widely used of these instruments is the Short Form-36 (SF-36), a product of the Rand Corporation's Medical Outcomes Study. This 36-question survey asks patients about their physical functioning, pain, ability to work and participate in social activities, and emotional state. Condition-specific surveys target people with chronic diseases or people who have undergone certain procedures, like hip replacements. The most common condition-specific measures are the 18 Technology of Patient Experience (TyPE) surveys developed by the Health Outcomes Institute.

Geographic Location

As an MCO negotiates contracts with employers, often the result is enrollees who are concentrated in certain geographic areas of the community. Or, an MCO's growth plan may target neighborhoods with unique demographics. If you do not practice in the desired geographic location, you may have no value to the MCO. Certainly, if the MCO simply has excess physicians, this becomes an easy, nonthreatening rationale for dropping some of them.

Preventive Care

Under managed care, the goal is to provide as few medical services as possible, while still maintaining the patient's health at optimum levels. One of the ways of satisfying that apparent contradiction is preventive health measures carried out by your office. Modern MCOs will be expecting you to install procedures in your office to ensure that patients receive appropriate preventive screenings and services such as immunizations, mammograms, Pap smears, hemocults, cholesterol level checks, and early detection measures. They will want to see evidence of an effective recall system to ensure follow-ups after surgery and other treatments. Also consider offering patient education materials (video libraries, newsletters, and pamphlets) and programs (dietary, exercise, smoking cessation, risk screening, and stress reduction), and supporting community groups that do the same things. Your practice will stand out in the MCO's eyes.

> **Case Study:** An OB-GYN practice set up an incentive program to encourage prenatal patients to come in early in their pregnancies for checkups, with bonuses for those who never missed appointments. When the physician panel for the practice's primary MCO was reduced, this group stayed. For this reason alone? Maybe not. But it certainly provided an added reason for the MCO to keep them.

Attitude toward Managed Care

There are a couple facets to this criterion that MCOs use. On one hand, they are very concerned that none of their physicians criticize their organization or managed care concepts in general—certainly not to patients and also not in the media. They have a legal right to prevent their affiliates from disparaging their business reputation. Some MCO contracts will state this prohibition explicitly. Physicians have been dropped from MCO panels for openly attacking the organization.

This behavior must be clearly distinguished from a physician's right to explain to patients how a plan's particular brand of managed care differs from traditional fee-for-service medicine, and how it limits her clinical decision making. This can include disclosing incentive schemes, utilization control mechanisms, and benefit limits imposed by the MCO.

Many MCOs do not want to have their enrollees hearing this information any more than outright criticism. Some have included "gag" provisions in their contracts with physicians. There has been so much resentment (by doctors and their patients) of this stifling of communication in the physician-patient relationship that several states are considering laws prohibiting such gag language in contracts.[*]

One of the largest nationwide MCOs, U.S. Healthcare Inc., did include such contract language—until they canceled the contract of a well-known physician and prompted the AMA Council on Ethical and Judicial Affairs to declare gag clauses "unethical interference in the physician-patient relationship." A week later, the MCO announced elimination of all such contract provisions.

> **Practice Tip:** When evaluating a managed care contract, check for any language that inhibits your dialogue with patients. If necessary, have your attorney review it. If such provisions are included, determine if there is a law prohibiting them. If there is, raise the issue with the MCO. If the language is legally permissible, attempt to negotiate its softening or total elimination. If you cannot persuade the MCO to back off on its gag rule, reconsider affiliating with them.

On the other hand, MCOs are especially attracted to physician groups that appear to actually embrace the idea of managed care. They will notice this enthusiasm in statements the doctors make about the positive aspects of managed care, in the group's demonstrated proficiency in managing care, its implementation of a practice infrastructure that supports managed care, and its expressed desire to work with the MCO in a team and as partners. The absence of such eagerness may be just enough to tip you into the class of physicians to be deselected.

> **Note:** There is a positive side to knowing the likely criteria for deselection. By emphasizing and improving your performance along each of those parameters, you can boost your chances of gaining acceptance by an MCO physician panel and, once you are on, staying there.

A full list of the criteria used by MCOs might include the following:

Quality and Competence

- professional credentials
- failure to comply with quality assurance, peer review, and utilization procedures
- unprofessional conduct determined by the state physician licensing agency

---

[*]In January 1996, Massachusetts enacted a law that bars insurers and managed care companies from terminating or refusing to contract with a doctor solely because that physician has talked with patients about treatment options and/or terms of coverage. The law does not prohibit "disparagement" clauses, which bar doctors from denigrating an HMO to an enrollee, but provider groups think it offers them sufficient protection.

- dismissal by Health Care Financing Administration (HCFA) from Medicare or Medicaid participation
- failure to meet the MCO's separate credentialing requirements
- revocation or suspension of hospital privileges
- discrimination against plan members
- drug or alcohol abuse

Business and Economics

- cost-effective practice patterns
- subscriber access
- time schedules
- referrals
- consultations
- medication costs
- patient satisfaction measures
- use of emergency department
- patient disenrollment
- billing patterns

Data on these factors are gathered continuously and summarized in report cards or profiles for each physician. Exhibit 23–1 discusses board certification as a credentialing criterion.

COMMON SITUATIONS IN WHICH A PHYSICIAN MIGHT BE UNFAIRLY EXCLUDED FROM A PROVIDER OR MCO PANEL

The physician has a contract with the MCO that permits either party to end the contract without giving a reason. In a few egregious cases, the contract (dictated by the MCO) grants this right only to the MCO. As long as the MCO represents a relatively small fraction of the physician's revenues, the ability to leave without cause has some value, even if it is rarely exercised. Once the physician becomes largely dependent on the MCO, she has little incentive to withdraw her participation. On the other hand, an MCO is rarely so reliant on a particular physician that it cannot live without him. In other words, an apparently "evenhanded" right to terminate without cause really gives power primarily to the MCO.

Some physicians have been deselected by more than one of their plans. In areas heavily penetrated by managed care, this can leave a physician with virtually no patients—since none are available outside of the MCO.

If it becomes necessary to drop some physicians, many wish that the choice could be left to the patients. This is not likely to happen. Although the wiser MCOs measure and pay attention to patient satisfaction, that is not their leading criterion for judging doctors. Cost is.

In some cases, the MCO sends word of the deselection to the physician and his patients simultaneously. This is certainly a breach of simple professional and business courtesy that prevents the physician from breaking the news and explaining it to her patients. A few plans also have shown a penchant, when the patients call to ask why they can no longer see their doctor, for giving misleading reasons. Some have reported, falsely, that the physician has retired or is no longer in practice. This is grounds for a lawsuit for defamation or interference with business opportunity or pursuit of one's profession.

Although it is nearly impossible to get accurate data from the MCOs on their reasons for dropping physicians, the growing anecdotal evidence points to cost or economic efficiency as far and away the primary factor. There are frequent stories of physician deselection by MCOs that collected thorough economic information on their physicians but knew almost nothing about the quality of care they delivered.

In one case, an MCO bent on deselection ignored protests from employers and patients, and eventually accepted a loss of substantial premiums. When five physicians in Houston, Texas, were cut by a Prudential-owned MCO, the employer of many of their patients, the Apache Corporation, told Prudential that it would drop the insurer unless the doctors were reinstated. In response, Prudential gave up its contract with Apache and the $1 million in annual premiums it produced.

There is some evidence that physicians are invited into plans that consume their practices,

Exhibit 23–1 Board Certification as a Credentialing Criterion

A rapidly growing number of MCOs are including board certification by the American Board of Medical Specialties among their physician credentialing criteria. This is being done largely at the urging of employers and consumer groups, wishing to ensure maximum quality of care for enrollees.

Although some MCOs require board certification as an absolute prerequisite of physician panel membership, most simply accept "board certification or board eligibility" as one factor among others demonstrating clinical competence. For those physicians who are not certified, the "board eligible" option has some complications. Its meaning is unclear, sometimes referring to a physician who has been accepted to take the certification exam and, at other times, to any physician with enough experience to apply for certification. All specialty boards have ceased issuing the official designation "board eligible."

The courts have been generally willing to allow hospitals to use board certification as an alternative indicator of ability to provide quality care. It is best done by expressly relating it to care quality, writing it into organization bylaws, following a formal procedure that avoids arbitrary decisions, and being willing to accept alternatives where certification may be unreasonable (in a rural setting, for instance). The failure to take any of these precautions can be the basis for a physician's legal challenge of the requirement.

drain off their patients, and then discard the doctors.

A common pattern of the way MCOs contract with physicians is emerging. When an MCO moves into a new market, it signs up almost any interested physician without examining or questioning her credentials and experience (see Exhibit 23–2 for information on signing an exclusive contract with an MCO). The goal is twofold—to have sufficient physician resources to provide a full range of medical services and to be able to assure employers that their employees will have access to a wide selection of physicians, perhaps the employee's very own. Once the MCO is established in the marketplace, once it feels that it has solid relationships with the employers, and once the managed care competition heats up, the fine-tuning of the physician panel begins.

Sometimes the tuning is not so fine. Physicians have been dropped in such large numbers that it is hard to believe that the choices were based on thoughtful evaluations. For example, in 1992, MetLife dropped 1,100 physicians from its plan in southern Florida. The following year, when Blue Cross/Blue Shield in Washington, D.C., set up its first managed care entity, a physician provider organization (PPO), it excluded a third of the 8,800 physicians participating in its indemnity plan.

Deselection is also heightened as an issue by the heated competition among HMOs. They are conducting price wars to grab market share, and their profit margins are squeezed in the process. They are looking for every opportunity to cut costs.

It is not just profit-obsessed MCOs that are terminating physician contracts. Once the health plans get their "incentives aligned" with an affiliated physician group, that group is often drawn into the winnowing process. When TakeCare of Colorado wanted to cut its 1,400 specialists in the Denver market back to a 1,000, they turned to the Columbine Medical Group, a physician-run IPA contracting with the plan to provide health care. They collaborated in devising a set of deselection criteria that then were applied by the physicians themselves to their colleagues.

ACCREDITATION REQUIREMENTS FOR CREDENTIALING PROCEDURES

Left to their own devices, some MCOs might make their selection and deselection decisions on the basis of impulsive, ad hoc reasoning. Most will use accurate data, rational business-related grounds, and systematic procedures to arrive at those decisions. Up until now, however, very few

Exhibit 23–2 Signing an Exclusive Contract with an MCO

As managed care competition increases, health plans will want to concentrate on relationships with their most loyal and cost-effective providers. The way they will do this is through exclusive arrangements with physicians and physician groups. They will put pressure on their contracted IPAs to form very tight, closed, and controlled panels. The end goal of the MCO is to minimize costs; it hopes to achieve this through an exclusive arrangement with a group of physicians in particular specialties. In return for exclusive access to the MCO's members, the group subjects itself to fairly rigorous cost controls.

For the physicians, there are benefits and hazards in these arrangements. A big plus is the sheer administrative simplicity and economy of dealing with a single organization rather than several. Frequently, because the physicians are giving up all opportunities with other MCOs, the primary health plan is willing to pay extra for the exclusive relationship with them. This normally will take the form of higher capitation or other reimbursement. Some other possible "goodies" to look or ask for are

- shares of stock in the MCO

- electronic hookups that reduce the delay in precertifications
- on-line services to verify patient eligibility and benefits

However, these benefits last only as long as the contract. And, if the MCO fails to renew a couple years later, the physicians will be in a real predicament. They will have lost all their other MCO contacts and may find that the other plans have signed up all the physicians they need.

The exclusive arrangement should be viewed as the codification of a true strategic partnership between the physicians and the MCO. It should have a term of at least three to five years, with strong inhibitions on early termination by either party.

If this new relationship is a long-term partnership, it is important to ask some key questions at the very start—before you sign. What are the long-range strategic objectives of the MCO? How does the exclusive arrangement serve those objectives? Who are the lead decision makers in the MCO? What is their experience and reputation for working with physicians?

MCOs have been willing to disclose their decision making processes to anyone, least of all the physicians affected by them. Instead, physicians were told on short notice that they had been deselected. If they were given a reason, it was too late to do anything about it. Finally, some relief is in sight.

There are three private organizations vying to be the primary authority for accrediting MCOs. They are the National Committee for Quality Assurance (NCQA), the Joint Commission on the Accreditation of Healthcare Organizations (the Joint Commission), and the Utilization Review Accreditation Commission (URAC). Each has published standards that an MCO, or any other qualifying entity, must satisfy in order to be accredited. All three sets of standards address the issue of physician credentialing in very similar and responsible ways.

These accrediting standards help physicians in two ways. If the MCO desires the increasing essential accreditation, it must implement the credentialing procedure and criteria requirements. Those requirements then inform the physician of how he can expect to be treated by the MCO and what rights he will have if deselected. Most of these credentialing standards are included in the section below in the "Model Physician Credentialing Procedure."

STATE LAWS DEFINING CREDENTIALING PROCEDURES

In response to physician complaints about unfair credentialing procedures, several states have enacted laws stipulating how such procedures must operate. Here are some typical provisions:

- Upon request, HMOs and PPOs must disclose to physicians their written application procedures and qualification requirements for contracting with them. (Texas)[4]
- Carriers offering managed care plans must credential physicians on the basis of objective standards disclosed to physicians when they apply. (Maine)[5]
- Upon request, an insurer must give a physician a written statement of the terms and conditions upon which it will enter into an agreement with her. (Indiana)[6]
- Upon the request of a current or prospective physician member, a health care service contractor must explain the criteria it uses for contracting with physicians for medical services. (Oregon)[7]
- A health plan's credentialing criteria must be based on input from providers credentialed in the plan. (Rhode Island)[8]
- In New York State
  - MCOs must consult with "appropriately qualified" health care professionals in developing their qualification standards.
  - MCOs must regularly inform physicians of data used to evaluate them.
  - MCOs must consult with health care professionals in developing methodologies to analyze provider profiling data.
  - If an MCO uses profiling data to measure physician performance, it must compare them with stated criteria and an appropriate group of physicians using similar treatment modalities serving a comparable population.
  - MCOs must reveal the profiling data to the affected physicians.
  - MCOs must give physicians the chance to explain aspects of their practices that might affect the profiling data and to collaborate with the MCO to improve performance.[9]
- If an MCO uses economic factors in credentialing, it must make adjustments for case mix, severity of illness, patient age, and other variables that might explain cost variations. (Rhode Island)[10]
- An MCO must publicly notify physicians within its geographic service area of its intention to expand its physician network so they may have the opportunity to apply for membership. (Rhode Island)[11]

The National Association of Insurance Commissioners (NAIC) has published a model law that would affect MCOs—the Health Care Professional Credentialing Verification Model Act. As a model act, it has no effect unless and until it is adopted by the legislatures in individual states. The act requires that MCOs:

1. Establish written policies and procedures for credentialing verification of health care professionals.
2. Apply those policies and procedures consistently.
3. Set up a credentialing verification committee composed of physicians and other licensed professionals to review the verification information gathered and make decisions on the basis of it.
4. Keep records of the credentialing process for a period specified by each state.
5. Give physicians the opportunity to review and correct information submitted in support of their applications.

These model laws are frequently the basis for legislation in specific states. Look for activity on this issue in your state's legislature. If you are more concerned or ambitious, use the model act in a lobbying effort with your representatives.

SOURCES OF CREDENTIALING INFORMATION

There are some critical questions about the sources of credentialing information used by MCOs in making their decisions. When gathering this information, an MCO can consult either primary or secondary sources. Primary sources have the original data on the physician's particular credential—for instance, the medical school that granted his medical degree, or the insurance company that provides his malpractice insurance coverage. Secondary sources collect the required information from several primary sources, package it, and pass it on to the MCO. Primary sources are inevitably more accurate than secondary.

Historically, hospitals checked with primary sources when they checked at all. With a renewed concern for quality, the thoroughness and accuracy of credentialing information are an important matter for MCOs. A new industry of aggressive credentialing organizations has sprung up to meet the needs of MCOs for this kind of information. In addition to conducting the traditional background checks on a physician's education, training, licensure, and malpractice history, these for-profit companies are also looking into physicians' personal bankruptcies, child support payments, and tax records. One of the largest of these credential verification organizations is Healthcare Credentials Management Services, Inc. in San Diego, California.

These private organizations add to the number of places where sensitive and potentially damaging information about doctors is stored. There are also the AMA's Physician Master File and it's new American Medical Accreditation Program (AMAP) (see Exhibit 23–3), the several state medical licensure boards, the two programs operated by the Federation of State Medical Boards— the Federation Credential Verification Services and the Action Data Bank, the federal government's National Practitioner Data Bank, and the Official Directory of Board Certified Specialties maintained by the American Board of Medical Specialties. In addition, there is a major push to make at least some of these data available to the public. Basic credentialing information on physicians in Florida and Massachusetts is available on the Internet.

Today, an MCO is likely to go to one of these outside organizations for a basic package of credentialing information. It then adds its own internal data on patient satisfaction, performance evaluation, utilization rates and clinical out-

comes, complaints, and any other factors it considers relevant. On the basis of all this material, the MCO decides whether to initially contract with, later renew the contract with, or deselect a physician.

With so much vital information passing through so many different hands, there is a potential for errors being made and inaccurate data entering a physician's file. The disclosure of confidential information to the wrong people is also a possibility. A savvy physician will take steps to minimize these risks.

1. If an unpleasant event is about to occur in your career, such as disciplinary action by a hospital, try to negotiate a resolution that will keep it from showing up in your record. Quality-related discipline must be reported to the National Practitioner Data Bank (NPDB). Consider resigning from the medical staff before the peer review investigation begins. Persuade the peer review/disciplinary committee to sanction or suspend you for less than the 30-day minimum that triggers the NPDB reporting requirement.

2. When something negative does appear in your record, do not try to hide it. Certainly do not lie about it. Tell the MCO about it before they discover it through their credentialing research. Seek a personal interview with their medical director or chief contracting officer to explain your side of the story.

3. When a permanent unfavorable report is to be entered into your record in the NPDB, you will receive 30 days' notice. Take full advantage of the opportunity to challenge or correct this decision. The NPDB has, on occasion, committed errors, such as confusing two physicians with the same names. Even if the report entry cannot be prevented, you will be permitted to include in the record your version of the events.

4. Most of the organizations that collect personal information for credentialing purposes allow physicians to check the

Exhibit 23–3 American Medical Accreditation Program (AMAP)

There is a more physician-friendly alternative that gives the individual doctor a bit more control over the information-gathering process. In 1997, the AMA rolled out the American Medical Accreditation Program (AMAP), designed as an all-purpose source of accreditation for physicians. Its aim is to be for doctors what the Joint Commission is for hospitals and the NCQA is for MCOs. Here's how it works:

A physician joins the program voluntarily and pays a fee of between $50 and $150. The AMA begins with the information on the physician that it already has in its 90-year-old master file. Next, AMAP officials visit and examine the physician's practice setting. While there, they review a mix of patient charts. The physician's record then can be filled out with information on economic ratings, participation in peer review, self-assessment exams, and findings from the site visits. If the physician has had her license revoked, suspended or

surrendered, or been the subject of other disciplinary action, this fact is noted in the record. However, no details are offered. If someone accessing the record wants more information, he or she is directed to the organization that provided the original information.

When a physician seeks admission to an MCO's provider panel, she is able to cite her AMAP accreditation standing and refer the MCO to AMAP for further details.

The goal of the AMAP program is twofold. One is to offer a physician accreditation service performed by a relatively disinterested party (the AMA) rather than the organization (an MCO or large group practice) that is considering employing or contracting with the physician. The other is to promote a new accreditation model—one that demonstrates how "good" a physician is instead of focusing solely on his mistakes and bad qualities.

contents of their records and to take steps to correct errors. It would be a good idea to contact these sources periodically to find out what information they are keeping on you.

5. When you first contact, or are contacted by, an MCO or other contract partner, along with other information requests, ask about the criteria and procedure that will be followed in deciding whether to admit you to its provider panel. Once you have this information, figure out how to position your practice most attractively in light of the criteria and look for procedural opportunities to present your case to the decision makers. If you have some time before you will actually apply, use the criteria as guidelines for upgrading pieces of your practice.

6. Once you are seriously negotiating for admission to the MCO, ask further about the criteria and procedure by which the MCO will decide whether to renew your

contract and, possibly, deselect you during the term of the contract. Express a strong interest in building a long-term partnership with the MCO by always exceeding its expectations of you.

7. After you have become a member of the MCO's provider panel, strive to do two things: (1) Through formal performance evaluation or other means, learn how well you are meeting the MCO's expectations and work to correct identified shortcomings, and (2) on your own initiative, look for ways to make greater contributions to the MCO's success, rendering yourself indispensable.

ACCREDITATION REQUIREMENTS FOR DESELECTION PROCEDURES

The accreditation standards issued by the NCQA, the Joint Commission, and URAC all address the issue of physician deselection, though rather more briefly than the broader issue of credentialing. The NCQA standards are a good example. According to them, an MCO must

- Have policies and procedures defining how they may change a physician's conditions of participation as a result of quality-related performance, including ending participation entirely.
- Define the corrective actions it will take before deselection.
- Offer the affected provider a process for appealing the deselection decision.
- Give the physician notice of quality-related deselection decisions and available appeal process.

Unfortunately, the NCQA has made clear that these requirements apply only in cases of quality-related issues with a physician. It explicitly does not forbid "without cause" deselection of physicians.

DESELECTION PROTECTIONS OF THE HEALTH CARE QUALITY IMPROVEMENT ACT

Some valuable protections are available under the Health Care Quality Improvement Act (HCQIA) for physicians disciplined or deselected for reasons concerned with "competence or conduct affecting patient care." In order for other physicians to qualify for limited immunity from lawsuit for helping conduct professional peer review, that review must be carried out

- in the reasonable belief that it was in furtherance of quality health care
- after reasonable effort is made to learn the facts of the matter
- after adequate notice and hearing have been given to the affected physician, as well as any other procedures that are fair to him under the circumstances
- in the reasonable belief that the final action taken is justified by the facts learned and the hearing procedures conducted

If the physicians responsible for the peer review do not care about immunity, they are free

to ignore these procedural requirements. The entire act, and these requirements in particular, apply only to actions taken on the basis of quality-related issues. It has not been established whether the HCQIA should also pertain to matters such as outcome measures, credentialing criteria, and compliance with utilization standards or recordkeeping requirements, which are less directly related to "competence or conduct affecting patient care."

Where the HCQIA does apply, it requires the following specific procedures:

- A physician must receive written notice when a professional review action against him has been proposed.
- The notice must include a statement of the reasons for the proposed action.
- If the physician requests a hearing, he must be notified on the place, date, and time of the hearing, which must occur within the next 30 days, as well as the names of witnesses expected to testify in support of the proposed action.
- The health care entity has a choice of a hearing before an arbitrator mutually acceptable to it and the physician, a hearing officer appointed by the entity, or a panel of individuals appointed by the entity.
- During the hearing, the physician my be represented by anyone of his choosing including an attorney, may have a record made, may call and examine witnesses, may present relevant evidence, and may present a written statement.
- After the hearing, the physician must be given the written recommendation and reasons of the hearing official(s) and the written decision and reasons of the entity.

STATE LAWS REGULATING NON–QUALITY-RELATED DESELECTION DECISIONS

Quality-related credentialing and deselection is pretty well covered by the accreditation standards of the NCQA, the Joint Commission, and URAC, and the terms of the HCQIA. Where a physician runs into trouble is with deselection for reasons unrelated to quality, usually what would be called business or economic reasons. This is where the concept of "economic credentialing" becomes an issue.

There is little dispute over the desirability of removing physicians delivering poor quality care. There is a great deal of controversy over the practice of dismissing physicians from provider panels for excessive utilization or costs, or admitting them to the panel in the first place on the basis of likely financial performance. Numerous MCOs have attempted to minimize the fuss by simply giving no reason for a physician's dismissal—a so-called "without cause" termination. Let's see what protections are available to physicians in those situations.

First, your relationship with the MCO is primarily a matter between two private parties. As such, it is defined almost entirely by the language of the explicit written contract that you signed with the MCO. Any problems that come up must be resolved within those terms. If an issue arises that is not covered by the contract, the parties are generally free to act unilaterally.

Every MCO-physician contract, however, does cover the selection/deselection process—to one degree or another. Normally, it describes two methods of contract termination. The MCO may terminate its relationship with the physician "with" or "without" cause. The "with cause" provision defines the acceptable causes. The MCO usually has to give longer notice when terminating without cause than when it has a good reason—say, 90 days versus 30 days. The physician may end the contract without cause under the same terms as the MCO. The physician customarily is not given the option of terminating for specific causes; though, as a practical matter, any substantial contract breach by the MCO will justify the physician's withdrawal from the contract.* If the equity in this language seems unbalanced, in favor of the MCO, it is because the MCO has all the economic and bargaining power. Only if you are a large group of physicians critical to the MCO's market success do

you have a chance of negotiating a mutually fair deselection process.

This kind of contract language permits you to challenge a deselection on the grounds that the MCO failed to follow the terms of the contract. If it attempted to deselect for cause, the cause it used was not legitimate or not one of those stated in the contract. In deselecting you, it did not give the required advance notice.

When deselecting physicians simply to shrink their provider panels, MCOs usually really on the "without cause" option. They have little to lose. The physician is bound by her ethics and other provisions in the contract to continue treating patients currently in her charge. Meanwhile, the MCO has at least 90 days to restructure assignments for its physician panel.

Second, if the business-related deselection can somehow be tied to quality concerns, the physician may be able to take advantage of all the pro-

---

*This is the termination language from a typical MCO-physician contract:

Termination by Physician or MCO without Cause. Either Party may terminate this agreement without cause at any time upon ninety (90) days prior written notice given to the other party.

Termination by MCO for Cause. MCO shall have the right to terminate this agreement for cause upon thirty (30) days prior notice given to the physician under any of the following circumstances:

a) for physician's material noncompliance with any policies and procedures established by the MCO regarding the remittance of any fees, dues, or assessments received from enrollees for covered services;

b) for physician's failure to meet the qualifications and requirements established in the MCO's articles of incorporation, bylaws, or policies and procedures created by the MCO for its physician providers;

c) for physician's material noncompliance with this agreement;

d) for physician's having engaged in conduct inconsistent with or potentially detrimental to the delivery of good quality patient care or contrary to the best interests of the MCO; or

e) for physician's excessive or inappropriate pattern of utilization, which may be contrary to the delivery of cost-efficient, good quality medical care.

> **Practice Tip**: If meaningful contract negotiations with an MCO are possible, press for termination only for certain stated reasons. Seek to prevent the MCO from terminating you for no reason at all. Whatever the termination terms, ask for the longest advance notice period possible. Six months would be great. No matter what, make sure that you are familiar with the details of the MCO's deselection procedure before you sign the contract. And remember, if it is not included in the contract directly or by reference, the procedure can be changed unilaterally by the MCO at any time.

tections described above. Often this is possible. For instance, it might be argued that utilization requirements are employed under capitation to make sure that there are adequate funds to provide quality care to the entire patient population covered by the capitation fee.

Third, while the courts have generally approved credentialing and exclusive contracting decisions by hospitals on purely economic grounds, they simultaneously insist that the decisions treat physicians fairly and follow established procedures.

Fourth, if an organization has defined procedures for deselection or nonrenewal in its bylaws or contracts with physicians, it is absolutely bound to them. The bylaws or contracts may serve as the legal basis for a court action by physicians against the organization.

Fifth, approximately half the states have enacted "any willing provider" (AWP) laws. Generally, these require that an MCO admit to its provider panel any provider who agrees to its terms and conditions of participation. As a practical matter, these statutes offer little help to physicians fearing MCO rejection. Most of them are designed to provide relief for pharmacists and few actually include physicians. The "terms and conditions" that a physician must satisfy to gain participation through the AWP plans can easily be read to encompass the kinds of economic credentialing that bothered physicians in the first place.

The majority of the courts that have considered the question conclude that the Employee Retirement Income Security Act (ERISA) preempts the enforcement of these statutes.[12] While there was a surge of legislative enthusiasm for AWP laws in the early 1990s, only two were enacted in 1995 and one in 1996. Attention has turned from the use of such laws to statutes promising patients direct access to desired physicians and due process for physicians in danger of deselection.

Sixth, in a case involving a New York State surcharge on hospitals,[13] the U.S. Supreme Court, for the first time, showed a willingness to limit the scope of ERISA preemption. If this trend is followed, there may be greater freedom for attempts by state legislatures to protect the livelihood interests of physicians.

Seventh, there are common law doctrines that may afford some protection for deselected physicians. It is a basic rule of contract law that the parties to an agreement must exercise "good faith and fair dealing" in their behavior under the contract. In the case of *Harper v. Healthsource New Hampshire, Inc.,*[14] the New Hampshire Supreme Court interpreted this rule to mean that a physician deselected, with or without cause, is entitled to a review of the MCO's deselection decision. If there is a reason for the deselection, the physician may argue that he does not truly satisfy the reason. If no reason is given for the deselection, the physician may question whether the decision was in bad faith or actually for reasons contrary to public policy. Not all states' courts are as eager to extend the rule of "good faith and fair dealing" to new areas like economic credentialing of physicians by MCOs. But, when a bellwether state like New Hampshire starts, other states are more likely to follow.

A smaller number of states recognize a common law right to due process where important economic interests are at stake. The landmark court decision in this area was the case of *Delta Dental Plan of California v. Banasky.*[15] There, after the plan unilaterally modified the fee schedule of two dentists, the court held that they had a right to fair procedures protecting them from arbitrary exclusion or expulsion from private organizations that control important economic interests.

ANTITRUST IMPLICATIONS OF AN MCO'S EFFORTS TO HIRE THE BEST PHYSICIANS

MCOs can usually choose whether or not to contract with a particular physician or physician group, without risk of violating the antitrust laws. Nonetheless, there are several scenarios in which antitrust problems could develop.

- If an MCO is the primary competitor in the local managed care market and excludes a physician because she participates on another MCO panel.
- If the MCO or network is sponsored by a hospital that is dominant in its area, with an overwhelming market share. It might run into problems if it tried to exclude a physician from its plan who also operates a clinic or other health care facility that competes with the hospital.
- If the MCO is controlled by independently practicing physicians, either because they own it or dominate its board. If that organization excluded a physician for arbitrary or anticompetitive reasons (because he competed with some of the controlling doctors), it could run into an antitrust challenge. However, for the challenge to succeed, the MCO would have to be so large that the exclusion would make it nearly impossible for the physician to practice medicine in the community.
- If the MCO is thoroughly controlled by local physicians, has enrolled a majority of all physicians in the area, and excludes a physician primarily because she also participates in another MCO, it will be at greatest legal risk.
- If a physician group dominates its specialty in the market and participates in several MCOs there, its demands for exclusive relationships with those MCOs may be viewed

as monopolistic exclusion of other physicians in that specialty.
- If the same physician group signed a long-term exclusive contract with a single MCO that represents a large share of the market's potential enrollees, antitrust concerns could also arise.

These are a few of the most likely antitrust physician exclusion scenarios. These cases are very fact specific, depending on how the market is defined, the size of the MCO or physician group in that market, the actual power that it wields, ease of entry into the market, and motives for the actions being challenged.

The antitrust implications of the deselection of a MCO panel physician (in contrast with the initial deselection) emerge under similar circumstances.

As a general rule, antitrust law does not require that an MCO observe any sort of due process when terminating a panel physician. Unless it has agreed by contract to do so, the MCO is not required to give advance notice of the termination, have a good reason for the termination, disclose the reason, or allow an appeal of the termination decision. These are some of the situations that may set off antitrust alarms:

- If a market-dominant MCO drops a physician for joining another plan.
- If a hospital-owned MCO deselected a physician because he competed with the hospital for patients not covered by managed care.
- If an MCO gives in to threats from a group of its physicians and drops one of their competitors, it has participated in an antitrust conspiracy.

Practice Tip: If you are rejected or deselected by an MCO or physician group under circumstances that resemble any of these scenarios, consult an attorney skilled in antitrust law. If you are a leader in an MCO or physician group with substantial market power, talk with an antitrust attorney when you start designing a deselection process.

RECOMMENDATIONS TO ENSURE SELECTION AND PREVENT DESELECTION

It is obvious that many of the above legal protections are not currently available in all states. Furthermore, it is preferable to avoid the expense and trauma of prolonged litigation if at all possible. Therefore, the wisest course of action for a physician is to be admitted to the provider panel of the MCO she wishes, to repeatedly have her participation contract renewed, and to never be considered for deselection. Easier said than done. Here are some tips for becoming and staying affiliated with an MCO.

Before Applying for MCO Panel Membership

1. Start preparing yourself and your practice for a life under managed care (see Chapter 7, "Step One: Preparing Your Practice for Operation under Managed Care"). Make as much progress as you can in setting up new systems, gathering relevant data, and modifying your practice style.
2. With the best data you can put together, prepare to demonstrate your effectiveness at delivering medical care in the high-quality, cost-effective style sought by most MCOs. In particular, try to provide objective evidence of your utilization rates, clinical outcomes, patient access, and patient satisfaction.
3. When you have focused on a particular MCO, obtain as much information as you can about the physician selection criteria and procedures it uses. Get this from the MCO, government regulatory and financing agencies, and other providers who have dealt with the MCO.
4. Get a sense of the kind of physician the MCO seems to be looking for and plan how to present or package your practice to fit the MCO's requirements as closely as possible. If there is too great a gap between what the MCO wants and the kind of practitioner you know yourself to be, you probably should skip that MCO if you can.
5. Before doing anything else, prepare a strategic plan of which a key component is the decision to build long-term relationships with MCOs and adapt your practice style to the needs of managed care.
6. Prepare a well-researched list of the reasons why you wish to join this particular MCO. Consult with colleagues and advisors about the kinds of reasons that appeal to MCOs. Rehearse your presentation of those reasons until it is persuasive and believable. Do not pretend. If you cannot see good reasons for partnering with an MCO, it may be time for a new career direction.

During Contract Negotiations

1. Explain the features of your practice that make you valuable to the MCO and that distinguish you from other similar physicians.
2. Fully express your positive, constructive attitudes toward managed care, your desire to develop the skills of a proficient care manager, and your desire to build a partnership with the MCO.
3. Discretely raise the issue of what criteria and procedure the MCO uses in selecting physicians for its provider panel and under what circumstances it might choose to deselect you or not renew your contract. This will sound more palatable if put in the context of your wish to meet the MCO's needs from you in order to develop a long-term working relationship.
4. Under no circumstances let the negotiations or the subsequent association evolve into anything like an adversarial relationship. Get clearly in your mind that you and the MCO are partners, collaborators, a team, seeking win-win solutions to any problems that arise.
5. Read the contract with great thoroughness. Be sure you understand what you are

promising to do for the MCO. For instance, if you agree to perform services for which you are not qualified, you may end up performing them ineptly or incurring excess cost through overuse of specialists.

After Admission to the MCO Provider Panel

1. Look for opportunities to accept new responsibility, acquire new skills, and in any way make yourself indispensable to the MCO.
2. Look for and welcome feedback from the MCO on how well you are meeting its various performance expectations. If it is not forthcoming, ask for feedback until you understand clearly how you stand with the MCO. This is essential. It must be ongoing. The goal is never to be surprised by an MCO decision to deselect or nonrenew.
3. Meet as regularly as you can with the medical director. Learn what he likes to see in his physicians and what he feels about your performance. Communicate to him your enthusiasm and commitment to the organization.
4. Seek assignment to peer review, utilization management, or quality assurance committees. Not only does this demonstrate your desire to be a member of the MCO "team," it also gives you an inside look at the systems that lead to deselection and nonrenewal decisions.
5. Whenever a shortcoming is called to your attention, jump on it. Look for every possible way to correct and improve your performance. Request advice from your superiors. Ask to attend continuing medical education (CME) programs that will help upgrade your skills. The MCO will be more forgiving of a physician who is going all out to meet its expectations.
6. In the course of trying to satisfy the MCO, do not compromise your own principles, particularly with regard to patient care and patient rights.

7. Arrange to receive from the MCO copies of the same data it relies on to evaluate you. Review them promptly and point out any inaccuracies or discrepancies you discover.
8. Give high priority to maintaining high patient satisfaction, as measured in whatever survey instrument the MCO uses. Very high patient approval ratings will make it more difficult for the MCO to dismiss even a high-utilizer physician.
9. When you have problems with the MCO (as you surely will), present your case in a cooperative, professional manner with the intention of finding a joint solution. Do not simply complain; offer solutions. Aim to build a reputation as a team player.

After Notification of Imminent Deselection or Nonrenewal of Contract

1. Begin to take notes about everything you and the MCO do.
2. Keep and read carefully every communication from the MCO about the deselection or nonrenewal.
3. Reread carefully the relevant language of the contract with the MCO and any other materials describing the deselection or nonrenewal criteria and procedure, particularly the appeal process.
4. Review the reasons given for your dismissal and compare them with your understanding of your performance. Check to see if the MCO is using the same data that they have been sending to you.
5. Make a basic decision about whether the dismissal is justified. If it seems unjustified, decide whether it is such a miscarriage of justice that you will appeal the decision.
6. Closely track the MCO's actions to make sure it follows all the terms of the dismissal and appeal procedure that was described to you.

7. Make note of the procedural steps that require or allow action on your part.

8. In conversations with appropriate MCO officials, decide whether it might be possible to resolve the matter through informal negotiations.

9. If it appears that there is a major conflict between you and the MCO, one that requires implementation of the formal appeal procedure, seriously consider hiring an advisor to work with you in planning and executing the appeal. This person may or may not be an attorney and may or may not represent you at the hearing.

10. Plan a step-by-step strategy for reversing the MCO's decision, including possible legal action if the internal appeal fails.

11. Take full advantage of every opportunity for persuasion afforded you by the appeal procedure. Present a written statement of your position and arguments. Call witnesses who will support your arguments. Question the witnesses called by the MCO. Introduce any other evidence that might strengthen your case. Insist that written notes be taken of all proceedings. Demand written statements of the decisions and reasons at each level of appeal. Pursue the appeal process as far as it will go, or as far as it makes sense.

12. Once you have exhausted all the avenues of remedy and lost, put the matter as completely behind you as possible, avoid carrying grudges against the particular MCO or managed care in general and move on to the next best options for your career.

13. If the MCO's case for dismissal against you is a close one, attempt to negotiate an outcome that does not stigmatize you in subsequent efforts to join other MCOs. Moderate the seriousness of the allegations about your performance. Characterize the dismissal rationale to make reporting to the NPDB unnecessary. Do not try to threaten or bribe; do not ask the MCO to lie about what happened.

MODEL PHYSICIAN CREDENTIALING PROCEDURE

What follows is a nearly ideal credentialing/deselection mechanism to be implemented by an MCO, hospital, or large group practice. It is ideal from the viewpoint of the physician. There is probably not a single delivery organization in the country that currently operates a system like this, although the law and public and physician pressures are pushing in that direction.

This model can be used in several ways. It is a benchmark against which to measure the credentialing systems of organizations you are considering joining. The key features of the model might be good bargaining points in negotiations with the organization. Be aware that, without any external statutory mandate, the willingness of the MCO to include provisions like this in the contract depend on its general good will, its view of its "partnership" with its physicians, and the bargaining power of particular physician groups. As a practical matter, the MCO is not likely to agree to these protections for only a few of its physicians. Either it will see the value in offering due process to all its doctors or none of them will receive it. Of course, it is possible that a single, substantial physician group—perhaps a large IPA—could be so important to the MCO's strategy that it would accept its demands for some due process procedures. If, someday, you are in a position of leadership or influence in a provider organization, the model features could serve as guidelines for the credentialing you will have to do.

At the Time of Application to the Provider Panel

1. The acceptance or rejection of application to join the physician panel is based on objective criteria related to a physician's ability to meet the organization's expectations for quality care, resource utilization, personal interaction, and other reasonable performance standards.

2. The process of applying these criteria follows a rational, systematic procedure that ensures uniform treatment of all applicants.

3. Upon written request from anyone, including interested physicians, the organization provides a full description of the criteria and procedure employed in credentialing physicians.

4. In preparing and approving the criteria and procedure, the organization seeks and considers input from a committee of its participating physicians.

5. The criteria and procedure are approved by the appropriate governing body of the organization.

6. The organization discloses the sources, primary and secondary, it uses to verify credentials in order to permit affected physicians to challenge and correct erroneous information found there.

7. The organization informs the physician when it learns of information about her which does not meet its credentialing criteria.

8. The credentialing procedure includes site visits to all otherwise unaccredited sites where medical care is provided (i.e., separate physician medical offices).

9. The physician has an opportunity to contradict information or reports that disqualify him from admission to the provider panel. This opportunity does not consist of a formal appeal procedure.

10. Physicians are given the reasons when their panel applications are rejected.

During the Term of the Physician's Participation with the Organization

11. After a physician is admitted to the provider panel but before he has signed a participation contract, the organization discloses to him the following features of the system it uses to evaluate his performance and decide whether to renew his contract

or even deselect him during the term of the contract:

- the criteria and performance measures that will be the basis of ongoing evaluations
- how and where the data will be gathered to support those criteria and measures
- how frequently the physician will receive copies of the data being used by the organization
- how frequently, in what format, and from whom the physician will receive formal feedback from the organization on how well she is meeting its expectations
- the minimum standards the physician must meet in order to ensure renewal of the contract
- the minimum standards the physician must satisfy to avoid midcontract deselection
- specific performance levels or scenarios that are likely to result in contract nonrenewal and deselection
- the opportunity that the physician will have to respond to claims that he has not met the organization's standards or criteria
- the appeal procedure available to the physician whose contract is not renewed or who is deselected during the term of the contract
- the corrective measures the organization may take to improve the physician's performance before deselecting him or failing to renew his contract

12. The organization relies on written, objective criteria in deciding whether to deselect physicians or refuse to renew their contracts.

13. The organization employs a vigorous and systematic internal decision-making procedure in deselecting or nonrenewing its physicians.

14. In preparing and approving the criteria and procedure, the organization seeks and con-

siders input from a committee that includes participating physicians.

15. When deselection or nonrenewal seems imminent, the organization provides the affected physician with adequate notice of the fact, the reasons for the contemplated dismissal, and, where feasible, the opportunity to correct the problem behavior and retain his or her position on the provider panel.

16. The organization does not deselect or nonrenew a physician without having a reason and being willing to explain that reason.

At the Time of Deselection or Nonrenewal of the Contract

17. Once the organization has made the decision to deselect or nonrenew a physician, it notifies her of the fact, states the reasons for the decision, and explains the procedure by which she may appeal the decision.

18. The organization offers a procedure of at least two steps that a physician may use to appeal deselection and nonrenewal decisions. This appeal procedure includes the following features:
    • The physician receives a full explanation of the procedure.
    • If the physician requests a hearing, he receives notice of the place, date, and time at least 30 days before the scheduled date of the hearing.
    • The physician is informed of all his rights at the hearing.
    • The physician is informed of the nature of the hearing (e.g., arbitrator, hearing officer, panel of individuals) and the steps that will be followed.
    • The physician receives advance notice of the persons who will appear as witnesses for the organization.
    • The physician has the opportunity to call his own witnesses and to question the organization's witnesses.

    • The physician may be represented at the hearing by a person of his choosing, including an attorney.
    • The physician may present relevant evidence at the hearing.
    • The physician may insist that a written record of the hearing be prepared.
    • The physician receives a written statement of the decisions reached at each stage of the appeal procedure, along with the reasons for those decisions.

19. These rights and procedures apply whether the deselection or nonrenewal is for quality or economic reasons.

20. These rights and procedures may be abridged in cases of imminent harm to patients, a licensing board's action that restricts the physician's authority to practice, or fraud or malfeasance.

21. The organization does not deselect or nonrenew a physician in retaliation for her exercise of her rights, including advocacy on behalf of a patient's welfare.

CASE STUDY: MEDICA CHOICE

This 5,000-physician IPA in Minneapolis accepts almost any physician with a clean record unless she belongs to a group whose other members do not wish to join. All the doctors in the IPA are paid on a discounted fee-for-service (FFS) basis with a 15 percent withhold. They earn the withhold by staying within 20 percent of the utilization norm for all the IPA doctors for that year.

If a doctor's utilization pattern is more than 20 percent outside the norm for others in her specialty for three years running, she is required to pay a stiff financial penalty each year until she brings her utilization back within the acceptable range. If a doctor cannot accomplish that, she would usually resign rather than continue to pay the penalty.

This IPA implements a number of other progressive utilization management procedures, including

- It reviews the utilization of primary care physicians annually.
- Outlier physicians receive a copy of their utilization profiles.
- An IPA administrator also visits them to discuss improvement strategies.
- Physicians are dismissed only for fraud and abuse, or failure to "correct their errors."
- Dismissed physicians can appeal to an IPA board, half of whom are doctors.

- Credentialing, utilization review, and disputes with administration are peer reviewed.

> **Lesson:** If you have a choice and all other factors are equal, choose to affiliate with a traditional MCO over one owned by an insurance company.

REFERENCES

1. American Medical Association, *Economic Credentialing (193)* (Report of the Hospital/Medical Staff Section Governing Council Report Q, Chicago, 1993).
2. 211 N.E.2d 253 (1965), *cert denied*, 383 U.S. 946 (1966).
3. 604 A.2d 1053 (Pa. Super. Ct. 1992).
4. Tex. Admin. Code tit. 28, § 11.1601 (1996).
5. Me. Rev. Stat. Ann. tit. 24-A, § 4303.
6. Ind. Code Ann. § 27-8-11-3 (Burns Supp. 1996).
7. Or. Rev. Stat. §§ 743.801, 743.803 (Supp. 1996).
8. R.I. Gen. Laws § 23-17.13-3.
9. Act of 9 October, 1996, §§ 3, 15, 1996 N.Y.S. 7553.
10. R.I. Gen. Laws § 23-17.13-3.
11. R.I. Gen. Laws § 23-17.13-3.
12. Federal courts in Texas and Virginia held that AWP laws in those states are saved from preemption because they regulate the business of insurance: *Texas Pharmacy v. Prudential Ins. Co. of America,* 907 F. Supp. 1019 (W.D. Tex. 1995); *Stuart Circle Hosp. Corp. v. Aetna Health Management,* 995 F.2d 500 (4th Cir. 1993).
13. *N.Y. State Conference of Blue Cross and Blue Shield Plans v. Travelers Ins. Co.*, 131 L. Ed. 2d 695 (1995).
14. 674 A.2d 962 (N.H. 1996).
15. 33 Cal. Rptr. 2d 381 (Cal. Ct. App. 1994).

RESOURCE LIST

"Cincinnati HMOs To Set Surgical Quotas for Specialists," *Managed Care Week*, 24 April, 1995.

Credentialing, Information Exchange #4015 (Englewood, CO: Medical Group Management Association).

"How To Avoid Deselection," *Medical Economics*, 15 April, 1996.

"No-Cause Terminations: Will They Go Up in Flames?" *Medical Economics*, 12 January, 1998.

Choosing the Best Strategic Partners for Your Group Practice, Physician Hospital Affiliation, or Integrated Delivery System

INTRODUCTION

A few of the recommendations in this book can be carried out by physicians or physician groups practicing just as they are now. They can conduct an environment assessment (Chapter 14, "Assessing the Market for Managed Care and Integration Opportunities"); prepare their practice for managed care (Chapter 7, "Step One: Preparing Your Practice for Operation under Managed Care"); and negotiate managed care contracts (Chapter 9, "Strategies for Negotiating with a Managed Care Organization") without adding new members. However, the main thesis of the book, and most of the strategies that it recommends, asks physicians to grow their practices and expand the settings in which they deliver care. You are urged to increase the number of physicians in your practice and form joint ventures, affiliations, and outright mergers with other physicians, other providers, and managed care organizations (MCOs). This is all done in the interest of putting you in the best strategic position for success in a managed care world.

These recommendations require that you create strategic partnerships with these other individuals and organizations. It is not a simple matter to find the right parties to join you in a long-term commitment that may decide the fate of your career.

This chapter examines the challenge of finding and selecting strategic partners for new health care ventures. It begins by reviewing the scenarios in which strategic partnerships play a role. There is a quick look at the mistakes to avoid in choosing a partner. Then, we answer the question, "How to find and identify good candidates for strategic partnership?" This includes places to look for candidates and methods for recruiting them. The chapter next offers criteria for actually selecting candidates in several categories. Finally, there are a few additional tips for making a strategic partnership work.

The intended result of this chapter is to raise the consciousness of physicians and groups about the great care they must take in selecting their allies in implementing their strategic plans.

WHO SHOULD READ THIS CHAPTER

If you are going to be involved at all in choosing or just voting on the persons or organizations your group affiliates with, it would be a good idea to read this material. It is not long. You might think that you could get by without it, that your experience and common sense will lead you to a sound decision. Others have taken that attitude and lived to regret it. More than a few mergers or affiliations have fallen apart because of basic incompatibility among the parties. This chapter will remind you of the right characteristics to seek in partners and give you a systematic way of making the choice.

So, if you are a member of a small physician group adding new members for strategic reasons, read this. If your group is looking for the best MCO to contract with, read this. Or, if they are contemplating a joint venture or merger with another group, read this. If your group has been invited to join a physician-hospital organization (PHO), independent practice association (IPA), or physician network, read this. If you are on the strategic planning committee of a large multispecialty group practice seeking other provider organizations to form an integrated delivery system (IDS), read this. If you are simply a voting member of a large physician group considering some strategic partnering decisions and will have a say in the final choices, it will serve you to read this chapter.

There are two categories of physicians who can get by without reading this. The chapter will have no value for someone belonging to an organization that has no strategic partnerships in its future—either because it is already as large and well connected as it needs to be or it somehow has found a way to grow internally without interacting with outside organizations. A physician who belongs to a group that has delegated strategic partnering to a separate, small committee may never be concerned with these matters. She can skip this chapter as well.

SCENARIOS REQUIRING A CHOICE OF STRATEGIC PARTNER

There are a surprising number of situations throughout a physician's career in which he or his group will be in search of a strategic partner (See Exhibit 24–1 for a definition of strategic partner). These are the most critical ones:

1. Recruiting a New Physician into the Practice

This may seem like a fairly mundane operational task. "Our business is growing or our rent is going up, so we need another physician in the group to handle the patients or cover the overhead." That kind of logic for a new hire is no longer sufficient.

The addition of new physician members to a practice must be based on strategic considerations. Even if the immediate need is to pay increased operating expenses of the office suite,

that new person will impact the strategic moves the group must make in the future.

For instance, if the group is trying to develop a modest multispecialty capability, there may be one or more obvious specialty gaps the new physician could fill. If the group aims to become the preeminent group in its single specialty in its market, the new doctor would be selected to enhance the group's position in that role. If the group is pursuing contracts with a particular MCO, it may prefer a new physician with a positive managed care attitude, demonstrated ability to control utilization and costs, and a patient base that matches the MCO membership.

Whether you want her to be or not, a new physician member is part of your strategic moves. You might as well make explicit plans for it.

2. Merging with Another Practice

The significance of a full-blown merger with another practice should alert you that there are probably strategic implications. The primary question is, how does this new group of physicians, with their unique specialties, skills, attitudes, culture, and location fit with the long-range ambitions of the current group? The choice of merger partner has at least the following implications:

- Another entire practice brings not one, but several sets of specialties, clinical skills, administrative skills, interpersonal skills, and attitudes toward patients, quality, money, and managed care into your practice. (Will these best serve your strategic plans?)
- When you merge with one practice, you may be passing up the opportunity to merge with another practice—at least in the short run.
- It is hard to reverse or back out of a merger (though it can be done). It is much easier to dismiss a physician who is not working out.
- When you merge with a practice, you prevent anyone else from merging with it.
- A merger with another practice makes the resulting group larger. Now, you can handle more patients and bring in more revenues, you are likely to have more capital to

Exhibit 24–1 What Is a "Strategic Partner"?

Two qualities distinguish a potential partner of any organization—the type of entity and its relationship to the organization. The entity could be one physician, several physicians, a formal physician group practice, a hospital, other nonphysician providers, or an MCO, among the most obvious examples. The relationship could be a legal contract or even an informal, unwritten agreement sealed with a handshake. Your organization could acquire the other one, or vice versa. The two of you could merge into a new, third organization. A good corporate lawyer can use a variety of organizational forms and legal contracts to create just about any kind of relationship the parties can imagine.

What makes the relationship "strategic" is the purpose that it serves. Generally, a strategic partnership is one created in pursuit of the objectives laid out in the organization's strategic plan. Such plans are designed to realize a long-range vision for the organization through projects that usually take several years to complete. They aim to build or rebuild the very core of the organization; their effects last for years if not decades. Your group will select a strategic partner for the long-term impact he, she, or it will have on the basic elements of your operations (i e., its structure, operating methods, revenue sources, financing sources).

It should be obvious that a well-conceived strategic plan is a prerequisite to the selection of strategic partners. Read the sections on strategic planning in Chapter 14, "Assessing the Market for Managed Care and Integration Opportunities," before attempting to carry out the recommendations in this chapter.

develop your internal systems and to add still more practices, you will carry more weight in future negotiations (contracts, mergers, joint ventures), and you are more likely to scare some other industry players.

- It may make you more attractive or, possibly, less attractive to MCOs, employers, hospitals, other physician groups, other future strategic partners, lenders or capital investors, and even patients.
- The new group can help plug holes in the clinical or administrative competencies of your group.
- If you do not choose a partner with whom you are compatible and the partnership collapses, you will lose time and perhaps credibility with possible future partners.

3. Joint Venturing with Another Practice or Provider

This action is a little like hiring a new physician. It seems to have merit in its own right, without worrying about strategic implications. That may be true, but consider this. It will take time

(yours and others') and money to initiate and sustain the joint venture. Those are precious resources that will not then be available for other projects that are part of the strategic plan. This is a challenge that will bedevil health care organizations from now on—how to allocate limited resources of all kinds.

In addition to consuming these resources, joint ventures can actually make a contribution to the strategic goals of the group. Through the venture, two or more entities can jointly develop skills or systems that permit them all to manage care more effectively. By combining services or resources in a joint venture, several providers may achieve cost savings that will make them all more competitive. During the implementation of a joint venture, the participants may become comfortable enough with each other to want to integrate still more closely, even merge. A joint venture can be a test working relationship.

4. Agreeing To Participate in a PHO

The choice to accept an invitation to participate in a PHO certainly has strategic motives, but would seem to be pretty cut and dried. Either you participate or you do not. However, it can get a little more complicated than that.

The initial reason for creating a PHO is usually to gain access to managed care contracts (because the new entity can provide nearly all the health care services required by MCO members). But, what if the MCO whose contracts are sought likes the physicians and not the hospital, or would prefer another oncology group or a higher ratio of primary care to specialist physicians? Maybe it would be better if the PHO was not automatically composed of a hospital and its entire medical staff. Maybe some thought should be given first to the combination of providers that would be most appealing to the MCOs to be targeted by the PHO.

Furthermore, if the PHO is to succeed in the long run, it must immediately begin to integrate the operations of its participating providers and to develop their skills in managing care. It makes sense, therefore, to assess, in advance, the willingness of prospective participants to embrace managed care, learn new skills, and collaborate closely with other providers. Prior experience with integration and managed care should also be taken into account.

5. Deciding To Join an IPA

The IPA is a model that can advance the strategic goals of each of its participating physicians. To do so, they must be selected carefully and their managed care skills developed aggressively. The IPA must have a long-range vision for itself.

For some time, the common wisdom has been that an IPA could only be a transitory form on the way toward development of a more fully integrated group practice (because the IPA physicians tended to remain in their separate practice settings and resist adopting more cost-sensitive practice behaviors). Recently, there has been some evidence that properly motivated physicians can learn to manage cost and quality in an IPA framework and compete successfully for managed care contracts.

Several strategic concerns come into play when forming or joining an IPA.

- Do the numbers and specialties represented meet the mix requirements of potential MCO contract partners, particularly with regard to primary care physicians?
- Are the practice locations of the participating physicians convenient to the MCO's enrollees?
- Are the participating physicians willing to adjust their practice styles sufficiently, especially with regard to quality and utilization, to keep the entire network competitive?
- Are the physicians also willing to integrate their practices just enough to do two things—make care received through them more seamless and satisfy the Department of Justice to allow them to negotiate prices as a group without actually merging the practices?
- If market conditions demand it, will the physicians consider integrating still more closely, perhaps merging into a centrally managed, multispecialty group practice?
- Is there agreement on the services that the IPA will provide to the physicians—contract negotiation, billing and collection, utilization management, quality assurance, general marketing and business assistance?
- What will be the response of other players in the local market to the consolidation of so many physicians into a single delivery organization?

6. Selling Out to and Working for a Physician Practice Management Company (PPMC)

This scenario gets more serious. Once you have sold your assets to a PPMC, there is little alternative but to be satisfied with its policies and procedures. If you become truly unhappy with your choice, it may be necessary to leave not only the PPMC, but also the practice of medicine. A careful analysis of the PPMC's strategic intentions and their impact on your career should precede a decision to sell out. Some of the issues to look for are

- Which of your practice assets are you expected to sell—intangible as well as tangible assets? Will the PPMC assume the liabilities along with the assets? How will the assets be valued and what price will you receive for them? Will your payment be in cash, stock, or a combination?
- What are the terms under which you will continue to practice for the PPMC? Will you stay in your original practice location? For how long? To accommodate the needs of payers, PPMCs often relocate their physicians. Will you be subject to utilization and quality management measures with which you have no experience? Are the cost and quality controls likely to be tightened in the future? Some PPMCs have asked their physicians literally to change specialties to fit into their strategic staffing plans. What will be your level of reimbursement and how does it compare with what you are earning now? Some PPMCs use complex formulas to calculate physician compensation that, under certain circumstances, can result in lower income.
- In exchange for a physician's practice assets, many PPMCs give some of their own stock, rather than cash. This automatically makes the physician a partner with a vested interest in the company's strategic future. You will be counting on appreciation in the value of the PPMC's stock.
  - Is the PPMC's stock publicly traded?
  - Ask to see the PPMC's strategic plan.
  - What are the plan's goals for growth in revenues, income, and stock price?
  - What are the plan's goals for expanding its physician network?
  - What are the plan's goals for developing or joining full-service, integrated systems?
  - What are the implications of the plan for the way you will be able to practice medicine?

- How long has the PPMC been in business? How many physician practices does it operate in how many states? What is its reputation for treatment of physicians after they have joined the PPMC? (Be sure to interview some of them.) What is the state of the PPMC's finances and does it have the funding to support its strategic plans?
- Who are the executives and managers of the PPMC? What is their experience in managing physician practices? Do they appear to have the expertise to carry out their strategic plans? What is their attitude, if not formal policy, toward physician autonomy and clinical decision making?

7. Accepting an Invitation To Become Part of a Multispecialty Group Practice

An advantage of this option is that most physicians set out to build a multispecialty group practice because they clearly see it as one of the best strategic moves they can make in a managed care environment. They know that it will have strategic implications. However, that does not mean that they have the ability to carry out their strategic plans or that their strategic plans coincide with yours. Proceed thoughtfully in deciding whether to accept even an invitation like this.

- Ask a lot of questions of the group's founders. Ask to see a copy of their strategic plan. (They better have one!) Exactly what is their vision for the group practice three or four years from now? Will they be a major contract partner of one or more MCOs, or will they be leaders in forming an IDS? Do their plans make sense in light of what you know about the local market and competition (as a result of your environmental assessment)?
- Do the group's leaders appear to have the business savvy to carry off their plans? Do you have confidence in them? Do they have the wisdom to know the limits of their own managerial abilities and when to rely on professional managers?

- Does the group appear to be assembling the right mix of primary care and specialty physicians? (Although few groups have achieved it, the common wisdom still calls for a 50–50 breakdown.) How selective are they in the physicians they invite to join? Will you be part of an elite group or a grab bag of available physicians?
- Is the group committed to acquiring the systems and developing the procedures (for cost control and quality assurance) necessary to be competitive in the local marketplace? Are the group's financial projections realistic? Does it have sufficient capital funds to implement its strategic plans and maintain day-to-day operations until it reaches break-even? Does the group seem well enough connected with key stakeholders (like hospitals, other providers, employers, and MCOs) to receive their support in its strategic endeavors?
- Review the questions under the PPMC option about your personal involvement in and expected benefits from the organization. Especially do this if you will be giving up existing practice assets to join the group.

It is important to your future that the founding physicians have aspirations that go beyond simply creating a group practice of physicians in multiple specialties. They must be willing to evolve and change as the marketplace shifts. There must be a constant willingness to develop new skills and to invest money in new systems, new ventures, and new relationships.

8. Signing a Contract with an MCO

In some markets, entering into managed care contracts is so easy that some physicians have 20 or 30 of them. It hardly requires a second thought. But it should.

If your practice is going to rely more and more on revenues from managed care contracts, they must become the focus of your strategic plans. The MCOs you contract with must be viewed as strategic partners. Chapter 8 "Step Two: How To

Analyze and Evaluate a Managed Care Contract," proposes most of the questions that should be answered before signing such a contract. What needs to be emphasized here is the importance of a full assessment of the MCO behind each contract.

- What is its track record and reputation?
- What are the credentials of its leaders and managers?
- What are their long-range plans for the MCO in the local market?
- Do they view their relationships with physicians as long-term partnerships?
- Do they have the fiscal strength to sustain themselves and grow?

The number and kinds of MCOs you contract with is also very much a strategic decision. Too many contracts and you may not be an important enough provider to any of the MCOs. Too few contracts and you may be overly dependent on one or two MCOs. Pick the wrong MCO (because it offers the wrong kinds of plans or has contracts with the wrong employers) and you may suffer the consequences when they lose business.

9. Negotiating a Direct Contract with an Employer

This represents a bold strategic move, not one to be taken lightly. Carefully planned, it can reap great rewards to the physicians. If mishandled, it can alienate the physician group's current MCO partners and leave the employer dissatisfied.

For physicians (or any providers) to contract directly with an employer (the end payer) requires a radical restructuring of the traditional employer-MCO-provider-patient delivery/financing chain. It means eliminating the MCO middleman, taking over the functions it performs (marketing, enrollment, claims processing, provider contracting), and pulling in the profit it has been earning. If the physician group has evolved into a complete IDS, this step is a very plausible option. But, first, it must consider several factors.

- Has the employer initiated the discussion about a direct contracting relationship? If so, the physicians' MCO contract partners will have less reason to complain, since they are going to lose that employer's business anyway.
- Is the direct contract arrangement being proposed by an employer coalition (several large area employers in combination) rather than a single employer? A coalition will offer a larger population of enrollees to be served (sometimes numbering in the hundreds of thousands) over which to spread risk and on which to earn net income. More employers also mean more resources that can be devoted to making the arrangement work.
- Look very carefully at the requirements laid out by the employers for provider participation in the direct contracting arrangements. They normally will be specified in an request for proposal (RFP), and will include the formation of an integrated system (the employers are unlikely to contract with individual physician groups), focused on primary care, with data systems for measuring the quality of care. The smartest employers will want to see evidence that the system reduces lost work time and inefficiency due to injury or illness.
- Will the employer coalition work with a provider group to develop a system that will meet the RFP requirements? Most will do so; it is in their best interests. They will share data, assumptions, and concerns sufficient to help the group get started.
- To how many prospective provider systems has the RFP been issued? How many of them are likely to be accepted as direct contract partners of the employers? Each provider system will be in competition with others—the employers are counting on the benefits from this. Poor relative performance could result in a system losing its contract.
- How will the providers be paid if they win a contract? A common practice is to use an resource-based relative value scale (RBRVS) fee schedule for physician services, a diagnosis-related group (DRG)–based per diem schedule for inpatient hospital services, and a negotiated fee schedule for most other services. However, there are other control measures in place to ensure that costs are minimized and kept within budgets. Be sure that you can live with and prosper under the reimbursement scheme.

There are other variations on the direct contracting model. The best overall advice is to view the employers with whom you contract as long-term strategic partners—and expect them to treat you the same way.

10. Selecting Other Physicians and Groups To Collaborate with in Forming an IDS

When a physician group (typically already organized as a multispecialty group practice, an IPA, a group practice without walls (GPWW), or even a PHO) reaches the point of putting together a true IDS, it will make numerous selections of other providers to join with them in this bold venture. The size and scope of an IDS, as well as its dramatic impact on the local market, require that it be approached as nothing but a strategic undertaking. If it is successful, every one of the other providers selected to participate will be a partner and workmate for the rest of your career.

To get to the stage where an IDS seems like a plausible next step, the physicians will be formed into a fairly large group, will be well on the path toward integration, and will have significant experience in choosing others to work synergistically with them. The selection of strategic partners should not be a new concept. Nonetheless, there are unique features of IDSs that bear keeping in mind.

Reread the discussion and questions in the sections on Merging with Another Practice, Agreeing to Participate in a PHO, Deciding To Join an IPA, and Accepting an Invitation To Become Part of a Multispecialty Group Practice. They raise many strategic considerations that are just as applicable to the IDS formation process.

Prospective partners must be willing to engage in certain activities that may be a change for them.

- They must embrace, not resist, managed care.
- They must commit to constant adaptation in the ways they provide care—as the market evolves, as competitive forces pressure them, as their customers demand, as better practices and procedures become apparent, and as new technologies become available.
- They must be willing to try to work effectively with a wide variety of other providers who are part of their system.
- They must accept new forms of reimbursement, the assumption of new levels of financial and clinical risk, and the constant measurement and analysis of their performance.
- They must accept that the IDS is a competitive business that can never rest in its efforts to improve.

Whatever scrutiny you may have given to partner candidates in other organizations, raise the evaluation and critique to still higher levels in selecting IDS partners.

11. Choosing a Hospital for Affiliation with Your Group of Physicians, To Form a PHO, IDS, or Other Multiprovider System

The possibility of the physicians affiliating with a hospital occurs obviously under several of the previous scenarios. A PHO requires a hospital participant from the beginning, as does an IDS. Other types of physician organizations may hook up with a hospital at almost any stage of their integration process. Any sort of funding affiliation with a hospital must be viewed as a strategic partnership. It is usually a large, well-organized, well-financed entity that has the potential to overwhelm or dominate a physician organization. In a worst case scenario, it can doom the doctors' chances of gaining a competitive advantage in the marketplace. Consider these distinctions of a hospital partner:

- It often initiates negotiations with physicians, particularly to form a PHO. That in

itself can give it a dominant voice in the proceedings.
- It is composed of a more formally organized and professionally managed corporate infrastructure. Its executives and managers have more experience analyzing business issues, evaluating deals, and thinking systematically about new opportunities. This affords the hospital a further edge over relatively inexperienced physicians.
- Some of the strategic options involve creating an entity to which the physicians sell their practice assets. If that entity is controlled by a hospital, there always is a risk that its primary purpose is to increase the flow of inpatients to its beds. That contradicts one of the essential goals of managed care.
- If there are several qualified hospitals in town, the one initiating the strategic proposal may or may not be the best one for the physicians' own strategic goals. In particular, this hospital may not be most favorably received by other, later, strategic partners—such as MCO contract partners.
- Even if this hospital is best suited to the purposes of your physician group, there may be serious political problems if it insists on bringing into the venture all the members of its medical staff. A key success ingredient for integrating organizations is rigorous selectivity of all its providers.
- In addition to whatever desires it may have to maintain its bed occupancy rate, hospitals often have a general preference for specialist over primary care physicians. It continues to be the common wisdom that delivery organizations appealing to managed care must emphasize their primary care physicians and capabilities.
- Many enlightened hospitals fully comprehend the requirements of managed care and are willing to commit their substantial managerial and financial resources to creating appropriate partnerships with physicians. Your group needs to seek out such institutions. If ideal candidates are not available,

connect with the best, most adaptable one you can find. In some cases, where all the hospitals are unsuitable, it may be necessary to hold off until they feel greater market pressure and adjust their thinking.

The hospital selected as strategic partner can empower a physician group or destroy its efforts to compete. Be as circumspect as possible in making this choice.

MISTAKES TO AVOID IN CHOOSING A STRATEGIC PARTNER

One way of making good strategic partner choices is to examine mistakes others have made in the process and try to avoid them. Here are the most common:

- Reaching tentative agreement prematurely—usually by signing a memorandum of understanding or letter of intent (difficult to back out of this)—before deciding what benefits should result or needs be met from the partnership and before determining what issues will make or break the deal.
- Figuring out only superficially the forces driving the partners into affiliation—the "spread of managed care" is not enough. How are or will the physicians be suffering as a result of the spread of managed care and how might a strategic partnership address this?
- Getting clear on the needs to be met by a partnership, but not translating them into criteria for the partner to be sought.
- Formulating partner selection criteria, and then ignoring them, in order to select a person or organization for social ("we've known them for a long time") or political ("they will be upset if we pass them by") reasons.
- Focusing too much on the mechanics of the deal and not giving enough attention to the objectives that the deal is meant to achieve.

- Allowing an individual, group, or organization to dominate the negotiations and virtually dictating the terms while others remain silent and are dissatisfied with the resulting agreement. Eventually this leads to failure or collapse of the partnership.
- Failing to realize that the form of the partnership can be just as essential to success as the selection of the partners.
- Selecting good partners, constructing an appropriate partnership relationship, and assuming that is all that is necessary to ensure success—failing to take into account the need for
  - a plan of implementation of the partnership agreement, particularly when it involves considerable integration
  - continued nurturing and development of the partnership arrangement
- Using consultants and attorneys to make the partnership decisions rather than facilitating the decisions made by the physicians.
- Being flat-out ignorant of the issues that may require a strategic partnership, and otherwise joining in just because everyone else seems to be doing it.
- Partnering for the wrong or illegal reasons ("by sticking together, we can prevent the managed care plans from assembling a large enough provider network to succeed or from beating us down individually on reimbursement rates").
- Each group wanting its executive to have a leading role in the new organization that is created and not agreeing on who will go and who will stay.
- Talking too much before the partnership deal has been consummated. Sometimes, negotiating privately and quietly with the preferred partners minimizes antagonizing those left out who might disrupt the proceedings.
- Misperceiving the differences in values or culture among the prospective partners. This can happen with any combination of entities, but is most likely when for-profit and not-for-profit corporations, or religious and non-religious organizations, try to come together.

HOW TO FIND AND IDENTIFY GOOD CANDIDATES FOR STRATEGIC PARTNERSHIP

Once having defined good criteria for the persons or organizations you seek as strategic partners, the question remains whether you can find any who will satisfy those criteria. These are some thoughts on how to find the best candidates.

In some cases, there will be absolutely no choice. If there is only one hospital in the market area, and it meets most of the high-priority criteria, then that is the one to choose. If your group is attempting to expand in a particular specialty and there are only a few physicians available in that specialty, you will have to take one of them.

> **Note**: Sometimes, any deal is better than no deal at all. Other times, no deal is better than what is available. The hard part is figuring out which situation you are facing.

Normally, there will be a healthy number of choices—sometimes many, sometimes just a few, but usually enough from which to pick and choose an excellent team.

Generally, health care providers are out in the open—not hiding or trying to avoid attention. You may not know about all of them, but their identities and descriptive data are available with a modest amount of searching. Here is how to go about it.

Providers You Know

These are the physicians, hospitals, clinics, health centers, and other providers you have dealt with in the course of your practice. You know them and something about their values and abilities. They are a good starting point in the search for good partners. They must be augmented with other candidates, so that you can make a genuine choice.

Rigorous Lists

It is increasingly easy to obtain, from outside sources, lists of every provider in a particular category. And they are accompanied by more and more background information on each person or organization. The sources are medical societies, hospital associations, professional associations for ancillary providers, state licensing agencies, mailing list brokers, private directories, and, in a growing number of states, the Internet.

Personal Database

Before you are actively looking for a strategic partner, that is, right now, begin to build a database of names and information on very good (and very bad) potential provider candidates for partnership. Whenever you come across a piece of relevant data, grab it and store it. Then when you need it, it will be ready. It really does not have to include every provider in town. Concentrate on those you feel that you might especially want to work with and those you absolutely want to avoid. In compiling the database, use all the other sources mentioned in this chapter, plus

- Constantly seek opinions and recommendations of others, especially those whose candor and objectivity you trust.
- Note relevant items from the news media.
- Keep track of your own experiences with other providers personally and professionally.

If you operate in a very large market area—say, an entire metropolitan area—it is not necessary to gather information on every single provider active there. You need only enough to feel confident that you have a good cross-section, a representative group, of the people and institutions available.

If you are operating in a smaller market, it probably does make sense to research all the providers. It will be a more manageable task. It also is more important that you pair up with the very best of the small number available and not be left with also-rans.

Issue an RFP

If you are in a strong bargaining or leadership position (and even if you are not, but can pretend you are), consider issuing an RFP. An RFP is a description of the provider qualifications you are seeking in strategic partners for the type of integrated system you intend to create—with an invitation for providers to submit proposals describing themselves and why they should be considered. RFPs are used regularly by contractors seeking partners in many other fields (e.g., construction, military, government). Employer health care coalitions have used them in their quests for integrated systems to contract with. They offer several advantages to physicians.

- RFPs are a rational, businesslike way to find qualified prospective partners.
- If well publicized, they could bring out some providers you might otherwise miss.
- RFPs give the physicians an opportunity to define clearly what they are looking for in a strategic partner.
- It is possible to issue an RFP without revealing the identity of the physician group or its strategic intentions.
- Work with a good attorney to draw up the RFP. Either mail it out to preselected providers or publish it in a medium (for example, a medical society newsletter) likely to reach the best candidates. Use an anonymous name or your attorney's name if you wish to withhold the name of your group. Of course, in a small market, it may be difficult to stay hidden.

What the group wants to avoid at this stage is choosing its partners from too limited a pool or because they are conveniently known to the group. The goal is to bring together the best people and organizations in each provider category and specialty, to form the best integrating system in the area.

APPLYING CRITERIA IN THE CHOICE OF A STRATEGIC PARTNER

Any choice is more rational and likely to succeed if the standards or criteria against which

each alternative is measured are determined in advance. This ensures that the decision makers will apply the same standards to each candidate and will not be swayed by the idiosyncrasies of any particular candidate. The following are the general criteria that physicians should apply to any strategic partner:

- understanding of and commitment to the integration process
- compatibility in goals, culture, and experience
- likelihood of building trust
- ability to make decisions and act expeditiously
- market and financial strength
- capability to contribute expertise and sophistication to IDS business management functions
- cost limitation and control mindset
- ability to collaborate with other provider parties with very different psychologies and motivations
- quality of leadership—to lead own entity and interact with leaders of the other entities
- openness to reeducation and changing attitudes toward the delivery and financing of health care
- ability to attract other desirable provider partners

These may be sufficient for a rough cut at choosing a partner. You can probably use your common sense to expand on them in order to select a certain kind of partner. The next several sections list more detailed criteria for evaluating four particular categories of partner candidate: individual physicians, physician organizations, hospitals, and MCOs.

Here is a simple procedure for applying those criteria:

1. Remove from the criteria list any that are irrelevant or unimportant to you.
2. Add to the criteria list others that you want to consider.

3. Assign a weight to each criterion so that, altogether, they add up to 100 percent.

4. Allow a score or rating of 1 to 10 on each criterion, with 1 meaning that the candidate completely lacks that quality, and 10 meaning that he or she fully possesses the quality.

5. Draw up a standard scoring sheet incorporating the criteria, weights, and scoring ranges.

6. Complete the scoring sheet after investigating and interviewing each candidate.

7. Multiply the score for each criterion by its weight.

8. Add up those results to get a total score for the candidate.

9. Make the partner choice on the basis of those scores, or adjust them for other subjective factors that could not be quantified.

CRITERIA FOR SELECTING AN INDIVIDUAL PHYSICIAN AS A STRATEGIC PARTNER

Your first experience in choosing a strategic partner is likely to occur when your group invites a new physician or physicians to join them. Because of the very personal and individual nature of this decision, the following criteria may be easier to understand:

- quality of the medical care
- value (cost and quality) of the medical care
- style of interaction with patients
- style of interaction with other physicians
- style of interaction with ancillary providers and staff
- ability to fit into the prevailing culture of your group
- efficiency (utilization of resources) with which medical care is provided
- attitude toward managed care, in general
- attitude toward practicing under capitation
- attitude toward accepting risk and taking risks

- attitude toward money—how much does she want to earn and how willing is she to invest in the organization and her future
- attitude toward the prerequisites to success under managed care, namely
  - review of his utilization of resources
  - review of the quality of medicine practiced
  - review of the clinical outcomes of his practice decisions
  - review of the satisfaction levels of his patients
  - willingness to adapt his practice style to clinical protocols or guidelines
  - willingness to adjust his referral patterns to specialists on MCO panels or otherwise identified premium practitioners
- willingness to subject his performance (in all aspects) to regular review by the larger organization
- agreement with the principle that the organization must be selective in all the people who work for it, including providers and physicians, must rigorously evaluate their performance, and must dismiss those who do not meet its standards
- commitment to work primarily for the good of the organization and secondarily for the good of the individual, in the belief that the individual will gain more in the long run if the organization succeeds
- ability or willingness to work in teams with other physicians, other providers, and staff
- commitment continually to upgrade her skills, adjust her practice behaviors, and reexamine her attitudes
- previous experience with practice under managed care contracts
- previous experience with practice under capitation contracts
- previous experience with practice under other kinds of risk-sharing arrangements
- previous experience with practice under common managed care mechanisms for managing quality, costs, and patient satisfaction

- demonstrated ability to practice high-quality medicine
- demonstrated ability to deliver high-level clinical outcomes
- demonstrated ability to maximize the satisfaction of patients served
- demonstrated ability to minimize the cost and utilization of resources consumed in delivering a unit of medical care
- desire and/or demonstrated ability to serve in supervisory, leadership, or governance roles

Not all of these criteria may be relevant to a particular candidate or important to your group. Use the ones that seem most useful to you.

CRITERIA FOR SELECTING A PHYSICIAN GROUP AS A STRATEGIC PARTNER

Apply the same criteria for individual physicians to the physician members of the physician organization or group, although perhaps not with quite the same thoroughness. If your group is relatively small, and the group proposed as a partner is also (say, no more than 10 doctors), it probably is a good idea to apply the individual criteria to all of them. Because of the relative sizes, they are going to have a major impact on the way your group operates. If you are a much larger group joining with a smaller physician practice, the impact will not be as great, and you can afford to be a little less rigorous.

In addition to the scrutiny of individual physicians, check the overall organization against these criteria:

- has been operating as a group at or near its present size for a long enough time to have demonstrated both abilities and deficiencies
- reputation, as a group, for delivering high-quality, patient-friendly care
- demonstrated ability to practice as a group under managed care contracts
- demonstrated ability to practice as a group under capitated contracts
- demonstrated ability to practice as a group under other risk-sharing arrangements

- demonstrated ability to manage its operations in a fiscally responsible way (as reflected in financial statements)
- has taken steps to integrate the practices of its member physicians
- has begun to scrutinize the performance (in all aspects) of its member physicians, has taken steps to improve it and ultimately to remove those physicians who do not meet group expectations
- has shown a general willingness to invest net income in the infrastructure of the organization, rather than pay it all out to member physicians
- has begun to make investments in the kind of information systems needed to support the various care management mechanisms
- has begun to make investments in the care management mechanisms necessary to control quality and cost
- demonstrates, through word and deed, a willingness to embrace, rather than resist, the concepts of managed care
- demonstrates, through word and deed, a desire and ability to work with your group as a strategic partner
- apparent ability of the group's physicians and staff to mesh with the prevailing culture of your group
- willingness to adjust virtually any aspect of its operations to meet the requirements of MCOs, other payers, patients, and other stakeholders
- accepts the view that health care delivery and the physician organization are businesses and must be managed appropriately
- accepts the view that physicians must consolidate and grow into larger, more efficient, physician-run integrated organizations
- accepts generally the strategic vision that your group has outlined and is willing to contribute to its development and implementation

These are the general criteria for physician organizations as strategic partners. They are in addition to the more specific requirements you will have with regard to size, specialties, and locations. They also do not include the checks you would naturally perform for licensing, accreditation, or any legal infirmities.

CRITERIA FOR SELECTING A HOSPITAL AS A STRATEGIC PARTNER

Selecting a hospital as a strategic partner involves factors more related to organizational structure and operations than individual qualifications and performance—although some of the latter are relevant. Here is what to look for:

- a reputation, both in the community and among physicians, for delivery quality health care
- a demonstrated ability to manage its operations in an efficient, fiscally responsible manner (as reflected in a financial statements for at least the last three years)
- is governed by a board of directors familiar with ongoing developments in the health care delivery/financing marketplace, both nationally and locally, and committed to appropriate strategic positioning of the hospital in that marketplace
- is directed by executives and managers who
  - are experienced in hospital management
  - are committed to managing their organizations in a more businesslike fashion
  - possess solid, traditional business management skills
  - are capable of strategic thinking
  - are respected by all who work at the hospital, including the physicians
  - have a track record of tight, efficient management of hospital operations
  - are capable of accepting secondary managerial roles in any larger physician-run organization they might join
- is marked by an organizational culture that encourages growth and change
- a medical staff amenable to the partnership, even if all the physicians will not be able to

participate in the integrating system that emerges
- a strong fiscal foundation, perhaps including capital that might be invested in the strategic venture that the hospital forms with your group
- a record of investing in modern information and control systems required to manage operations efficiently and compete successfully for managed care business
- a recognition of the diminished role of hospitals and the ascendant role of physicians, particularly primary care physicians, in the new American health care system
- a willingness to cede authority, both formally and informally, to physicians, particularly primary care physicians, in the strategic venture they create together
- if the partnership will be something less than legal absorption of the hospital into a new entity with your group (in other words, an arm's-length contractual agreement such as a joint venture) it is important to know
  - whether the hospital is part of a chain
  - how independent its decision making is of the chain's main office
  - the reputation and track record of the entire chain

The implications of a strategic partnership with a hospital, especially if it involves a merger of entities, are more far-reaching than the combination of one small physician group with another—and much more difficult to unwind. This review deserves as much time and resources as you can devote to it.

CRITERIA FOR SELECTING AN MCO AS A STRATEGIC PARTNER

There is good information in Chapter 8, "Step Two: How To Analyze and Evaluate a Managed Care Contract" on assessing MCOs as candidates for strategic affiliation. In some ways, this is the trickiest relationship of all to measure. The relationship could take the form of a contract and last for a year. Many physicians have numerous contractual relationships like that. Are they all worth the same investigation and analysis you would carry out if the MCO were about to purchase your practice assets? Of course not.

If you are merely contracting with an MCO for a limited period to provide services to its members, if you have no special reason to believe that this might grow into a close long-term relationship, and if this is just one of several such relationships, it should be enough to apply the criteria suggested in Chapter 8. On the other hand, if the deal you are about to do with an MCO involves any of the following:

- a contract with long-term potential, and you and the MCO have been talking about building a "partnership" together
- the joint creation by your group and the MCO of an IDS with your group in a leadership role
- the acquisition by the MCO of your group's assets for any reason
- your entering into an employment relationship with the MCO
- the investment of significant funds by the MCO in your group, perhaps accompanied by the surrender of some control of your group to the MCO
- any other joint venture between you and the MCO that either is expected to last for five years or longer, or will seriously preclude your group from taking advantage of other attractive strategic opportunities

then consider these additional criteria:

- the MCO's experience in executing similar deals in the past and the results achieved
- the MCO's experience in long-term relationships with physician groups, particularly ones like yours
- the MCO's reputation in all of its dealings with physicians
- the MCO's business plan for the venture proposed with your group
- your personal comfort and trust with the MCO executives who will manage its role in the venture

- the MCO's acknowledgment of the primacy of physicians in clinical decision making and its willingness to allow physicians, and particularly your group, an appropriate role in the governance and business management of the joint venture

The strategic arrangement you negotiate with an MCO could lead to the emergence of a health care delivery and financing combination that dominates your market. It would be highly desirable to be part of such a powerful, forward-looking entity. Seize the opportunity if it becomes available. Keep in mind, though, that not every MCO has that potential. It may lack the vision, the resources, the leadership, the imagination and perseverance, and the luck to pull it off. Your job is to find the ones that do have all that.

TIPS ON MAKING STRATEGIC PARTNERSHIPS WORK

1. Have the wisdom to know when a relationship you are contemplating has strategic import and implication.
2. When it does, scrutinize both the proposed partner and the relationship according to the criteria laid out in this and other chapters of the book.
3. During your prior assessment of the prospective partner, pay attention to your subjective feelings about its people and organization, the compatibility of the two organizations' cultures, the tenor of the negotiations and how conflicts were resolved.
4. Whatever your prior dealings with the partner, decide that in the future they will be based on trust, collaboration, and sharing. The one thing they must not be is adversarial. If you cannot do this, do not enter into the relationship.
5. From the start, establish a broad channel for the two-way flow of information between your group and your partner. Do not stint. Err on the side of providing too much information rather than too little.

This includes information on operations, plans, problems, and anything else bearing on the partnership. The goal is to avoid confusing or surprising either one of you.

6. Especially during the first year or two, representatives from both parties should meet very regularly for the sole purpose of reviewing the state of the partnership— what has gone well, what has gone poorly, dissatisfactions or gripes of either party, and what needs to be changed or adjusted.

7. At the very beginning, set two or three goals for each of the first three years by which you will measure the success of the partnership—the relationship between the parties. These may be different from the goals used to determine the operating success of the organization.

8. In the give-and-take that is part of any relationship, do not simply give your 50 percent and wait for your partner to give his. Instead, both commit to giving 60 percent or 70 percent; the overlap will enrich and nurture the partnership.

9. Build into the initial agreement some mechanism for disassembling the partnership if the relationship becomes totally unworkable. It should not be too easy to access the mechanism, but just enough to minimize the disagreement and acrimony at the time of separation.

RESOURCE LIST

"Alliances in Health Care: What We Know, What We Think We Know, and What We Should Know," *Health Care Management Review*, Winter 1995.

"Enticing a New Doctor to Your Practice," *Medical Economics*, 27 March, 1995.

"Finding a Partner—Not a Predator," *Family Practice Management*, September 1997.

"Partnerships with a Purpose: Health Care Providers, Managed Care Companies, and Insurers," *Physician Executive*, November 1994.

Physician Recruitment and Retention Guidebook (Washington, DC: American Health Lawyers Association, 1997).

CHAPTER 25

The Kinds of Physician Reimbursement Systems You Can Expect under Managed Care

INTRODUCTION

The first and often the only provision physicians read when evaluating a managed care contract is the one describing the terms and amounts of their reimbursement. This is a critical piece of the managed care relationship for a number of reasons. A physician moving from predominantly fee-for-service (FFS) to capitation-based reimbursement will be concerned with maintaining or improving her income under the new scheme. She also will wonder if she must alter her practice style in order to maximize her income through that system. The managed care plan or integrated delivery system (IDS) is interested in a reimbursement mechanism that encourages just the right kind of practice behavior by its providers. Within a physician group, an inequitable, misunderstood compensation plan can create conflict and disagreement.

This chapter examines in some detail the primary formulas by which physician and group compensation is determined in a managed care environment. Several models of physician compensation systems are described. The legal constraints on physician compensation are laid out in detail.

The intended result of this chapter is that physicians be able to understand the reimbursement/compensation systems they encounter, evaluate how well each system will work for them, and perhaps design a better one if necessary.

WHO SHOULD READ THIS CHAPTER

One of your most important concerns as you begin to find your place in the world of managed care is the compensation paid to physicians—both you and others in your organization. This chapter provides a solid introduction to the systems, policies, procedures, and formulas used to determine the reward given physicians in return for their services. As the recipient of that reward, you need to understand how it is calculated and what you can do to maximize it. You will also be concerned with the effect on your medical practice style of certain incentive payment plans used by managed care organizations (MCOs). If you choose to become part of a physician-sponsored organization, this chapter will help you understand the options available for compensating all categories of physicians employed by the group. In some cases, you may be the member of a committee that defines the compensation plan.

If you already are a member or employee of a well-established delivery organization, fully comprehend the basis for setting your reimbursement (perhaps you are paid a straight salary), and do not expect that basis to change in the near future, you may be able to skip this chapter. Of course, you may be interested in learning what you may be missing by practicing in another setting.

COMPENSATION FROM MCO TO GROUP TO PHYSICIAN

In a classic managed care relationship, compensation takes place at two levels. At the first level, the MCO compensates the providers (physicians and hospitals) with which it has contracts. The physicians are often, though not always, organized into groups. The group may be an independent practice association (IPA), preferred provider organization (PPO), management services organization (MSO), group practice without walls (GPWW), or simply a fully integrated group practice. The MCO compensation flows to the group. (In some cases, MCOs are willing to contract directly with individual physicians, so the first level of compensation does not really occur in those cases.) At the second level, the group sets up compensation arrangements with its individual physicians. It is important to understand how the compensation is structured in both these cases.

FIRST LEVEL: HOW MCOs USE COMPENSATION TO SHARE RISK WITH PHYSICIAN GROUPS

MCOs obtain their revenues from employers who pay a fixed premium per member to cover services from providers within the MCO system, services from out-of-area providers, reinsurance costs, administrative and marketing expenses, and profits. Services from the system providers are the largest cost items and are split among primary care physicians, specialist physicians, and hospitals.

Some MCOs are still reimbursing at least some of their providers on an FFS basis. Usually, they negotiate a discounted fee schedule with the physicians and simultaneously subject them to resource utilization review procedures. Under these systems, the physicians continue to file the claims traditionally required by indemnity insurers. The paperwork overhead for the MCO and provider is tremendous. The doctors resent the intrusion of utilization review into their clinical autonomy. As a cost control device, this approach is only slightly more effective than straight FFS. It is outmoded and declining in use.

The overwhelming trend is in the direction of substantial sharing of the financial risk with the physicians. This can be accomplished by a variety of means. What is described here is a fairly typical combination of capitation payments and risk or performance funds or pools. Another common risk-sharing mechanism is a risk withhold.

Table 25–1 shows the costs and utilizations for the services in an average managed care benefit package.

The MCO takes the premium revenues from the employers and sets up two performance pools, one for the specialist physicians and one for the hospitals. It also pays the primary care physicians a capitation fee, which puts them at risk for the cost and utilization of services they prescribe. A portion of that fee is withheld and placed in a risk fund.

The *primary care risk fund* may contain 10 percent of the total primary care capitation fee. (In the hypothetical case in Table 25–1 this would be $10.73 per member per month [PMPM].) What happens with the fund depends on how well the primary care physicians manage their use of the hospitals and specialists. If their utilization of hospital and specialist referral services exceeds predetermined target levels, they will receive none of the fund. All money in the fund will go back to the MCO. If, however, they utilize hospital and specialist services at less than the target levels, the primary care doctors receive the withheld risk amounts.

The *hospital performance pool* is credited monthly with the predetermined (by actuarial methods) amount for each member and debited for the actual amount of members' hospital charges. The credit amounts may be risk adjusted to account for the differing expected hospital usage of different demographic groups. In addition, to protect the compensation system against unpredictable catastrophic charges, the pool credits per member may be limited to a figure like $25,000 per year.

Using the numbers from Table 25–1, a total of $46.78 PMPM is accounted for by hospital-related services—inpatient services worth $31.15 and outpatient services worth $15.63. That total is reduced by 20 percent to cover the costs that

Table 25–1 Costs and Utilizations in a Managed Care Benefit Package

Service	Frequency/1000	Cost per Service	PMPM Cost[a]
Inpatient	325 days	$1,150	$31.15
Outpatient	625 cases	300	15.63
Primary care	3,680 visits	35	10.73
Specialists	3,050 visits	120	30.50
Radiology	650 procedures	90	4.88
Lab and Pathology	1,550 procedures	25	3.23
Other	60 procedures	300	1.50
Total			$97.62
Administration			11.71
Grand total			$109.33

a. The per member per month (PMPM) cost is calculated by multiplying the number of service units ("frequency/1000") times the cost per service unit ("cost per service"), then dividing by the number of members (1,000) and the number of months in a year (12).

Source: Adapted with permission from Establishing Parameters to Measure Success, *Integrated Health Care Delivery Systems Manual*, p. 6, Section 1011.1, © 1993, Thompson Publishing Group.

come in over the $25,000 limit. That leaves $41.63 (.80 × $46.78) to be allocated each month per member to the hospital pool.

Credits and debits to the pool are reconciled once a year. Any surplus in the hospital pool is applied first to any deficit that exists in the specialist pool. Any remaining surplus is divided between the MCO and the primary care physicians. A deficit in the hospital pool is first reduced by any surplus in the specialist pool, and then by the money in the primary care risk fund. Any deficit remaining after that is absorbed entirely by the MCO.

To see how the primary care physicians, as a group, benefit from this risk sharing, look again at the table figures. If they can reduce inpatient service utilization by 10 percent, the actual PMPM debit to the hospital pool (after 20 percent is included for costs over the stop-loss limit) is $28.66. This represents a $2.50 surplus over the predetermined PMPM credit. If it is split 50/50 with the MCO, the primary care doctors realize a $1.25 PMPM increment over their standard $10.73 allocation—an efficiency bonus of 12 percent.

The *specialist performance pool* works in exactly the same way as the hospital performance pool, with offsetting of surpluses and deficits reversed. The risk adjustments for demographic variations in utilization of specialist services, as well as the stop-loss protection for excessive charges for an individual member, will be somewhat different than for the hospital pool.

Once you have a good understanding of how this capitated system works, think about its various features that could be adjusted to create different levels of risk sharing and different kinds of incentives for the providers. There is the number and size of the performance pools, the number and size of the risk funds, the procedure and ratios for deficit recovery and surplus distribution.

The above example showed one risk fund and two performance pools that offset surpluses and deficits. To alter the impact of the compensation arrangement, the pools could be joined into a single pool or could function quite independently of each other. The risk fund could be eliminated, accompanied by a smaller capitation payment to the primary care physicians and larger allocations to the performance pools. The specialists could also be put on a capitated risk-sharing basis, with their own risk fund and offsetting surpluses and deficits with the primary care doctors.

There are many permutations and variations possible. Each MCO's compensation approach will be unique.

SECOND LEVEL: HOW PHYSICIAN GROUPS DISTRIBUTE THEIR REVENUES TO INDIVIDUAL PHYSICIANS

For the individual physicians in a large group practice, the method of reimbursement from an MCO to the group is almost irrelevant. Whether capitation payments or discounted fees accompanied by a risk withhold, the monies all flow into the group's gross revenues. What interests the individual physician is how those revenues are distributed to him or her. This is the second level of physician reimbursement/compensation.

The internal method of physician compensation within a group has far-reaching consequences. First, if it does not provide adequate compensation, current physicians will leave the practice and new ones cannot be recruited. Second, monetary payments have a powerful motivational function. It is important that they be tailored to encourage desirable forms of physician behavior. Third, if the compensation methodology is confusing, complex, and generally hard to understand, it will create dissension and upset among the physicians. Fourth, a compensation scheme that satisfies the physicians and offers the right kind of incentives must also comply with significant legal restrictions.

Ingredients of the Physician Compensation Package

It is a small point, but important to keep in mind. A typical physician compensation package consists of three components. The largest piece is usually a fixed salary, which the physician receives regardless of her performance or the organization's performance. Increasingly, a part of the physician's monetary reward is dependent on the achievement by her, her team or department, or the entire organization of certain predetermined performance objectives. The often-overlooked third component is the employee benefits paid by the organization to its physician employees.

What percentage of the total package is accounted for by each component? Of course, this varies from one organization to another. Of the two direct compensation pieces (salary and incentive), the share designated as an incentive is usually 10 to 20 percent and the salary is 80 to 90 percent. As the number of employee benefits offered has increased, they have come to take up as much as 30 percent of the entire package. So, a typical physician compensation bundle might look like this:

Salary Compensation	$120,000
Incentive Compensation	$ 20,000
Employee Benefits	$ 50,000
Total Compensation	$200,000

As provider organizations come under greater pressure to deliver even more cost-effective medical care, the incentive portion is rising as high as 40 percent of direct compensation in some cases.

What sorts of employee benefits might be included in a good physician compensation package? These are some benefits you are likely to see:

- medical, dental, and prescription insurance
- disability and life insurance
- retirement and savings plans
- paid vacations and holidays
- business expense reimbursement
- medical malpractice insurance
- professional expense reimbursement (continuing medical education (CME), licensure, memberships, subscriptions)
- deferred income benefits

Two especially desirable features of a benefit package are flexibility of choice and well-crafted retirement options. Because each physician's life circumstances are different, her needs for particular benefits will vary. Progressive employers accommodate these needs by offering "cafeteria style" benefit plans, in which each physician gets to spend the same lump sum on her preferred combination of benefits. Many physicians coming out of solo or small group practice have not had the opportunity to prepare or fund a good retirement plan. They will be particularly interested in satisfying this need when they accept employment.

The organization is restricted by antidiscrimination laws from giving physicians certain of these benefits in greatly more generous amounts than the nonphysician employees receive.

Factors Affecting Physician Compensation in Group Practices

If physicians are dissatisfied with some aspect of their compensation, they often blame the group's compensation system. This is only one of several possible causes, both internal and external. The outside forces include

- physician supply in the local market
- local market competition for the group's services
- local and national state of the economy
- population case mix of the group and its individual physicians
- managed care penetration in the local market
- reimbursement methods of local MCOs and other payers
- competition among local MCOs and payers

These internal group elements can also affect the compensation plan:

- leadership and management capabilities
- organization structure
- organization governance
- payer mix
- physician specialty mix
- group size
- group tradition and culture

MODELS OF PHYSICIAN COMPENSATION SYSTEMS IN THE TRANSITION FROM FFS TO CAPITATION

Under FFS arrangements, a physician's income increased according to the volume of revenue-producing charges he could generate. More and larger charges produced higher profits. Naturally, compensation plans in such settings tend to reward that kind of "productivity." Discounted FFS payments from PPOs and other noncapitated payers spur exactly the same kind of behavior. In fact, they may even encourage physicians to increase the number of patient visits of services provided per visit in order to offset the reduction in fees. This is one of the leading reasons for the rush to managed care and capitation.

Medical practices normally do not shift abruptly from FFS payer arrangements to capitation. The percentage of capitated patients seen increases steadily over time, allowing the physicians time to adapt their practice styles to the new demands of managed care. Capitation does require very different behavior on the part of physicians, and the compensation system must be re-engineered to support that. Experience shows that compensation formulas begin evolving from pure productivity-based incentives to salaries with utilization and quality incentives when 25 percent to 35 percent of a practice's revenues come through capitation.

Once the practice is attracting significant capitated revenues, the compensation evolves to emphasize the group's goals and performance over the interests of its individual physician members. Under capitation, more services and higher-cost services mean expenses that are deducted from group profits. Group practices with a high percentage of capitation must retune their definition of productivity to reflect an optimal use of health care resources, offering incentives for increased workloads and accessibility and using clinical quality and patient satisfaction as the bases for income distribution.

Physician groups in markets experiencing heavy managed care competition are concentrating on these goals in order to survive:

- increase market share (number of covered lives)
- control utilization (units of service delivered)
- minimize expenses (cost of service units)
- optimize quality (clinical outcomes and patient satisfaction)

They use their compensation systems to stimulate member physicians to pursue the goals.

As they move from FFS to capitation, physician groups tend to use a combination of compensation methods, such as a hybrid productivity-capitation formula. An individual physician's FFS income would be based on charges, collections, or visits for FFS patients while her capitated income would reflect the number of plan enrollees assigned to her.

There is a continuum of proven compensation methods for steering the course from productivity-based incentives to capitation.

Separate FFS and Capitation Compensation

This approach is just one step removed from straight FFS reimbursement. The FFS revenues still coming into the practice are tracked and compensated in traditional fashion, separate from capitation revenues. A utilization review committee establishes a monthly budget that takes into account expected capitated revenues and expenses necessary to treat the lives covered by those revenues. Individual physicians are credited with an FFS equivalent for each prepaid patient visit. At the end of the month, the credits for all physicians are totaled and then adjusted to fit within the budget. For example, assume three physicians with the following hypothetical billings for the month:

Physician A	$42,000
Physician B	$53,000
Physician C	$37,000
Total	$132,000

Also assume a budget for that month of $110,000.

The adjustment factor will be 110,000/132,000 = .83

The resulting compensation for the physicians will be

Physician A	$42,000 × .83 = $35,000
Physician B	$53,000 × .83 = $44,167
Physician C	$37,000 × .83 = $30,833
Total	$110,000

The physicians have the comfort of seeing their services charged in a way they understand and are accustomed to. Yet, there is a firm limit on the total payout to all the physicians, and there is no direct correlation between each doctor's income and his individual patient decisions. The physicians are really in competition with each other for the largest slice of a pie fixed in size. For that reason, the prepaid budget approach does not offer incentives for primary care physicians to seriously control utilization. It is possible for the committee to use physician-specific cost and referral data to limit inappropriate billing and practice patterns through peer pressure and utilization review.

Transitional Merger of FFS and Capitation Compensation

In this system, FFS and capitation revenues are combined in a single pot and then distributed to individual physicians in one of two ways. Capitation dollars are allocated directly on the basis of FFS equivalents, or they are simply divided evenly among the primary care doctors. Expenses are either deducted from the pot before the distribution or apportioned to each physician according to the mix of FFS and capitation patients she sees.

These kinds of transitional mechanisms require a fairly sophisticated information system to track patient visits, service units, and expenses. An effective utilization review program is also necessary to manage the capitation revenues.

One problem with the transition from FFS to capitation is that, if care is not taken, different treatment patterns may develop for the two kinds of patients. The easiest solution is to push through to full integration and nearly 100 percent capitated revenues as quickly as possible. Most physician groups find that, as their capitated revenues exceed roughly one-third of the total, it is easier to begin managing all patients under the same practice guidelines, utilization controls, and quality assurance protocols. In other words, treat all patients as though they were capitated.

Full Capitation Compensation

Under a predominantly capitated payment system, the compensation formula is based on covered lives per physician for both primary care and specialist doctors. All remnants of FFS reimbursement are gone. This has a couple advantages for the physician group. First, the doctors are put at financial risk and, therefore, pushed to build stronger utilization management and quality assurance capabilities—to move more aggressively toward integration. Second, in order to achieve those ends, the individual doctors must begin thinking in terms of group interest, over personal interest.

One methodology used by more highly integrated groups to allocate capitation revenues among their members works this way:

1. The services to be provided by each specialty within the group, as well as other responsibilities each will assume, are clearly defined. This prevents attempts by one specialty to pass patients on to another specialty in order to minimize costs.
2. On the basis of historical patient utilization data from within the group and comparable data from the local market, determine how revenues from various capitated payers will be allocated to each specialty.
3. Total the revenues for each specialty from all capitated payers.
4. Subtract overall group administrative overhead and physician expenses from the revenue allocations to calculate the amount available for physician compensation in each specialty.
5. Subtract a contribution to a benefit reserve for items like group health insurance, professional liability insurance, and CME support.
6. Subtract an amount to cover services for which the group is at risk but that must be provided outside the group.
7. Define a formula by which total net revenues for each specialty will be allocated to individual physicians. The usual approach is to give varying weights to the several qualities the group wants its physicians to emphasize. Actual compensation is deter-

mined by multiplying those weights times each physician's ratings for the qualities and applying this to the net revenues allocated to that specialty. Table 25–2 shows an example of the qualities and weights a specialty department might choose.

A physician organization has great leeway in manipulating these variables to create exactly the kind of compensation it wants, encouraging just the kinds of physician behavior it values. There are three basic choices to make: what qualities will be stressed, what weights they will be given, and how each physician's performance will be measured. The choices should be made by each specialty department and are likely to vary from one department to another.

Compensation by Salary Plus Bonus

The final step in the evolution from an FFS-based compensation system to one based on primarily capitated revenues is a combination of salary plus bonuses or a profit-sharing plan. This arrangement offers a guaranteed compensation base for physicians, coupled with incentives toward productivity and profitability goals that serve the group interest. To succeed with this level of sophisticated compensation system requires

• a substantial degree of operational integration in the group
• a modern, well-developed information system
• something close to consensus on the group's vision, values, and principles
• stable, bold, and informed physician leadership
• a knowledgeable task force to administer the system

The first step in putting together a system like this is to set salary levels. Here is how to do that:

1. Add all group revenues together—FFS, discounted FFS, and capitation.

Table 25–2 Model Criteria and Weights for Determining a Physician's Compensation

Quality	Weight	Measurement Criteria
Productivity	40%	Net collections based on relative value units
Utilization management	20%	Length of stay, usage of generic drugs, referral patterns, out-of-group usage
Patient satisfaction surveys	10%	Periodic questionnaire and in-person survey
Quality of care	10%	Clinical outcomes assessments, committee reviews
Group focus	10%	Meeting attendance, coverage, supervision (scored by the compensation committee)
Efficiency	10%	Cost per visit

2. Decide on a minimum base salary for each specialty.

3. Develop minimum "work effort" requirements for each specialty. These are the work contributions expected of each physician simply in order to earn her base salary. One group practice defined the following work effort requirements for its internal medicine physicians:

AVAILABILITY

- 45 weeks per year
- 36 hours per week (4.5 days)
- 1,620 hours per year

PRODUCTIVITY

- 19 office visits per day (10 on a half day)
- 2.4 office visits per hour
- 86 office visits per week
- 8.5 hospital/skilled nursing facility visits per week
- 32 hospital/skilled nursing facility visits per month

4. Calculate the funds available for performance bonuses—on top of the base salaries. Generally, this involves subtracting all expenses, including physician salaries, from all revenues. The remainder is the group's income, available for paying bonuses. The income can be left in a single pool for allocation to all physicians or divided into separate FFS and capitation pools. The division would be based on the ratio of FFS revenues to capitated revenues.

5. Choose the criteria on which the income will be allocated to participating physicians. If you are just starting with a salary/bonus compensation system, consider a simple, easy-to-understand formula. For instance, you might base the FFS bonus on each physician's share of total FFS revenues and base the capitation bonus on each physician's share of capitated enrollees. It is not a very sophisticated approach, but it gives the group's doctors a chance to acclimate to sharing overhead expenses.

6. Eventually, and as quickly as the group's proportion of managed care revenues warrants, move to more focused bonus criteria that spur the kinds of physician behavior that managed care requires. Think about covering areas like availability, productivity, efficiency, clinical outcomes, patient satisfaction, community service, utilization management, referral patterns, administrative responsibilities, and participation in group activities. Here are just some of the criteria you might want to include:

- *clinical outcomes*—percentage of hospital readmissions, repeat surgeries, infections or poisonings during treatment, cases with adverse reactions, deaths following care, and completeness of patient recovery of functioning
- *appropriateness of care*—percentage of care performed in questionable settings, questionable care in a short-stay setting, unnecessary Caeserian-sections, expense for lack of self-care, expense for preventive treatment, and expense for experimental treatments
- *patient satisfaction*—travel time, waiting time to schedule an appointment, waiting time during appointment, and total time spent per visit

The base salary ensures physicians of a comfortable level of personal income. That amount can be augmented by achievement of goals important to overall group success. Those goals, as reflected in the incentive criteria, can and should be regularly adjusted as

- The physicians become more comfortable practicing with incentives.
- The proportion of the group's revenues from capitation increases.
- The competition for managed care contracts or affiliations heats up.
- Employers and MCOs demand specific capabilities or performance from the group.

BASIC FOUNDATIONS OF A GOOD PHYSICIAN COMPENSATION SYSTEM

Physician compensation has implications that go beyond simple remuneration for services provided.

- The plan for compensating the physicians must reflect the organization's goals and objectives. It is a powerful tool for achieving the sought-after "alignment of incentives" among different specialties and kinds of providers in the organization.

- The compensation plan should be tailored to the organization's structure.
- All the payments to physicians—salary, incentives, and benefits—must be honestly correlated with available financial resources. Committing to payments that will compromise the organization's financial integrity is no good for any one.
- The compensation plan will take into account the organization's size and progress toward full integration. More mature organizations can offer more sophisticated arrangements than smaller entities just learning to operate under managed care.
- The nature of each physician's practice will partially determine her compensation arrangement. If it has been acquired intact by the organization, a different pay method will be warranted than if it is being started from scratch.
- The compensation plan must be sensitive to local supply and demand, and compensation levels for physicians with comparable skills and experience.

It may seem obvious, but the overall physician pay plan should be a "system." Compensation packages should be relatively consistent and predictable for all individual physicians and across physician groups. Do not expect to negotiate a special deal for yourself that is noticeably different from what your colleagues are receiving. Variations in compensation are acceptable only as a reflection of relevant factors like experience, specialty, level of responsibility, work schedule, and productivity. (More about productivity a little later.)

It is essential that physicians have prominent roles on the committee that sets compensation policies. If the organization is physician run, that should not be a problem. Just be sure not to delegate the bulk of the responsibility to nonphysician financial people. When the organization is owned by nonclinicians and run by professional managers, look more closely at how the compensation plan was conceived. It is fair to ask this very question during contract discussions. The plan will have more credibility with doctors if some of their own served on the compensation committee.

LESSONS LEARNED BY PHYSICIAN GROUPS IN DESIGNING THEIR COMPENSATION SYSTEMS

Many groups have been well along the path toward integration and practicing under managed care for several years. In that time, their experience in developing appropriate compensation systems has produced some useful guidelines.

- Decide where the group is going strategically before starting work on a compensation plan.
- Develop a coherent group culture and build trust in order to focus on group incentives.
- Minimize complexity in the compensation plan—make it as easy to understand as possible.
- Adjust each physician's capitation for the coming year on the basis of her prior year's performance.
- Link base salary or fixed compensation features with explicit work effort requirements.
- Create incentives that amount to at least 20 percent to 30 percent of total compensation.
- Base bonuses primarily on outcomes, patient satisfaction, and financial performance.
- Provide physicians with guidelines and protocols to support them in performing within the incentives.
- Give the physicians prompt and thorough feedback on individual and group performance.

LEGAL LIMITS ON PHYSICIAN COMPENSATION ARRANGEMENTS

The potential legal problems with physician compensation systems lie in three areas: fraud and abuse, taxes, and corporate practice of medicine. The fraud and abuse restrictions apply to all groups receiving any reimbursement under Medicare and Medicaid. This means virtually every group. The corporate practice of medicine problem comes up only for provider groups that are incorporated and only in states that enforce a "corporate practice" doctrine. The tax issues affect only charitable tax-exempt organizations.

Fraud and Abuse

There really are two federal fraud and abuse laws that apply to the compensation physicians receive from an organization to which they make referrals. The "antikickback" law[1] prohibits the knowing solicitation, receipt, offer, or payment of any kind of remuneration in return for referring a patient for a product or service that is wholly or partially paid for by a federal health program. If a physician makes referrals to an organization that makes payments to him as either an employee or an independent contractor, at least part of the compensation might be viewed as payment for the referrals.

The physician's relationship with the organization avoids this dire consequence by qualifying for one of the exceptions or "safe harbors" under the law. There is a safe harbor for physicians with a bona fide employee relationship with the organization.[2] The validity of the relationship is measured against the Internal Revenue Service (IRS) criteria listed in Exhibit 25–1. The safe harbor for payment by a group practice to an independent contractor physician[3] requires that

1. There be a written agreement signed by the parties.
2. The term of the agreement be no less than one year.
3. The agreement delineates the services the physician will provide.
4. If the physician will deliver services on a periodic, sporadic, or part-time basis, the agreement specifies the exact schedule of these periods, their precise length, and the payment for each period.
5. The total compensation paid over the term of the agreement be set in advance, be consistent with fair market value determined in arm's-length transactions, and not take

Exhibit 25–1 Special Case: Employees vs. Independent Contractors

More and more physicians are being employed by provider organizations of one kind or another. There are still many others who have and prefer independent contractor relationships with the organizations. The distinction is an important one. Employers must withhold taxes and meet IRS reporting requirements for their employees, but not for their independent contractors. Employees qualify for certain exceptions or "safe harbors" under the fraud and abuse, and Stark laws, while contractors qualify for others. A corporation that actually employs physicians may violate a state "corporate practice of medicine" doctrine.

Whether a physician is an employee or an independent contractor is determined by the IRS on the basis of the facts of the relationship rather than the way it may be described in a contract. These are factors that suggest a physician is an employee:

- The physician does not have a private practice.
- The physician is paid a straight wage.
- The organization provides supplies and professional support staff.
- The physician's services are billed through the organization.
- The physician's fees are shared on a percentage basis with the organization.
- The organization controls or has the right to control the physician's work activities.
- The physician works specified hours for the organization.
- The physician wears a coat bearing the organization's name.

These factors will imply an independent contractor relationship:

- The physician is responsible for hiring and paying associates.
- The physician has not agreed to a definite and fixed work schedule.
- The physician is independent of the direction or control of the organization's medical director.

- The physician is not granted the same rights and privileges as employees of the organization.
- The physician has a major investment in the facilities used to provide her services.
- The physician assumes any financial risk inherent in providing the services.
- The physician offers her services to the general public.

The overriding criterion used by the IRS is the degree of control the organization has over the physician's work activities. Furthermore, the IRS has stated that it will give greater weight to the control over the physician's business operations than his professional decisions. Factors to be considered in assessing the physician's control over the business aspects of medical care delivery are

- The physician is trained by the organization.
- The physician has a continuing working relationship with the organization.
- The physician works essentially full-time for the organization.
- The physician works on the organization's premises.
- The physician works according to priorities and sequences set by the organization.
- The physician submits regular reports to the organization.
- The physician is paid on the basis of work time spent rather than results achieved.
- How far the physician has become integrated into the organization's structure and operations.
- The nature, regularity, and continuity of the physician's work for the organization.
- The organization's authority to demand the physician's compliance with its policies.
- How closely the physician enjoys the rights and privileges of regular employees.

into account the volume or value of any referrals made between the parties.

The Stark law[4] prohibits a physician from making a referral for a "designated health service" to an entity with which he has a financial relationship and prohibits the entity from billing Medicare or Medicaid for the services provided under the prohibited referral. A financial relationship includes a compensation arrangement or an investment interest. The designated health services include:

- clinical laboratory services
- physical therapy services
- occupational therapy services
- radiology services
- radiation therapy services
- durable medical equipment
- parenteral and enteral nutrients, equipment, and supplies
- prosthetics, orthotics, and prosthetic devices
- home health services
- outpatient prescription drugs
- inpatient and outpatient hospital services

This law, too, has exceptions that cover certain physician compensation arrangements. The compensation of a physician-employee is protected if there is a bona fide employment relationship and

1. The employment is for identifiable services.
2. The compensation is consistent with the fair market value of the services and does not take into account the volume or value of the physician's referrals.
3. The agreement would be otherwise commercially reasonable without the referrals.

There is also an exception for independent contractors whose arrangement with the entity (the group practice) meets these requirements:

1. There is a written agreement, signed by the parties and specifying the services it covers.

2. The agreement covers all the services the physician will provide to the group.
3. The services contracted for are not more than are reasonable and necessary for the legitimate business purposes of the arrangement.
4. The agreement term is at least one year.
5. The compensation to be paid over the term of the agreement is set in advance, does not exceed the fair market value of the services, and does not take into account the volume or value of any referrals between the parties.

A physician compensation scheme can come close to paying for referrals by giving a physician either (1) a share of the overall profits of the group or (2) a productivity bonus based on services personally performed or incident to personally performed services. But the share or bonus may not be directly related to the volume or value of that physician's referrals.

There is one situation in which compensation may actually take into account referrals. This applies to physician incentive plans that meet the following conditions:

- It may not include a specific payment designed to induce the limitation of medically necessary services provided to a specific patient or enrollee of the organization.
- The organization is prepared to provide the Secretary of Health and Human Services with a good description of the plan.
- If the plan places a physician or physician group at substantial financial risk, it must comply with other requirements the Secretary may impose. Such requirements have been imposed on certain MCOs, in the shape of the Health Care Financing Administration (HFCA) rule described in the section below, "HCFA Rule Regulating Incentive Plans To Protect Physicians and Patients."

An incentive plan is defined as any compensation arrangement that directly or indirectly may have the effect of reducing or limiting services provided to patients of the group.

Under the Stark law, we have some idea of which compensation arrangements will work and which will not.

- Compensation may not take into account one physician's referrals to another physician in the same group.
- Compensation may not be based directly on ancillary services ordered by the physician.
- Ancillary service revenues should be shared equally among group physicians or distributed on the basis of each physician's personal productivity.
- Incentive compensation may be paid on the basis of adjusted gross revenues from services personally performed by each physician.
- Incentive compensation may be based on achievement of nonproductivity goals, like staying within budget limits.
- Incentive compensation may be based on a version of a resource-based relative value scale (RBRVS) measurement of personally performed physician services.

Federal Tax Law

These compensation issues arise only for organizations that have gained tax-exempt status under the Internal Revenue Code § 501c(3). To qualify for such status, the organization must satisfy certain requirements. The ones most relevant to physician compensation are the prohibitions against private benefit and private inurement. Any private benefit that a person receives through the activities of a tax-exempt organization must be incidental to the accomplishment of the organization's public benefits. In addition, no part of the net earnings of a tax-exempt organization may inure to the benefit of a private individual or shareholder. A "private individual" refers to a person with a personal and private interest in the activities of the organization, often called an "insider." As an example, the IRS considers physicians to be insiders if any of the following are true:

- They are employed by a hospital.
- They have privileges to admit and treat patients at the hospital.
- They are engaged in a partnership or joint venture with the hospital.
- They have a close, professional relationship with the hospital.

By extension, all physicians in similar ways related to a tax-exempt provider organization are potential recipients of prohibited private inurement.

The IRS believes that certain compensation arrangements are especially likely to result in private benefit or inurement and studies them more closely. These are income guarantees, incentive compensation, office space and ground leases, provision of support staff or practice management services, loans, outright cash assistance, purchase of specialized equipment, and subsidizing of malpractice insurance. To avoid these kinds of problems with compensation plans, the IRS asks that

- The compensation be reasonable.
- The compensation plan be consistent with the organization's exempt purpose.
- There be a ceiling on total compensation based on objective data regarding the value of the physician's service.
- The compensation levels be set by an independent committee following arm's-length negotiations with the physician.

To maintain consistency with an organization's exempt purpose, a compensation plan should meet the following criteria:

- Maximize efficiency.
- Shift risk away from the organization.
- Reduce the cost of providing health care.
- Improve patient care.
- Vary the amounts paid to individual physicians according to success in meeting organizational goals, rather than contributions to gross revenues.

- Avoid encouraging admissions or referrals to the organization as a means of generating income for the physicians.
- The plan does not have the effect of a joint venture.

Do not be surprised if the IRS requirements are not entirely compatible with the fraud and abuse requirements. Do not try to resolve these issues independently. Consult a good health lawyer experienced in these matters.

Corporate Practice of Medicine

This legal doctrine prohibits corporations from practicing medicine, either directly or through employed physicians. This is a state law doctrine. A few states do not even have it on their books. The doctrine exists in quite a few states that do not regularly or vigorously enforce it. Some states, like California and Texas, are passionate enforcers of the doctrine.

Most states have created special clear exceptions to the doctrine by allowing the formation of professional service or medical corporations. Usually, the corporation must be owned entirely by licensed physicians.

Follow these precautions to avoid attention in those states that are ambivalent about enforcement of the corporate practice of medicine doctrine:

- Allow physician-employees to exercise independent clinical medical judgment.
- Do not allow interference with the physician-patient relationship or patient confidentiality.
- Provide for continuity of patient care if a physician-employee leaves for any reason.
- Ensure that the medical record management system supports continuity of care.
- Do not inhibit the patient's freedom of choice in any way.
- Allow physician-employees to be responsible for determining whether the fees charged for their services are reasonable.

HCFA RULE REGULATING INCENTIVE PLANS TO PROTECT PHYSICIANS AND PATIENTS

An effective incentive program incorporates a few simple principles. It is tied to events or tasks clearly within the physician's control. Payments connected to the volume of patients seen serve no purpose if the patient flow is determined by the managed care plan. The incentives encourage behavior that fits the current payment basis from the MCO (capitation, FFS, or in between). Certain incentives may work to shape physician actions in capitated settings while very different incentives make sense in FFS practices. The program is easily understood by those that it is designed to influence—the physicians. If you cannot figure out how you will adjust your behavior to maximize your incentive pay, it is not a good plan, and you should ask for a simplification.

Patients also have shown concern about the effects of compensation incentives they do not understand or, even worse, do not know about. They are interested in whether the physician treating them has a "hidden agenda" to minimize the care they receive. Legislators and government regulators have stepped in to protect the concerns of both patients and physicians.

The federal HCFA issued a final rule,[5] establishing requirements with respect to physician incentive plans, on March 27, 1996, followed by an additional notice on September 3, 1996. The rule applies to provider organizations receiving reimbursement under the Medicare and Medicaid programs. Several states have indicated their intentions to apply the terms of the rules to commercial managed care contracts with private employers and subscribers outside Medicare and Medicaid. For this reason, and because the rule offers physicians a reasonable degree of protection against extreme cost-cutting mandates by MCOs, it is worth understanding how it works.

Health Plans Covered by the Rules on Physician Incentives

The HCFA rules apply to federally qualified HMOs, competitive medical plans (CMPs), and other health insuring entities with Medicare or Medicaid risk contracts. They apply as well to any MCO that bills Medicare or Medicaid and intends to rely upon the physician incentive plan exception to the Stark II self-referral prohibitions. The rules have an indirect impact on physicians, physician groups, and other entities (IPAs and physician-hospital organizations (PHOs)) that contract with MCOs. They restrict incentive plans affecting Medicare and Medicaid enrollees, but not commercial enrollees.

Requirements of the Rule

To operate a physician incentive plan, some basic requirements must first be met.

- No specific payment may be made directly or indirectly to physicians as an inducement to reduce or limit medically necessary services.
- If the incentive plan places a physician or physician group at substantial financial risk for services not provided by the physician or physician group, the health plan must provide stop-loss protection to the physicians.
- The health plan must also conduct periodic surveys of past and present enrollees to determine access to services and satisfaction with the quality of services.
- Certain of the information gathered must be disclosed to permit the government to determine whether an incentive plan complies with the requirements.

The rule states that "substantial risk" occurs when the incentive plan places the physician or physician group at risk for amounts over 25 percent of potential payments to the physician or physician group if the risk is based on the use or cost of referral services (i.e., specialty, inpatient, outpatient, or laboratory services that a physician

or physician group orders or arranges for, but does not furnish directly). Potential payments include the maximum anticipated total payments, based generally on the most recent year's utilization and experience, that could be received if use or costs of referral services were low enough.

The rule states that the following arrangements create substantial risk when a group's panel size is less than 25,000 patients:

- withholds greater than 25 percent of potential payments
- withholds less than 25 percent of potential payments if the group is potentially liable for amounts exceeding 25 percent of potential payments
- bonuses greater than 33 percent of potential payments not including the bonus
- withholds combined with bonuses that are more than 25 percent of potential payments
- capitation arrangements if the difference between the maximum and minimum possible payment is more than 25 percent of the maximum possible payment
- capitation arrangements where the maximum and minimum possible payments are not clearly explained in the contract with the physicians
- any other incentive arrangements that have the potential to hold a physician or physician group liable for more than 25 percent of potential payments

When and to Whom Stop-Loss Protection Must Be Provided

Health plans must provide all physician groups at substantial financial risk with either *aggregate* or *per patient* stop-loss protection. If the protection applies to all patients on the panel as a group, it must cover 90 percent of the costs of referral services that exceed 25 percent of potential payments. If the protection is defined on a per patient basis, it must cover 90 percent of the referral costs that exceed specified per patient limits. The limits are based on the size of the patient panel. They are lowest for smaller panels and increase as the size of the panel increases. For panels over 25,000, no stop-loss protection is required at all.

In determining the size of its patient panel, a health plan can "pool" several physician groups' patients and may also pool Medicare and Medicaid patients with commercial patients. In the latter case, the rules then apply to the commercial patients as well. Otherwise, the rule does not apply to physician incentive plans related to the service of non-Medicare or non-Medicaid patients.

In addition to protecting physicians whom they place at substantial financial risk, health plans must also offer stop-loss coverage to

- individual physicians, if any physician group with which the plan contracts places its individual members at substantial financial risk
- physicians or physician groups whose contract with an IPA or PHO or similar entity places them at financial risk, and the entity has contracts with the health plan to treat Medicare or Medicaid patients

Patient Surveys Required of Health Plans

The rule requires that health plans conduct enrollee surveys under three circumstances.

1. When its physician incentive plan places a physician at substantial risk.
2. When the plan contracts with a physician group that places its own members at substantial risk.
3. When the plan contracts with another entity (such as an IPA or PHO) that places the physicians or physician groups with which it contracts at substantial financial risk.

The survey must include at least a sample of all Medicare and Medicaid patients who are currently enrolled or were enrolled during the previous 12 months. It must gather information on the enrollees' satisfaction with the quality of service provided and their level of access to the service. The surveys must be conducted no later than one year after the effective date of the incentive plan and at least every two years after that.

Information Disclosure Required of Health Plans

If the incentive plan applies only to services furnished by the physician or physician group in question (in other words, it does not apply to referral services), the health plan need disclose just that fact to HCFA. If the incentives do cover referral services, the following specific information must be disclosed to HCFA:

- the type of incentive arrangement (withhold, bonus, or capitation)
- the percentage of any withhold or bonus
- the amount and type of stop-loss protection
- the patient panel size and, if it is the result of pooling, the components of the pool
- capitation payments to primary care physicians for the most recent year broken down into primary care and referral service by type of provider
- results of the enrollee surveys

When Medicare or Medicaid patients request it, the plan must tell them the type of incentive arrangement, the existence of any stop-loss protection, and a summary of the survey results.

Under this rule, or a state variation of it, health plans have three choices: (1) They may choose to eliminate their physician incentive plans rather than comply with the stop-loss and disclosure requirements. (2) They may structure their incentive plans to avoid placing physicians and physician groups at substantial financial risk. (3) They can carry out incentive plans that trigger the regulations and take steps to comply with them by

- purchasing or providing the necessary stop-loss protection
- designing and conducting the required enrollee surveys
- filing the required information disclosures with HCFA

Using the Terms of the HCFA Rules

The mere publication of the HCFA rules, the furor around them, and the media attention focused on them makes them quite useful for physician groups. In contract negotiations with MCOs, physician groups can reasonably demand that protections of this sort be incorporated into any incentive schemes applied to them. Even if the full package of protections is not accepted, these demands can be used as powerful bargaining chips on other contract provisions.

SOURCES OF COMPARISON DATA ON PHYSICIAN COMPENSATION

Whether you are sitting on a compensation committee charged with setting pay levels for physicians in your group or just trying to compare a compensation package you have been offered with what other doctors are getting, knowing where to obtain reliable comparative data is useful. Compliance with several of the legal limits on compensation plans (e.g., determining the "fair market value" of a physician's services or negotiating compensation in an arm's-length transaction) is facilitated by access to good figures on physician compensation. Here are the best sources.[*]

American Group Practice Association (AGPA)

The Alexandria, Virginia,-based AGPA, which recently merged with the Unified Medical Group Association of Seal Beach, California, conducts an annual compensation survey of physicians employed in group practices. The AGPA's most recent data are from 1995 and are based on a survey of 346 organizations. The results include data from 24,306 physicians representing 70 medical

---

specialties or positions. The survey results cost $225. Contact Ryan O'Connor at 703-838-0033.

American Medical Association (AMA)

The Chicago-based AMA collects income data, not compensation data, from about 4,000 physicians annually. Data come from a mix of employed, self-employed, and independent-contractor physicians. Data represent net income after practice expenses but before taxes. The data are published each year in the AMA's annual *Socioeconomic Characteristics of Medical Practice* report. The report costs $75 for AMA members and $120 for nonmembers. Contact the AMA at 312-464-5000.

Ernst & Young

Ernst & Young, a national accounting and consulting firm, conducts an annual compensation survey of physicians employed in hospitals, group practices, and managed care plans. It also has a category of physicians employed by integrated delivery systems. The firm's data from April 1995 were based on a survey of 89 organizations. Some 38 percent were hospitals; 32 percent were integrated delivery systems; 21 percent were group practices; and 9 percent were managed care plans. The results include data from 10,520 physicians representing 42 medical specialties or positions. The firm did not disclose the price of the report. Contact Janel Patterson at 212-773-2154.

Hay Group

The Philadelphia-based benefits consulting firm conducts an annual compensation survey of physicians employed by hospitals, group practice, and managed care plans. Hay's data from July 1995 were based on a survey of 158 organizations. Some 58 percent were hospitals; 24 percent were group practices; and 18 percent were managed care plans. The results include data from 20,801 physicians representing 65 medical specialties or positions. Survey results are free to participating organizations. The cost of participation ranges from $975 to $1,475 depending on the size of the organization. Contact Marla Badenhop at 510-945-8220.

Hospital & Healthcare Compensation Service (HHCS)

The Oakland, New Jersey,-based consulting firm conducts an annual compensation survey of physicians employed by hospitals, group practices, and managed care plans. It also includes data from federally employed physicians. HHCS' data from January 1996 were based on a survey of 303 organizations. Some 78 percent were hospitals; 17 percent were group practices; and 5 percent were managed care plans or other types of employers. The results include data from 9,600 physicians representing 43 medical specialties or positions. The survey results cost $250. Contact Tom Cioffe at 201-616-5722.

Medical Group Management Association (MGMA)

The Englewood, Colorado,-based trade organization for group practice administrators conducts an annual compensation survey of physicians employed primarily in group practices. The MGMA's data from 1994 were based on a survey of 1,409 organizations. Some 91 percent of those were group practices. The results include data from 25,696 physicians representing 70 medical specialties or positions. The survey results cost $150. Contact Lisa Pieper at 303-397-7895.

Merritt, Hawkins & Associates

The Irving, Texas,-based physician search firm collects income data on physicians it places in all types of health care settings. Merritt's data are gleaned from its physician placements made during the 12-month period ending each April. In the 1996 survey, some 1,352 placements at 495 organizations were included in the survey. The data cover 33 medical specialties or positions. The survey results are free. Contact Phil Miller at 214-868-2220.

Physician Executive Management Center (PEMC)

The Tampa, Florida,-based physician search firm conducts an annual compensation survey of physicians employed by group practices and managed care plans. PEMC's data from the fall of 1995 were based on a survey of 31 organizations. Some 85 percent of the organizations were group practices; 15 percent were managed care plans. The results include data from 1,179 physicians representing 10 medical specialties or positions. PEMC didn't disclose the price of the report. Contact David Kirschman at 813-963-1800.

Physician Services of America (PSA)

The Louisville, Kentucky,-based physician search firm conducts an annual survey of salary expectations of physicians whom the company is trying to place. PSA's data from August 1995 are based on responses from 33,000 physicians representing 32 medical specialties. The survey results are free. Contact Jennifer Wild at 502-423-9622, extension 220.

Sullivan, Cotter and Associates

The Detroit-based human resources consulting firm conducts an annual compensation survey of physicians employed by hospitals, group practices, managed care plans, and other types of employers. Sullivan's data from January 1996 were based on a survey of 192 organizations. Some 62 percent of the organizations were hospitals; 27 percent were group practices; 9 percent were managed care plans; and 20 percent were other types of employers. The percentages do not add to 100 because of multiple response categories. The results include data from 13,752 physicians representing 79 medical specialties or positions. The survey results cost $350 for organizations that agree to participate in next year's survey; $600 for health care organizations; and $1,200 for non–health care organizations. Contact Kimberly Mobley at 313-872-1760.

Towers Perrin

The Parsippany, New Jersey,-based management consulting firm maintains a database on physician compensation data from a variety of sources, including previous customized research projects, confidential client information, and published survey data. The data included in its annual physician compensation reports represent solely hospital-employed physicians. Towers did not disclose the price of information available through its database. Contact Kathryn Hastings at 201-331-3546.

William M. Mercer

The Detroit office of the national benefits consulting firm conducts an annual compensation survey of physicians employed by hospitals, group practices, and managed care plans. The data from 1995 were based on a survey of 210 organizations. Some 58 percent of the organizations were hospitals; 18 percent were managed care plans, 14 percent were group practices, and 10 percent were other types of employers. The results include data from 14,712 physicians representing 87 medical specialties or positions. The price of the survey results to nonparticipating organizations is $750. Contact Carol Breen at 313-877-7303.

REFERENCES

1. 42 U.S.C. § 1320a-7b.
2. 42 C.F.R. § 1001.952 (i).
3. 42 C.F.R. § 1001.952 (d).
4. 42 U.S.C. § 1395nn.
5. 42 C.F.R. § 417.479.

RESOURCE LIST

"Capitation Is for Specialists, Not for Primary Care Physicians," *Managed Care,* August 1997.

"Developing an Incentive System for PHO Physicians," *Healthcare Financial Management*, February 1996.

"How Capitation Turned Red Ink to Black at Harris Methodist Health Systems," *Managed Care,* August 1997.

Income Distribution, Information Exchange #4890 (Englewood, CO: Medical Group Management Association, 1996).

Income Distribution? Prepaid Component, Information Exchange #3474 (Englewood, CO: Medical Group Management Association, 1997).

Income Distribution? Stark II, Information Exchange #4738 (Englewood, CO: Medical Group Management Association, 1995).

"Making the Transition from Productivity Compensation to Capitation," *Managed Care*, August 1997.

"MD Payment Plans Continue To Evolve under Capitation," *Capitation Management Report*, June 1997.

Physician Compensation and Production Survey: 1997 Report Based on 1996 Data, Survey #4986 (Englewood, CO: Medical Group Management Association).

Physician Compensation Systems (Chicago, American Medical Association).

Physician Incentive Plans, Super Search Packet #4893 (Englewood, CO: Medical Group Management Association).

"Strange Bedfellows: Paying Fee for Service to Primary Care Physicians while Capitating Specialists," *Managed Care Week*, 29 September, 1997.

## CHAPTER 26

Managing Risk in the Practice of Medicine

INTRODUCTION

There is a lot of talk about "risk sharing" in the delivery of health care. The risk involved is the one initially assumed by a managed care organization (MCO) or insurance company when it agrees to provide a range of health care services to a business's employees who enroll with it, in return for a monthly premium paid by the business for each of those employees. The premium is calculated as carefully as possible to cover the costs of all the services those enrollees are likely to demand from the MCO. The risk is that the enrollees will be sicker than anticipated and will require more services, costing more money than the premium will cover.

The MCO shares that risk with provider organizations and individuals by paying them a fixed amount per month (a capitation fee) per enrollee in return for their delivery of a defined package of services to each enrollee. The same risk problem exists here—it may cost the organization more money to meet the enrollees' service needs than are anticipated by the capitation figure. The organization will have to bear the additional cost and perhaps incur a net loss as a result. If the problem persists, the organization will fail.

The risk sharing can go even further if the provider organization chooses to subcapitate its individual participating physicians—either primary care or specialists. The same potential for mismanagement of the risk exists there.

This chapter defines the primary variables in the risk that physicians face under managed care. It then proposes a variety of strategies for coping with that risk. The ultimate goal is to give physicians greater control of one of the most worrisome and unpredictable aspects of managed care, to increase the likelihood of their professional success.

WHO SHOULD READ THIS CHAPTER

This chapter is required reading for the physician who may be entering into a risk-sharing arrangement for the first time. There is a potential for considerable financial loss if the risk is not assessed and managed properly. Here, she will learn the basic principles of doing that.

Even those physicians who have been practicing under noncapitated managed care contracts for some time need to acquire the kinds of risk management skills described in this chapter. Managed care, often discounted fee for service (FFS) with MCO-directed utilization management, does not necessarily involve capitation payments to a physician who must manage his own utilization. The time to become adept at managing the financial risk is before it impacts a large percentage of your revenue stream.

Many of the risk management strategies outlined here are carried out even more effectively by large groups of physicians. A physician may belong to such a group without personally bearing risk for the volume and cost of services provided. He still may want to use the ideas in this chapter for informing and guiding that group.

The chapter may be skipped by any physicians who are absolutely confident in their ability to practice profitably under risk sharing or who are part of a large, well-managed organization that compensates them on a relatively no-risk basis (i.e., salary plus a simple incentive bonus).

DIFFERENT KINDS OF RISK YOU MAY ENCOUNTER

There are four variables in the equation that determines whether physicians will prosper under a capitation arrangement.

- number of enrollees ("covered lives") for which they are responsible
- number of units of service provided to those enrollees
- intensity, severity, or complexity of each of those service units
- cost of each unit of service

The extent to which the physicians cannot predict or control any of those variables is a measure of the risk they face under that arrangement.

For instance, if an unusually small number of enrollees choose to receive their care from the physicians and several of them have catastrophic illnesses, the resulting expenses could very quickly exceed the capitation rate. On the other hand, so many enrollees may be drawn to the physicians' group practice that they cannot handle them all. The physicians may have to subcontract with other physicians for their care—at much greater expense. If the physicians provide more units of service to their patient-enrollees than are really medically necessary (in other words, if they do not manage their utilization of resources), they will incur greater costs than contemplated by the capitation rate. If they provide fewer units than the patients truly need, the patients will be sicker longer and feel greater dissatisfaction. Providing service that is more complex or intense than the patient actually needs is

almost always more expensive than necessary. If the physicians' practice is generally not well managed, if they have not developed streamlined, integrated processes, all their costs of operation will be higher. Most capitation rates assume an efficient, tightly run practice.

Risks can become a problem for a physician practice in three generic ways.

1. Through mismanagement, poor practice styles, and overutilization, the physicians are simply unable to deliver the contracted services at a cost less than the capitation rate.
2. Although individual members of the practice may practice cost-effective quality medicine, the inefficient behaviors of a few may incur excessive costs borne by the entire group.
3. Provisions in the managed care contract put the physicians at risk for events over which they have no control or for which they are not compensated. A poor description of the services to be delivered may obligate the group to do more than it is capable of. Midcontract changes by the MCO in copayment requirements or assignment of enrollees or reporting burdens on the physicians can alter the cost/profit equation for the group.

Risk management is about minimizing or eliminating all these risks.

SITUATIONS IN WHICH A PHYSICIAN WILL BE AT RISK

Physicians are at some degree of risk in the following situations:

- They belong to a physician group that receives a large proportion of its revenues from capitated contracts. The risk for individual physicians is aggravated when the group is small enough in size that poor overall risk management can have a direct impact on the income of each one of them.

- The physicians in a group are compensated through a lump sum base payment plus a withhold amount, which they receive only if it is not consumed by excessive utilization.
- The physician group receives a lump sum base payment plus bonuses earned for achieving certain performance goals (utilization, quality, patient satisfaction, etc.).
- A solo practicing physician is party to a managed care contract that pays him on a capitated, salary plus withhold, or salary plus bonuses basis.
- The physicians are under contract with an MCO that pays them on a discounted FFS basis, but also enforces utilization management measures against them. If certain utilization criteria are not met, the physicians are at risk of being deselected.

The only situations in which physicians are not at serious financial risk are when they are paid on a straight FFS, discounted FFS, or salary basis with nothing contingent on their performance, utilization, or practice behaviors. Such situations are diminishing in number.

BASIC STRATEGIES FOR MANAGING THE RISK IN THOSE SITUATIONS

Strategies for dealing with risk are not complicated. There are three basic alternatives—bear the risk, share the risk, or shift the risk.

Bear the Risk

These strategies include everything the physician group can do internally to reduce the likelihood of risks occurring and their impact when they do occur.

Utilization Management Procedures

These are assertive measures for limiting the use by physicians of valuable resources, such as materials, pharmaceuticals, lab tests, specialists,

and even the physicians' own time. They must be balanced with other measures to ensure that quality and patient satisfaction are not compromised in the process. Carried out consistently, these procedures will make it more likely that the physician group can provide just the right care required by its enrolled patients at a cost within the fee schedule or capitation rate paid by the MCO. The group might simply copy the procedures traditionally used by MCOs—preauthorization of hospital admissions and major procedures, concurrent review of ongoing hospital stays, retrospective review of completed hospital stays, second opinions on expensive medical procedures, and mandatory outpatient surgery for defined medical problems. Or, it might adopt some of the following more sophisticated strategies.

Gatekeeper Systems Controlling Access to Specialists

Service costs really begin to mount when patients are referred to the care of specialists. So-called "gatekeeper systems" require that a specially trained and designated primary care physician (PCP) authorize most, if not all, patient contacts with specialists. The more responsible gatekeeper systems do not try to restrict patient access to certain kinds of physicians or care, but rather aim to make sure that the patient is directed to the "right" kinds of care. This can be an important distinction. In their broad role as choreographers of patient care, the PCPs also will monitor and regulate utilization of almost the full range of resources a patient might need in addition to the specialist referrals.

Two additional mechanisms help the PCP carry out her duties most effectively. She is quite likely to be reimbursed on a capitation basis. This gives her a strong incentive to minimize the costs of treating the patients assigned to her; she will realize any savings that result. This must be offset by incentives that keep her from cutting treatment and costs so far that the patients suffer. Traditional quality assurance procedures help prevent dramatically excessive cost cutting. Even better are countervailing incentives like withholds or bonuses tied to the achievement of quality or patient satisfaction criteria.

Other Systems for Managing the Use of Resources (Case Management, Disease Management, Demand Management)

Still other methods have been developed for managing the consumption of resources by patients. Under *case management* a single person is made responsible for coordinating the full continuum of care (personnel and procedures) required to treat a patient's symptoms during a single case episode. The net effect is to avoid wasted time and wasted expense. The patient is likely to be more satisfied with a more streamlined treatment pathway. *Disease management* takes a systematic approach to actively managing patients with a specific disease. Using the concepts of clinical guidelines, outcomes management, and total quality improvement, this strategy tailors the treatment plan to the patient and the disease. On the other hand, *demand management* attempts to reduce the patients' need to access the health care system at all. It accomplishes this through early detection and treatment, preventive care, patient education on self-diagnosis and treatment, telemedicine consultations that avoid facility visits, and initial contact with physician extenders and midlevel providers.

Dissemination of Comparative Physician-Specific Utilization Data

One of the simplest, least threatening methods of helping physicians cut back on inappropriate utilization is to show them the data that reveal how high their utilization is. This is a listing of the relevant utilization rates for all the physicians in the group practicing comparable medicine. Initially, it may be useful to hide the identities of the physicians except for the one receiving the list. If the numbers are small, however, it may be difficult to disguise identities. Once the physicians become comfortable with comparing themselves to their colleagues, it may not be necessary to hide the names. Evidence has shown that mere

awareness of these data can often spur significant changes in physician practice behaviors.

Peer Review of Physician Outliers in Utilization

As an alternative to revealing the comparative data, other physicians in the group, often part of a formal peer review team, may meet with a physician identified as an excessive utilizer. At this stage, their goal is to call attention to what looks like a problem and hear whatever explanations he may have. A common response from the physician is that he is seeing higher-risk patients. The team will verify this. It probably will offer some mild suggestions for curbing the physician's utilization.

Mentoring and Counseling of Physician Outliers in Utilization

If the problem of excessive utilization persists after the sharing of comparative data or the peer review and there is no good explanation for the variation, one or more physician colleagues may engage in more aggressive mentoring and counseling of the high utilizer. It may be made mandatory that the physician spend time working with, consulting with, or practicing under the tutelage of a physician more experienced in managed care. The goal is to assist the physician in developing new, natural clinical skills that meets the organization's needs.

Discipline of Physician Outliers in Utilization

In very rare cases, where a physician is utilizing to excess for no good reason and refuses to make adjustments, the group may take some disciplinary measures against him. The most common would be monetary penalties. The group might also limit other privileges or perquisites important to the physician. Rather than engage in such punitive practices, however, most groups will work with an outlier physician for a more than reasonable length of time and then go straight to dismissal.

Dismissal of Physician Outliers in Utilization

If a physician cannot bring his utilization rates within acceptable norms (because he has tried and cannot make the necessary changes or has not wanted to try at all), it ultimately may be necessary for the group to dismiss him from its ranks. Most physician-run organizations will be loath to do this. Nonetheless, when the one physician's behavior begins to cost the entire organization money and impact the earnings of others in the group, dismissal is the only sound business decision.

Thorough Credentialing of Physicians Joining the Group

Every group, organization, or facility of true professional integrity conducts a thorough review of the competence-related credentials of every physician who will be practicing for it. This initial check and subsequent rechecks become even more essential when an incident of malpractice can impact the entire organization—because it ends up bearing the cost or is named as a defendant in the litigation. Thorough credentialing is the first step in ensuring that the organization delivers nothing but quality medical care.

Careful Screening of Physicians Joining the Group

Physician groups must also look at other characteristics besides clinical competence in evaluating new physician members. Effective managed care physicians must be able to minimize utilization of resources while maintaining quality, satisfy patients, produce optimal clinical outcomes, comply with clinical guidelines, work in teams with other physicians and clinical practitioners, cooperate productively with nonclinical personnel, respond to quantitative and qualitative feedback, and demonstrate at least a modest amount of enthusiasm for managed care. Failures in too many of these areas can lead to unnecessarily high costs, lower physician incomes, patient unhappiness and disenrollment, MCO unhappi-

ness and contract cancellation, high employee turnover, lower group morale, medical malpractice lawsuits, and lost strategic opportunities. Competitive physician groups seek these attributes in their new physician members and dismiss those members when they fail to demonstrate them.

Traditional Quality Assurance Measures (Tissue Review, Records Review)

A responsible delivery organization continues to monitor the quality of care provided by its physicians through traditional quality assurance procedures such as tissue/surgical reviews, records reviews, infection control, pharmaceuticals usage, and blood utilization. In addition to these basic functions, there may also be a general risk management committee as well as a variety of other programs designed to minimize the risk of untoward clinical events. Nearly all of them can be implemented by a physician group or integrated provider organization.

Development and Application of Clinical Protocols and Pathways

By encouraging their members to follow clinical protocols or pathways, physician groups are trying to minimize unwarranted variation and steer their practitioners toward the clinical practices that are most likely to be effective. The idea is not to force physicians to adhere rigidly to a "recipe" of treatment choices. Instead, the pathways show them what works best most of the time. Physicians have the discretion to deviate from the pathways whenever their clinical judgment dictates. They will be challenged if the deviations become commonplace and cannot be justified by the patients' conditions.

The larger groups are developing their own protocols or pathways, based on study of their own experiences with the patients actually enrolled with the group. Smaller groups normally cannot afford such a research and development effort. They must turn to the specialty societies, insurance companies, and government agencies that are creating more generic protocols. In such cases, it is important to evaluate the scientific origins and foundations of the protocols. They must be based on clinical data that are relevant to the physician group that will be using the protocols.

Evaluation of Treatment Decisions and Practice Styles through Measurement of Clinical Outcomes

When the clinical outcomes of treatment decisions can be measured with some accuracy, they provide the basis for translating the best of those decisions into protocols and pathways. In more advanced practice environments, they may be used to evaluate the clinical performance of individual physicians. Although outcomes measurement technology is still in a very primitive stage, it offers organizations the potential for fine-tuning the selection and retention of the most quality-conscious physicians.

Centralized and Standardized Purchasing of Commonly Used Supplies, Materials, and Equipment

It is a no-brainer to consolidate the selection and purchase of the wide variety of supplies and equipment used in the delivery of medical services. The organization can standardize on a few brands and models to be used and acquire them in more economical volumes. The benefits are reduced costs of operation and fewer chances of delay or error in finding the right item when it is needed.

Financial Incentives Encouraging Optimal Clinical Decision Making (Capitation, Risk Withholds, Performance Bonuses)

These are the most powerful and profound tools for encouraging physician behavior that minimizes the risks faced by the group. In the simplest terms, the doctors are given monetary rewards for acting in ways that satisfy the needs of the overall organization or its payers. These needs usually include keeping costs as low as possible without compromising quality, and keeping the patients healthy and satisfied. When a physician is capitated, she has an incentive to use as few costly resources as possible in treating her patients, since she (or her organization) will reap the savings if costs are kept below the capitation fee and will bear the expense if they exceed the fee. Capitation has proven to be an effective device for aggressively cutting costs; there are questions about its simultaneous negative effects on quality. Under a risk withhold arrangement, physicians receive a certain percentage of their compensation (typically 10 to 30 percent) only if the amount is not consumed by excessive utilization or they otherwise meet performance targets. Performance bonuses are additional compensation paid to physicians who reach predetermined performance goals. The bonuses may be tied to absolutely any behavior the group wishes to encourage, including combinations of cost cutting and quality improvement.

Tracking and Responding to Patient Complaints

One of the best indicators that things are going awry in the way a physician group delivers care is the volume and nature of the complaints that patients make. Savvy organizations establish and promote accessible, patient-friendly complaint mechanisms. They encourage patients to complain about almost anything that bothers them. Many of the complaints are frivolous or inconsequential. However, the organization can sift through those to concentrate on the more serious patient concerns. Often, it can catch a problem before it escalates into a major quality issue and even a malpractice lawsuit. By responding sensitively to the most trivial grievances, the organization can build good will among its patient-enrollees. Potential contract partners, especially MCOs, will be impressed by the availability of an effective patient complaint procedure.

Patient Satisfaction Surveys

Instead of waiting for patients to have problems and come to complain about them, the best physician groups actively conduct regular surveys of their patients on a variety of topics. They are looking for evidence of what works and what does not work. The findings can identify emerging problems before they grow into major crises. They can help the organization allocate its resources to carry out improvements. The positive results can be used in negotiations with payers and as selling points in marketing. MCOs frequently want to see a regular patient survey program in operation. The patients themselves will simply appreciate the interest in their opinions.

Maintain Adequate Cash Reserves

To the extent that the organization faces the risk of unpredictably high expenditures (because of a higher incidence of catastrophic illnesses or excessive utilization by its physicians), it must act in some ways like an insurance company. Primarily, it can make sure that it has adequate cash reserves on hand to cover those expenditures. The money held back under a risk-withhold contract is, in effect, a kind of reserve against such contingencies. With adequate reserves, it is less likely that a sudden surge in expenses will sink the organization.

Sound Cash Management

The corollary of maintaining sufficient cash reserves is competently managing all the cash used by the organization in its operations. This starts with maintaining enough liquid working capital to support day-to-day operations without sacrificing too much of the interest that could be earned through less-liquid investments. It means generating additional revenues through placement of temporarily excess cash in money market accounts and other short-term investment opportunities. Ultimately, it includes shaping a structure of capital sources (short- and long-term debt, lines of credit, retained earnings, public and private sales of stock, physician-member dues) that balances risk and cost to provide investment capital when it is needed.

Experiment with Investments in Early Detection and Preventive Care

The best way to minimize the actuarial and financial risks of sickness in a group's patient pool is to prevent the sickness entirely. There are a variety of preventive care initiatives that physicians are taking with their patients. These include prophylactic treatments (immunizations) and encouragement of patient lifestyle changes (smoking cessation, weight reduction). Early detection of some illnesses (Pap smears) may catch them at a stage of lower severity when they can be addressed through less costly treatments. What is uncertain is whether these detection and prevention strategies are cost-effective; that is, whether the money invested in them is offset by the savings in treatment costs later on. It may turn out to be cheaper to just wait and see if the illness develops at all, then treat it as aggressively as possible. Larger organizations can test the viability of these strategies.

Other Measures To Reduce Clinical Variation

There is a growing feeling in delivery organizations that, for the most common and simple diagnoses, dramatically different treatment of similarly situated patients cannot be justified clinically. Studies have found a remarkable degree of clinical variation that cannot be explained by patient risk differentials. Such unwarranted variation can result in the added expense of unnecessary treatment choices. Furthermore, inappropriate care can cause a detriment to the patient's health status.

Provider groups are taking a number of aggressive initiatives to reduce clinical variation. Physician profiling permits a group to identify physicians with unusual clinical patterns. Measurement of clinical outcomes indicates which physicians are producing less desirable clinical results. The development and application of clinical guidelines and protocols steer physicians toward treatment progressions that evidence shows to be the most effective. Implementing measures like these is a major step toward managing the risk providers must assume under managed care.

Implement Total Quality Management (TQM) and Reengineering of All Process (Clinical, Administrative, Logistical, and Operational)

The development of clinical guidelines and protocols is often part of a much broader program of reengineering any relevant processes, procedures, or systems within the organization. The goal always is to streamline operations and remove impediments to improving quality and lowering costs. Reengineering and the closely related concepts of TQM or continuous quality improvement (CQI) involve more than incremental "changes" or "improvements" to the existing processes. In their more advanced forms, they call for the redesign of those processes, from the ground up, as though they were being created for the first time. This technology is applied not only to clinical processes, where it can dramatically cut costs while maintaining quality, but also to every other area of operations (administrative, logistical, financial). Ideally, the reengineering never stops; the organization is constantly transforming itself.

Look for New Ways To Employ Physician Extenders

The risk element is moderated when physicians concentrate on performing the most highly skilled tasks for which they have been trained. The most sophisticated managed care providers strive to push all tasks down to the lowest level person qualified to perform them. This entails pervasive use of physician extenders or midlevel providers. These are people such as physician assistants, nurse practitioners, registered nurses, nurse midwives, social workers, psychologists, behavioral health counselors, and community health workers. This philosophy extends to using a qualified primary care physician to handle duties otherwise referred to a specialist. The emphasis is on being confident of the less highly paid practitioner's ability to assume the higher level responsibility. If she cannot handle it, the responsibility is not delegated. If she can, the patient does just as well, sometimes better (mid-level providers sometimes bring unique interpersonal skills to the treatment equation), at lower cost. Forward-looking groups are constantly looking for new ways to safely leverage their nonphysician practitioners. A good example is the experiments by a few MCOs using registered nurses to carry out some primary care functions.

Install Information-Gathering Equipment and Procedures To Track Key Risk Variables

The largest capital investments being made by physician organizations are in information systems—the hardware, the software, the proprietary systems, the new personnel categories, and the retraining of existing personnel. These systems are needed to support the complex decision making that must take place in the wide gray area where clinical and financial issues intersect. These are just some of the topics on which information must be gathered and analyzed:

- physician utilization rates—by patient group, by payer
- treatment patterns—by physician, by patient, by payer
- costs incurred—by physician, by patient, by payer
- overall physician profiles
- patient satisfaction ratings—by physician, by patient group, by payer
- profitability—by department, by facility, by health plan, by payer
- clinical outcomes—by physician, by patient group, by payer
- other quality indicators—by physician, by patient group, by payer
- patient data—medical records, plan membership, enrollment data, demographics, complaints
- claims processing and follow-up—by health plan, by payer

- treatment and service authorization—by patient, by health plan
- physician credentialing—by physician
- management of clinical protocols—by protocol, by physician, by patient
- physician compensation and incentive accounting—by physician, by specialty
- competitive intelligence—by competitor, by payer

There are numerous other topics that are encompassed by a modern management information system. These systems do not come cheaply; large provider groups are spending several millions of dollars annually for several years on them. The best systems give an organization a competitive advantage by enabling it to deliver "value" care more efficiently; satisfy its stakeholders more fully; negotiate more rewarding managed care contracts; respond more quickly to new legislation, new payer policies, and new strategic moves by competitors; and, most of all, better manage the risks it must assume under managed care.

Diversify the Services Offered

Individual investors are advised to diversify their stock portfolios to minimize or spread the risk inherent in equity investing. The same logic applies to the service offerings of a physician organization. A single specialty physician group that serves primarily a single demographic group (the elderly, children) is more vulnerable to actuarial miscalculation, catastrophic illnesses, or new market competition than a multispecialty group whose patient pool encompasses more diverse demographics. The diversification strategies are fairly obvious.

- Add physicians in one or two new specialties to a single specialty practice.
- Continually expand the variety of physician specialties available in the group—commensurate with market demands.
- Grow steadily toward becoming a multispecialty group able to provide a full spectrum of care required by the group's patient pool.

- Enter into strategic affiliations with other provider entities (such as hospitals) in order that the group may accept and manage the risk of global capitation.
- Add the capability to provide ancillary services (diagnostic laboratory, pharmacy, rehabilitation, high-tech imaging) that are currently contracted out.

Learn and Adapt to the Risk Characteristics of the Patient Pool (Utilization Experience, Epidemiologic, Geographic, and Demographic Characteristics Obtained from the MCO)

One of the biggest risks faced by a physician group is the possibility that the patients who enroll with them will be sicker and require more care than they anticipated when they agreed to a capitation rate. In addition, the risks presented by a group's patient pool can change over time, as the composition and demographics of the pool changes. The alert group is constantly tracking the risk characteristics of its patients, noticing significant changes, and adapting its personnel and their training, its services, and its facilities. These characteristics show up in factors like the patient's demographics, their places of residence and work, and the occurrence and distribution of conditions they present. Even before a change in the patients' risk profile becomes evident, some shifts may be apparent in the physicians' utilization patterns as they treat the patients.

Renegotiate Contract Terms as Risk Experience Develops

When a physician group begins accepting risk-sharing arrangements with MCOs for the first time, it may not have much experience in managing that risk. If an MCO is entering a market or serving a particular patient population for the first time, it too may not have an accurate appreciation of the risk it is undertaking. The better MCOs recognize this and are willing to renegotiate their provider contracts, often in midstream, as both they and their provider partners gain experience. Raise this contingency when the contract is first being negotiated. In any event, if the group at any point finds itself facing far more risk than it can handle, it should start talking with the MCO involved. At least make the MCO aware of the situation. Propose a risk adjustment to the originally agreed to reimbursement scheme.

Careful Evaluation of Each Managed Care Contract Executed To Understand Clearly the Risk Level It Presents

One of the most unfortunate, and avoidable, downside risks that groups encounter is that resulting from a misreading (or failure to read) the managed care contract in the first place. There are many ways that a contract may commit a group to perform tasks and services that they are either unqualified or unprepared to do.

- They may agree to provide medical services for which they do not have the skills, requiring them to contract with more expensive outside physicians to do the work.
- They are committed to treating all the patients who enroll with them, without regard to the practice's capacity for handling patients.
- While the group may be capable of delivering all the medical services specified in the contract, they have not determined whether their costs of doing so are covered by the capitation rate or fee schedule.
- Under the contract, the group is expected to perform utilization management, credentialing, reporting, and other administrative tasks without calculating the cost of doing so or incorporating that cost into the capitation rate or fee schedule.
- The contract may imply a number of risk elements for which the group deserves additional compensation, which may not have been included in the capitation equation.

Managed care contract terms can vary widely. Every contract should be scrutinized, the responsibilities and risks being assumed by the group should be listed and costed out, and those costs should be carefully compared to the reimbursement promised under the contract.

Avoid Open-Ended "Consult and Report" Referrals

Physicians who tightly manage their own utilization of resources may still lose control of medical expenditures when they have to refer a patient to a specialist outside the group. This is more likely to happen when the referral is made on a "consult and report" basis, giving the specialist free rein to do almost anything he sees fit with the patient. As long as he reports back regularly to the referring physician, he is in a position to incur almost unlimited expenses—all borne by the capitated physicians who make the referral. Avoid this situation by making more specific referrals. Wherever possible, authorize referral services at the code level. Even better, consult often and closely with the specialist about his treatment plans, and be willing to exercise a veto when necessary.

Seek Consistency among Managed Care Contracts in Their Procedural Demands on the Physicians

When physician organizations sign managed care contracts with numerous MCOs, each of which may include several health plan options, it is common for each plan and each MCO to make different administrative and reporting demands. The plan coverages vary, copayment and deductible features are different, the physicians may be subject to different utilization management procedures, and different forms and procedures must be used in filing claims. Each MCO may require the physicians to assume a different range of administrative duties and different kinds of data must collected and passed on to the MCO in different formats. There are two problems with this potpourri of contract requirements. It costs the physicians a great deal more to keep track of and follow all the different procedures. If a procedure or requirement is inadvertently ignored, the patient may be discomforted, the group may have to incur even further expense, and ultimately the renewal of the contract may be jeopardized.

The physicians may not have a lot of leverage over the MCO's administrative requirements and other contract terms. They can, however, limit the number of contracts they sign in order to emphasize and cultivate their relatio-nships with a smaller number of MCOs. They may also attempt to negotiate adjustments in the contracts to make them more consistent with regard to all operating procedures, claims processing, credentialing, utilization review, quality assurance, information reporting, and other terms. The MCOs can only say "no."

Share the Risk

These strategies reduce the risk exposure of individual physicians or groups by spreading it among multiple physicians or groups.

Physicians Come Together in Larger Groups

Join with other physicians to form larger groups. The risk borne by individual physicians is decreased by being spread over a larger number of physicians. The odds of an actuarial miscalculation, a concentration of catastrophic illnesses, or seriously excessive utilization by several physicians causing major financial harm is less likely in a larger group than in a practice of a few physicians. This, the primary strategic recommendation of this book, puts physicians in the position of being able simultaneously to assume much greater risk and to manage it more effectively—to their advantage and profit.

Physicians Affiliate with Other Physicians through Independent Practice Associations (IPAs)

The same risk-spreading benefit accrues, to a more superficial extent, when physicians ally

with each other through the vehicle of an IPA. If the IPA as a whole is capitated and then pays its individual members a discounted FFS (which is often the case), any unpredictably high expenses tend to be shared by the entire group. What the IPA misses out on are the risk management advantages of tighter clinical and financial integration, which is usually avoided by IPAs. The best IPAs see themselves as a transitional form moving with all due speed toward exactly that level of integration.

Physicians and Physician Groups Affiliate with Nonphysician Entities (e.g., Hospitals in a Physician-Hospital Organization (PHO))

The risk of managing care is dispersed even more broadly if the physicians also ally themselves with other nonphysician providers. The primary candidates are hospitals. The new entities they often form are PHOs. This strategy facilitates risk management in a couple of new ways. Besides being just another player with whom the risk can be shared, hospitals bring a wealth of experience in managing clinical risk within their facilities that can be applied to a managed care setting. Furthermore, they typically have capital resources to invest in the personnel and systems necessary to support sophisticated risk management. When hospital services are included under a global capitation arrangement between a physician group and an MCO, the physicians take on still more risk but are proportionately even better prepared to manage it successfully.

Physician Ownership in the For-Profit Entity

For-profit provider organizations have the option of offering their physician-members ownership interests in the organization. This can be negotiated in several ways. If the organization purchases the physicians' practice assets, it may pay them at least partially with shares of stock in the organization. In order to capitalize its formation and subsequent growth, the organization may require investment from its participating physicians and give them stock in return. Even where it does not need the capital, the organization may allow the physicians to purchase stock shares as a form of personal investment. In any case, this option becomes especially appealing when the stock shares are publicly traded, the organization is growing and thriving, the value of the shares is increasing, and the physicians see the opportunity someday to cash out their much appreciated investments.

The risk management benefit of physician ownership comes through the new alignment of the physicians' interests with those of the organization. When the organization prospers (through lower costs, higher quality, greater patient satisfaction, more patients, and more managed care contracts), the physician sees her ownership interest grow in value. She begins to see a connection between her professional behavior, the organization's success, and ultimately her own monetary reward. This connection becomes a powerful incentive for each owner-physician to adopt those behaviors that minimize risk and further the organization's interests.

Development of a Teamwork Culture and Mentality

There is little question about the value of a team approach to many aspects of health care delivery, whether it involves a clinical procedure, quality process improvements, or resolving administrative snarls. There is also a broader, more abstract benefit. As a cooperative, collaborative mood or culture begins to develop in the organization, physicians are more and more likely to identify their satisfaction and success with that of their colleagues and the organization to which they all belong. They will increasingly see the importance of their role in risk management initiatives. A teamwork mentality is worth encouraging for either of these reasons.

No Capitation until a Minimum Number of Patients Are Enrolled

When a physician group first accepts patients on a risk-share basis, it may take some time—

months, if not a year or two—before its patient pool reaches the size where the actuarial probabilities on which its capitation rate was calculated come into play. There are some rough estimates of the minimum number of patients for which physicians in each of the specialties must be responsible in order to feel reasonably safe from the risk of a higher-than-expected demand for their medical services. Enlightened MCOs are willing to agree with physician groups in this situation that their capitation payments will not begin until the size of their enrolled patient pool has reached a predetermined minimum. Until that time, the MCO pays the physicians according to a previously agreed-upon discounted FFS schedule.

In some cases, it also makes sense for the group and MCO to set a ceiling on the number of patients the group will be required to accept. There are limits to the group's patient capacity (measured in space and number of physicians). If exceeded, much higher expenses and rapid fall-off in quality can be expected.

Increase the Size of the Risk Pool

More providers (through merger or acquisition), serving more patients and handling more contracts, spreads the risk and allows the law of large numbers to work. The larger the size of the pool of risk patients, the wider the possibility of catastrophic events and expenses is spread, and the easier it is for the statistical odds to work in the group's favor. Physicians have every incentive to increase the number of patients they are serving under a risk arrangement. This is accomplished in a few basic ways.

- Add more physicians to your staff so that you can serve more patients.
- Add more physician extenders so that your existing staff can see more patients.
- Merge with, integrate with, or acquire another physician group and get both its physicians and patients.
- Open more facilities, such as satellite clinics, to allow more room for seeing patients.

- Enter into more contracts with more MCOs so that more patients will be directed toward your group.

Lease Rather Than Buy Equipment, Space, and People

A very simple way to reduce financial exposure is to invest less money in fixed assets. The group still needs the assets; it just leases them rather than buys them. This is certainly true of real estate and major equipment items. But it also applies to personnel. Instead of committing to pay a person a full-time salary and benefits for sporadic work, contract with the person on a freelance basis, either directly or through an agency. In some cases (e.g., maintenance, messenger, laundry), it is possible to close down an entire in-house unit and outsource the entire service.

Shift the Risk

It is possible through these strategies to transfer the risk, or a specific piece of it, to other people or entities.

Exclusions and Carve-Outs

Sometimes, a group desires and obtains a managed care contract to provide a full range of medical care under a global capitation rate. However, there may be a few select services that the group is unqualified or unprepared to deliver. To accept responsibility for those services would place the group at a much heightened risk. The answer is to negotiate with the MCO for an exclusion or "carve-out" of the services. This means that the MCO will contract separately with another, more qualified, group of physicians to handle just those services. It might also be provided that, as the first group gains experience or hires physicians in new specialties, the excluded services will be brought back within its global contract.

Subcontracting and Subcapitating with Other Providers

Rather than let the excluded services go to another group, even temporarily, the primary physician organization may accept responsibility for them and simply do its own subcontracting with other physicians. It may even choose to subcapitate them as well, depending on the likely volume of services involved. It will take this route only if it feels confident in the abilities of the other group of physicians and can obtain their services at a reasonable cost. The advantage of this arrangement is that the physicians retain control of as much of the premium dollar as possible. The larger the premium share they are able to manage efficiently, the more savings there are for them to keep.

Stop-Loss Insurance

The best actuaries in the world cannot predict every string of catastrophic illnesses that might befall a group's patients. There is always a slim possibility that expenses will be incurred that far exceed the capitation payments. To protect against this, it is common for groups to purchase stop-loss insurance, which kicks in with monetary payments whenever expenses exceed a predetermined level. The terms of stop-loss policies can vary. The trigger may be the expenses incurred for one patient or for all patients enrolled with one health plan. It may be the expenses incurred during one episode of care, during one month, or over the course of a year. The dollar level of expenses that triggers the policy is variable too. Most MCOs offer such stop-loss coverage to their provider risk partners who pay a premium for it. Because the coverage is going to all the providers serving the MCO, the premiums may be much less than if the physicians purchased the policy separately from an insurer.

On the other hand, if the physician group has contracts with several MCOs, it may be purchasing stop-loss coverage from several different sources. The terms of those coverages may vary considerably (for instance, the attachment points, the services to which the insurance will apply, the coinsurance percentage split between the group and the MCO, and the actual payment rates for each stop-loss case). In the interests of uniformity and predictability, the physicians might be better off buying a single umbrella policy from a single source, probably an independent carrier.

Malpractice Insurance

Adequate malpractice insurance coverage is a prerequisite for physician practices in almost any setting—hospital staff privileges, membership in a group practice, or direct employment. The intent is to provide a financial life net in the event of a clinical misstep by a physician that causes injury to a plaintiff. This is certainly one of the possible risks that might arise in a managed care setting. Perhaps the need is even greater with so many pressures and incentives for physicians to limit care in order to minimize costs. The MCO normally will demand certain levels of malpractice coverage of both the entire group enterprise and of its individual physician members. The group may decide that it wants even greater protection for itself. In any event, good, solid malpractice insurance coverage is a key risk management strategy.

Other Reinsurance

Insurance is the classic method for protecting against risk. If a physician group finds itself facing any other risks that it feels unqualified to manage or for which it is not adequately compensated, it might explore with insurers the options for purchasing some manner of insurance protection. This could include the risk of lawsuits from various parties (e.g., patients, employees) or damages from unpredictable events (e.g., power outages, flooding, strikes).

Accept No Risk That Cannot Be Controlled

The golden rule of risk-sharing is not to assume any risk that the group cannot manage. This does not mean reducing the likelihood of a risky event to zero. It means having a full appreciation of the dimensions of the risk, implementing some good strategies for moderating that risk, and arranging contingency protection for the financial implications of the risk. If those elements are not present, it is extremely dangerous, even foolhardy, to proceed under a cloud of risk.

Do Not Hesitate To Drop Contracts That Pose Risks That Are Too High or Unmanageable

If a physician group is to avoid uncontrollable risks, it must be willing in the appropriate circumstance to turn down or refuse to renew the managed care contract that imposes such risks. It may be very difficult to give up a contract that seems to bring a steady patient flow and stream of revenues. Just remember that the cost of the risks occurring may more than offset the revenues being earned. If a contract seems so risky that the physicians are thinking of dropping it, the first step is to raise those concerns with the MCO. If they agree with the physicians' assessment, they may be willing to take steps to reduce the risk (by assuming more of it themselves), provide the physicians with additional information to enable them to manage the risk, or increase the capitation rate or other risk-sharing reimbursement to compensate for the risk. The absence of understanding or sensitivity on the MCO's part may be just another reason to terminate the contract.

Most physicians reject the loss of autonomy that goes with traditional MCO-dictated methods of utilization management. The main way for physician's to retain control over their clinical decision making is to take the responsibility, and the risk, of directly managing the cost and quality of care they provide. Use these strategies to keep that risk under control.

RESOURCE LIST

1998–99 Guide to Patient Satisfaction Survey Instruments, 2d ed., Atlantic Information Services, (800) 521-4323.

D. Abbey, *Ultimate Patient Satisfaction* (Westchester, IL: Healthcare Financial Management Association, 1997).

"Aligning Incentives Using Risk-Sharing Arrangements," *Healthcare Financial Management*, February 1997.

D. Balestracci and J. Barlow, *Quality Improvement: Practical Applications for Medical Group Practices*, 2d ed., (Englewood, CO: Medical Group Management Association, 1996).

V. Bradford, *The Total Service Medical Practice, 17 Steps to Satisfying Your Internal and External Customers* (West·hester, IL: Healthcare Financial Management Association, 1997).

Clinical Practice Guidelines Directory (Chicago: American Medical Association, 1998).

Clinical Process and Outcome Measurement Directory (Chicago: American Medical Association, 1998).

"Determining Costs Associated with Quality in Health Care Delivery," *Health Care Management Review*, 22 June, 1994.

"Disease Management: Program Design, Development, and Implementation," *Healthcare Financial Management*, June 1997.

"Four Techniques for Managing the Risk of Capitation Contracts," *Healthcare Financial Management*, January 1997.

C. Guinane, *Clinical Care Pathways—Tools and Methods for Designing, Implementing, and Analyzing Efficient Care Practices* (Westchester, IL: Healthcare Financial Management Association, 1997).

Health Care Report Cards 1998-99, Atlantic Information Services, (800) 521-4323.

"Influencing Physician Practice Patterns," *Topics in Health Care Financing*, 22 June, 1994.

"Is Your Organization Ready To Share Financial Risk with HMOs?" *Healthcare Financial Management*, August 1994.

R. Kirk, *Managing Outcomes, Process, and Cost in a Managed Care Environment* (Gaithersburg, MD: Aspen Publishers, Inc., 1997).

P. Kongstvedt, "Use of Data and Reports in Medical Management," in *The Managed Health Care Handbook* (Gaithersburg, MD: Aspen Publishers, Inc., 1993).

P. Kongstvedt and D. Plocher, *Best Practices in Medical Management: An Expert Guide to Care Management in a Managed Care Environment* (Gaithersburg, MD: Aspen Publishers, Inc., 1998).

S. MacStravic and G. Montrose, *Managing Health Care Demand* (Gaithersburg, MD: Aspen Publishers, Inc., 1998).

"Managing Risk in a Changing Health Care System," *Journal of Health Care Finance*, Spring 1996.

"Managing Utilization: The Old Way and the New Way," *Health Care Strategic Management*, 1 October, 1996.

"The Marriage of Risk Management and the Process of Patient Care," *Physician Executive*, July 1995.

C. Murer and L. Lenhoff-Brick, *The Case Management Sourcebook* (Westchester, IL: Healthcare Financial Management Association, 1997).

Nelson et al., *Improving Patient Satisfaction Now* (Gaithersburg, MD: Aspen Publishers, Inc., 1998).

"New Strategies for Clamping Down on Referrals," *Medical Economics*, 10 April, 1995.

Nurse Practitioners and Physicians Assistants, Super Search Packet #2685 (Englewood, CO: Medical Group Management Association, updated annually).

Outcomes, Information Exchange #3269 (Englewood, CO: Medical Group Management Association, 1996).

Outcomes Management and Practice Guidelines, Super Search Packet #3501 (Englewood, CO: Medical Group Management Association, updated annually).

"Outpatient Critical Pathways: Five Advantages for Physicians Who Act Now," *Physician Executive*, April 1996.

Physician Productivity and Profiling, Super Search Packet #2101 (Englewood, CO: Medical Group Management Association, updated annually).

Physician Services Practice Analysis (PSPA) Ver. 6.5 for Windows, Software #4632 (Englewood, CO: Medical Group Management Association).

Physician Work Profiling: Handbook for Group Practices, Book #5070 (Englewood, CO: Medical Group Management Association, 1998).

Physicians Assistants, Information Exchange #3304 (Englewood, CO: Medical Group Management Association, 1996).

Practice Guidelines - Development, Information Exchange #4031 (Englewood, CO: Medical Group Management Association, 1997).

Practice Guidelines - Implementation, Information Exchange #4096 (Englewood, CO: Medical Group Management Association, 1997).

Provider Risk Sharing and Provider Sponsored Organizations (Washington, DC: American Health Lawyers Association, 1998)

Quality Assurance, Super Search Packet #1729 (Englewood, CO: Medical Group Management Association, updated annually).

"Risk Management in an IPA Setting," *Physician Executive*, May 1994 (Part 1), June 1994 (Part 2).

J. Saxton and T. Leaman, *Managed Care Success: Reducing Risk while Increasing Patient Satisfaction* (Gaithersburg, MD: Aspen Publishers, Inc., 1998).

S. Schramm, *Global Capitation: Strategies and Techniques for Assuming Full Risk* (Westchester, IL: Healthcare Financial Management Association, 1998).

D.H. Stamatis, *Total Quality Management in Healthcare* (Westchester, IL: Healthcare Financial Management Association, 1996).

Telemedicine, Information Exchange #4458 (Englewood, CO: Medical Group Management Association, 1998).

Telemedicine: The Rise of Digital Healthcare, (Alexandria, VA: Capitol Publications).

Utilization Management & Review, Super Search Packet #1859 (Englewood, CO: Medical Group Management Association, updated annually).

Utilization Review, Information Exchange #3011 (Englewood, CO: Medical Group Management Association, 1996).

"Where Disease Management Is Paying Off," *Medical Economics,* 14 July, 1997.

Zimmerman et al., *The Healthcare Customer Service Revolution: The Growing Impact of Managed Care on Patient Satisfaction* (Westchester, IL: Healthcare Financial Management Association, 1996).

CHAPTER 27

Financing Strategies To Support Your Integration Plans

INTRODUCTION

All the strategic moves described in this book require funding to implement—sometimes in significant amounts. It often is possible to get started in the planning phase with out-of-pocket contributions from the original founding physicians. However, their pockets are not bottomless. Eventually, it will become necessary to lay out much more money—upward of a million dollars in many cases—which means turning to others for funding.

This chapter explains

- what financing will be needed for and the approximate amounts involved
- where the financing can be sought at each stage of an organization's development and the pros and cons of each source
- how to prepare your organization for seeking financing
- the impact of nonprofit versus for-profit status on the available financing options
- steps to take to make a provider organization more attractive to financing sources

The intended result of this chapter is that group and system organizers appreciate the considerable costs of forming such complex systems and recognize the limits on securing funds to cover the costs. They also will know where to go to find needed financing and how to get it on the best terms.

WHO SHOULD READ THIS CHAPTER

The physicians most interested in the information in this chapter are the leaders in the formation of a new provider organization, either early in the planning process, when the availability of financing options may influence the organizational form chosen, or later, after they have settled on a particular structure and want to know where to go for financing. Reading this chapter also is a good way to prepare for negotiations with individual funding sources—to understand what terms they offer and to compare them with the terms you might be able to obtain elsewhere.

You can skip this chapter if you trust the leaders and planners of an organization you are considering joining.

WHAT CAPITAL FINANCING IS USED FOR WHEN PHYSICIANS INTEGRATE AND AFFILIATE

It probably is obvious that the formation of new provider organizations requires significant amounts of capital to support new asset purchases and start-up operating costs. It is important to know precisely how much money may be needed and what it will be used to purchase.

Broad Categories of Sound Investment Projects

A modern, well-conceived provider organization aims to spend capital on the following broad categories of projects:

- acquisition and development of physician practices, mainly in primary care
- acquisition and installation of sophisticated electronic clinical and management information systems
- conversion of acute care inpatient facilities to outpatient and long-term care facilities
- creation of strategically located ambulatory primary care satellite facilities
- funding of health care financing products such as health maintenance organizations (HMOs) and preferred provider organizations (PPOs) (including necessary financial reserves)
- creation and growth of new integrated delivery entities
- obtaining of working capital to support growth in scope of operations
- establishment of reserves to protect against new risks being assumed
- modernization and updating of current facilities and equipment
- creating of new ancillary service profit centers

These types of investments have been shown to contribute effectively to making a physician organization more competitive in a managed care marketplace.

What Not To Spend Money On

Planning strategic capital expenditures is usually a judgment call, based on thorough environmental analysis and prior executive experience. Two reasonable strategic planners can reach different conclusions about how to spend millions of dollars to advance a business's fortunes. In the development of integrated health care delivery entities, there is some common wisdom on what are undesirable capital projects.

- Do not spend money expanding inpatient capacity.
- Do not invest in a significant new physical plant or equipment ("bricks and mortar").
- Do not buy physician practices if you can achieve the same ends through contract affiliations.
- Do not buy physician practices unless you are sure you know how to manage them.
- Do not invest in any venture unless you know how to manage it.
- If you do buy physician practices, do not overpay for them.
- If you do buy physician practices, pay in stock, rather than in cash.

Use your capital investments to implement your long-range organizational strategy. The investments themselves are not a strategy (Exhibit 27–1).

There are occasional exceptions to these rules, but, in most cases, such investments will be a waste of money that saddles the organization with an unproductive debt load.

Start-up Costs for Common Physician Organization Models

In thinking about forming or even joining a new provider organization, it is smart to ask how much it all is likely to cost just to get started. It is impossible to state precise figures for particular organizational models. There are too many variables, and a physician-hospital organization (PHO) combining one hospital and one group of doctors in one city can take much more to establish than a PHO in another city. It is possible to make some rough estimates. The following figures are from 1995[1] and were conservative even then. They probably should be doubled or tripled now.

- Independent Practice Associations (IPAs) and other physician networks—$1.2 million

Exhibit 27–1 Virtual Integration Requires Less Capital

Avoid asset-based integration in favor of "virtual integration," which achieves coordination through patient-management agreements, provider incentives, and information systems. The early models of IDS assumed that a central organization would own and control all of the necessary provider components—physician practices, hospitals, laboratories, pharmacies, and rehabilitation and long-term care facilities. This was thought to be the only way to achieve desired operating efficiencies. There is a shift toward creating systems that are integrated through contractual agreements and electronic data links—a sort of "virtual integration." It is still to be proven that such structures can function as efficiently as the more tightly "owned integration" models. One thing is clear. This kind of integration normally requires less capital investment. Practices do not have to be acquired, and physical structures do not have to be built. Considerable sums must be spent on sophisticated information systems, but they are necessary anyway. Look very seriously at following the path of virtual integration.

- PHOs $2.2 million
- Staff-model physician organizations—$7.8 million
- Management services organizations (MSOs)— $9.6 million
- Freestanding medical groups—$19.7 million
- Foundation-model medical groups—$20.0 million

Typical Start-up Financing Scenario

What follows is a more detailed look at the implementation steps and associated costs in the formation of a PHO. Startup costs consist of legal and consulting fees, organizational expenses, and the cost of participants' time spent in planning. Start-up expenses for the most rudimentary form of provider integration—a PHO—can approach $500,000. A typical budget for a PHO composed of a hospital and 200 members of its medical staff might look like Exhibit 27–2.

The budget very quickly exceeds $500,000, and this does not include the cost of the time spent by the hospital and physicians in meetings over this issue. The costs increase almost geometrically as the planned organization becomes more complex.

- larger size
- more comprehensive information system

Exhibit 27–2 Typical PHO Budget

Introductory Phase	
Initial feasibility study	$40,000
Preliminary design of organizational structure	30,000
Early legal advice	10,000
Education of prospective participants	20,000
Actual Implementation	
Attorneys (corporate, health care, tax, antitrust)	$90,000
Management consultants	70,000
Early Operations (Until Break-Even Point Is Achieved)	
Physical plant	$100,000
Working capital ($100,000/year for two years)	200,000

- tighter integration
- addition of a financing component
- acquisition of physician practices
- building of primary care clinics
- addition of professional management staff

Consider these cost estimates for adding a few of these components.

Acquiring Physician Practices

The cost of buying a single physician's practice can vary from almost nothing to close to $1 million. The actual amounts depend on the numbers of physicians in various specialties, the extent of managed care market penetration, and the state of competition in the immediate area. To assemble a multispecialty network of 100 physicians, count on spending at least $30 million on acquisitions costs alone. The actual cash outlay can be reduced if the acquiring organization has publicly traded stock to exchange with the physicians for their practice assets. [*]

Building Primary Care Clinics

Rather than purchase existing practices, some delivery systems try to create their own networks of primary care practices. This involves recruiting primary care physicians (PCPs), finding clinic locations for them, staffing and equipping the clinics, and bearing the operating costs until the clinics reach a break-even point. The experience

---

[*]In 1995, the Prudential Health Care System in Cincinnati gave up plans to build its own physician network when it realized that the average first-year cost would be over $400,000 per physician. The Johns Hopkins Health System was considering spending just under $400,000 per head to acquire a 60-physician group practice. Over the last two years, Intermountain Health Care in Utah has absorbed 250 physicians at a total cost of approximately $50 million (data from D. Coddington, K. Moore, and E. Fischer, *Making Integrated Health Care Work*, Center for Research in Ambulatory Health Care Administration, Englewood, CO, 1996, p. 168).

of systems that have gone this route, including constructing new clinic facilities, indicates a cost of approximately $3 million to get a 10-physician practice off the ground.

Comprehensive Information Systems

The sophisticated electronic information systems for gathering the management and clinical data that is critical to market success do not come cheaply. The larger integrated delivery systems (IDSs) are spending between $5 million and $10 million annually to computerize data collection. These are some specific cases: [2]

- Lovelace Health Systems—$50 million over 5 years
- Intermountain Health Care—$10 million annually
- Scott & White—$7.5 million in 1995
- Baptist Health System—$4.7 million in 1995
- HealthSystem Minnesota—$5 to $10 million annually for several years
- Advocate Health Care—$15 to $20 million annually for several years

Adding a Financing Component

When an IDS adds a financing component, it becomes a managed care organization (MCO) capable of contracting directly with payers such as employers. This step is not taken until a comprehensive, smoothly functioning system is well in place. It is an expensive step, involving feasibility studies, consultants' and attorneys' fees, initial opening costs, equipment and software, required financial reserves, an introductory marketing campaign, and operating funds until a break-even point is achieved. There are none of the asset purchases connected with building the delivery system. Adding a financial component is largely a paper exercise.

To establish managed care plans in rural or less populated areas (markets of fewer than 500,000 people), groups and systems usually spend at least $5 million. For plans serving wider geographic areas or more densely populated markets (over 1,000,000 people), the initial costs are likely to exceed $10 million.

SOURCES OF CAPITAL FINANCING FOR NEW PROVIDER ORGANIZATIONS

There usually is little difficulty in settling on strategic projects worthy of capital financing. The problem lies in identifying good sources of that financing. These are the best places for physician groups to look. They are a combination of traditional financers of business ventures and others that have sprung up specifically to serve the interests of provider organizations.

- salary concessions by specialist physicians
- retained earnings of your organization (enhanced by your more effective management of care)
- public investor community (capital markets)—debt
- public investor community (capital markets)—equity
- local hospitals interested in coventuring or buying practices
- local IDSs desiring to fill out their physician networks by acquiring, merging with, or affiliating with physician groups
- local health plans wishing to keep providers open to seeing their enrollees
- local physician practice management companies (PPMCs) intending to acquire physician practices, build them into networks, and increase the value of their stock

There is a wide and diverse range of institutions ready to provide financing to deserving provider organizations. Some of these institutions are traditional (such as banks and pension funds), and others are specific to health care organizations (such as hospitals, practice management companies, and some venture capital firms).

The financing instruments that they use fall into two broad categories: debt and equity. Sources of debt financing usually "lend" their money to a needy organization. In return, they ask for a legal commitment to receive a fixed annual interest payment. Also, at the end of the loan period, they also want all of their money back. To compensate for the risk that the organization may be unable to pay either the interest or the principal, the lender may require that the borrowing organization provide certain of its assets as security for the loan.

Sources of equity financing are said to "invest" their money in a needy organization. They do this by purchasing shares of common stock in the entity. In return, they expect that the value of their investment will increase or that they will receive dividend payments. Unlike interest payments, there is no legal obligation for the organization to pay the dividends and no guarantee that the stock price will go up. Equity investors take into account the risk of their investments through the price they are willing to pay for the stock (the higher the risk, the lower the price).

The specific type of financing (debt or equity and types within each category) and the types of institutions willing to lend or invest will depend on numerous factors. Foremost among these is the stage of the organization's development and the scope and nature of the activity to be financed. An organization that is well along in its development will have an established financial track record that lenders or investors can study. It also is likely to be larger and better able to bear the costs of any financing. Certain types of financing are best suited to certain kinds of activities with certain life spans.

Traditional Debt Sources of Financing

The following are the primary traditional sources of debt financing available to any kind of business organization, including physician-sponsored delivery organizations:

- loans and credit provided by commercial lending institutions
- lines of credit
- commercial paper
- conventional bonds and notes (taxable)
- tax-exempt bonds
- seller financing

Commercial Loans

Short-term loans are used to meet temporary need for quick cash infusion or as bridge financing until a longer-term debt can be negotiated. They are less than a year in duration. Long-term commercial loans usually run from 3 to 10 years. Interest rates may be either fixed or variable.

These loans are obtained from commercial banks. Although the loan may be made to the overall integrated entity, the bank may require that the most substantial, financially strong component (typically, the hospital) participate as a guarantor or as the primary debtor. This is less likely to happen if the total entity has a solid track record and the bank has experience dealing with integrated provider organizations.

The lenders will usually ask the borrower to pledge some security to protect their loans. For short-term loans, a bank may seek a security interest in the organization's accounts receivable or may simply require that it maintain compensating account balances with the bank. The more substantial security demanded for long-term loans can include the following:

- mortgage or deed of trust in the organization's real estate
- security interest in gross revenues, equipment, or personal property (of physicians in a group practice)
- separate guarantee of the loan by a party component of the organization or by a parent corporation
- securities owned by the organization

There will be additional conditions attached to these loans. The bank may charge a commitment fee on top of the interest payments. The borrower may have to comply with certain affirmative and negative covenants. This may involve keeping minimum balances in certain ledger accounts, maintaining certain financial ratios, and giving the lender periodic reports on financial condition. The borrower may have to promise not to borrow additional money, to further encumber the pledged security, or to grant security interests to other parties.

The advantages of commercial loans are that they can be negotiated on fairly short notice, especially if the bank already knows one of the participants in the borrower entity, such as the hospital. The cost of negotiating and processing the loan is relatively small. The banks are usually flexible on the loan terms that they are willing to accept: duration of the loan, interest rate charged, and type of security required.

The disadvantages of commercial loans are that banks may be reluctant to make them to new ventures with no financial history. If they are willing to make a loan, it may be under arduous terms. The primary shortcoming of this kind of financing is that it is somewhat more expensive than some of the alternatives.

For many organizations, commercial loans can be a useful, if not dominant, part of their financing strategy, filling in when other, more permanent financing is not immediately available.

Lines of Credit

Under a line of credit, a bank agrees to lend constantly varying amounts of money up to a predetermined maximum. The amounts lent vary because the borrower's money needs vary. For instance, if a group practice's payroll must be distributed on the first of each month but the majority of its capitation revenues are not received until the middle of the month, it may use a line of credit to tide it over. The total line of credit may be $500,000 but the group usually draws down only $350,000 of that amount and only for two weeks each month. Around the holidays of each year, the group may take close to $450,000.

The special attractions of a line of credit are that the borrower pays interest only on the exact amount of credit being used and for the exact period of time that it is used. In the above hypothetical, the interest on $350,000 for 2 weeks, 11 times a year, plus $450,000 for 2 weeks once a year is considerably less than the interest on $500,000 for 52 weeks a year.

Lines of credit are most useful to start-up ventures or organizations that otherwise expect to experience cash flow fluctuations. Commercial banks are the most common issuers of lines of credit. They are less likely to demand security for the credit line than for a commercial loan and, when they do, it will take the form of accounts receivable, bank accounts, or other liquid assets. The interest rate charged is usually variable and tied to the prime rate. A commitment fee is typically added. Lines of credit run for terms of one year or less, though they are frequently and easily renewed.

The covenants demanded by the banks tend to be less onerous. They take these forms:

- maintaining certain debt coverage ratios
- maintaining certain account balances with the bank
- making regular financial reports to the bank
- avoiding making any loans by the organization
- avoiding further encumbering secured assets
- paying the credit loan off completely for at least 30 consecutive days each year

Seriously consider lines of credit if (a) your organization is just starting, (b) your organization does not have a financial track record, (c) your organization does not include a participant with an independently solid credit rating, (d) you have cash needs that fluctuate from week to week or month to month, or (e) you need quick cash to keep you going (for less than a year) until you are able to negotiate longer-term, more permanent financing.

Commercial Paper

The borrower engages an investment banker to locate interested lenders in the market. The offering memorandum describes the terms of the loan and the borrower. Your obligation to repay is documented in a note. Large institutional lenders are most likely to buy commercial paper. They may require a guarantee from a parent corporation or a participant with a more extensive financial history. You will need to hire a specialist attorney to review the memorandum and other related documentation, and to provide legal opinions on the validity and enforceability of the note. A bank may even be drawn into the arrangement as a depository for the required security.

The security offered by the borrower will greatly affect the marketability of the notes. The preference is an asset than can be liquidated quickly and easily, such as securities.

The interest rate on commercial paper is usually fixed and due at the time of the note's maturity. Commercial notes are legally restricted to rather short terms but may be "rolled over" at maturity. Somewhat like lines of credit, commercial credit is often used as a stopgap measure until more permanent financing can be arranged. The covenants attached are usually less onerous than for commercial loans or credit lines, often consisting of financial reporting and debt coverage requirements.

The features of commercial paper that are so appealing to borrowers include the following:

- The "marketing" of the notes often results in the most attractive interest rate.
- The covenants agreed to may be the least demanding of any debt form.
- Under favorable market conditions, commercial paper debt can be arranged rather quickly.

Among the disadvantages of commercial paper are the substantial processing fees involved (for the investment bank, the outside attorney, and the depository bank) and its sensitivity to the vagaries of the public market for such debt.

Taxable Bonds

Perhaps the most permanent long-term debt form is taxable bonds. They have the potential for being the lowest-cost capital source as well. Bear in mind that a tax-exempt organization also has the option of issuing taxable bonds if, for some reason, it or its capital project does not qualify for tax-free bond financing.

Taxable bonds require extensive documentation, extensive disclosure to prospective investors, a trust indenture mechanism (which establishes the funds and accounts into which the bond proceeds will be deposited and managed, in particular, accounts for holding the funds from which principal and interest payments will be made), and an offering memorandum (describing the bond terms and the bond issuer).

Depending on the financial track record of your organization, a parent corporation or more financially experienced participant may be asked to guarantee the bonds or to serve as the legal issuer. The issuance starts with an investment banking firm attempting to market the bonds to likely lenders. These are most often large institutional investors. Sometimes, one of them may be persuaded to purchase the entire issue.

In addition to the borrower, the lender, and the marketer, a bond transaction requires the involvement of a trustee for handling the funds loaned under the indenture and an attorney to provide necessary legal opinions.

Taxable bonds are secured debt—usually by real estate, accounts receivable, securities, or the guarantee of a parent corporation. Their interest rates may be fixed or variable. Their maturities are quite long term, up to 20 or 30 years. The covenants required of the borrower are perhaps the most burdensome of any debt form, including the following:

- maintaining specific financial ratios
- limiting further long- and short-term borrowing
- limiting liens and encumbrances on security assets
- limiting loans, leases, or gifts of affected assets
- pledging gross revenues to the lender
- assuring compliance with environmental laws relating to affected assets

There are several bond-rating services whose assessment of the risk presented by your bond issue can have a dramatic impact on their marketability and the interest rate that you will have to pay. Numerous factors may influence that rating. There is one way to overtly improve the rating—by purchasing bond insurance or a letter of credit that further assures payment of the bonds upon maturity. This protection is expensive, however, and may exceed the interest savings realized by the higher rating. It also may be completely unavailable to organizations with a limited credit history.

The primary advantages of corporate bonds are their generally lower interest rates and their ability to support very large dollar-value debt financing. The disadvantages are the length of time and the amount of effort necessary to execute a bond issue, the substantial cost of the preparation process, and the large minimum dollar-value of a bond issue required to justify all this time, effort, and expense.

Taxable bonds should be considered by your organization in the following circumstances:

- as a source for a very large financing package, generally exceeding $10 million
- as a source of long-term (20 to 30 years), near-permanent debt
- when your organization has a long financial track record and an excellent credit rating
- at a time when the capital markets are looking favorably on bond issues—as reflected in ease of marketing and lower interest rates

Taxable debt has fewer restrictions than does tax-free debt.

- Borrowers do not need to issue the debt through a special financing authority or governmental agency.
- Borrowers do not need a legal opinion on their tax-exempt status from a bond counsel.
- Borrowers are not limited in their ability to refund in advance.
- Borrowers have no restrictions on the yield realized from the borrowing proceeds.
- Borrowers need not limit the average maturity of the debt to the average life of the assets financed by it.

- Borrowers are not restricted in how they may use the proceeds.

Tax-Exempt Bonds

There is a special form of debt financing available to nonprofit organizations with § 501(c)(3) tax-exempt status available through the combined efforts of the federal and state governments. The federal tax law provides that lenders do not have to pay federal income taxes on the interest from "qualified 501(c)(3) bonds" issued by state or local governments for the benefit of such organizations. It works this way.

If it wishes, a state creates a public agency with a name such as Health and Education Facilities Authority. Its mandate is typically to finance projects for institutions of higher education, hospitals, and cultural organizations. The agency issues bonds in the open market. The purchasers of those bonds (the "lenders") accept a lower interest rate in return for the exemption from income taxes. The agency then lends the proceeds of the sale of the bonds to the qualifying non-profit organizations (the "borrowers"). The agency acts as a conduit between the lenders and the borrowers. The agency usually is committed to repay the principal of and interest on the bonds solely out of the repayments it receives from the nonprofit organizations.

These agencies may be set up at the state, county, or municipal level. It is optional, but most governmental units see a real benefit in being able to offer this low-cost financing to local nonprofit entities. They usually include exemption from state income taxes in the deal with the private lenders.

The federal government, through the Internal Revenue Service (IRS), imposes some strict requirements on the use of these tax-exempt bond financings.

1. At least 95 percent of the bond proceeds must be used for the exempt activities of the §501(c)(3) organization. No more than 5 percent of the proceeds may be used in the trade or business of a nonexempt per-

son. The IRS has issued guidelines[3] on the use of exempt facilities, such as a hospital, by a physician or other nonexempt person who is not an employee of the nonprofit entity. If the guidelines are followed, it is possible, for instance, for a nonemployee physician to use a medical suite provided by an exempt hospital.

2. Generally, no single § 501(c)(3) organization may benefit from a total of more than $150 million worth of these tax-exempt bonds. This rule does not apply to qualified hospitals, and the sum is so large that it is unlikely to affect any other interested nonprofit health care entity.

3. The proceeds of the tax-exempt bonds may be used to refinance other tax-exempt bonds, taxable bonds, or other forms of conventional financing.

4. The average maturity of these bonds may not exceed 120 percent of the average reasonably expected remaining life of the facilities being financed. This requirement does not apply to bond proceeds used to finance working capital expenditures.

The state or local legislation creating the financing agency may impose additional requirements that must be satisfied before the bonds can be issued or the proceeds spent. It is likely to specify the types of projects that may be financed and to define eligible project costs.

The following types of projects are more suitable to financing by means other than tax-exempt debt:

- acquisition of physician practices, group practices, or practice assets for ownership by an entity that is not tax-exempt
- acquisition or capitalization (formation) of an existing MSO, PHO, or MCO, with its attendant required financial reserves
- acquisition, construction or renovation of a facility, or conversion of an existing facility to provide private physician office space, unless the physician is an employee of a 501(c)(3) organization

- assets that the 501(c)(3) organization can reasonably predict may be used for private business use, such as a multipurpose facility that may be exclusively or primarily used as office space for physicians in their private practice

Organizations that use taxable debt are able to get their money from the market faster and with lower borrowing costs (aside from the interest rates) and have much greater freedom in how the money is used. Taxable debt borrowers have access to a wider range of investment sources. They include the huge pension fund market, as well as international investors. Tax-exempt money is available only from special tax-exempt bond funds.

Most tax-exempt bond transactions are done on a negotiated basis with an investment banker involved from the beginning in preparing the disclosure and structuring the financing. The borrower determines the term of the bonds and the amortization schedule. The interest rate may be one fixed rate for the entire term of the bonds or, in the case of serial bonds, a series of fixed, possibly differing rates for each maturity. Bonds may also be issued as commercial paper, with the interest rate set for a period of up to 270 days, after which they must be purchased and perhaps reissued at potentially different rates. The bonds may, but are not required to, be rated by a nationally recognized bond-rating agency, such as Moody's or Standard & Poor's. The bonds are likely to sell better at a lower interest rate if they are backed by some form of security (bond insurance, letter of credit, pledges of revenue, guarantees, debt service reserve fund, mortgage on real property, or security interest in personal property).

These bonds offer a couple of advantages to the entities that can meet the qualifying standards. Nonprofit organizations gain access to a much wider world of capital financing sources than do the local banks or hospitals they normally must deal with. When they do secure necessary capital, it comes at interest rates lower than the commercial market charges. The downside is that the planning and negotiation of a tax-exempt bond financing is a complex, time-consuming process. It probably is worth pursuing only for the largest nonprofit health care organizations.

Seller Financing

An often overlooked source of capital is seller financing—the willingness of the vendor or institution selling an asset to your organization to allow you to pay the purchase price over time on an installment basis. Sellers of real estate or large-ticket capital equipment frequently offer their own financing arrangements. Be prepared for the following possible terms: high interest rates, down payments, relatively short payment periods (no more than three years or so, except in the case of real estate), and required personal guarantees from individuals if the organization has a minimal credit history (Exhibit 27–3).

Debt financing and leasing are the most common capital sources for physician groups. They are relatively easy to arrange and resemble the kinds of financing most doctors have done in their personal lives (i.e., auto loans, house mortgages). There are a few guidelines to keep in mind when going the debt route.

- It is a viable alternative to surrendering ownership and control by selling out to a hospital, PPMC, MCO, or health plan.
- Using debt financing allows the group to postpone choosing a long-term strategic capital partner.
- Depending on the group's size and its strategic ambitions, debt financing may not provide enough capital to meet all of the group's needs.
- Compared with equity financing, debt usually is less expensive and more risky. It also is easier to restructure. One form of debt (for example, a line of credit) can be rolled over into another (such as a long-term loan) or into equity.
- Taking out a loan, even if personally secured by the physicians, can be an important first step in establishing the group's creditworthi-

Exhibit 27–3 Credit Ratings for Physician-Owned Organizations

There are several commercial services (e.g., Dun & Bradstreet) that examine the creditworthiness of businesses likely to seek debt financing and give them objective ratings heavily relied upon by potential lenders. Physician-owned organizations have been at a disadvantage in this process because the traditional services did not seem to appreciate how an organization that pays out most of its net earnings to its physician-owners could also cover the cost of debt.

Fitch IBCA has published a special report on six unique credit factors that should be considered when assessing physician group practices.[*] These are the factors and the rationale behind them. They are worth paying close attention to as guidelines for making your group more attractive to lenders.

1. **Productivity-linked compensation.** Under managed care, profitable group operation requires financial incentives for physician practice efficiency. This should take the form of a link between physician compensation and physician productivity and utilization of resources. It also is essential that the compensation is viewed as a controllable expense, determined ultimately by the group's management. When warranted, salary draws should be adjusted up or down. Potential bonuses should be payable only after debt service payments have been made.

2. **Free cash flow.** When there are controls on physician salary draws and a commitment to retention of earnings within the business, standard accounting principles reveal a clearer picture of the unencumbered cash flow available to service the debt. The organization's ability to generate significant free cash flow is a critical measure of its credit standing. A solid history (five or more years) of keeping capital within the organization, through retained earnings and prudent distri-

butions to owners, can earn it an investment-grade rating.

3. **Proper mix of physicians and facilities.** Under managed care, revenue volume is determined by the number of covered lives served by the organization. In turn, the number of covered lives that an MCO will entrust to a provider organization depends to a large degree on the number and geographic distribution of delivery sites (practice offices or clinics) and on the number and specialties of the organization's physicians, with special emphasis on primary care doctors.

4. **Practice experience under capitation.** Under capitated managed care, the most profitable physician groups are those most adept at "managing" care appropriately—controlling costs while maintaining quality. Lenders look more favorably on groups with a positive capitation track record that has permitted them to sustain profitable operations. Without such experience, the group's ability to generate income necessary to cover loan costs will be in doubt. One way of assessing the group's care management experience is to look at its existing payer mix.

5. **Experienced, diverse management team.** Most desirable is a blend of administrative and medical management, with demonstrated strength in clinical and financial controls. Special attention is given to a clearly defined managed care strategy, expertise in managed care contracting, sophisticated information systems, and medical practice protocols. These all contribute to generating operating efficiencies that allow management to maintain acceptable physician salary levels while providing sufficient earnings and free cash flow for equity retention and debt service.

6. **Traditional factors.** A physician group's creditworthiness will also depend on more traditional factors such as service area, competition, debt issue details, and legal provisions.

_____
[*]Find a copy of this report at www.fitchibca.com on the Internet. Also check out the Standard & Poor's rating criteria for Physician Groups and Faculty Practice Plans, to be found at www.ratings.com.

Courtesy of Fitch IBCA, Inc., New York, New York.

ness. This puts it in a better position to seek other forms of financing, such as equity.

- It usually is a good idea to build up a reserve of retained earnings before approaching a lender. This will demonstrate the physicians' commitment to the business, give the lender confidence in the group's financial strength, and probably garner a slightly lower interest rate.

- Debt financing is best used for the development or purchase of hard assets, rather than as general funding of operations. Good examples are new physicians in needed specialties, primary care satellite clinics, ancillary service ventures, sophisticated information systems, and modernization of facilities and equipment.

- The type of debt financing should be matched to the use of the funds: short-term loans (repayment in less than one year) for working capital and other short-term uses; medium-term loans (one to eight years) for equipment purchases, leasehold improvements, and market expansion; and long-term loans (more than eight years) for acquisition of buildings, real estate, and other long-lived assets.

Traditional Equity Sources of Financing

The following are the primary traditional sources of equity financing available to any kind of business organization, including physician-sponsored delivery organizations.

Sweat Equity

More than half of all the financing for early and expansion stage businesses (in all fields, not just health care) comes from the founders in the form of personal investment and forgone salaries. Contributions from friends and family are often invited. Many businesses then strive to survive by living and growing off the earnings from operations.

Equity Generated Internally

A business generates equity internally whenever it earns a net profit and retains that money in the business. It becomes a component of the entity's net worth. The use of retained earnings as a capital source is discussed later in the section on financing sources unique to provider organizations.

Equity Obtained from External Sources— Donations and Grants

A provider group that has chosen to organize as a nonprofit charitable entity may have access to donations from individuals and organizations. The tax-exempt, tax-deductible quality of such donations makes them attractive to private persons or foundations wishing to support the group's beneficent purposes. It may also be possible to win grants from foundations and government agencies for research, education, and community-oriented activities of the group.

Equity Obtained from External Sources— Private Placements

Investment banks and financing agents raise equity capital for new entities by "placing" their unregistered stock with private, accredited investors. The main advantage of this funding source is that it usually results in less loss of control for the existing shareholders than does venture capital financing. On the downside, the timetable to complete a private placement is often long and uncertain. The private investors who receive the stock can offer little or no sound business advice and have minimal patience for losses and underperformance.

Closely related to the private investor is the wealthy individual willing to act as an "angel" for a new business. If his interest stems from previous experience in the field—an older physician with a successful history in medicine—he may be able to offer some useful business counsel. This kind of investor is often able to make quick investment decisions, but there are limits to the extent of his resources. He also is likely to be intolerant of losses and to have a shorter investment horizon than do most venture capitalists.

Equity Obtained from External Sources—Public Stock Offerings

Few physician organizations will qualify for access to public equity markets on their own. The transaction costs are very high, requiring offerings of rather large size. Once its stock is established in the public marketplace, the organization will find itself subject to shareholder emphasis on short-term performance results. This sometimes can make it difficult for a business to focus as much as it would like on longer-term strategic objectives. There also is an element of legal exposure when stocks are publicly traded. Generally, the only way a physician group will participate in a public stock offering is in collaboration with a larger entity, such as a PPMC or an IDS.

Equity Obtained from External Sources—Venture Capitalists

When physician groups that are not ready for public stock offerings look for large equity capital infusions, they increasingly are turning to venture capital firms. There are over 600 active institutional venture capital firms managing over $35 billion available for investment in companies at early, expansion, and late stages of growth. Many of them have a special interest in businesses delivering health care. These are some of them:

- Acacia Venture Partners (San Francisco, CA)
- Accel Partners (San Francisco, CA)
- CGJR Health Care Services Group (Nashville, TN)
- Edison Venture Fund (Lawrenceville, NJ)
- Essex Woodlands Healthcare Ventures (Chicago, IL)
- Hickory Venture Capital Corporation (Huntsville, AL)
- Pacific Venture Group (Encino, CA)
- Sequel Venture Partners (Boulder, CO)

The best single listing of venture capital firms, their areas of interest, how they operate, and where to contact them is found in *Pratt's Guide to Venture Capital Sources.*[4] To learn more about the special connection between venture capital firms and health care businesses, look into "Venture Capital & Health Care," a monthly newsletter published by Asset Alternatives, Inc. in Wellesley, Massachusetts.

- Venture capital firms are not a capital financing panacea. Bear in mind these facts about how they operate before you approach them.
- Venture capital firms tend to focus on projects of a certain dollar size and in certain regions of the country. They rarely look at projects requiring less than $500,000. Those interested in smaller-scale investments typically think in terms of $1 to $5 million. Some will concentrate their investments in New England, the Mid-Atlantic states, the Deep South, or the Far West.
- These firms are much tougher than strategic health care partners in the valuation they place on a group's equity or the percentage ownership interest they will demand. Early-stage investors typically seek 40 to 60 percent total ownership in the organization.
- The less developed the venture, the greater the risk to the firm, and the larger the equity share the venture capital firm will want.
- The large ownership interest taken by the venture capitalists is quickly translated into seats on the board of directors. They will use those seats to participate actively in the group's decision making and governance processes.
- The firms will be looking for annual rates of return on their investment on the order of 30 to 60 percent.
- All of these demands serve to dilute the physicians' ownership interest and governing control. Is the trade-off worth the capital investment the firm will make?
- In assessing investment opportunities, venture capitalists look for a sound business plan, an experienced management team, a

strong earnings growth potential, and a potential appeal to the stock market. There are four big questions you are likely to hear from these people:

– How big is your market? (its size and the competition)
– Who is on the management team? (experience, credibility, and know-how)
– What is the service? (stage of development, unique qualities)
– How much will it cost? (uses of the capital invested)

• The ultimate goal of the average venture capital firm is to push the venture—your physician organization—in the direction of an initial public offering (IPO) within five years. It will use its authority on your board of directors to move you along that path with all due haste.

• Despite all this criteria and restrictions, venture capitalists have a definite interest in the field of health care delivery. Overall, they see it as having high growth potential; they are looking for those niches and ventures with exceptionally high potential.

Equity Obtained from External Sources— Strategic Partners

Hospitals and health systems are traditional sources of capital funding for physician groups and networks. They often are willing to invest significant amounts of capital to form integrated links with the physician practices. They tend to be less demanding than are venture capital firms in the amount of ownership and control they want in return for the dollars they invest. These options are discussed separately, in more detail, in the next section.

Financing Sources Unique to Provider Organizations

Provider-sponsored organizations can turn to some special sources of financing that are available to only them. The financing arrangement may employ some of the debt and equity devices described above. The difference is that the lender or investor may have a specific interest in and knowledge of such health care organizations. These are the most common of these sources:

• ancillary service revenues
• retained earnings of the organization itself
• specialist compensation concessions
• local area hospitals
• self-owned managed care plan revenues
• for-profit practice management companies
• independent managed care plans and IDSs
• health insurance companies and health plans

Ancillary Service Revenues

Good, reliable sources of cash flow to support continued growth are the ancillary services that many provider organizations offer. These include laboratory services, pharmacies, various imaging services, rehabilitation services, and the like. The larger and more integrated the organization, the more likely it is to develop its own ancillary service capability. More aggressively managed businesses operate their ancillary service units as profit centers. One of the advantages of provider integration into more rational delivery systems is that the same volume of ancillary services can be furnished in a more coordinated, efficient fashion.

Retained Earnings of the Organization Itself

Eventually, your organization will reach a break-even point and begin to generate net income that can be used to further grow the business. One of the primary motivations for forming the organization may be the belief that you and your physician colleagues can practice more cost-effective medicine when you are in charge. If this is true, you may, in fact, be able to utilize fewer resources in delivering the same volume of medical care and to invest the savings in the assets, activities, and affiliations necessary to compete in managed care. Be conservative, however, in estimating how much more efficient you will be until you are well experienced in managing care.

For an organization to retain earnings for capital investment purposes, the physicians must resist the temptation to immediately withdraw any net profits as personal income. Here are some rules and principles for doing that:

- Very few physician groups have been able to fund their capital plans entirely through retained earnings and without taking on a financial partner. The Marshfield Clinic is one.
- A substantial net worth on a balance sheet can inspire lenders to charge one or two points less in interest rates on loans to the group.
- The group's ability to finance a project entirely through retained earnings gives it leverage, even when negotiating for outside financial support from a capital partner. When you have alternatives, you have more freedom of action, and the prospective partner will see that. Do not expect a lender to believe more in your business than do you and your colleagues.
- Retained earnings are best used to complement or leverage financing from other sources, rather than to pay for the entire project by themselves.
- A group that tries to rely on retained earnings to finance all its strategic initiatives may end up underfunding them.
- Retained earnings are best invested in projects that produce an immediate income stream. Seeing the return right away encourages group physicians to allow the earnings to be retained. Ancillary service programs are ideal for these investments—diagnostic laboratories, outpatient surgery, outpatient rehabilitation, imaging equipment, and a pharmacy.
- Anticipate great resistance from many physicians in the group who have grown accustomed to receiving all the group's income left over at the end of the year. Deal with that opposition in these ways:

  - Tie the retention of earnings to the implementation of the group's strategic goals.
  - Be prepared to report in greater detail about the calculation and spending of the retained earnings.
  - Propose to use the retained earnings, in lean years, to smooth out ups and downs in physician income.

- Simply retaining the earnings is a more expensive proposition in partnerships and professional corporations, where any net profits are taxed as personal income to the physicians before being reinvested. Look into restructuring the organization so that it, rather than the physicians, pays the taxes.
- Because their greatest value is just sitting on the balance sheet, strengthening it, many organizations make every effort to rebuild retained earnings if they become depleted.
- The group usually requires strong leadership to persuade all of its members to adopt a policy of retaining earnings and sticking to it.

Specialist Compensation Concessions

When primary care and specialist physicians come together in a unified organization of truly integrated and aligned interests, a wonderful synergy can emerge. The participants become willing to make individual short-term sacrifices for the long-term welfare of the entire organization. One form this takes is willingness by the specialists to accept lower annual compensation than they might be able to receive if they remained in private practice. The reason this makes sense to them is that, as the health care system is changing, they will not have the option of continuing to practice privately. Furthermore, any compensation shortfall today will be more than made up by later gains from a more competitive integrated entity.

Consider this hypothetical situation. Two good-sized multispecialty group practices join forces to begin assembling an IDS. Together, they account for nearly 300 physicians, 200 of whom are specialists. If each of those specialist doctors forgoes $25,000 a year in earnings, the overall organization has an additional $5 million each year in investable capital to work with.

Local Area Hospitals

Local acute care hospitals have been a source of funding for new physician groups of all sorts for several years. The ventures they have been willing to finance range from simple group practices to PHOs, MSOs, medical foundations (MFs), even full-blown IDSs. Historically, under fee-for-service reimbursement, hospitals were able to generate considerable excess cash flow to use for purposes such as these. Furthermore, charitable hospitals have access to tax-exempt bond financing (whose proceeds may be restricted in their use).

It is well to be aware of a hospital's likely motives for financing the strategic ventures of their affiliated physicians. Some hospitals may be trying simply to capture a stream of patient admissions in order to maintain their bed populations. In a managed care environment, this strategy is shortsighted and destined for failure in the long run. Be particularly sensitive to this hidden agenda if your financing arrangement with the hospital gives it significant influence over your organization's strategic direction.

More enlightened hospitals see their futures inextricably intertwined with those of their physicians—in a tightly integrated entity committed to controlling both cost and quality. In fact, in most communities, the hospital needs the physicians more than they need it. Take advantage of this knowledge in negotiating financing terms with the hospital. This does not mean strong-arming the hospital. It requires working together to create an organization that can compete as effectively as possible for managed care contracts.

Outside of commercial loans and leases, hospitals have been the primary source of external financing for physician groups. This financing usually takes one of three forms.

1. The hospital buys the practice assets and employs the physician.
2. The hospital forms an MSO that takes over management of the physician practice and employs its staff, though not the physician.
3. The hospital enters into a strategic partnership with the physician practice—through acquisition, merger, or contract—on the way to forming a larger integrated system.

Because this capital source has been so popular, there is a lot of information about the good and the bad of relying on hospitals.

- Hospitals frequently are more generous in the salaries they pay their physicians than are PPMCs or groups that acquire practices.
- An estimated 80 percent of hospitals are losing money on the physician practices they have acquired—as much as $100,000 per physician per year. These are the reasons:
  - After initially acquiring practices for their referrals and as the basis for a managed care network, the hospitals began to look to them for profits.
  - The hospital's administrative and benefit overhead is loaded onto the practice.
  - The hospitals pay too much for the practices.
  - When the employed physicians go on salary, their productivity drops by as much as 10 to 15 percent.
  - Employed physicians may be more conservative in their coding.
  - The hospital often makes expensive capital investments in projects such as information systems and medical office buildings for the physicians.
  - Hospitals do not have competence or experience in managing practices.
  - The hospital's brusque, insensitive attitude alienates the physicians.
- The only hospital financing model that shows signs of working is the strategic partnership, probably because larger physician groups are involved, and the hospital allows

their physician members into leadership positions within the hospital.

- Hospitals are outstanding sources of large amounts of capital, derived from their great cash flow. Tax law inhibitions may keep non-profit hospitals from passing through as much of this money to physicians as they might like.
- Hospitals often provide the most attractive financing terms.
- Hospitals usually allow the least control and flexibility to the physicians.
- A hospital is a natural partner with physicians in forming an integrated multiprovider system that is so popular in managed care circles. In almost all other ways, it is an undesirable strategic partner.

Self-Owned Managed Care Plan Revenues

This is a capital source normally available to only well-established, thoroughly integrated full-service delivery organizations that have taken the final step of creating their own managed care plans. When this is done successfully, the plans can produce a steady flow of cash for investment in further growth. When you reach this point in your organizational evolution, you will know it. It will seem to be the logical next thing to do. Many IDSs make this move specifically for the capital that it generates.

For-Profit Practice Management Companies

Second only to local hospital financing, practice management companies have been a leading source of growth capital for ambitious physician groups. These are for-profit, publicly traded entities that acquire physician practice assets (usually for stock rather than cash), then invest significant sums in their information systems and ancillary service capabilities. In a sense, they offer indirect access to the public equity markets for smaller provider organizations. They are discussed in much greater detail in Chapter 16, "Step Seven: Partnering with a Management Services Organi-

zation or Physician Practice Management Company."

Independent Managed Care Plans and Integrated Delivery Systems

It is in the interest of independent managed care plans, such as group model HMOs, to encourage the development of physician groups and networks with which they can contract for medical services. Toward this end, many have entered into capital partnerships with growing integrated systems, both physician and hospital-dominated. The integrated systems themselves aggressively seek to affiliate with physician practices to expand their networks. These are some of the lessons that have been learned about physician partnering with these entities:

- True integration is an important and necessary competitive tool, but a system is not integrated just because it describes itself as such. Check to see whether it really has tied its components into a more synergistic whole.
- If the integrated system is already in existence, you can interview the current physician members to learn how they have been treated and feel about the experience. On the other hand, a late-joining physician group will have less influence over the direction of the system and may receive less money in the transaction.
- Be sure to consider how well you will relate to and work with the physicians who are already part of an existing system.
- The risks are greater in joining a newly forming IDS, but the physicians are likely to have a greater say in how it is structured and managed. To help get it off the ground, they may be able to negotiate higher acquisition prices and employee salaries.
- Most integrated systems and MCOs maintain substantial financial reserves, accumulated from hospital operations and managed care enrollments. These constitute a significant nest egg for capital investment purposes.

- When considering a financing-motivated affiliation with an IDS, gather information on its finances and flow of funds.
- Do the necessary environment analysis to determine whether this particular IDS is going to be a winner in the competitive marketplace.
- Ask the system representatives about their business and financial plans, as well as their expectations for your group. If they do not have any, offer to help create them.

Health Insurance Companies and Health Plans

When they saw their fee-for-service indemnity business melting away under the pressure of managed care, the old-line health insurance companies made some strategic adjustments. Most created their own capitated managed care products. A few have gone further and invested directly in various sorts of integrated delivery organizations. The leaders in this movement are Aetna, Prudential, CIGNA, and many of the Blue Cross/Blue Shield plans. The insurance companies have huge war chests of cash; they are spending it lavishly to acquire physician practices and build networks to contract with their managed care plans. In dealings with these companies, it is essential to learn their long-term motives before making any commitments. They will end up controlling your destiny, and it had better be one you like.

- Old-line insurance companies have been as effective at managing physician practices as have hospitals, which is to say that they have not done very well at all.
- Many companies tried to set up physician networks as a defensive strategy to make sure that they would have a provider system to use their services as much as the MCOs. They did not have long-term vision for the networks or a sensitivity to the concerns of physicians practicing in a large bureaucracy.
- Some of the most successful insurance institution investors in physician groups have been the Blue Cross/Blue Shield plans. The

reason seems to be that the plans were willing to let the physician groups manage themselves and invest enough capital to instill a sense of economic security, as well as to allow them the freedom to explore other strategic relationships.

DETERMINING WHICH FINANCING OPTION IS AVAILABLE AND APPROPRIATE

Once you have identified the examples of these financing sources that seem to be available in your area, how do you decide which ones might be interested in you and which would be suitable to your present circumstances? These are the critical factors in finding answers to that question.

Type of Organization

Your choice of capital financing source will depend on what kind of organization you are and how long you have been in business. The type of organization is relevant because some lenders or investors understand the nature of your proposed business activities and some do not. Many of the organizational forms and interorganizational affiliations described in this book are recent innovations of the last 5 to 10 years. MSOs, IPAs, MFs, group practices without walls (GPWWs), and IDSs were foreign terms before the mid-1980s and remain confusing for many people, including financiers unacquainted with the modern health care industry. Money institutions are less willing to provide funding to enterprises they do not understand. This problem is disappearing as the workings of managed care and its related institutions become more widely recognized outside the industry. For the time being, do not be surprised if you have to do a lot of explaining and educating to prospective lenders or investors.

One short-term way around this problem is to focus the attention of the financiers on the separate components that may make up your organization. For instance, bankers or venture capitalists probably have a better grasp of the functions of the hospital or the physician group practice that are the two primary founders of a burgeoning IDS. In addition, they certainly will have longer financial histories, which can be scrutinized by prospective funding institutions. The downside is that a debtor lending money may insist that the component organizations guarantee or individually bind themselves to the loan agreement.

Stage of Growth

Students of the creation and development of businesses often view them as moving through several growth stages, which bear directly on the kind of financing they can expect to obtain.

At the *start-up stage*, during its first year or so of existence, your organization will have little or no revenues, no profit history to entice investors, few assets with which to secure a loan, and no credit history to reassure lenders. As a result, do not expect to be able to obtain unsecured bank or other commercial debt financing during this period. Your primary sources of capital financing will be contributions from you and your physician colleagues (using your own assets or personally guaranteeing loans), equity funds from venture capitalists or private stock placements, and investments from strategic partners (such as hospitals).

To justify the risk of placing money in a start-up venture, equity investors will be looking for an annual return on capital of at least 20 percent and payback of the entire invested amount within five years. It will be a challenge to meet these requirements while still earning traditional physician salaries. Those who can, however, will find the equity markets increasingly interested in funding even physician groups with a good revenue stream.

The strategic partner is often the most plausible financing source. Look first to a local hospital. Its expectations for return on capital will be far less than a venture capitalist. The trade-off will be the conditions it attaches to its participation—primarily in the form of influence over the strategic direction of the organization. Too often, the terms will be intolerable to a group of visionary physi-

cians. The other strategic alternative is a for-profit practice management company (such as Phycor, MedPartners, and Caremark), which tend to have a more "physiciancentric" point of view.

In the *emerging organization stage*, the organization has developed as a recognizable IPA, MSO, GPWW, or multispecialty group practice. It has an operating history of three years or so, rapidly growing revenues, marginal profits, some assets that might secure a loan, and a fledgling credit history. Such an entity can expect to obtain financing on the following terms:

- three- to five-year loans at fixed interest rates 2 to 3 percent above the prime rate
- repayment schedules tailored to projected revenue growth
- credit backing from more established participants in the venture (e.g., hospital)
- if there are no such participants, a request for equity participation (20 to 30 percent) by the lender for the duration of the loan
- accounts receivables pledged as security for the loan

By the time the organization has reached the *early maturity stage*, it has built a substantial balance sheet showing significant assets, growing retained earnings, and a capital structure balance between debt (two-thirds) and equity (one-third). It will now have access to almost the full range of financing options described above. An initial public offering of stock may even be possible. Prior financing can be renegotiated on more attractive terms. On the basis of a longer, stronger credit history, loans will be available at lower interest rates and with less security.

Financial History

Every organization except the rawest start-up has some kind of financial history. The income statements, balance sheets, and cost records go a long way toward revealing the efficiency of its operations. They will indicate how well managed the group has been in the past and, by extension, how well it might employ capital entrusted to it by an outside investor. Investors feel more comfortable placing their funds in the strong financial structure that usually results from several years of positive financial performance. Compile your financial statements for at least five years in the past. Ask a financial analyst or investment banker to scan them and give you a reading on their soundness and appeal to the average lender or investor.

Systematic Financial Planning

Good financial planning requires that you lay out the uses of capital funds that you would like to make over the next three to five years to carry out the objectives of the group's strategic plan. You then postulate a series of capital infusions, from any and all sources (debt and equity), necessary to finance those uses. The capital uses or expenditures will come at regular intervals, depending on your ability to manage the projects and to acquire the necessary financing. On a year-by-year basis, the expenditures should be matched exactly with financing sources of the appropriate size.

The master financial plan will be composed of capital budget projections and pro forma income statements, balance sheets, and cash flow statements. Alternative operating scenarios should be laid out. The actual capital sources used will be the result of negotiations.

Development of a master financing plan will permit participants (who are asked to make capital contributions) to plan their own finances further ahead. Such a plan also ensures that necessary funding will be available when capital expenditures are most needed. A multistage plan permits the organization to steadily evolve a capital structure that is optimally balanced between debt and equity. Well-planned and carefully balanced financing is also likely to incur the minimum cost of capital.

The ability to carry out a systemwide financial strategy is another long-term competitive advantage of operating through an integrated health care system. Such a system is large enough to acquire the capital to make needed investments—

at advantageous terms—and able to deploy the capital where there is the most to gain. The greater size usually means greater financial stability, which is encouraging to investors and lenders. Larger entities also require larger capital infusions, which gives them access to capital sources that entail lower costs of capital.

> **Primary Goal of Any Capital Financing Strategy:** Obtain all the capital you need at the most attractive terms. Invest in those projects that meet your strategic objectives and cover your costs of capital by the widest margin. Anything you do to serve this goal is to your advantage. A formal capital financing plan is one of those things.

Under its AMA Solutions subsidiary, the American Medical Association (AMA) has a couple of new programs to support physicians in their quest for capital financing. AMA ConsultingLink is a national referral network for financial consultants and business advisors. Call them at (800) 366-6968 for a free referral to a consultant in your area. The AMA CapitalLink program is designed to provide direct access to a wide variety of financing options. They include small business loans (for up to $1 million), "mezzanine" financing for projects costing from $1 million to $5 million, and venture capital investment for projects over $5 million.

MAKING A PROVIDER ORGANIZATION MORE ATTRACTIVE TO FINANCING SOURCES

Capital partners are selective in deciding where to invest their money—whether by loan or equity. There are several proven steps you can take to make your organization more attractive to investors:

• Prepare and present a thorough, well-thought-out business plan.

- Provide evidence of the physicians' willingness, in the past and future, to risk their own money in making the venture succeed.
- In particular, build a record of allowing retained earnings to accumulate in the business, rather than drawing them all out at the end of the year.
- Demonstrate the steps you have already taken to enhance the group's ability to manage utilization, reduce costs, improve quality, and maintain patient satisfaction.
- Regardless of your group's state of development or capital needs, start now to develop relationships with potential investors.
- Be realistic and exact in your financial projections. Unrealistic projections may impair your credibility on first impression.
- Seek advice from investors, even if they reject your first proposal. Change your business plan or approach on the basis of the feedback you receive.
- Develop an in-depth knowledge of your market and competition before talking to investors.
- Find out in advance everything that the investors are likely to discover during their due diligence process.
- Talk to your prospective customers (e.g., patients, MCOs, employers) to make sure that there is a market for your services. Obtain references and testimonials while you are at it.

MISTAKES TO AVOID IN SEEKING CAPITAL FINANCING

Start-up businesses with no prior operating experience regularly make mistakes in financing strategy that can compromise their very survival. Physician-sponsored organizations are no different. These are the most common examples. They can all be avoided.

Financial Planning Not Based on Strategic Planning

It is necessary to have a carefully crafted strategic and business plan that outlines in detail your projected activities and expenditures before trying to raise capital. The strategic plan will ensure that the new venture is headed in a rational direction, minimizing wasted effort and wasted spending. The business plan will specify how much financing is needed, during what periods of time, for what types of expenditures—all essential information to make sure that you have the capital you need at the least cost. These plans will impress the investors or lenders and increase the chances of getting the money you need from them.

Without this kind of advance planning, there is a good chance that your venture will not have the right amount of money when it needs it and that it will pay too much for the financing it does obtain. The ultimate result may be the failure of your undertaking.

Failure To Prepare a Formal Financial Plan

Once the strategic and business plans are in place, you must prepare a formal financial plan. A responsible lender or investor will not give you money without seeing one. This plan projects the organization's financing needs for the next three to five years. It should be composed of the following elements:

- estimate of the one-time start-up or transition costs
- cash flow projections on a monthly basis for the first three years
- projected income statements and balance sheets on a quarterly basis for the first three years
- projected capital expenditures budget for the first three years
- proposed timing and source of capital infusions for the first three years
- statement of assumptions upon which the projections are based
- description of alternative financing scenarios if primary assumptions prove inaccurate

Such a plan will streamline the fundraising process and minimize the costs of capital obtained.

Failure To Adapt the Business and Financial Strategies to Changing Market Conditions

A long-term strategy, a business plan, and a financial strategy will seem like major accomplishments. However, they will start to become obsolete the moment you adopt them. You already know how rapidly the health care industry is transforming itself. No one is sure where this tumultuous change will end. For competitive businesses, this means paying close attention to the market and regulatory environment so that you can shift or adjust almost any strategic aspect on very short notice. There is a fine managerial art to knowing when to stick stubbornly to a strategic direction you believe will succeed in the end and when to abandon a strategy that events have passed by. The wrong choice can result in wasted spending on useless projects or the failure to spend on needed projects.

Overestimating Revenues and Underestimating Expenses

Until you have planned and started one or two business ventures, you may not understand the natural tendency of founders to exaggerate the revenues that will be generated and to minimize the expenses that will be incurred. This is not done consciously; it just happens to enthusiastic entrepreneurs who believe avidly in their business visions. Obviously, it can have disastrous effects on the scheduling of loans and investments, and on the allocation of resources. The common wisdom is to halve the estimated revenues and double the estimated expenses. That contingency may not occur, but you will be in a lot better financial shape if you prepare to handle it.

Assuming That Growth Can Be Financed Internally

Perhaps a natural outgrowth of inflated revenue estimates is the belief—more a hope—that the organization will not have to turn to external financing sources at all, but rather can fund all of its growth internally. In some less capital-intensive, slower-moving industries, this occasionally is possible. It is out of the question for a new physician organization that will be spending hundreds of thousands of dollars, if not millions, within a rather short period of time on medical practice acquisitions, primary care network construction, and information system development. Count on having to go to outside capital sources—sooner rather than later.

There are measures you can take to reduce your reliance on such sources. Start now diverting some of the revenues from your practice to a capital growth and expansion fund. Once you begin operating in your new venture, commit all physicians to accepting the minimal compensation they need now to subsist, defer additional compensation to later or pay it in the form of stock, and pour the savings into capital investment. This will not preclude outside financing, but it will postpone it and perhaps limit the control you have to cede to nonphysician investors. An added benefit is that your self-discipline will impress lenders and investors, possibly lowering your capital costs.

Failing To Assess the Strategic Motives of the Capital Partner

This is primarily a problem with equity investors. In return for their investments, they will receive ownership interests in the organization and perhaps even seats on the board of directors. One of the objectives of a good financing strategy is to minimize the share of the business you must trade for a given chunk of financing. As hard as you try, you are likely to wind up with a hospital, insurance company, venture capitalist, or other nonphysician party as a capital partner.

Assuming Capital Costs That Exceed the Organization's Ability To Service Them

Perhaps surprisingly, it sometimes is possible to persuade or allow a lender to give your organization financing at an interest rate and under terms that it ultimately cannot support. If the use of the financing does not generate the revenues and cash flow necessary to pay its cost, the organization may end up sacrificing other strategic goals to meet interest and principal payments. Finally, default, forced bankruptcy, sale of secured assets, or lender involvement in operational matters may result. This risk is minimized by careful financial planning and informed negotiation of loan terms.

FINANCING AN INTEGRATED SYSTEM MADE UP OF SEVERAL DISTINCT COMPONENTS

Because of their different operating characteristics and business, the several components of an integrated provider system are likely to be viewed differently by capital markets.

Consider a system composed of a hospital organization, a physician group, and a health care plan. These entities face distinctly different business risks, reflect varying financial operations, and are built on rather divergent capital structures. Each manages quite different assets: Hospitals have large physical plants, physician organizations rely on human resources, and health plans manipulate monetary funds.

The capital markets assess these varying characteristics and assign them different interest rates and security requirements. For instance, the building and grounds of a hospital might seem to offer solid protection to a lender. Yet, if the demand for the hospital's services is declining and there is no other use to which the hospital assets could easily be put, capital markets might rate it as a relatively high risk.

In determining how great a debt load an organization can handle, financial analysts tend to apply a multiplier to the cash flow available for debt service. In the case of physician groups, it is assumed that the debt service is paid for before physician compensation is withdrawn. As a result, the same cash flow will support significantly more debt in a physician organization than in a hospital organization.

What this means for capital financing strategies is that it sometimes is better to seek separate financing for the individual components of an integrated system rather than for the entire system as a whole. The figures in Table 27–1 illustrate why.

The ratios between cash flow and debt load may vary from these figures but are relatively accurate. This hypothetical system could raise 28 percent more capital ($17.5 million) through separate, as opposed to joint, financing.

This is likely to be temporary phenomenon. The separate provider components are rated differently and specifically because the markets are familiar with the concept and structure of hospitals, physician groups, and health plans. Within five years, they will be just as familiar with integrated systems and will value them as highly, or more highly, than their individual components. This will be reflected in lower interest rates and higher permissible debt loads.

Table 27–1 Integrated vs. Individual Cash Flow and Debt Load Comparison

	Cash Flow Available for Debt Service	*Debt Load Supported by That Cash Flow*
Hospital Organization	$10 million	$50 million
Physician Group	$2.5 million	$30 million
Hospital-Dominated Integrated System	$12.5 million	$62.5 million
Separate Hospital and Physician Components	$12.5 million	$30 million

REFERENCES

1. R. Coile Jr., "Assessing Healthcare Market Trends and Capital Needs: 1996–2000," *Healthcare Financial Management 49*, no. 8 (1995): 60.
2. D. Coddington, et al., *Making Integrated Health Care Work* (Englewood, CO: Center for Research in Ambulatory Health Care Administration, 1996).

3. *Revenue Procedure* 82-15, 1982-1 C.B. 460.
4. S.E. Pratt and D. Bokser, eds., *Pratt's Guide to Venture Capital Sources,* 22d ed. (Newark, NJ: Venture Economics Investor Services, 1998).

RESOURCE LIST

S. Becker et al., "Taking the Provider-Driven Company Public: A Primer on Business and Legal Issues," *Journal of Health Care Finance 22*, no. 4 (1996): 71.

M. Blecher, "Capital: Who's Got It? How To Get It?" *Hospitals & Health Networks 71*, no. 12 (1997): 38.

Capital Survey of Emerging Healthcare Organizations, Second Annual Report 1996, Survey #4872 (Englewood, CO: Medical Group Management Association).

D. Coddington et al., *Capitalizing Medical Groups: Positioning Physicians for the Future* (copublished, Burr Ridge, IL: McGraw-Hill Healthcare Education Group, and Westchester, IL: Healthcare Financial Management Association, 1998).

P. DeMuro. *The Financial Manager's Guide to Managed Care and Integrated Delivery Systems, Strategies for Contracting, Compensation and Reimbursement* (Westchester, IL: Healthcare Financial Management Association, 1996).

Financial Management of the Medical Practice (Chicago: American Medical Association, 1996).

J. Greene, "Starting Up the Upstarts," *Hospitals & Health Networks 71*, no. 24 (1997): 16.

R. Lowes, "Try a Do-It-Yourself Public Offering," *Medical Economics 74*, no. 8 (1997): 50.

J. McCally and M. LaFond. *Physician Practice Management Redefined, the Move to Integrated Practice Organizations* (copublished, Burr Ridge, IL: McGraw-Hill Healthcare Education Group, and Westchester, IL: Healthcare Financial Management Association, 1998).

E. Pavlock, *Financial Management for Medical Groups: A Primer for New Managers and a Refresher for the Experienced* (Englewood, CO: Medical Group Management Association, 1994).

C. Payne, *Strategic Capital Planning for Healthcare Organizations* (Westchester, IL: Healthcare Financial Management Association, 1995).

S. Preston, "Deal a Hospital a Minority Stake in Your Doctor Group," *Medical Economics 74*, no. 8 (1997): 46.

S. Preston, "Issues Bonds Backed by a Letter of Credit," *Medical Economics 74*, no. 8 (1997): 66.

J. Sterns and D. Johnson, "Financing Alternatives for Medical Group Practices," *Medical Group Management Journal 42*, no. 1 (1995): 58.

J. Vaughn and J. Wise, "How To Choose the Right Capitalization Option—Finance Options for Physician Group Practices," *Healthcare Financial Management 50*, no. 12 (1996): 72.

The physician who becomes especially interested in or responsible for matters of financial management would be well advised to join the Healthcare Financial Management Association (HFMA). An HFMA member receives a subscription to the magazine *Healthcare Financial Management*, and can earn certification in financial management, participate in local chapter activities, attend seminars and conferences, and purchase HFMA publications. Nonmembers may subscribe to the magazine and purchase the books. The magazine articles and books address many of the issues raised in this book, and do it in language that does not require an MBA or CPA to understand. The HFMA can be reached at the following address:

HFMA
Two Westbrook Corporate Center, Suite 700
Westchester, IL 60154-5700
(800) 252-4362
http://www.hfma.org

## CHAPTER 28

Collaborating with Other Physicians without Legal Risk

INTRODUCTION

As physicians are working to develop the optimal strategy for managed care success, they must inevitably collaborate with other physicians. In most cases, this takes the form of strategic consolidation through affiliation, merger, and acquisition—followed by integration of practice behaviors at the operational level. However, physicians may also collaborate without a particular strategic purpose in mind, perhaps to achieve some short-term gain unrelated to managed care. They might simply want to talk with colleagues in anticipation of embarking on a joint managed care strategy.

This chapter describes a few of the ways in which physicians might choose to collaborate with each other—short of outright affiliation. This is accompanied by an examination of the legal risks that crop up when competing physicians start talking to each other. Suggestions for minimizing these risks are included. There is also a special section on physician unions—an alternative collaboration strategy being studied and adopted by a growing number of physicians.

WHO SHOULD READ THIS CHAPTER

This is a good chapter for physicians who have in mind some kind of joint venture with other physicians for the purpose of adding another revenue stream or simply to gain experience in working with other like-minded professionals. The chapter might also give some ideas and incentives to other physicians who have never before considered joint efforts with colleagues.

It is also a chapter worth reading by physicians who are beginning to realize that they must join with other physicians to form larger, integrated entities and who feel an impulse to discuss the possibilities with them. This chapter offers guidance on how to do that safely.

The physicians who can skip this chapter are those who are well on a path toward consolidation and integration with their peers and are totally engrossed by the process. They are well beyond the stage of "just talking" and may already have lawyers to explain the legal nuances of joint ventures.

LEGAL BACKDROP FOR PHYSICIAN COLLABORATION

The primary restraint on physician collaboration is the federal antitrust laws and how they are enforced. These laws are enforced by the Department of Justice (DOJ) and the Federal Trade Commission (FTC). The language of the laws is rather broad. To help health care organizations better anticipate how the laws might be applied to them, the two agencies have issued guidelines, called the *DOJ/FTC Statements of Enforcement Policy in Health Care*.[1] They have been revised several times, most recently in August 1996, each time making it slightly easier for providers to collaborate with each other. Here is the latest word on when and how physicians may talk and work together.

The general rule is that physicians in competition with each other may not collude or conspire with each other to restrain trade or to monopolize a market. There are two standards of illegality of these kinds of behavior. Certain types of restraints on trade are so damaging to competition and so unjustified that they are conclusively presumed to be illegal—without any inquiry into their actual effects on competition. These are called *per se* violations of the antitrust laws. The sorts of behavior included in this category are price fixing, group boycotts, division of markets, and tying arrangements.

All other kinds of collusive behavior are analyzed under the "*rule of reason*" approach. This is a structured process used by the agencies or courts to define the relevant product or geographic market, to evaluate the purpose of the restraining activity, to evaluate the effects of the activity on competition in the defined market, and to balance this against any pro-competitive effects that may exist. If the activity favors competition more than it discourages it, there is no antitrust violation.

Some courts have taken a third approach midway between the first two. In circumstances where a court feels that a rule of reason analysis should be applied to behavior that is otherwise a per se violation, it will take a "*quick look*" at the pro- and anticompetitive effects of the behavior. This is much less than the in-depth inquiry of a full-blown rule of reason analysis.

If they cannot avoid an antitrust accusation entirely, organizations and individuals will prefer to be charged with a rule of reason violation, a quick look violation, and a per se violation—in that order.

For at least 20 years, the courts have been quite reluctant to apply the per se rule to defendants who are health care providers. The reasons given are the lack of judicial experience necessary to characterize many health care activities as plainly anticompetitive and the fact that they often are carried out in the public interest rather than for commercial gain. That bias of the courts is likely to change as they accumulate the necessary experience and as they conclude that certain activities have no redeeming value.

Price Fixing

The most dangerous form of collusive behavior by physicians would be any sort of agreement that relates in any way, even indirectly, to the prices they charge for their services. Historically, criminal prosecutions by the DOJ have focused almost exclusively on agreements among competitors related to pricing. Prohibited activities include not only the basic fixing of prices but also any collusive activity that does the following:

- establishes minimum or maximum prices
- creates pressure to increase prices
- stabilizes prices
- interferes with a competitor's freedom to make price changes independently
- establishes uniform terms of sale, discount policies, or some other agreed-upon approach to the prices charged (such as a fee schedule)
- prevents competitors from advertising prices

On the other hand, group purchasing agreements will pass legal scrutiny if properly constructed and implemented. They are viewed as traditional means of creating economic efficiencies for the participating members, as long as there is no evidence of substantial anticompetitive effect.

Group Boycotts

Another form of collusive behavior likely to get health care providers into serious trouble are concerted refusals to deal with, or outright group boycotts of, a third party such as a hospital or a managed care organization (MCO). This is likely to be a per se violation when the boycott is horizontal—as in the boycott of one group of physicians by another group of physicians. A vertical agreement (for example, between an MCO and a contracting physician group) not to deal with a third party (such as another MCO) has been analyzed by several courts recently under the rule of reason approach.* Some examples of health care activities that might constitute prohibited boycotts follow.

- denial of hospital staff privileges
- restrictive membership requirements into, or expulsion from, an organization in which membership is economically desirable (such as membership on an MCO's physician panel)
- refusal to deal or contract with certain or all MCOs
- denial of accreditation or certification

Joint Ventures and Networks

As physicians pursue joint ventures or networks designed to move them toward the formation of the organizations recommended in this book (i.e., large, multispecialty integrated groups), they must eventually engage in price fixing, boycotts, and other actions that normally would be considered per se antitrust violations.**
The critical question is how closely integrated they have become, how far they have progressed toward becoming a single business entity rather than a collection of many separate and competing business entities.

---

*This was the position of the U.S. Court of Appeals for the First Circuit in the case of *U.S. Healthcare, Inc. v. Healthsource, Inc.*, 986 F.2d 589, holding that Healthsource had not conspired with its participating physicians to exclude U.S. Healthcare from the New Hampshire market.

**It is clear that all the physicians belonging to a unified, integrated group practice may set a common fee schedule, may contract jointly with external payers, and may choose to avoid business relationships with certain payers, with other physician groups, or with any other third parties. It also is clear that these activities are entirely legal.

The enforcement agencies (DOJ, FTC) have provided excellent guidelines on this point in their *Statements of Antitrust Enforcement Policy in Health Care* issued on August 28, 1996.[2] Generally, they recognize additional forms of integration that will permit physicians to engage in otherwise illegal collusive action.

Under the *Statements*, all "physician joint venture networks" and "multiprovider networks" fall into one of three categories.

1. those with sufficient financial integration to place them in an antitrust "safety zone"
2. those with insufficient financial integration but sufficient nonfinancial integration to subject them to a rule of reason analysis
3. those with insufficient financial and nonfinancial integration which will be deemed to be committing per se violations

Joint Ventures in the Antitrust "Safety Zone"

If the characteristics of a physician joint venture place it within this safety zone, the DOJ and FTC promise that it will be immune from antitrust prosecution. The physician members will be permitted to collaborate on pricing, services, contracting strategies, and membership in their group. Two requirements must be met to qualify for this safety zone.

First, the participating physicians must share substantial financial risk. Most often, this will take the following forms:

- capitation payments from the MCO to the group
- payment to the group of a predetermined percentage of the premiums earned or revenues received by the MCO
- offering to the participating physicians, as a group, of significant financial incentives, such as substantial withholds of payment (15 to 20 percent) until specified cost containment goals have been met or a program of penalties and rewards for the overall group's achievement of utilization targets

- payments to the group on the basis of global fees or all-inclusive case rates

Other policies and procedures that have the same risk-sharing effect may qualify as well.

Second, the group may not include more than 20 percent of the physicians in each specialty in the local market area on an exclusive basis or 30 percent of those physicians on a nonexclusive basis.

Joint Ventures Subject to a Rule of Reason Analysis

By integrating in other nonfinancial ways, physician joint ventures that do not qualify for the safety zone (insufficient financial integration or too many physicians in a particular specialty) may avoid per se violations and subject themselves to no more than the more flexible rule of reason analysis. The *Statements* ask for "an active and ongoing program to evaluate and modify practice patterns by the network's physician participants and create a high degree of interdependence and cooperation among the physicians to control costs and ensure quality."[3(p.1309)] The enforcement agencies will find evidence of such a program in elements such as these:

- mechanisms to monitor and control utilization
- selectivity in choosing group physicians who are likely to further these efficiency objectives
- significant investment of capital, both human and monetary, in the infrastructure and capability necessary to realize the claimed efficiencies

However, they also are open to other forms of integration that might achieve the same efficiencies.

Joint Ventures Engaged in Per Se Antitrust Violations

A physician joint venture that lacks significant financial risk sharing or significant clinical or other nonfinancial integration, or one that includes more than the maximum percentage of physicians in each specialty will be committing per se antitrust violations if its physicians attempt to collaborate on prices or any other competitive parameter. It can expect to be the target of a federal prosecution, which it will lose.

Joint Ventures to Which the Physician Makes Referrals

This is a category of physician joint venture and collaboration that is not governed primarily by the antitrust laws. The Medicare "anti-kickback" law,[4] enacted in 1972, and the so-called Stark II law,[5] enacted in 1993, directly determine the terms under which physicians may participate in these joint ventures.

The Medicare Anti-Fraud and Abuse Statute was enacted in 1972 to deal with abuses of the Medicare reimbursement system. It made it illegal to offer, pay, or receive a kickback or bribe in connection with furnishing services covered by Medicare or Medicaid. In its simplest form, a prohibited kickback involves a payment by one entity, such as a clinical laboratory or a specialist physician, to a physician for referrals he makes to the entity. The statute also applies to investments made by physicians in an entity (such as a clinical laboratory) to which they make referrals, where the return on their investment is tied to the volume of their referrals or is disproportionately high.

In 1989, the Office of the Inspector General (OIG) in the Department of Health and Human Services (DHHS) issued a Fraud Alert describing the kinds of joint venture financing arrangements that would raise suspicions under the Fraud and Abuse law.

- nominal initial capital contributions from physician-investors
- initial capital contributions from physicians funded by loans from the joint venture
- profit distribution arrangements that promise physicians unusually high returns on unusually small investments

- extremely high returns paid to physicians on their investments in comparison to the risks involved
- physician-investors chosen for their ability to make referrals
- especially lucrative return on investment offers made to physicians expected to make a large number of referrals
- the joint venture actively encourages physician-investors to refer patients to it, limits their ability to transfer their investment interest, requires divestment of their investment interest if they leave the area, or records and publishes the number of referrals by each physician-investor
- the joint venture owns very little of the inventory and equipment necessary to conduct its business
- the joint venture is managed and operated fully by one of the joint venture partners

In 1991, the OIG issued regulations[6] defining a set of "safe harbor" exceptions from the Fraud and Abuse law.

- A physician may refer patients to a facility that is part of a large corporation (publicly traded and over $50 million in assets).
- A physician may refer patients to a smaller entity, no more than 40 percent of which is owned by persons in a position to make referrals and no more than 40 percent of whose referrals come from investors.
- Under either of those safe harbors, a physician's return on investment cannot be based on the volume of her referrals but only on the amount of her capital investment, investment opportunities must be offered on the same terms to both referring and nonreferring investors, and the joint venture cannot make loans to physicians to finance their investments in the venture.
- A physician may make referrals to a group practice in which he is an "active" investor.
- A joint venture may make payments to a physician for furnishing services reimbursed

by Medicare or Medicaid under a bona fide employment relationship with the venture.
- A physician may make referrals to a joint venture with which he has a personal services or management contract, so long as the contract is written and signed, specifies the services to be provided, has a term of one year or more, sets the compensation in advance consistent with fair market value determined in arm's-length negotiations, and is not based on the volume of referrals.

In 1993, Congress enacted the Comprehensive Physician Ownership and Referral Act, more commonly known as *Stark II*. This law prohibits physicians from making Medicare or Medicaid referrals to entities that furnish clinical laboratory or other designated health services and with which the physician (or an immediate family member) has a financial relationship (includes ownership or investment interests and compensation arrangements). The "designated health services" include the following:

- physical therapy services
- occupational therapy services
- radiology or other diagnostic services
- radiation therapy services
- durable medical equipment
- parenteral and enteral nutrients, equipment, and supplies
- prosthetics, orthotics, and prosthetic devices
- home health services
- outpatient prescription drugs
- inpatient and outpatient hospital services

There are numerous exceptions to the Stark II prohibitions.

- A physician may refer for services to an owned entity if she or a member of her group practice provides the services personally or supervises the person providing them.
- A physician may refer to an owned entity where the services are provided by certain types of MCOs to their enrollees.

- A physician may refer to a publicly traded entity with assets of at least $75 million.
- A physician may refer for services furnished in a rural area if substantially all of the services go to residents of the area.
- A physician may refer for services provided by a hospital in which he has an ownership or investment interest (in the hospital itself, not merely a subdivision of it) and where he has staff privileges.
- A physician may refer for services in the context of a bona fide employment relationship or a personal services arrangement.

Keep in mind that Stark II applies only to referrals that will be reimbursed under Medicare or Medicaid.

POTENTIAL OPPORTUNITIES FOR PHYSICIAN COLLABORATION

There are a great many ways in which physicians might combine their resources and ideas to adapt their medical practices to the onrush of managed care and MCOs. Some of these are quite acceptable under the current laws, and some of them will create serious legal problems. These are some of the most common forms of physician-to-physician collaboration and their legal implications.

Physician Activities Intended To Impede the Establishment of MCOs

Many physicians would prefer to never have to deal with MCOs. Some would like to prevent them from entering the local marketplace at all. The natural impulse is to collaborate with other like-minded physicians to plan resistance strategies. A limited number of joint activities are acceptable under the law—mainly those having to do with the exercise of the physicians' rights to free speech and political action. For instance, a group of independent doctors could do the following:

- Form a political action committee to raise funds for a candidate who would advance their interests in the health care marketplace.
- Communicate publicly, with one voice, their grievances and criticisms about the effects of care management on their practice of medicine.
- Jointly lobby key legislators to enact laws protecting physician clinical autonomy, patient choice, or the physician-patient relationship.

What they cannot do is take any joint action regarding the terms under which they offer their services to their customers or their treatment of customers, payers, patients, competitors, or suppliers. They cannot agree on the following:

- the prices that they will charge for their services (whether in the form of fee schedules, capitation rates, or risk withholds)
- other terms of the managed care contracts they are willing to enter into
- which MCOs they will contract with and which they will not
- which government programs (Medicare and Medicaid) they will participate in
- which specialists to whom they will make referrals
- which hospitals to which they will admit patients
- where they will locate their practices
- which physicians will see which patients from different managed care plans
- which specific services they will offer

Physician Joint Conduct Designed To Keep Competitors Out

The implicit goal of competitors in a free market system is to drive each other out of business. The law does permit this when it is accomplished through the provision of new products or services, at lower prices, or at more convenient times and locations—in general, giving the customer more of what he or she wants. That is the essence of real competition.

There is an entire range of other competitive strategy and tactics that are prohibited by the law. Some of those are capable of being implemented by a single, dominant competitor. Most require the collaboration or conspiracy of numerous smaller competitors, as in a physician joint venture.

To maintain their own market positions, a group of unintegrated physician practices may not agree to

- Use their influence on the medical staff of a key local hospital to deny staff privileges to competing physicians.
- Withhold referrals from physicians who compete in some ways with them.
- Refuse to deal with any party (noncompeting physicians, hospitals, MCOs) that chooses also to deal with the group's competitors.
- Charge fees or prices designed to make it impossible for other physicians to compete.
- Alter the terms of their market behavior to punish and drive their competitors out of business.
- Require that customers dealing with one or more of them must also deal with the others in the group.

Except for the medical staff option, all of these activities may be carried out by individual group practices.

Physician Organizations Operating as Covers for Collective Decisions on Fees and Access to Health Care Facilities

The DOJ, FTC, and other government enforcement agencies are concerned solely with the collusion activities of competing physicians. What the physicians claim to be doing, the superficial structure of joint organizations they may form, or the labels they give to their organizations or activities are of less interest. It will make no difference that the physicians try to create the impression that they are clinically integrated or sharing risk if, in fact, they are not. They will be at high risk of an antitrust legal action. (See also the section below, entitled "Special Case: 'Sham Networks'—Don't Try To Fool the Feds.")

Price Fixing among Providers or Provider Associations

This is a per se violation of federal antitrust laws by any combination of physicians or physician organizations that do not meet the prerequisites of *the DOJ/FTC Statements of Antitrust Enforcement Policy in Health Care*. Do not even think about doing it.

Physician Participation in a Professional Review of a Physician's Clinical Competence or Practice Efficiency

This is a trick subheading because a physician may avoid liability for his participation in a properly conducted professional review of another physician's clinical competence but not for his practice efficiency.

The problem arose when physicians deprived of hospital staff privileges brought antitrust and other lawsuits against the participants in the professional review or credentialing process that made the decisions. As a result, other physicians became reluctant to sit on professional review or credentialing committees. In the interests of encouraging a fair process for weeding out incompetent physicians, Congress enacted the Health Care Quality Improvement Act of 1986[7] (HCQIA).

The HCQIA provides limited immunity from legal liability to physicians who participate in properly structured professional review procedures. To qualify for this immunity, the review procedure must be focused on the "competence or professional conduct of an individual physician (which conduct affects or could affect adversely the health or welfare of a patient or patients), and which affects (or may affect) adversely the clinical privileges, or membership in a professional society, of the physician."[8] A review proceeding that is concerned with any of the following matters will not qualify.

- a physician's association or lack of association with a professional society or association
- a physician's fees, advertising, or any competitive acts to solicit or retain business
- a physician's participation in prepaid group health plans, salaried employment, or any other manner of delivering health services, whether on a fee-for-service or other basis
- a physician's association with, supervision of, delegating of authority to, support for, training of, or participation in a group practice with a member or members of a particular class of health care practitioner or professional
- any other matter that does not relate to the competence or professional conduct of a physician

Participating physicians will be immunized from liability, not from a lawsuit itself. They still can be sued; but they will win. These are the kinds of liability that they can and cannot avoid:

- immunity from monetary damages under all federal laws, including antitrust laws but excluding civil rights laws
- no immunity from injunctive and other equitable relief under federal laws
- immunity from state law liability unless the state specifically chooses to opt out of the HCQIA's protections
- no immunity from malpractice suits brought under federal or state laws by patients against health care providers for negligent care
- no immunity against federal or state government actions to enforce antitrust laws
- immunity for witnesses who provide information in professional review proceedings unless they were aware that the information was false

Historically, the greatest threat to professional review physicians has been antitrust lawsuits from deselected physicians seeking monetary damages for loss of their ability to pursue their careers. The HCQIA effectively removes that threat under certain circumstances.

1. The peer review actions were undertaken in the reasonable belief that they furthered the quality of health care.
2. There was a reasonable effort to discover the facts in the case.
3. Procedural due process protections were available to the physician involved.
4. The review participants reasonably believed that the action taken against the physician was warranted by the facts.

The Act goes into even greater detail about the elements of the required procedural due process.

1. The physician must be given notice of any proposed action against her, the reasons for the proposed action, and notice of her right to request a hearing.
2. If a hearing is requested, the physician must be given 30 days' notice of the time, place, and date of the hearing and a list of the witnesses expected to testify on behalf of the review committee.
3. The hearing must be held before an arbitrator mutually acceptable to both the health care entity (e.g., hospital, group practice, independent delivery system) and the physician or before a hearing officer or panel of individuals appointed by the health care entity, provided that such persons are not in direct competition with the physician.
4. At the hearing, the physician must have the right to (a) be represented by an attorney or other person of the physician's choice, (b) have a record made of the proceedings, (c) call, examine, and cross-examine witnesses, (d) present evidence, and (e) submit a written statement at the close of the hearing.
5. Following the hearing, the physician must have the right to receive the written recommendation of the review committee and

the final written decision of the health care entity.

There are a few narrow situations in which even these due process requirements need not be observed:

- where no professional review action is actually taken
- where a physician is suspended or otherwise restricted for less than 14 days while an investigation is conducted
- where failure to suspend or restrict privileges immediately "may result in an imminent danger to the health of any individual," as long as notice and a hearing are eventually given to the physician

Physician Participation in Exchanges of Information and Fee Surveys with Competitors

It may come as a surprise to learn that, under certain circumstances, physicians can share information about price and cost information without running afoul of the antitrust laws. Specifically, physicians may contribute to written surveys of their prices for health care services or the wages, salaries, and benefits earned by their health care personnel if the following conditions are satisfied:

- The survey is managed by a third party.
- The information provided by the physicians is based on data more than three months old.
- There are at least five providers reporting the data upon which each shared statistic is based, no individual physician's data represents more than 25 percent (on a weighted basis) of that statistic, and any information shared is totaled in such a way that it is not possible to identify the prices charged or compensation paid by a particular physician.

The idea is to permit the physicians to make adjustments in their prices and costs in response to changes in market conditions as reflected in average, not physician-specific, figures. They must not be able to coordinate those adjustments with individual physician competitors.

Physician Investments with Others in Ventures to Which They Refer Patients

It may seem natural for a physician to invest in a venture providing services that are especially familiar to him and that will be useful to his patients. However, the Fraud and Abuse statute and the Stark II law place major restrictions on these kinds of ventures. The most important message from these two laws is to avoid any arrangement that even suggests that a physician is receiving benefits, monetary or otherwise, for the patient referrals that he makes. Here are some other points to keep in mind when planning a venture like this:

- A physician may always invest in a large, publicly traded company providing "designated health services," although this is probably not what most physicians have in mind when they contemplate a joint venture.
- A physician will be free to invest in ventures to which she refers when they are located in rural areas.
- A physician can always refer patients to a venture that he co-owns if he provides the services personally or supervises the people who do. It also is acceptable for members of the physician's group practice to provide, or supervise the provision of, the services.
- A physician may make referrals to a group practice in which she is an active participant and investor.
- The physician's initial investment in the venture should never be funded by a loan from the venture.
- The joint venture should offer identical investment terms to investors who are and are not in a position to refer patients to the venture.
- There should be absolutely no discussion, promises, or requests concerning referrals

between physician-investors and the joint venture.

- The returns earned by physician-investors should not be disproportionately high, compared with the size of their initial investment and the financial risks involved.
- A physician may make referrals to an organization providing "designated health services" or she may have an investment or ownership interest in such an organization, but she may not do both.

If evidence continues to show that fraud and abuse is consuming a significant portion of the national health care budget, do not be surprised if laws are enacted to ban absolutely any financial connection between physicians and entities to which they might refer patients.

Group or Joint Purchasing of Equipment, Materials, or Services by Physicians

The antitrust enforcement agencies will not challenge a joint purchasing arrangement among a group of physicians as long as they meet two conditions.

- Their joint purchases account for less than 35 percent of the total sales of the product or service they are purchasing in the local market.
- The cost of the products or services purchased jointly represents less than 20 percent of the total revenues earned from all health care services by the physicians participating in the joint purchasing agreement.

These arrangements are more likely to pass legal muster if the physicians do the following:

- Make clear that the participating physicians are not required to use the arrangement for all of their purchases of a particular product or service.
- Make sure that any negotiations necessary to carry out the arrangement are conducted by

an independent third party who is not an employee of any of the physicians.

- Communications between the third party and each individual physician are kept confidential and not shared with the others.

Mergers, Acquisitions, or Joint Ventures That Tend To Lessen Competition or Create Monopolies

Even where the physicians in a joint venture integrate their practices enough to satisfy *the DOJ/FTC Statements*, they may still have antitrust problems by virtue of their sheer size. The legal question is whether this would appear to be a restraint of trade, monopolization, or an attempt to monopolize. The enforcement agencies and the courts generally use the rule of reason to analyze the anticompetitive effects of the venture on the basis of its history, stated purpose, market power, and market behavior.

Activities that typically constitute a "restraint of trade" follow.

- straight price fixing
- collusion intended to establish minimum or maximum prices, create pressure to increase prices, stabilize prices, interfere with a competitor's freedom to change prices independently, or establish uniform terms of sale, discount policies, or other price-related factors
- agreements not to advertise prices at all
- allocation or division of markets among actual or potential competitors
- concerted refusals to deal or full-blown boycotts
- denial of hospital staff privileges
- restrictive membership requirements in or expulsion from an organization in which membership is economically desirable
- ethical code prohibitions or other restrictions limiting the scope of medical practice
- denial of accreditation or certification
- denial of insurance

The offense of monopolization requires (a) the possession of monopoly or market power—that is, the power to control market prices or to exclude competition and (b) the willful acquisition or retention of that power—as distinguished from natural development of the power through a superior product, business savvy, or good luck.

Monopoly power is measured by reference to the relevant product and geographic markets. The definition of the relevant product market is based on concepts such as "reasonable interchangeability," "cross-elasticity of demand," and "cross-elasticity of supply." The relevant geographic market is based on a court's definition of the area in which sellers of a particular product or service operate and to where customers go to acquire that product or service.

As a general rule, 70 to 90 percent of the market is enough to constitute monopoly power; a two-thirds market share is probably just on the borderline; and anything below 50 percent is usually quite safe. Market share is the most obvious, but not the only, indicator of monopoly or market power. Other factors that may have a bearing follow.

- maintaining market share with an inferior product or service
- technological superiority resulting in cost advantages, price leadership, and substantial economies of scale
- relative size of the competitors
- competitors' performance
- barriers to entry or expansion
- pricing trends and practices
- homogeneity of products
- potential competition
- stability of market shares over time

The existence of monopoly or market power by itself is not illegal. The power must be exercised through anticompetitive, predatory, or unreasonably exclusionary behavior. The restraint of trade activities listed above are examples of such behavior.

"Attempted monopolization" involves anticompetitive behavior carried on by a firm that has less than monopoly power in a relevant market.

Monopolization is such an important issue that the *DOJ/FTC Statements* "safety zone" requirements include a maximum 20 percent of physicians (by specialty) in an exclusive joint venture and 30 percent in a nonexclusive one. The agencies, however, have been willing to approve arrangements that exceed those maximums when it can be shown that a large, nonexclusive physician group does not have sufficient market power (despite its size) or that it will not be able to exercise the power it has.

There are two strategies that a large physician-run organization might follow to best protect itself from antitrust enforcement scrutiny. The first is to forget entirely about financial risk sharing and do business with third party payers solely on the basis of the messenger model. It's awkward, but it is very safe. Alternatively, the physicians could form what was called a *qualified managed care plan* by the DOJ in the consent decree it executed with a PHO in 1996. In such a plan, physicians are included as risk-sharing members up to the 20 percent (exclusive) or 30 percent (nonexclusive) limits. Then the plan may contract with additional physicians, as long as it accepts "significant financial risk for the payments to and the utilization practices of the subcontracting physicians" and did not "compensate those subcontracting physicians in a manner that substantially replicates membership or ownership in the organization."[9] Under either strategy, the organization will be better off if it accepts physicians on a nonexclusive basis, allowing them to join other organizations at the same time if they wish.

Of course, the bulletproof safest course of action is to keep the number of physicians under the maximums set forth in the *DOJ/FTC Statements.*

Collective Efforts by Competing Physicians To Resist MCO Cost Control Efforts

Individual physicians can do almost anything they want to fight the efforts of an MCO to control costs through interventions in their clinical decision making. They may refuse to renew their contracts with the MCO. They may appeal or challenge the utilization management decisions. They may perform the procedure, prescribe the medication, or make the referral, despite the MCO's denial of reimbursement. Of course, the physician or the patient will probably end up paying for it.

A group of physicians can resist an MCO in most of the same ways, as long as they are gathered into a single entity that meets the integration criteria of the *DOJ/FTC Statements*.

A group of physicians in separate private practices, with no integration links among them, may jointly engage in political action to limit the authority of MCOs to influence their practice behavior. This kind of action is described in the section below on "Jointly Lobbying for Legislation To Prevent MCO Abuses or Empower Physicians."

Attempts by a group of separate, unintegrated physicians to coordinate their business decisions, their market actions, and, in particular, their dealings with MCOs with the intention of forcing the MCOs to halt their efforts to invade physician clinical autonomy are not permissible.

Selection of Physicians To Participate in Alternative Delivery Systems at the Exclusion of Other Physicians

This is a tough issue for physicians. To be efficient and successful under managed care, even physician-run organizations must accept only those physicians who can deliver cost-effective, high-quality care. On the other hand, the physicians excluded are not too happy about such selective policies. Some have even brought lawsuits challenging the decisions to exclude them.

As a general rule, fair and objective policies for choosing and retaining as organization members only those physicians able to satisfy legitimate business-related criteria are acceptable in the law. For years, hospitals have been free to enter into exclusive contracts with physician groups to staff hospital-based specialties such as radiology, pathology, and anesthesiology. In many jurisdic-

tions, this authority has been expanded to include what is often called *economic credentialing*.

It now is rather well established that MCOs, and almost certainly other provider organizations, have a legal right to select, deselect, or retain physicians on the basis of practice efficiency and economic criteria. Some organizations further protect themselves by giving no reason to a physician when they reject or deselect him. This generally is not a good idea. In the absence of a given reason, the physician's imagination can run wild. He and his attorney may suspect motives that violate the antitrust or employment discrimination laws and may challenge the decision in court.

The best course of action is to do the following:

1. Tell physicians in advance that they will be evaluated on the basis of the economic efficiency of their practice methods and what exact criteria will be used.
2. Tell them that their performance will be regularly measured and how that will be done.
3. When a physician first begins to show signs of poor efficiency, call the matter to his attention.
4. If the problem persists, counsel him with increasing intensity, offering appropriate continuing medical education opportunities and mutually setting improvement goals.
5. If the physician is unable to improve sufficiently, dismiss him from the organization.
6. If a committee is involved in making the dismissal decision, make sure that no direct competitors of the physician participate.
7. Tell him the exact reasons for the dismissal.
8. Have the necessary documentation to back up those reasons.
9. Offer at least two levels of appeal procedure, equivalent in scope to traditional due process procedures.
10. Make sure that no direct competitors of the physician are involved in the appeal process.

11. Avoid using a no-cause termination clause as the authority for dismissing a physician.

SPECIAL CASE: "ANY WILLING PROVIDER" LAWS, NOT A PANACEA

Under some pressure from physicians who have been rejected or deselected by MCOs, at least half of the states have enacted what are called *any willing provider laws*. In their simplest form, these laws state that any physician willing to comply with a fee schedule and other requirements of an MCO has a legal right to join its provider panel. In practice, they are not as useful to physicians as they might seem.

In the first place, many of the laws apply only to certain nonphysician providers, such as pharmacists. They also usually are directed primarily at MCOs and may not be binding on physician organizations or integrated systems. Where physicians are covered, the statutory language typically requires that an MCO have an annual period during which all physicians can apply to join its panel and use explicit selection criteria in judging those applications. Those criteria may include economic or utilization standards, and a physician who cannot satisfy them will not make it onto the panel.

To minimize the legal risk in selecting and deselecting physician participants or members, follow these guidelines:

- Define and publish specific, business-related criteria for selection and deselection.
- Do include criteria for poor performance, failure to meet organization requirements, or inability to meet the needs of patients, payers, or fellow physicians.
- Develop the criteria with the input of other physicians in the organization.
- Define and publicize a due process procedure for appealing selection or deselection decisions.
- Encourage fellow physicians to participate in the appeals procedure or to attend the hearings.

Physician Membership in Professional Associations That Address Matters of Common Concern

Physicians already engage in this kind of activity through their membership in national, state, and local medical societies. Through these organizations, physicians may speak with one voice on virtually any issue that affects their professional lives. They may complain about the contract terms or capitation rates offered them by MCOs. The associations may survey their members' views on managed care and publish the results. They may highlight the worst abuses of MCOs and propose corrective measures. Those measures may include new legislation for which the associations and their members actively lobby. An association may form a political action committee to lend support to physician-friendly candidates for public office.

The association may not be used as a forum for discussing and comparing the competitive strategies of individual physicians. Through their association connections, the physicians may not coordinate their strategies.

Joint Negotiation or Other Collective Action in Dealings with Third-Party Payers

To survive, physicians must contract with MCOs that are much larger than the majority of physician practices. This puts them at a severe disadvantage in the contract negotiations and any other dealings with the MCOs. Collective negotiation is one obvious way to achieve rough parity in dealings with an MCO. Unfortunately, it is quite unlawful. This kind of collaboration on the terms under which competing physicians will offer their services to customers like MCOs is exactly what the antitrust laws were designed to prevent.

Until a group of physicians has achieved the kinds and levels of integration specified by the *DOJ/FTC Statements*, it must refrain from any collective action in dealing with MCOs or other third-party payers.

Jointly Lobbying for Legislation To Prevent MCO Abuses or Empower Physicians

This is a constitutionally protective exercise of the physicians' individual rights to engage in political action. They are free to work together with other parties, including directly competing physicians, to persuade and pressure state and federal legislators to enact just about any kind of law. The physicians may have very selfish motivations for seeking the new legislation. Their ultimate purpose may be to protect their incomes or to tightly restrict MCOs. Their goal may be a more altruistic one of enhancing the physician-patient relationship. These are all acceptable.

Again, what is not acceptable is any attempt by the physicians to share information about their operations or practice strategies, or to plan jointly how they will compete in the marketplace. There is a clear distinction between anticompetitive conspiracies and group lobbying efforts.

SPECIAL CASE: "SHAM NETWORKS"—DON'T TRY TO FOOL THE FEDS

If a physician joint venture or network does not fall within the safety zone of the *DOJ/FTC Statements* and appears to have been organized for the primary purpose of restraining trade, it will not qualify for analysis under the rule of reason. These are often referred as *sham networks*, made to look superficially like an integrated network, but in fact engaged in significant anticompetitive activity. They will be judged under the per se rule.

The following factors are often cited as evidence that a joint venture or network has prohibited, anticompetitive motives:

- statements indicating an anticompetitive purpose
- a recent history of collusion or anticompetitive behavior in the market, including efforts to obstruct the development of managed care
- an obvious anticompetitive structure of the network

- the absence of any mechanism or procedures designed to create new efficiencies or otherwise to increase competition through the network vehicle
- the existence of anticompetitive collateral agreements
- the absence of procedures to prevent anticompetitive spillover effects outside the network

The lesson here is never try to use a joint venture as a false front for what are known to be violations of the antitrust laws.

SPECIAL CASE: THE MESSENGER MODEL, A LEGITIMATE MEANS OF PRICE FIXING

There is one safe way for a group of competing physicians to negotiate prices more or less jointly with a single payer—use the "messenger model." In the most traditional variation of this model, the physicians appoint an independent third party as an intermediary agent between them and the payer. The agent receives from each physician an individual fee schedule proposal and delivers these to the payer or obtains an opening offer from the payer and communicates this to the physicians. The agent takes offers and counteroffers back and forth between the payer and physicians until enough physicians have agreed to the payer's terms to create a large enough panel of physicians. At no time does the agent negotiate with the payer on behalf of the physicians, nor does she share each physician's offers and counteroffers with the other physicians. The messenger is purely a conduit for information. The individual physicians never know or talk to each other about the separate deals they are striking with the payer.

Sometimes, the physicians may give the messenger a range of prices that they will accept and the authority to accept a payer price offer that falls within that range. Any offer not within the range is passed on to the physician for acceptance or rejection. The messenger may not exercise discretion in deciding which payer's offers will go to the physicians.

The messenger may also give the physicians objective information about a payer's offer, such as the meaning of contracts terms and comparison with offers from other payers. The messenger may not recommend accepting the offer or not and may not tell which physicians have or have not accepted.

To facilitate setting their individual prices, the physicians as a group may conduct a survey of the prices charged and costs incurred by the group members. They will avoid antitrust risks if they meet certain requirements. These are explained in the above section, "Physician Participation in Exchanges of Information and Fee Surveys with Competitors."

There are a few variations of this traditional model that give the physicians a little more flexibility in negotiating with a payer without violating the antitrust laws. They are all still pretty ponderous ways of doing business with a customer. The only alternative is for the physicians to further integrate their practices, financially or clinically, along the lines of the *DOJ/FTC Statements*.

To be absolutely safe in implementing the messenger model, do the following:

- Select as messenger a third party, preferably not an employee of any of the involved physicians, and certainly not someone involved in negotiating or making contracting decisions for them.
- Formally adopt guidelines instructing the messenger on how he is to carry the offers back and forth, and prohibiting him from negotiating on behalf of any of the physicians or from sharing information among them.

SPECIAL CASE: PHYSICIAN UNIONS— LEGITIMATE COLLABORATIONS AMONG EMPLOYED PHYSICIANS

The desire of physicians to speak with "one voice" in their dealings with MCOs is natural.

The antitrust prohibitions against their doing that are clear. The response of a small but growing number of physicians to this impasse is to organize themselves into labor unions.

Of the 700,000 practicing physicians in the United States, there currently are about 30,000 physicians (primarily residents, interns, and physicians employed by hospitals and MCOs) who are members of eight physician unions. There is vigorous organizing activity, as well as legal action, going on in the states of California, Florida, and New Jersey.

Most of the current barriers to the formation of physician unions are legal. The antitrust laws prohibit competitors in any industry, including health care, from talking together about the terms under which they will sell their services to customers. In this case, the "customers" the physicians are most concerned with are MCOs. There is an exception to the antitrust laws for employees of a single organization. Because they are employees of one entity, they are presumably working toward a single goal and are no longer considered to be in competition. They are free to discuss with their employer their wages and other conditions of employment. To do that in a more systematic way, the employees may attempt to form a labor union.

There are three reasons why not every physician in the country can expect to immediately become a member of physician-focused collective bargaining unit:

1. A person doing work for an organization generally either contracts independently with the organization or is employed by the organization. Only employees are permitted by the labor laws to form unions. Independent contractors may not, and their attempts to bargain collectively will run afoul of the antitrust laws. In fact, the majority of unionized doctors are employees, usually of hospitals, but also of MCOs in a few cases.

The key question, therefore, is whether a particular physician qualifies as an employee. It should not be hard; nearly 50 percent of all physicians in the United States are now employed by a separate entity. The problem is that most of the physicians interested in the possibility of union membership do not meet the strict definition of *employee*. They are primarily physicians in independent practice (solo or small groups) who feel at a disadvantage when negotiating a contract with an MCO and when the MCO subsequently tries to intervene in their clinical decision making.

There are two ways around this problem. Some physicians are arguing, in legal actions they have brought, that the degree of control exercised by the MCOs over the way doctors do their work is so extensive that they constitute de facto employees.[*] They claim that they are already employees under existing law. Other physicians and the American Medical Association (AMA) have proposed changes in the current laws, primarily antitrust and labor laws, to ensure that even physicians who do not meet the employee criteria would be able to bargain collectively.

2. Not all qualified employees are permitted to form unions to bargain collectively. Those employees engaged in policy making for the employer—that is, supervisors, managers, and executives—may not become union members. Logically, they are the employers. The key is deciding where the line gets drawn on the organizational chart between the members of management and the rank-and-file employees. Several health care organizations have

---

*The leading criteria for determining who is and is not an employee are those issued by the Internal Revenue Service (IRS). It is concerned primarily with the degree of control exercised by the employer over the time, location, and methods of the employee's performance of his work. These physicians argue that MCOs exercise so much control over the way they practice medicine that they should be considered employees and should enjoy the rights of employees.

claimed that, even where physicians might be considered employees, they have policy-making authority that prevents them from organizing a labor union.

3. Even where it could be established that certain physicians are indeed nonmanagement employees, it is a long, twisting path to organizing a union that is certified by the National Labor Relations Board (NLRB) and recognized by the employer. Some of the hurdles to be overcome: definition of the appropriate bargaining unit, collection of "expression of interest" cards from 30 percent of those in the bargaining unit, conduct of the election campaign with vigorous opposition from management, likely appeals of the election results, and adversarial negotiation of a contract between the union and management.

In a worst case scenario, if the physicians are unable to negotiate the contract terms they want, the traditional union response would be to withhold their services from the employer—that is, to go out on strike. It is an open question whether unionized physicians would be willing to take such an extreme step and, if they did, what the reaction of the public might be.

There is a somewhat less effective variation of the traditional labor union being considered by some physicians. It sometimes is referred to as a *guild*. Physicians come together to discuss only those issues that they are not prohibited from discussing by the antitrust laws. They are limited to talking about lobbying and nonfinancial matters, such as the hours a physician must work or the number of patients she must see. This is, in effect, the role that medical societies at the state and national levels have been serving for many years.

Physician Union Resources

Federation of Physicians and Dentists
Based in Tallahassee, Florida
Has been in existence for 12 years
Has 8,000 members in eight states

Committee of Interns and Residents

Has 9,000 members in six states and the District of Columbia

Recently affiliated with the Service Employees International Union (SEIU), the nation's largest health care union

First National Guild for Providers of the Lower Extremities

Represents podiatrists on the East Coast

Affiliated with the AFL-CIO's Office Professional Employees International Union

Union of American Physicians and Dentists

Based in Oakland, California

Has approximately 3,000 members

Doctors' Council of New York

Represents 3,500 attending physicians, dentists, podiatrists, and veterinarians employed by New York City agencies, hospitals, and clinics

Largest union of attending physicians

REFERENCES

1. "Department of Justice and Federal Trade Commission Statements of Antitrust Enforcement Policy in Health Care," Statement 8, Section B, Subsection 1, reprinted in *Health Law Reporter 5* (Washington, DC: Bureau of National Affairs, 1996).

2. "Department of Justice and Federal Trade Commission Statements of Antitrust Enforcement Policy in Health Care," *Health Law Reporter 5*.

3. "Department of Justice and Federal Trade Commission Statements of Antitrust Enforcement Policy in Health Care," *Health Law Reporter 5*, 1309.

4. 42 U.S.C. § 1320a-7b (1988 & Supp. IV 1992).

5. 42 U.S.C. § 1395nn (1993).

6. 42 C.F.R. 1001.95 et seq. (1991).

7. 42 U.S.C.A. § 11101 (1986).

8. 42 U.S.C.S. § 11151(9) (1986).

9. *United States v. HealthCare Partners*, 1996-1 Trade Cas. (CCH) P71,337 (D. Conn. 1996).

RESOURCE LIST

"Good News for Physicians: FTC and DOJ Revise Antitrust Guidelines for Networks," *Healthcare Business & Legal Strategies 5*, no. 22 (1996).

"Government Agencies Soften Stance on What Constitutes Price Fixing," *Healthcare Financial Management*, February 1997.

D. Mangan, "Will Doctor Unions Finally Take Hold?" *Medical Economics 72*, no. 14 (1995): 115.

H. Meyer, "Physicians, Look for the Union Label," *Hospitals 70*, no. 23 (1996): 69.

M. Todd, *IPA, PHO and MSO Development Strategies—Building Successful Provider Alliances*, (Westchester, IL: Healthcare Financial Management Association, 1997).

D. Van Duch, "Employed Physicians Unionizing—Price-Fix Risks," *The National Law Journal*, 21 July, 1997, A1.

D. Vavala, "Fighting Fire with Fire: Physicians Blazing New Paths to Autonomy," *Physician Executive 21*, no. 4 (1995): 3.

T. Vranjes, "Groups Debate Ethical Issues of Physician Unionization," *Medical Industry Today*, 29 January, 1998.

L. Williams, "Structuring Managed Care Joint Ventures," *Healthcare Financial Management 25*, no. 8 (1995): 32.

CHAPTER 29

Common Causes of Failure in Integrating Physician Organizations

INTRODUCTION

Roughly 19 of 20 new businesses fail within the first five years of their existence. The same few reasons for failure are repeated again and again by the founders of these businesses. They seem unable to learn from the mistakes of their predecessors.

The shift to managed care in the United States has been in progress for over 10, nearly 20 years. As managed care organizations (MCOs) have developed and spread, providers of all kinds (including physicians) have tried to form organizations in response. Some have prospered; some have failed. These organizations have been studied in considerable detail, often being written up in case studies. There is a long enough documented history of the development of provider organizations to begin to draw conclusions on why they have succeeded and failed.

This chapter looks at the most common reasons why physician organizations run into operating problems and sometimes fail completely. It also makes a few suggestions for avoiding those mistakes.

WHO SHOULD READ THIS CHAPTER

Any physician with ambitions to respond aggressively to MCOs by joining in the creation of a physician-run entity, as recommended by this book, would do well to anticipate the potential reasons for failure. Following the ideas in this chapter will not guarantee success of a physician venture. Avoiding the pitfalls noted here will minimize the chances of failure.

Certainly, if a physician has focused on a particular strategy involving the formation of one of the physician organization models, it is time to think seriously about a detailed implementation plan. The plan should take into account the problems that others have encountered in similar ventures. This chapter describes those problems and suggests ways around them.

If, after reading most of this book, a physician decides to accept employment with a larger group or provider organization, if he chooses not to get involved in the creation of a new organization, or if he simply decides to retire from the practice of medicine, the material in this chapter may seem irrelevant. In such cases, it probably can be skipped.

COMMON MISTAKES AND CAUSES FOR FAILURE IN THE FORMATION OF PROVIDER ORGANIZATIONS

Physician Discomfort with Investing in the Organization where They Practice

Some physicians have difficulty making a personal investment in a physician-run organization—and certainly in other kinds of organizations with which they may be affiliated. Physicians coming out of solo or small group practices usually have no history of investing for the long term—and little appreciation of the need to do it. They have never had to do it before. Yet, the new entity will not get very far without adequate start-up and growth capital.

A careful balance must be struck between the financial needs of the organization and the financial demands made on the physicians, particularly at the outset and during the early years. Well-researched financial projections should be made for the first three years of operation. Remember that these capital needs estimates are almost always too conservative. Draw on any other capital sources that may be available (hospital, venture capitalist, loans) without giving away too much control.

Eventually, however, it will be necessary to turn to the initial physician participants for significant capital contributions (whether in the form of stock purchases, member assessments, or annual dues). This will be a good thing, as a test of the physicians' commitment to the organization. It also will help bind them to the group and align its goals with theirs. Be prepared to reveal the research and projections behind the calculations of the contributions. Also, to the extent possible, keep the initial capital assessments as low as possible to avoid alienating too many potential participants.

Lack of Physician Experience in Accumulating Retained Earnings

In addition to the capital contribution problem, physicians historically have not needed to accumulate retained earnings in a corporate entity for reinvestment in the entity to support its growth. The common wisdom is that physicians in private practice take home whatever is left over after paying expenses. That will not work in a large, growing organization with a constant need to acquire new systems and capabilities.

Retained earnings are a major source of growth capital, though not the only one. Member physicians must understand this from the beginning.

They must be prepared to see net year-end income kept in the business for future investment.

Disagreements over Distribution of Organization Income

Income distribution programs can easily be a source of tension in physician organizations. If not handled carefully, they can disrupt the smooth functioning of the organization. This is especially true where primary care and specialist physicians are coming together in a single organization for the first time. Apart from whatever prejudices they may have toward each other, they are likely to be sensitive to how their respective salaries are determined by the organization. The primary care physicians (PCPs) are likely to focus on their new elevated roles in the health care delivery continuum and expect appropriately high compensation. The specialists may be focused on how much they could be making in solo practice (if they could still be in solo practice) and will resent any hint that they are subsidizing their primary care colleagues.

In time, this will sort itself out as everybody comes to realize that they all are better off when they work for the welfare of the entire organization. Until then, it probably will be necessary to pay the PCPs somewhat more than they were earning privately. However, those increases should not be funded by decreases in the pay of specialist physicians. Over the first few years, it probably makes sense for primary care compensation to grow faster than specialist compensation.

Selectivity or Lack of Selectivity in Accepting and Retaining Physicians in the Organization

The need, initially or eventually, to become more selective about which physicians will be permitted to participate in the organization often creates political and interpersonal stress. This selectivity can take different forms.

- The organization focuses on those physicians most likely to practice cost-effective quality medicine.
- Physician selection aims for a specialty mix appropriate to the population served.
- Customers and competitive forces may require board certification as a prerequisite for physician participation.

The hard facts are that the organization must become selective at some point or it will fail. The cost of its services will be too high and their quality will be too low. The only real question is whether the organization chooses its physician-members very selectively when it is first formed or waits until a year or two later to cull the physician panel.

If the organization admits every interested physician, it may alienate those high-performing doctors more committed to managed care. It will also be less attractive as a contract partner to MCOs. When the crunch does come and some physicians must be let go, the repercussions may be even more painful.

If the organization takes only those physicians with a record of delivering "value" medicine and an openness to change, it will immediately antagonize those who are left out. All in all, it is probably easier to deal with the upset physicians at the beginning, put that issue in the past, and get on with creating a lean, efficient delivery organization.

Failure To Follow a Systematic, Step-by-Step Approach in Creating the New Organization

Physicians who have never created an entity as complex as an integrated, multispecialty, multi-provider delivery organization may not appreciate the need to carry out formative tasks and functions in a rational sequence. For instance, they may try to negotiate groupwide managed care contracts before the group has been recruited and may find themselves committed to provide a volume of services without enough physicians to do it. They may try to begin operations before

necessary licensing has been secured, make monetary commitments to vendors before their own capital financing has been ensured, or start discussing a common fee schedule before their practices have been truly integrated. Taking any of these steps out of order can create life-threatening problems for the organization.

As soon as there is tentative commitment to proceed with forming the new entity, a fairly detailed stepwise plan and timetable should be prepared. Make clear to the participants that the schedule must be followed closely. Warn against any improvised deviations and place a single individual in charge of monitoring the progress in implementation.

Underestimates of Time, Money, and Energy Required To Create the New Organization

It is quite common for founding physicians to underestimate the time, energy, and initial capital required to get a new, complex organization off the ground and running smoothly and profitably—with the result that it collapses before it truly enters the marketplace. Starting any new business is a daunting task—doubly so in the current health care marketplace. It is not surprising when a modest group of physicians finds that it does not have the time and energy, after maintaining their existing medical practices, to simultaneously work on creating a new, even larger entity.

The work must be done. The doctors have two choices. They can take time away from their practices and their families to carry it out themselves or they can take money out of their own pockets to hire consultants to perform most of the necessary tasks. In the latter case, they still cannot delegate a lot of the key decision making and legal governance issues.

Underestimates of the Documentation and Other Procedures Required To Bring a New Physician into the Organization

Founding physicians may also underestimate the documentation required before a recruited physician can become an active practicing member of the group. Applications must be gathered, a multitude of credentialing data must be obtained and reports prepared, further background checks must be carried out, numerous interviews must be conducted, professional services or provider participation agreements must be negotiated and signed, and asset purchase agreements (if the physician's practice is being acquired), partnership agreements (if a partnership is being formed), or capital stock purchase agreements (if a stock corporation is being formed) must be prepared. Until all these prerequisites have been completed, a physician is not truly a member and cannot begin providing care.

Failure To Dedicate Enough Time to Recruiting New Physician Members

The foundation of any new delivery entity, particularly a physician-run organization, is its physician panel. As far as prospective payers are concerned, it does not exist until a physician panel with the right number and specialty mix has been assembled. The founding physicians may have trouble finding time to personally undertake the necessary physician recruitment. Though other nonphysicians can develop the lists of the best candidates, only the original physicians themselves will be able to persuade others to join. Until a critical mass of physicians has been brought on board, the organization is a nonstarter. Time must be allocated to accomplish that.

Time Demands on Physicians To Govern and Manage the New Organization

Many physicians founding or joining a complex physician organization may not be prepared for the substantial ongoing time commitments necessary for them to manage or oversee the management of the organization—the time required to build consensus, cultivate a suitable culture, deal with unanticipated problems (large and small), review the decisions of others, conduct strategic planning, and many similar tasks will seem endless. This is what it means to have an organization run by physicians. If they cannot find the time, critical decisions will end up being made by nonphysicians or not being made at all.

Reluctance To Hire Necessary Top Management and To Pay Them Appropriately

All but the most superficial physician organizations will need, very early on, to employ professional, paid top management. The first position to be filled is the medical director and, quite soon thereafter, a general manager or chief executive officer (CEO) (who may also be a physician). The medical director may be part time at first, but he must be compensated for his efforts. Surprisingly, many physicians are reluctant to pay one of their colleagues to be a medical director or to pay someone else to be a general manager—these may seem to them to be positions that they filled easily, without additional pay, in their previous small group practices. In a much larger organization, these are essential, full-time jobs. If the group stints on pay, it will see the effects in the way the organization is managed.

Inadequate Initial Capital To Sustain the Organization until It Reaches a Break-Even Point

One of the primary reasons that new businesses fail is insufficient initial capital to get the entity started and to keep it operating until it can thrive on its own. The new physician organization must start off with enough capital to form the organization and to sustain it until operating processes have been smoothed out, patient volume and revenues have picked up to an acceptable level, the entity has established itself in the marketplace, and a profit is being earned.

There are two steps to making sure there is enough start-up capital. Working with consultants experienced in creating physician organizations such as the one planned, prepare three- to five-year projections of financial needs. Do not rely on a template from another organization. The projections should be based on the current organization, with all its unique features, competing in its unique marketplace. Err on the side of projecting too high rather than too low. The common wisdom is to make the projections, then to double them.

The really hard part is attracting the capital called for in the projections. The very first money will come from the physicians who are the catalysts for the new organization. They will be the primary capital source for the first year or two. One possible alternative is to involve a hospital from the outset, perhaps in forming a physician-hospital organization (PHO). However, that means giving away some control of the entity and accommodating some of the hospital's wishes. Eventually, as the organization builds up an operating track record, it will attract the interest of other capital sources, such as banks, venture capitalists, and the stock market.

Basing of the New Organization's Business Plan on Unrealistic Projections

The only thing worse than no financial projections is inaccurate projections. One of the causes of undercapitalization is often overly optimistic projections about revenues, income, and cash flow. They may lead to a variety of other miscalculations that can limit the organization's success: insufficient or excessive personnel, equipment, and space to meet the demand for the organization's services. The organization can be sent off in all the wrong strategic directions. Its operations could be based on a wholly unrealistic business plan.

The environmental assessment discussed in Chapter 14, "Assessing the Market for Managed Care and Integration Opportunities," is an essential precursor to sound projections. Unless they have prior experience, the physicians should contract the projection work out to expert consultants in the field.

Inability to Cope with Sudden, Dramatic Growth in Revenues and Organization Size

It seems silly to worry about too much success. However, sometimes, a provider organization can enter a period of very rapid growth in patient demand and revenues that so outstrips its capabilities that service quality suffers. Attempts to compensate in the short term increase expenses dramatically. Patient and payer disappointment may lead to cancellation of contracts. Organizations can fail under these circumstances.

There are a few ways to protect against this outcome. Whether at the creation of the organization or later, when a new facility is being opened or a new product being marketed, make the best possible projections. It is probably better to have an excess in capacity than a shortfall. Have contingency plans in place to respond to sudden increases in demand—contract for beds, facilities, and providers to be available on an "as-needed" basis. When entering into new contracts with MCOs, ask to see estimates of the demand for your group's services. Negotiate a clause permitting the group to turn away enrollees when it has reached the limits of its capacity.

Organization Management That Is Stretched beyond Its Size or Competence

Any number of situations can stretch an organization's management beyond its competence level: sudden growth or just sheer size of the operation, operational system requirements for which the management has no experience (such as implementing a sophisticated financial/clinical information system, managing provider utilization, or instituting a quality assurance program), dealing with interpersonal problems with dissatisfied physicians, or negotiating with high-powered MCO executives. These kinds of problems can develop when a group stints on the caliber of management that it hires in the first place. If the physicians try to cut corners and save money by hiring a glorified bookkeeper as administrator of their group, they are likely to pay the price when serious challenges arise.

A good rule of thumb is to base the caliber of management hired on the organization's needs two or three years down the road. That kind of executive will help move the organization into a more prosperous future. If the organization hires its managers only for its current position, that is where it will stay.

Failure To Calculate Accurately the Costs of Performing under Managed Care Contracts

When an MCO proposes a discounted fee schedule or a capitation rate to a provider group, it is essential that the group knows whether those payments will cover its costs of providing the required services. Too many groups sign managed care contracts without carefully checking the promised payments against their costs of doing business, and sometimes that is because they do not have a clear fix on what those costs are. Their accounting systems cannot provide the necessary data in the necessary formats. The result is that the group may start losing money the minute it enters into the contract.

A variation of this problem is the failure to keep track of "incurred but not reported" (IBNR) expenses. These are the costs of services that have been delivered but not reported or billed for yet. If they are never properly reported, the group will have to bear the expense. If there is no provision for reporting such expenses after a contract has expired, the group will have to absorb them.

A modern provider organization cannot function without a sophisticated, computerized cost accounting and management system. This is an expensive necessity. Ideally, it also will interface with a clinical reporting system. When the systems are operational, be sure to use the data they generate to inform tasks such as contract analysis and negotiation.

Failure To Use Sound Underwriting Criteria when Assuming Financial Risk

Most groups welcome the opportunity to share risk in order to reap the savings if they can deliver medical services efficiently. However, some forget that there is risk involved in "risk sharing." The wise organization conducts a prior actuarial analysis of the population it will be serving to determine its likely service needs. It calculates its cost of meeting those needs, as well as the likelihood of the needs and costs being catastrophically higher. It balances that against the payments it will receive from the MCO and—most important for risk purposes—makes sure that it has adequate reserves or stop-loss insurance to cover any catastrophic expenses. This is the process of "underwriting" the risk.

Failure To Track Medical Costs and Utilization Accurately

It is almost suicidal to proceed very far into managed care—by letting such contracts become a significant part of revenues—without establishing the systems and procedures for managing care. The most essential of these is the ability to track and manage the utilization of resources and the resulting costs. It requires investment in computer hardware and software, proprietary control systems, personnel, and training to accomplish this. It also requires that the primary users of resources—physicians—be willing to adjust their behavior according to the data generated by these systems. Without a tight rein on costs, the organization will quickly become noncompetitive and will fail.

The value of good cost data for contract analysis has already been mentioned. Their importance is ongoing. Be prepared to demonstrate the cost management system to prospective contract partners. Use the system aggressively to discover ways to reduce costs without impairing quality. Communicate the cost data to clinical and non-clinical decision makers with the expectation that it will influence their behavior.

Failure of Management To Grasp the Implications of Reports They Receive

It seems tragic, but some organizations install modern and sophisticated management information systems whose output is not accurately interpreted by management. The best of these systems give comprehensive feedback on resource utilization and quality of care—factors critical to a group's success. If these reports are not read properly and if appropriate corrective action is not taken, serious financial complications and patient or payer dissatisfaction can result. The required action could range from counseling a physician who is an excessive utilizer to renegotiating a managed care contract with an unrealistic fee schedule or capitation rate.

Failure To Educate and To Continue Educating Providers

It seems an unavoidable fact that physicians must alter significantly both their attitudes and their practice patterns to succeed at managed care. It is difficult for them to do this on their own. The environment of an integrated system provides encouragement and resources to support them in this undertaking. The education must be broad based, covering many aspects of medical practice, including working in multidisciplinary teams, responding to performance data and organizational requirements, utilizing resources efficiently, maintaining quality of care, satisfying patients, and practicing under clinical protocols or guidelines. The education must be continuous, upgrading every physician's skills and behaviors as new techniques, technology, and competition warrant. If this physician education does not occur or lags behind the competition, the organization risks dissatisfying its customers—patients and payers—and losing its business.

Failure To Deal with Difficult or Uncooperative Providers

New physician organizations forming today include many members who entered the medical profession well before managed care came on the scene and have bitter feelings about it. Most are able to adjust their attitudes, and eventually their habits, well enough to be a contributing member of the organization. A very few hold on to their resentment and may become a disruptive force within the group. A few other physicians may simply be unable or unwilling to work cooperatively in a team or group. If their behavior is tolerated for political or social reasons, it can seriously impede group efforts to plan and implement the new venture. It can damage the morale of other physicians who must work with them. Prompt action must be taken to change their actions or to remove them from the organization.

Use of the New Organization To Resist Managed Care and MCOs

The purpose of forming a physician-run delivery organization is to succeed in an industry that has come to be dominated by managed care. To use the organization to fight against managed care is, at the least, a bit like tilting at windmills. At the worst, it can lead the participating physicians to violations of federal and state antitrust laws. Along the way, a lot of valuable time and resources will be wasted.

The health care delivery world has changed; there is no turning back. By creating successful physician-run entities, doctors have a chance to maintain influential roles in that new world, at least on a par with the hospitals, MCOs, and employers.

It is not necessary to like everything about managed care. There are plenty of things to dislike about it. If a group of physicians feels strongly enough, it may elect to support a lobbying effort to enact remedial laws. However, it is not worth dedicating the organization through which the physicians earn their livelihoods to defeating their primary customers.

Unwillingness or Inability To "Embrace" New Concepts in Health Care Delivery

In fact, a physician organization will do much better in the marketplace if its members can come to terms with the principles of managed care. It will do even better if they can work enthusiastically to implement these principles to their own advantage.

When originally conceived, utilization management seemed like an intrusion by nonphysicians on physician clinical autonomy. With the advent of capitated arrangements, physicians are in control of the utilization management levers.

They are in a position to neatly balance quality and cost while reaping the savings if they can do it efficiently. Other managed care concepts—such as quality assurance, clinical outcomes studies, practice guidelines, and patient satisfaction surveys—should have similar appeals to forward-looking physicians.

It is not enough to enter grudgingly into managed care contracts. MCOs are looking for strategic partners who appreciate the need to work constantly to satisfy the demands of the ultimate payers—employers and government funding agencies. This means not only becoming highly proficient at current care management mechanisms, but also adapting quickly to new techniques as they are developed.

Failure To Appreciate the Need To Gather and Use Comprehensive Financial/Clinical Information

Many of these potential strategic errors revolve around the misuse, failure to use, or failure to collect information about the organization's operations. The availability, analysis, interpretation, dissemination, and application of data on clinical and financial operations will be the backbone of an effective provider organization. Eventually, we will have the ability to subtly integrate clinical, financial, and other data types to make real-time adjustments in the way an organization delivers health care. Physicians seeking success must be willing to understand and must allow themselves to be influenced by these data.

Failure To Align the Goals of All Participating Providers

Consider the conflicts among providers under separate contracts with an MCO. The hospital wants to fill beds. The specialist physicians want a sufficient flow of referrals to maintain their income levels. The PCPs will do best by minimizing hospital admissions and specialist referrals. If these various providers bring these goals along when they combine themselves into a single organization, their cost profile will prevent them from winning a single managed care contract.

One of the first priorities of an integrating organization is finding ways to align the objectives of its disparate elements. The two primary tools for accomplishing this are the organization's selection criteria and its compensation formulas. It will help considerably if each provider joining the organization acknowledges that its traditional motivations are no longer valid and must be shifted. The recruitment and screening procedure should filter the best people in and out of the organization.

Money continues to be a powerful motivator. The compensation/reimbursement schemes used with different providers can very effectively steer their practice behavior in the desired direction. The alternatives are almost endless—fee for service, discounted fee for service, capitation, sub-capitation, specialty capitation, global capitation, case rates, diagnosis-related groups (DRGs), salaries, risk withholds, risk pools, other forms of risk sharing, profit sharing, monetary incentives, and bonuses. Careful design and combination of these mechanisms can go a long way toward producing the desired effects.

The ultimate aim is to persuade every provider affiliated with the organization that he, she, or it will be best served in the long run by working collectively for the benefit of the entire organization, rather than individually for each provider.

Spending of Money (Limited Capital Resources) Unnecessarily and Unwisely

There are a million ways to spend limited dollars in running a business, and it is easy to make misjudgments in those decisions. There is general agreement that certain kinds of capital expenditures should be avoided by most integrating organizations.

- Do not invest in "bricks-and-mortar" projects. Do not build a hospital or hospital expansion under any circumstances. Consider building a clinic or primary care facility that helps make the organization accessible to more patients in new market areas.

- Do not spend large sums in purchasing physician practices. Join them to the organization through contractual affiliations. If there is a desire to bind the physicians more closely to the organization, create a separate management services organization (MSO) under the organization's control. Let the MSO acquire physician practices in exchange for small amounts of cash and large amounts of MSO stock. Allow hospitals or venture capitalists to finance the MSO. Work ultimately toward a public offering of the MSO's stock.

- Avoid direct ownership of provider entities or other components of an integrating system if the same ends can be achieved through contractual links. Aim to create a "virtual" integrated system rather than an "owned" integrated system. Ownership usually entails greater expense.

Creation of an Organization Not Suited to the Local Market

Sometimes, physicians may decide to create a new type of delivery entity because they read about it in *Medical Economics* magazine, have colleagues in another city who have done it, or are being pressured by a local hospital. These are not good reasons to form any sort of organization. The magazine article is probably describing a physician group in a completely different part of the country. The colleagues are clearly operating in another market area. The local hospital may or may not have looked carefully at the local market area before generating its proposal.

Creating a new delivery organization is a major undertaking upon which many people will base their livelihoods. It must be the right kind of organization, at the right time, for the current marketplace. The decision to proceed should be based on a thorough analysis of the market's needs and demands, the current resources for meeting them, and the strategic intentions of other providers.

Creation of an Organization or Product That Fails To Take into Account Existing Relationships

A classic example of this mistake is the decision by an integrated delivery system (IDS) to create and market a managed care product that so upsets the system's existing payers that they refuse to renew their contracts with the system. Another example is when a hospital thoughtlessly forms a PHO with a subset of its medical staff, provoking the other physicians to split off and form their own competing multispecialty group practice.

Good strategic plans are aimed at anticipating how the competition will react to new initiatives. They also should take into account the impact of those plans on other of the organization's stakeholders. They will have reactions, too, which may be just as counterproductive for the organization.

Failure To Recognize the Difference between Simple Contractual Relationships and Strategic Partnerships

The hot item in the transformation of the health care industry is "strategic partnership." This is an affiliation between independent organizations meant to bind the organizations, endure for years, and serve strategic rather than operational purposes. Buying or merging with another entity is not forming a strategic partnership. That is outright ownership, with one entity now controlling the other.

On the other hand, although the legal links among strategic partners are usually contractual, it is a mistake to believe that whenever a contract is signed, a strategic partnership has been formed. All businesses have a multitude of contractual relationships. Only a small fraction of them carry strategic weight.

A strategic partnership implies substantial common interests between two organizations that they choose to explore together. The relationship usually involves more frequent communication among more personnel in the two organizations. There is more sharing of information. Preliminary attempts are made to do joint planning. Strategic partnerships are sometimes the precursors to merger or acquisition.

It is popular to say that MCOs want strategic partnerships with their providers, that they want relationships based on trust and common goals. This is probably true for most MCOs. However, do not confuse every managed care contract with a strategic partnership. It will take more work than that.

Continued Belief That a Physician-Manager Can Lead a Large, Complex, Growing Organization in a Competitive Ever-Changing Marketplace while Also Seeing Patients, Teaching Medical Students, and Conducting Research

In other words, running an ambitious physician organization is a full-time job. It requires an experienced business executive, often with formal management training, to lead a provider organization through the maze of other providers, payers, government agencies, financing sources, accreditation bodies, and competitors to success in the modern health care marketplace. This is not a responsibility that can be carried out by a well-intentioned physician using his common sense and working at it part time.

A new model of physician-manager, especially for physician-run organizations, is taking shape. It probably will require further management training after receiving an M.D. and gaining some experience in direct patient care. At some point, as the physician assumes greater and greater levels of managerial responsibility and eventually is offered an executive position demanding his complete attention, he will have to make a "turning point" decision whether to go down the clinical path or the managerial path.

The organization with physician-managers trying to wear several hats at once will suffer in the quality of its leadership, and eventually this will show up in the bottom line.

Failure To Set Priorities among Strategic Initiatives

A good strategic plan will have five to seven long-term objectives. Many organizations, partic-

ularly when they are just forming and beginning operations, can be pursuing many more goals of a strategic nature. In doing this, they must rely on a limited pool of resources—people, money, and time. Quite often, there will not be enough to support all the strategic initiatives properly. It is at this point that the group must be able to look to the priorities among those initiatives and to allocate the resources accordingly. The greatest tragedy is to pursue too many goals at once and, because no one of them gets adequate attention, fail at all of them.

Do have a modest number of specific, measurable strategic objectives. Concentrate on achieving those, and do not casually add others unless you remove some from the original list. From the beginning, set priorities among the objectives. It is fair to begin trying to implement all of the objectives simultaneously. However, eventually, snags will develop and limits will be reached. It will be necessary to pull back on some projects and to focus on those that are most crucial to the organization's mission.

Underestimating the Threat of Retaliation from Competitors

It is wonderful when people with little business experience—which includes a lot of physicians—begin to see the value of adopting specific strategies of competition for asserting their presence in the marketplace. After doing a careful internal and external environment assessment, they formulate a well-reasoned strategic plan that calls for recruiting more physicians, affiliating with a hospital, introducing a managed care product, or building a satellite clinic. These are perfect competitive moves for the current state of the market. If the market had stayed as it was, the group likely would be in a much more dominant position. The problem is that the market does not stand still.

When competitors become aware of an organization's new strategic moves, even mild ones, their impulse will be to respond and retaliate. They will adopt counter moves of their own. The organization should anticipate all possible market responses when it puts together its original strategic plan. It should prepare countermoves to the competition's countermoves. Still, there will be surprises that cannot be anticipated. Who could have guessed that a certain large group practice would sell out en masse to Phycor (a leading physician practice management company)? Who could know that the two primary teaching hospitals in town would merge? These are the challenges of competing in a volatile, highly charged marketplace.

Failure To Create the Right Mix of Physician Specialties

It has been said repeatedly that the ideal ratio of primary care to specialist physicians is 50/50. There is virtually no physician organization, PHO, IDS, or MCO in the country that has come close to achieving this ratio.

There is nothing magical or scientific about a 50/50 ratio. The rationale is simply that all provider organizations should be using more PCPs to perform triage for the specialists and, where they can do it without comprising quality, carry out more of the functions that a specialist might otherwise handle—at lower cost.

The question of physician mix is more complex than making sure the organization has enough gatekeepers. It means building a physician panel with the right specialties in the right numbers for the population to be served. This requires researching the demographics of that population and translating the findings into volumes of demand for different kinds of services. That, in turn, will reveal how many physicians in each specialty will be required per 1,000 patient enrollees.

There are standard physician/patient ratios published for most specialties in a managed care setting. Unfortunately, there are no standard patient populations. It is better to tailor a physician panel to the specific needs of the local patients that it will be seeing. Furthermore, the service demands on a physician organization can change over time as the patient population grows, evolves, and moves into new market areas; as

new managed care products and services are added; and as strategic affiliations are made with new providers and payers. Frequently, the physician panel composition has to be adjusted.

Without the right mix of physicians, the organization may find itself unable to meet demands for certain services. Specialists may wind up performing tasks that could be carried out just as well by lower-salaried PCPs. It may be necessary to contract with physicians outside the panel to meet excessive demand. The net result is much increased operating expenses.

Failure To Hold Physicians Accountable for Their Performance in All Dimensions

In solo or small group practice, physicians were normally accountable only to themselves. That worked fine in the absence of fierce competitive and customer pressure to minimize costs, maximize quality, and please patients. The modern integrating organization must establish procedures that hold participating physicians responsible for nearly every aspect of their practice performance (utilization, quality, patient satisfaction, teamwork, administrative service, rules compliance). The procedures can take several forms.

- monetary incentives implemented through the compensation program
- feedback to the physician of output from clinical/financial management information systems, clinical outcome reviews, physician profiles, and patient satisfaction studies
- one-on-one and peer counseling on unacceptable physician behaviors and methods for correcting them
- required attendance at continuing medical education events designed to teach new practice skills
- deselection of physicians who, despite all efforts, cannot perform at expected levels

Failure To Appreciate the Need To Modify Physician Practice Behaviors

It is quite possible that, 20 years from now, physicians will emerge from medical school and their residencies fully prepared to practice medicine in an environment of closely managed care. They will be immediately comfortable cooperating with the full range of quality and cost control mechanisms.

During the next 20 years, however, provider organizations will be working with a significant but declining number of physicians who received their training before managed care became a household term. They learned to deliver care with a less mechanistic concern for cost and quality. It is a practice style that is no longer viable.

Every physician participating in a modern IDS must be open to changing and adjusting her style of medical practice. This includes the clinical decisions, interactions with patients, and willingness to collaborate with team members. It means allowing others to comment on and influence practice behaviors that traditionally have been solely within the physician's discretion. Because it is likely that optimal practice techniques will continue to evolve for some time, physicians will have to remain flexible, too. Any organization whose physicians allow themselves to stay stuck in the present—not to mention the past—are bound to fall behind.

Ineffective Blending of the Cultures of the Integrating Organizations

Every organization and even departments within an organization have unique cultures—a commonly held set of values and beliefs. When different cultures come into contact, through a merger, for example, they can clash—with pyrotechnic results.

Think about the traditional cultures of specialists versus PCPs or urologists versus cardiac surgeons. The cultural differences are probably even more striking between hospitals and physicians. How about nonprofit versus for-profit entities, or secular nonprofits versus religious nonprofits? Compare a teaching hospital with a community hospital.

The point is to give a good deal of attention to the blending of cultures whenever two fairly large bodies of people are combined into the same organization. This usually means working with a consultant to audit the current cultures, determine their points of similarity and conflict, then devise interventions for smoothing the merger of the two groups.

## CHAPTER 30

How To Preserve the Good Things about Your Practice (Autonomy, Patient Contact, No Cost Pressure) as Long as Possible

INTRODUCTION

This book is based on the assumption that physicians must join together to form larger groups and to learn new skills in order to survive in a health care world increasingly dominated by managed care organizations (MCOs) of one sort or another. The MCOs will deal with only large, integrated provider organizations. Physicians in solo and small group practices will lose access to their sources of patients and revenues, and will eventually go out of business.

But wait a minute! Does it have to turn out this way for all physicians? Perhaps there are strategies that will allow them to preserve the good things about traditional medical practice—if not forever, at least for as many years as possible. There may be practice settings or areas of the country where the old ways will survive longer than in others.

This chapter looks at some of the more obvious measures a physician could implement to hang on to that preferable professional life style. Some are fairly simple, involving improvements in office operations; others are more complicated, requiring significant new medical education or relocation of the physician's practice. Not all the strategies will be fully available to all physicians. Still, there may be enough useful ideas here for many physicians to postpone for a while their jump to a managed care style of practice.

WHO SHOULD READ THIS CHAPTER

A physician probably buys this book because he realizes that he is going to have to make some strategic changes in his medical practice. If he was already committed to avoiding managed care entirely, he would never have picked it up in the first place. Still, it would be natural to wonder whether there were any alternatives, even temporary, to the managed care juggernaut. So if you believe that you will ultimately have to come to terms with managed care but would welcome an opportunity, safely and responsibly, to push that time as far into the future as possible, this chapter will interest you.

The physician who finds very little to like about managed care and is willing to think about the strategies described in this book only with great reluctance may leap at the possibility of avoiding it forever. This chapter offers to such doctors several plausible escape routes.

Even those physicians who are committed right now to consolidation, integration, and new ways of practice may be intrigued to see what options might be available.

Those physicians who want to concentrate on building organizations and developing skills that ensure their success under managed may consider a chapter such as this to be a distraction. They may see it as focused on the past, when all they want to do is prepare for the future. They should skip this chapter.

UNIQUE SPECIALTY OR SKILLS THAT WILL BE DEMANDED BY MCOs AND THEIR ENROLLEES ON ANY TERMS

If you have or can develop a specialty or skill that meets two criteria—it is absolutely required by a significant number of patients and it is available from relatively few other practitioners—you will be able to dictate (within reason) the terms under which you provide that care to an MCO or other organization. They will need your services and will have to accept your reasonable conditions. It is the simple economic law of supply and demand in operation.

This means that you can insist on working for the organization as an independent contractor, rather than as an employee, or under any other arrangement that makes sense to you. You can specify your reimbursement rates. It may be possible to demand exemption from the organization's utilization management procedures and application of its clinical guidelines. It would not be wise, however, to resist application of any quality assurance measures. No skill is unique enough to be worth a malpractice suit against the organization.

The easiest way to seize this alternative is to identify a procedure or area of sub-subspecialization within your current specialty to learn. It will take some extra work, probably involving intensive reading and some continuing medical education programs, but it can be accomplished within a reasonable time period. Common sense and familiarity with your specialty and the health care needs of the local community should tell you what procedure or subspecialty to target.

This option is a little more daunting if it requires that you learn an entirely new specialty. This normally would involve going back to school for a retraining course. However, it can be done. After all, specialists who have become redundant in their market areas are reported to be retraining in primary care specialties. The hard

question for the physician is whether he dislikes the principles of managed care enough to go to this effort to avoid them.

UNIQUE SPECIALTY, SKILLS, OR ACCESSIBILITY THAT PATIENTS WILL PAY FOR OUT-OF-POCKET

This is a similar alternative, in that it requires something so special about a physician's medical care that patients are willing to forgo insurance reimbursement or to step outside their managed care plan and pay for it out of their own pockets. In some cases, the special service offered by the physician may not even come under the patient's health care plan.

What kind of unique practice features would a patient be willing to pay for? The classic example is cosmetic surgery. Unless connected with an otherwise compensable injury, such procedures are never covered by traditional health care plans. If a patient desires those kinds of services, he must pay for them out of pocket. The cosmetic surgeon can charge what he wants and can practice where and how he wants. He will never have to worry about managed care restrictions.

The challenge then is to identify comparable specialties or subspecialties, to determine whether you already are trained them, and, if not, to acquire the necessary training.

Other variations of this alternative are to develop such a reputation in your field that patients will pay out of pocket to get care from you, even though virtually identical care is available from someone else under their health care plan. The reputation may be based on the superior quality of your care, a unique twist to your delivery of it (neater sutures when you close after an operation), or nothing at all. It is said that some people will pay extra to be represented by F. Lee Bailey in a legal matter, even if he loses their case. The opportunity to tell friends about the connection is priceless.

Sometimes, the unique location of a physician practice may be worth an out-of-pocket payment to some patients. If you have located your office in a Mexican resort town, American tourists with emergent health care needs may prefer to see you than a Mexican practitioner they do not know.

It is probably obvious that the only patients with the freedom to take advantage of these alternatives will have to be rather wealthy. Most people simply cannot afford to pay out of pocket for medical care that is covered by health insurance, no matter how special you are.

PRACTICE IN A LOCATION THAT WILL NEVER BE PENETRATED BY MANAGED CARE

There still are areas of this country that have not been substantially penetrated by managed care. Many parts of the Southeast and more rural areas in general fall into this category. However, they are declining in size and number all the time. Some commentators believe that, eventually, every single person in the United States will be receiving care through some part of a managed care system. That remains to be seen.

For the moment, there are clear opportunities to set up a solo practice in markets not yet invaded by MCOs, their plans, and their restrictions. An interested physician needs to do some research to identify the states, and areas of those states, where managed care penetration is especially low.* Then, look into the lifestyle and general amenities in the best areas and decide whether you and your family are willing to move to one of these areas to escape the threat of managed care. Just remember, one day some representatives from an MCO will show up in your small town in northern Wyoming and announce, "We're here!"

_____

*The "HMO-PPO/Medicare-Medicaid Digest" from the Hoechst Marion Roussel (800-529-9615) annual *Managed Care Digest Series* is a good, relatively inexpensive ($95) starting point. In 1996, the only states with penetration rates below 10 percent were Alaska (no managed care at all!), Alabama, Arkansas, Mississippi, Montana, Wyoming (also no managed care), and Idaho.

REFINE PRACTICE SKILLS TO REMAIN IN DEMAND BY MCOs ON A CONTRACT BASIS

For many physicians, one of the most uncomfortable aspects of managed care practice is the apparent need to become part of a large, often bureaucratic provider organization to acquire and demonstrate the ability to deliver high-quality, low-cost care. What if you could achieve the same utilization rates, patient satisfaction levels, and clinical outcomes—and show it—without joining such an organization? You might be able to remain independent in a solo or small group practice, contracting with MCOs and never formally joining them.

Unfortunately, for many physicians, the accomplishment of those goals would be like lifting themselves by their own bootstraps. It simply takes more time, self-discipline, and capital than most physicians can muster. That is not a criticism. It would be a challenge for anybody.

If you think you have everything that it takes, as well as an MCO willing to believe that a solo practitioner is capable of this, give it a try. There is not a lot to lose, as you will have to learn the skills eventually. If you can practice as efficiently and efficaciously as a physician in a tightly integrated group practice without actually being in a group practice, you may be ensured of your professional autonomy for quite a few years.

JOIN AN INDEPENDENT PRACTICE ASSOCIATION (IPA) IN A LESS PRESSURED MARKET

An IPA is the first, loosest, and most tentative level of physician consolidation. See Chapter 11, "Step Four: Joining an Independent Practice Association," for more detailed information on the formation and operation of an IPA. In its initial form," participating physicians remain independent, both legally and operationally. The IPA simply negotiates managed care contracts on their behalf and lets the revenues flow through to them. It makes no attempt to manage their utilization or quality, or to otherwise intervene in their business or clinical decision making. That is wonderful—as long as it lasts.

Once the MCOs with whom the IPA has contracted begin to feel competitive pressure, however, they will want to negotiate lower and lower reimbursement rates. To comply, the IPA physicians will have to start down the path of cost and quality management. Indeed, the common wisdom is that IPAs can be only transitional vehicles on the road to forming large, integrated group practices.

Until that happens, the IPA offers an opportunity for autonomous physicians to reap some of the rewards of managed care involvement without radically changing their practice styles or settings. When looking for an IPA to implement this alternative, be aware that some are committed to moving aggressively to develop managed care skills, even before they are forced to do so.

JOIN A GROUP PRACTICE WITHOUT WALLS (GPWW)

This option is very similar to the IPA one. The only difference is that, initially, the physicians do combine their practices into a single legal entity but keep them physically separate in their original locations. The same caveats apply here. When market forces start to develop, the GPWW will have to begin integrating and "managing" its member physicians if it wants to survive. Until that happens, membership in a GPWW can be a fine solution to the managed care "problem."

FORM AND JOIN A PHYSICIAN-RUN MANAGEMENT SERVICES ORGANIZATION (MSO)

This alternative follows the rationale and includes the limitations of the IPA and GPWW options above. An important distinction is that it is not just any MSO. It is one formed and controlled by the physicians who purchase their various practice assets, negotiate managed care contracts, and try to remain unentangled and unregulated for as long as possible.

SEEK OUT A MARKET WITH A LARGE MANAGED CARE PRESENCE BUT LITTLE COMPETITION

Under this strategy, the challenge is to find a market area that is heavily penetrated by managed care but is not experiencing the intense competition that forces MCOs to lower premiums and squeeze their providers to be more cost-efficient. In other words, a market area in which the MCOs are more relaxed when it comes to "management" of physician clinical decision making.

Competition is almost automatic when there are two or more roughly equal MCOs in operation. What you are looking for is an area dominated by a single MCO, almost in a monopoly situation. They are not easy to find, but they exist. For a while, Healthsource was the only MCO in the substantial southern New Hampshire market area. The downside of this option is that a competing MCO will eventually be drawn into the area by the unusually high premiums available. Their competition then will drive the premiums down and force tighter management of physician practice.

IF YOU CANNOT DO ANYTHING ELSE, JOIN A SYMPATHETIC PHYSICIAN-RUN ORGANIZATION

A physician-run organization, whether a large multispecialty group practice or a full-blown integrated delivery system (IDS), is more likely to be sympathetic to the physician desire for clinical autonomy than an organization dominated by MBAs. Nonetheless, faced with any sort of real competition or pressure from large employers, even these well-intentioned organizations will have to get tough with their physicians on utilization and quality. The enduring advantage you gain is that the physician-owners will almost always be a bit more gentle and understanding than will the professional managers—even when they are trying to influence your practice behaviors.

SEEK ORGANIZATIONS (REGARDLESS OF OWNERSHIP AND CONTROL) THAT WELCOME PHYSICIAN INPUT

More forward-looking organizations owned by hospitals, MCOs, insurance companies, or private investors have created opportunities for participating physicians to influence decision making at all levels. These are some forms that this may take:

- physician participation on the board of directors through guaranteed board seats, supermajority votes on physician-sensitive issues, separate majority votes of physician and non-physician directors on physician-sensitive issues, guaranteed seats on board committees addressing physician-sensitive issues (recruitment, quality review, managed care contracting, compensation)
- formal procedures for soliciting physician input to certain administrative decisions
- formal guarantees of physician control over primary aspects of clinical decision making
- routine involvement of physicians in designing the practice guidelines or clinical protocols to which they will be held

Clearly, a organization that is willing to implement policies and procedures such as these is probably going to be enlightened about physician concerns in other ways as well.

There are anecdotal reports of hospitals willing to invest in physician-hospital organizations (PHOs) and then give physicians dominant roles in running them. Some of the more progressive physician practice management companies (PPMCs), often investor owned, have seen the wisdom of allowing their physicians these kinds of authority. Among traditional insurance companies, CIGNA has gained a reputation for being particularly solicitous of physician views.

The challenge, of course, is to identify such an organization within your market area. This information does not get widely publicized. You should start by asking physician colleagues what they know or have heard, or have actually experienced, concerning the physician-friendliness of various integrating organizations in town. Ask if they have any written materials, including contracts they may have signed, describing the organizations' policies and procedures. Follow up by contacting the organizations directly to ask questions and gather more documentation. As you approach more serious negotiations with particular entities, your questions can become more focused and insistent.

CONTRACT DIRECTLY WITH EMPLOYERS TO DELIVER WHAT THEY REALLY WANT—VALUE

When MCOs attempt to regulate the utilization, quality, and other aspects of physician practice behavior, they are generally trying to interpret the wishes of the employer-payers (as well as to generate a profit for themselves). They may not read those desires accurately. Furthermore, why should the physician-patient relationship be restricted even more than it is to improve an MCO's bottom line?

One way to circumvent the restrictions and the MCOs is to develop, on your own initiative, the ability to give the employers what they really want—that is value, a balance between cost and quality. The next step is to enter into a direct contract with the employer to deliver medical care with that value. This means first doing several things.

1. An employer is unlikely to directly contract with solo or small group practice physicians. Some will deal only with rather comprehensive provider networks. Others are willing to create their own networks by contracting separately with several groups of providers. It will be necessary to form a modest critical mass of physicians sufficient to satisfy the particular employer you have targeted.

2. Assembling a slightly larger group of physicians will make available the resources (time, money, energy) needed to refine the practice skills to the degree expected by the employer.
3. Early in the process, serious discussions must be had with interested, supportive employers to learn exactly what they want from their health care providers in terms of cost, quality, patient satisfaction, accessibility, and data.
4. All of this carried must be out in a way that does not alienate your current MCO contract partners. It probably would not be a good idea to go after an employer presently served by one of those MCOs.

If you can successfully implement this option, you could end up with payer relationships that allow your group and its individual physicians considerable freedom to practice medicine the way they want—as long as they meet the employer's needs. In addition, you will not have to fight with those pesky MCOs.

SEEK OUT AFFILIATIONS/CONTRACTS WITH PAYERS THAT GIVE ABOVE-AVERAGE PRIORITY TO QUALITY OVER COSTS

The common wisdom has been that payers of all sorts, both employers and MCOs, are concerned with the costs of health care above all else. Quality and accessibility must be present, but they receive secondary attention. Whether this is true or not of most payers, there is the possibility that at least a minority of them is willing to pay something extra for care of above-average quality. If they exist, if you can find them, and if they are in an area suitable to you, they are more likely to allow you to practice more traditional medicine to satisfy their quality requirements.

It is not clear whether there are many payers with such a strong quality preference. One thing is certain—there are gradations of payer concern for cost and quality, and for sensitivity to physician needs for clinical autonomy. With a modest amount of research among colleagues and the payers themselves, you should be able to identify the more physician-friendly payers. They may not be ideal, they may not really allow you to practice the way you did 10 or 20 years ago, but they will be an improvement over any of the alternatives.

SEEK A SALARIED POSITION IN A DELIVERY ORGANIZATION (EVEN STAFF-MODEL HMOs) THAT INSULATES YOU FROM REGULATORY, COMPETITIVE, AND ADMINISTRATIVE PRESSURES

This may seem like the most perverse option of all. If you were trying to avoid a managed care lifestyle, why would you join an MCO?

Instead of looking for an escape from managed care, think more constructively—in terms of finding a practice setting that allows the kinds of professional freedom you really want. Be open to the possibility that you might find this in an MCO or in a larger provider organization.

A few years ago, Arnold Relman, former editor of the *New England Journal of Medicine*, commented in a talk at the Harvard School of Public Health that a lot of physicians who had joined the medical staffs of MCOs were earning just about what they had in private practice, were working regular hours without serious worry about on-call duty, had more time for their personal lives, and were generally quite content. Working for even the most beneficent large organization can never be anything like solo or small group practice. However, if your preference is to concentrate on delivering medical care without involvement in business matters or outside interference in your clinical decision making, the answer may be in a practice "oasis" within such an organization.

Here, too, it will take some searching to discover the MCO or provider organization that offers this sort of practice environment to its physicians. There may be none in your immediate area. You may have to relocate or simply join with some other like-minded doctors to create such an organization.

ADOPT MEASURES THAT WILL MAKE EVEN A SOLO OR SMALL GROUP PRACTICE MORE COST-EFFICIENT

Many physicians are in solo or two-physician practices (Exhibit 30–1). A responsible physician presumably accepts the notion that the care she provides should be as inexpensive as possible for the patient, without recklessly sacrificing quality. In addition to whatever other strategies she follows, or while she is deciding what those strategies might be, it makes sense to start now to develop the skills and support systems necessary for her to do that. Any improvements in this direction will immediately benefit the practice, the physician, and her patients. This superior practice ability will open up to the physician a wider range of strategic opportunities and will give her greater flexibility in negotiating with any organization she might join.

There are many routes to more cost-efficient, high-quality physician care. These are a few of the more obvious:

- streamlining procedures adopting established clinical guidelines
- improve patient scheduling and flow
- using midlevel providers to take over some of your responsibilities and lower-level ancil-

---

Exhibit 30–1 What Physicians Are in Solo and Two-Physician Practices?

63% of all doctors 66 years old or older
60% of all international medical graduates
54% of all non–board certified physicians
44% of all male physicians

Source: Adapted with permission from *American Medical News*, © 1995, American Medical Association.

---

lary personnel to take over the work of high-level ones (e.g., medical assistant for a registered nurse)
- linking computers of employees to avoid extra data entry and improve data accessibility
- tailoring work hours to patient needs (e.g., cut back on daytime work hours and replace them with evening hours)

FOLLOW THIS BOOK'S RECOMMENDATIONS IN BUILDING A PHYSICIAN-RUN INTEGRATED DELIVERY AND FINANCING SYSTEM

A large IDS will never be the same as a friendly, comfortable solo or small group practice. Under the pressure of market competition, it will probably end up making many of the same business decisions as those delivery systems owned and run by hospitals, insurance companies, and private investors. It certainly will find it necessary to institute utilization management and quality assurance measures, to report data comparing physicians' performances, and even to deselect some of its physicians. The big difference is that, if these steps have to be taken, they will be taken by other physicians, not by MBAs.

A physician-driven organization is likely to be more sensitive to the special concerns of doctors. It will do everything possible to protect physician autonomy, particularly over clinical matters. It will be more patient and supportive of a physician who is having trouble adjusting his practice style to managed care. It will dismiss a physician only as a last resort and with a clear explanation of the reasons. It will impose care management procedures that are the least invasive necessary to stay competitive in the marketplace. In a variety of subtle ways, the managerial style of its leaders and executives will acknowledge the unique role and tradition of physicians in the delivery of health care.

RESOURCE LIST

W. Guglielmo, "Roping Down Managed Care," *Medical Economics 74*, no. 13 (1997): 106.

Strategy Scenarios and Report Cards

INTRODUCTION

This book has described a wide range of possible strategies that a physician might pursue to deal most effectively with managed care. They vary greatly in their chances of long-term success and their likely impact on a physician's autonomy. A few doctors may see, very quickly, the one approach that makes most sense for them. The majority will wonder how to choose among all the strategic possibilities with all their features and nuances.

The purpose of this chapter is twofold. One is to describe a methodology for rating, scoring, or grading strategic scenarios. It is a methodology that a physician can use with her own scenarios and criteria. The chapter also spells out the most likely or popular scenarios, suggests some physician-based criteria, and uses them to grade the scenarios. The result is a fairly detailed comparison of the scenarios on those issues that are most important to physicians.

WHO SHOULD READ THIS CHAPTER

If you have read enough of the book's chapters to have a sense of the strategic alternatives available to you but are wondering how to pick among them, this chapter will help you do that. In fact, if you want to accept the book's grading judgments, they will tell you exactly which strategies to pursue. They follow the fundamental theme of this book—that physicians will do best in the long run by consolidating; forming larger, integrated organizations; and acquiring more discerning practice skills while maintaining as much physician control over their professional activities as possible for as long as possible

It is conceivable that a physician who wanted just to "cut to the chase" could jump straight to this chapter without reading the rest of the book. After finding a scenario that appealed to him, he could go back to those chapters that filled out the details of the strategies and organizations involved.

A different kind of physician might find exactly the strategy concepts she was looking for in one of the earlier chapters. That might provide sufficient information for her to adopt and implement her own personal strategy without turning to this chapter at all.

PHYSICIAN CRITERIA OR OBJECTIVES IN MAKING STRATEGIC DECISIONS

These are the criteria and objectives that are used later for evaluating the several strategy scenarios. They are intended to be a list of the various concerns that most physicians have about getting involved with managed care. There may be other criteria that have particular resonance for individual physicians. There is an explanation at the end of the chapter of how to incorporate those into the evaluation.

- **retention of assets**—each physician retains ownership of individual practice assets by each physician
- **physician control**—physician ownership or control of the organization
- **generation of capital**—ability to generate investment capital
- **legal risk**—degree of legal risk (primarily from antitrust and fraud and abuse laws)
- **original location**—continuation of practice at original location
- **risk sharing**—ability and willingness to share risk with a managed care organization (MCO)
- **capitation**—ability and willingness to accept capitation reimbursement
- **total capital**—total capital requirements to finance the strategy
- **required investment**—requirement of physician investment in the organization
- **investment opportunity**—opportunity for physician investment in publicly traded stock
- **physician leadership**—opportunity for physicians to assume leadership positions
- **care management**—vigorous application of care management measures
- **organizational viability**—long-term viability in its current form
- **physician revival**—likelihood of reestablishing physicians as major players in the health care delivery system
- **success odds**—probability of optimal long-term financial success in the health care marketplace
- **employment relationship**—likelihood of employment relationship with the organization
- **contract relationship**—likelihood of contractual relationship with the organization
- **maximization of income**—opportunity to maximize annual income
- **MCO appeal**—attractiveness to MCOs for contracting purposes
- **avoidance of domination**—general avoidance of domination by other entities such as hospitals, insurance companies, and MCOs

PHYSICIAN STRATEGY SCENARIOS FOR MANAGED CARE

These strategy scenarios represent different combinations of the strategic possibilities described in this book. They have been chosen because they are closest to what many physicians already are doing or because they offer particular promise. There is an infinity of strategies that physicians could follow to position themselves most advantageously in a managed care world. Physicians should not feel themselves restricted to this list. Think about the most appealing strategic features or concepts in the past chapters. Could they be combined in a way that is especially suited to your preferences and to the market area in which you practice? Take 15 minutes to sketch a brief description of it. Do that with any other possibilities that occur to you. Be imaginative and keep an open mind. What you are doing is the beginning of strategic thinking.

Seek practice settings that minimize involvement with managed care.

This scenario involves the implementation of any of the strategy alternatives outlined in the previous chapter (Chapter 30, "How To Preserve the Good Things about Your Practice (Autonomy, Patient Contact, No Cost Pressure) as Long as Possible"). It presumes that the physician will go to considerable lengths to avoid the constraints of managed care or to minimize their impact on his practice. Several of the alternatives are actually based on some of the more forward-looking strategies but attempt to adapt them to the physician's favor.

Join an independent practice association (IPA) that negotiates contracts for its members but does little integration or care management.

In this scenario, the physician joins an IPA with the most basic structure and aims. The physician remains legally and physically independent in his original practice setting. In the IPA, he joins numerous physicians—perhaps hundreds—in a wide variety of specialties. The primary and the only substantial service performed by the IPA is the negotiation of managed care contracts for the physicians. There are no additional administrative or care management services offered. The physicians hope to reap additional managed care revenues without altering their practice style.

Sell practice assets to a publicly traded physician practice management company (PPMC) and accept employment by it.

This is a simple, cut-and-dried scenario that appeals to many physicians who do not want to be continually involved in forming, managing, and developing organizations. They sell their assets to the most attractive PPMC available and practice medicine for that corporation for the rest of their careers. In the best case, the PPMC will be working to create a carefully crafted physician network, will "rent" it to MCOs, will go public with the corporation's stock, and will steadily grow the value of that stock.

Sell practice assets to a hospital or hospital-owned management services organization (MSO) and accept employment by it.

An MSO is a more primitive form of a PPMC. In this scenario, a single hospital (rather than a multistate PPMC) sets up an MSO for the purpose of acquiring and managing the practice assets of physicians on its medical staff. Sometimes, the hospital corporation itself buys them. The physicians become employees of the hospital or of the MSO. They do not have the opportunity to be paid for their assets with publicly traded shares of stock that will increase in value. The hospital may not manage their practice assets as professionally or effectively as might a PPMC.

Merge with other solo and small group practices, evolve into a medium-sized single-specialty or related-specialty group, and institute modest care management procedures.

This is a somewhat tentative scenario that still shows forward movement by the physicians. It might start with one small physician group merging with another, then bringing in other solo and small group practices over the next couple of years. It eventually grows to medium size but

without any special goal of becoming a large, multispecialty group practice, an integrated delivery system (IDS), or even of affiliating with a hospital. Along the way, the physicians begin to gather rudimentary data about the cost and quality of their care. They also take tentative steps toward using that data to modify their practice patterns.

Merge with other small and medium-sized group practices to form a large, multispecialty group practice. Begin accumulating capital, investing in information and management systems, streamlining patient flow, tightly screening and supervising physicians, integrating physicians' practices, and controlling costs and quality.

This scenario could start off like the previous one. Soon, however, the physicians see that they must grow faster and larger, and must develop more ambitious care management systems if they are to maintain some degree of autonomy. They adopt the specific goal of becoming a large, integrated multispecialty group practice.

Deliberately and aggressively take steps to form a physician-run IDS.

This scenario takes the previous two to their ultimate conclusion. Through affiliations with hospitals and other providers, the physicians assemble an IDS capable of providing a full spectrum of health care services to a targeted population. They are leaders in exploring and adopting the most modern methods for managing cost, quality, and patient satisfaction. Their ultimate aim is to be nothing less than the most productive, desirable health care delivery system in the market area. In addition, the physicians own and control the entity that accomplishes this.

Form an IPA that moves quickly to integrate its physicians' practices and to develop their care management skills in anticipation of further integration with other provider entities.

This is more ambitious than the baseline IPA scenario. The physicians acknowledge that they cannot remain independent, operationally and perhaps physically, forever. They also recognize that they must acquire the ability to control the cost and quality of the care that they provide, and that this means changing their practice behaviors. They accept the notion that they will eventually have to form strategic affiliations with other provider entities, but they are not sure which ones, and they do not have a timetable for carrying this out.

Form an IPA with the intention of developing eventually into a large, integrated, multispecialty group practice.

The founding physicians in this scenario view their IPA as just a transitional vehicle on their way to becoming a large, integrated, multispecialty group practice. They acknowledge this at the start. They have a specific, aggressive plan for moving in that direction. Along with growing and integrating, they will adopt all the modern, sophisticated mechanisms for managing all aspects of the care they deliver. Their ultimate goal is to become a powerhouse physician group that can remain strong and independent in its dealings with MCOs, other payers, and other provider organizations.

Form a large, sophisticated, integrated multispecialty group practice with the ultimate aim of contracting directly with employers.

Most of the other strategy scenarios are designed to better position physicians for their dealings and negotiations with MCOs and government payers such as the Medicare and Medicaid programs. This scenario is different. It can begin like some of the others—with an IPA, an MSO, a physician-hospital organization (PHO), or with the merger of physician practices. However, its final objective is the construction of a large, integrated, multispecialty group practice that contracts directly with employers to serve their employees. The physicians no longer deal through an MCO.

Accept an invitation into a PHO (composed of a hospital and its medical staff) that will negotiate managed care contracts on behalf of all its participating providers.

This is another of the entry-level scenarios for physicians who hope to attract some managed care revenues without having to consolidate, integrate, or change their practice behaviors. The PHO's sole function is to find and negotiate contracts with MCOs. The physicians and the hospital believe that MCOs will prefer the opportunity to sign a single contract with an assemblage of providers that can deliver most, if not all, the health care services required by the MCO's enrollees. The physicians have no plans for moving much beyond the simple PHO format.

Contribute to the formation of a PHO by a hospital and a group of physicians selected from both its medical staff and the community at large, with the intention of developing care management skills and evolving into a more integrated, comprehensive delivery system.

This scenario starts out like the previous one but uses the PHO only as a stepping stone toward the development of a more integrated, more comprehensive multiprovider delivery system. The physicians and hospital spend a short period of time in the PHO learning how to collaborate with each other. Pursuant to a formal strategic plan, they then move with all due speed to operationally link their practices, physically integrate some of them, acquire appropriate new information and management systems, develop new practice skills in managing care, and affiliate with the other provider entities needed to create the full-service system. The PHO itself disappears rather quickly.

After building a medium to large multispecialty group practice, create affiliations with other provider entities (particularly hospitals), through contracts rather than merger or ownership, to create a "virtual" integrated system.

This is an "electronic age" scenario in which physicians aggregate themselves, through mergers or an IPA, to eventually form a large state-of-the-art multispecialty group practice. From that point on, there are no further mergers with or acquisitions of nonphysician provider organizations. Instead, the physicians begin to assemble a delivery system that is "virtually" integrated through contracts, joint venture agreements, and other arrangements that do not involve ownership or capital expenditure.

WHAT THE RATINGS MEAN

Each scenario is given a rating or grade of A, B, C, D, or E for the degree to which it satisfies each of the criteria listed above. The grades are from the viewpoint of a hypothetical "average" physician, with "A" representing the most desirable position for that physician and "E" the least desirable. Specifically, certain things are assumed.

- A physician prefers to retain ownership of her practice assets.
- A physician prefers to own or control any organization that is formed.
- A strategy that generates investable capital is better than one that does not.
- Legal risk should be minimized.
- A physician prefers to stay at his original practice location.
- Risk-sharing arrangements with MCOs are desirable.
- Capitation arrangements with MCOs are desirable.
- Strategies with lower capital requirements are more desirable.
- A physician would prefer not to have to invest capital in a new organization.
- A physician would welcome the opportunity to receive or invest in publicly traded stock of the organization.
- A physician would prefer to see herself or other physicians in leadership roles.
- A physician would prefer to avoid care management measures.
- It is better that an organization exist for a long, rather than a short period of time, even though some of the organizations are clearly transitional entities.

- It is desirable that physicians be reestablished as major players in the health care system.
- It is desirable that the strategy succeed financially.
- A physician prefers not to be an employee of another organization.
- A physician prefers to have contractual relationships with other organizations.
- A physician desires to maximize his income.
- It is preferable that a strategy is more appealing to MCOs.
- It is preferable that physicians avoid domination by other nonphysician entities.

These assumptions may not hold for every physician. For instance, some may prefer direct employment over a contractual relationship. Keep the above assumptions in mind as you read the score cards that follow.

The overall grade is not an objective summation of the individual criteria grades. It is a separate rating of the total appeal of the strategy for the average physician. Appendix 31–A is a collection of strategy scenario report cards.

HOW TO MODIFY AND USE THE SCORE CARDS

There are several ways to adapt this method of rating strategy scenarios to fit a physician's unique interests and circumstances.

1. Define other strategy scenarios that you are thinking about or that occur to you as you read this book. Use the criteria here to rate them.
2. Define additional criteria that are important to you. Eliminate any criteria from the above list that are not relevant to you. Apply the criteria that are left to the scenarios in this chapter or to others that you create.
3. Apply the criteria in this chapter to the same strategy scenarios but assign your own grades where they differ from what is given.

4. To make the scenario ratings more comparable and slightly more scientific, change the grades to numbers (A=1, E=5). Assign weights to each of the criteria, depending on their importance to you. After giving quantitative grades to each criterion, multiply those grades by the weights you assigned, then add up the weighted grades for all the criteria. The result is your overall grade for the scenario, which can be compared with those for the other scenarios.

Strategy Scenario Report Cards

These are the grades assigned to the criteria for each strategy scenario. They are unavoidably subjective. Other reasonable people, particularly physicians, could assign very different grades.

Seek practice settings that minimize involvement with managed care.

Retain Assets	A	Physician Leadership	E
Physician Control	A	Care Management	E
Generate Capital	E	Organizational Viability	D
Legal Risk	B	Physician Revival	E
Original Location	A	Success Odds	D
Risk Sharing	E	Employment Relationship	A
Capitation	E	Contractual Relationship	A
Total Capital	A	Maximize Income	C
Required Investment	A	MCO Appeal	D
Investment Opportunity	E	Avoid Domination	E
Overall Rating	D		

Join an IPA that negotiates contracts for its members but does little integration or care management.

Retain Assets	A	Physician Leadership	B
Physician Control	A	Care Management	A
Generate Capital	E	Organizational Viability	E
Legal Risk	D	Physician Revival	D
Original Location	E	Success Odds	D
Risk Sharing	E	Employment Relationship	A
Capitation	E	Contractual Relationship	A
Total Capital	B	Maximize Income	D
Required Investment	B	MCO Appeal	C
Investment Opportunity	E	Avoid Domination	D
Overall Rating	D		

Sell practice assets to a publicly traded PPMC and accept employment by it.

Retain Assets	E	Physician Leadership	D
Physician Control	E	Care Management	C
Generate Capital	A	Organizational Viability	C
Legal Risk	A	Physician Revival	D
Original Location	C	Success Odds	C
Risk Sharing	B	Employment Relationship	E
Capitation	C	Contractual Relationship	E
Total Capital	D	Maximize Income	C
Required Investment	A	MCO Appeal	C
Investment Opportunity	A	Avoid Domination	E
Overall Rating	C		

Sell practice assets to a hospital or hospital-owned MSO and accept employment by it.

Retain Assets	E	Physician Leadership	C
Physician Control	E	Care Management	B
Generate Capital	D	Organizational Viability	D
Legal Risk	A	Physician Revival	E
Original Location	B	Success Odds	D
Risk Sharing	D	Employment Relationship	E
Capitation	D	Contractual Relationship	E
Total Capital	E	Maximize Income	D
Required Investment	A	MCO Appeal	D
Investment Opportunity	E	Avoid Domination	E
Overall Rating	E		

Merge with other solo and small group practices, evolve into a medium-sized single specialty or related-specialty group, and institute modest care management procedures.

Retain Assets	C	Physician Leadership	A
Physician Control	A	Care Management	C
Generate Capital	C	Organizational Viability	C
Legal Risk	A	Physician Revival	B
Original Location	B	Success Odds	D
Risk Sharing	C	Employment Relationship	A
Capitation	D	Contractual Relationship	A
Total Capital	B	Maximize Income	B
Required Investment	C	MCO Appeal	C
Investment Opportunity	E	Avoid Domination	B
Overall Rating	C		

Merge with other small and medium-sized group practices to form a large multispecialty group practice. Begin accumulating capital, investing in information and management system, streamlining patient flow, tightly screening and supervising physicians, integrating physicians' practices, and controlling costs and quality.

Retain Assets	E	Physician Leadership	A
Physician Control	A	Care Management	E
Generate Capital	A	Organizational Viability	A
Legal Risk	A	Physician Revival	A
Original Location	D	Success Odds	A
Risk Sharing	A	Employment Relationship	A
Capitation	A	Contractual Relationship	A
Total Capital	D	Maximize Income	A
Required Investment	D	MCO Appeal	A
Investment Opportunity	D	Avoid Domination	A
Overall Rating	A		

Deliberately and aggressively take steps to form a physician-run IDS.

Retain Assets	E	Physician Leadership	A
Physician Control	A	Care Management	E
Generate Capital	A	Organizational Viability	A
Legal Risk	A	Physician Revival[1]	A
Original Location	E	Success Odds	B
Risk Sharing	A	Employment Relationship	A
Capitation	A	Contractual Relationship	A
Total Capital	E	Maximize Income	A
Required Investment	D	MCO Appeal	A
Investment Opportunity	D	Avoid Domination	A
Overall Rating	A		

Form an IPA that moves quickly to integrate its physicians' practices and develop their care management skills in anticipation of further integration with other provider entities.

Retain Assets	E	Physician Leadership	A
Physician Control	A	Care Management	E
Generate Capital	D	Organizational Viability	D
Legal Risk	C	Physician Revival	B
Original Location	C	Success Odds	C
Risk Sharing	C	Employment Relationship	A
Capitation	C	Contractual Relationship	A
Total Capital	C	Maximize Income	C
Required Investment	D	MCO Appeal	B
Investment Opportunity	E	Avoid Domination	C
Overall Rating	C		

Form an IPA with the intention of developing eventually into a large, integrated, multispecialty group practice.

Retain Assets	E	Physician Leadership	A
Physician Control	A	Care Management	E
Generate Capital	B	Organizational Viability	A
Legal Risk	B	Physician Revival	A
Original Location	B	Success Odds	A
Risk Sharing	A	Employment Relationship	A
Capitation	A	Contractual Relationship	A
Total Capital	D	Maximize Income	B
Required Investment	D	MCO Appeal	A
Investment Opportunity	E	Avoid Domination	A
Overall Rating	B		

Form a large, sophisticated, integrated multispecialty group practice with the ultimate aim of contracting directly with employers.

Retain Assets	E		Physician Leadership	A
Physician Control	A		Care Management	E
Generate Capital	A		Organizational Viability	A
Legal Risk	A		Physician Revival	A
Original Location	E		Success Odds	C
Risk Sharing	A		Employment Relationship	A
Capitation	A		Contractual Relationship	A
Total Capital	D		Maximize Income	A
Required Investment	D		MCO Appeal	E
Investment Opportunity	E		Avoid Domination	A
Overall Rating	A			

Accept an invitation into a PHO (composed of a hospital and its medical staff) that will negotiate managed care contracts on behalf of all its participating providers.

Retain Assets	A	Physician Leadership	D
Physician Control	E	Care Management	E
Generate Capital	E	Organizational Viability	E
Legal Risk	D	Physician Revival	E
Original Location	A	Success Odds	E
Risk Sharing	E	Employment Relationship	E
Capitation	E	Contractual Relationship	E
Total Capital	B	Maximize Income	C
Required Investment	A	MCO Appeal	D
Investment Opportunity	E	Avoid Domination	E
Overall Rating	E		

Contribute to the formation of a PHO by a hospital and a group of physicians selected from both its medical staff and the community at large, with the intention of developing care management skills and evolving into a more integrated, comprehensive delivery system.

Retain Assets	A	Physician Leadership	D
Physician Control	C	Care Management	E
Generate Capital	C	Organizational Viability	A
Legal Risk	C	Physician Revival	D
Original Location	E	Success Odds	A
Risk Sharing	A	Employment Relationship	E
Capitation	A	Contractual Relationship	E
Total Capital	E	Maximize Income	B
Required Investment	B	MCO Appeal	A
Investment Opportunity	E	Avoid Domination	D
Overall Rating	D		

After building a medium to large multispecialty group practice, create affiliations with other provider entities (particularly hospitals) through contracts, rather than merger or ownership, to create a "virtual" integrated system.

Retain Assets	E	Physician Leadership	A
Physician Control	A	Care Management	E
Generate Capital	A	Organizational Viability	A
Legal Risk	A	Physician Revival	A
Original Location	E	Success Odds	B
Risk Sharing	A	Employment Relationship	A
Capitation	A	Contractual Relationship	A
Total Capital	C	Maximize Income	A
Required Investment	C	MCO Appeal	B
Investment Opportunity	E	Avoid Domination	A
Overall Rating	A		

Index

.